# HEALTH INFORMATION TECHNOLOGY

Nadinia Davis • Melissa LaCour

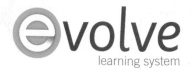 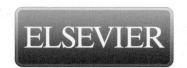
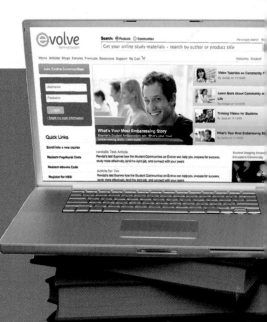

# HEALTH INFORMATION TECHNOLOGY

## THIRD EDITION 3

### Nadinia Davis • Melissa LaCour

**MBA, CPA, RHIA, CHDA, FAHIMA**
**Program Coordinator**
**Health Information Management**
**Delaware Technical Community College**
**Wilmington, Delaware**

**MHIM, RHIA**
**Dean**
**Distance Learning & Instructional Technology**
**Delgado Community College**
**New Orleans, Louisiana**

ELSEVIER

3251 Riverport Lane
St. Louis, Missouri 63043

HEALTH INFORMATION TECHNOLOGY, THIRD EDITION                 ISBN: 978-1-4377-2736-4

---

**Notices**

Knowledge and best practice in this field are constantly changing. As new research and experience broaden our understanding, changes in research methods, professional practices, or medical treatment may become necessary.

Practitioners and researchers must always rely on their own experience and knowledge in evaluating and using any information, methods, compounds, or experiments described herein. In using such information or methods they should be mindful of their own safety and the safety of others, including parties for whom they have a professional responsibility.

With respect to any drug or pharmaceutical products identified, readers are advised to check the most current information provided (i) on procedures featured or (ii) by the manufacturer of each product to be administered, to verify the recommended dose or formula, the method and duration of administration, and contraindications. It is the responsibility of practitioners, relying on their own experience and knowledge of their patients, to make diagnoses, to determine dosages and the best treatment for each individual patient, and to take all appropriate safety precautions.

To the fullest extent of the law, neither the Publisher nor the authors, contributors, or editors, assume any liability for any injury and/or damage to persons or property as a matter of products liability, negligence or otherwise, or from any use or operation of any methods, products, instructions, or ideas contained in the material herein.

---

**Library of Congress Cataloging-in-Publication Data**

Davis, Nadinia A.
   Health information technology / Nadinia Davis, Melissa LaCour.—3rd ed.
      p. ; cm.
   Includes bibliographical references and index.
   ISBN 978-1-4377-2736-4 (pbk. : alk. paper)
   I. LaCour, Melissa.   II. Title.
   [DNLM:   1.  Delivery of Health Care—organization & administration—United States.
2. Information Management—organization & administration—United States.   3.  Forms and Records Control—United States.   4.  Medical Informatics—United States.   5.  Records as Topic—United States.
W 84 AA1]
   610.285—dc23
                                                                              2012041703

*Content Strategist:* Linda Woodard
*Developmental Editor:* John Tomedi
*Publishing Services Manager:* Catherine Jackson
*Senior Project Manager:* Mary Pohlman
*Senior Book Designer:* Paula Catalano

Printed in China

Last digit is the print number:   9   8   7   6   5   4   3   2   1

*To Susan Cole, who made everything possible.*

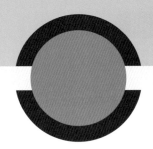

# PREFACE

The purpose of this text is to introduce the reader to health information management (HIM) both as a work-based, task-oriented function and as a contributing discipline to health care organizations, patients, and the health care industry. The third edition of Davis and LaCour's *Health Information Technology* has been revised, updated, and expanded to reflect the most recent changes in a very dynamic field.

Ever since physicians and other caregivers have been documenting their care of patients, they have had individuals working with them to help, at a minimum, store and retrieve that documentation. In the late nineteenth century and early twentieth century, the individuals who performed that function, most notably in hospitals, were the medical record librarians. (We like to imagine these people in the basement with cobwebs and dust mites, scurrying around trying to file and retrieve charts.) With each wave of change, HIM professionals have stepped up and embraced new challenges and opportunities: computerization, reimbursement, privacy and security, electronic health records, and the current transition to health information exchanges.

The health information management profession has grown over the last 75+ years as a result of health information management professionals, both individually and collectively, assuming increasing responsibilities as health care delivery has become a more complex industry. The field of health information management embraces a variety of individual functions and professional capacities, and a number of national and international professional organizations reflect the diversity of the profession in general.

Since the second edition of this title, the continued implementation of technology in this field has brought about major changes in the health information technology (HIT) landscape and the work performed by HIM professionals. *Health Information Technology* introduces the way the health care industry records, maintains, and shares patient health data, taking into account the evolving role of the Registered Health Information Technician (RHIT) from that of record filer and keeper to that of health care analyst, who turns data into useful, high-quality information for the purpose of controlling costs and furthering research.

The field of health information management today is so broad that its elements and the knowledge that individuals must acquire in order to successfully practice cannot be contained in one volume. This book is designed to meet the needs of students at the beginning of their course of study. It can easily fit into a one-quarter or one-semester course as an introduction to health information management, both in

degree programs and in certificate courses such as coding and tumor registry. It can also be used by individuals who wish to acquire some basic knowledge of health information technology and how it fits into the health care arena. To that end, we have endeavored to create a revision that is as current and comprehensive as it is user friendly, written in a style that is clear and concise, with concrete examples of the way the HIM profession works.

## Organization of the Text

*Health Information Technology* opens with a highly relatable vision of the way the modern health care operates. A thread of data collection is built from the health care encounter itself in Chapter 1 and carries through each subsequent chapter in a logical way: from health care delivery and data collection to data processing, from processing to storage, from storage to usage. In this way, the text invites the student to understand the importance of HIM professionals and the jobs they perform within the larger scope of health care delivery.

We have stressed accessibility and comprehension in every chapter of this text. A bright new design and layout have vocabulary terms and definitions in the margins, along with the meanings of acronyms/abbreviations, "Go To" cross-references, coding examples, and career tips. Each chapter begins with a list of learning objectives, vocabulary terms, and a chapter outline. Features within each chapter include interesting pieces of information (*HIT-bits*) pertaining to HIT, exercises in the form of questions, summary tables and figures, screen shots, and sample forms. End-of-chapter features include a Professional Profile highlighting a key HIM professional related to the topics discussed, and we have added a Career Tip instructing the reader on a course of study and work experience required for the position. We have also added a correlating Patient Care Perspective, which ties the HIM professional's role to tangible customer/patient care scenarios.

## New to this Edition

This edition presents a realistic, practical view of the technology and trends at work, right now, in the contemporary health care environment. Taking into account the latest advances in the discipline and valuable feedback from instructors and students who have used the second edition, we have made a number of changes, and broadened content in several key areas. Among them are the following:

- We have moved the electronic health record content from Chapter 12 to Chapter 3 to give this material a place of prominence; this chapter offers a complete picture of the hybrid/electronic health record environment, in addition to the purpose and impact of "meaningful use" requirements and the nature of health information security in electronic platforms.

- We present a detailed discussion of the landmark American Recovery and Reinvestment Act (ARRA) and Health Information Technology for Economic and Clinical Health (HITECH) Act and examine their impact across the discipline.

- Our treatment of HIM processes includes all-new content on records processing in electronic systems.

- We have devoted a full chapter each to coding and reimbursement, allowing us to emphasize the importance of coding in data collection as well as to provide a more coherent and detailed discussion of all facets of health care reimbursement.

- Chapter 9 introduces various electronic storage technologies, with a new focus on computer output to laser disk (COLD) and electronic document management systems (EDMS) (scanning/hybrid functions), an introduction to computing hardware and software, and digital storage technologies, including cloud computing.

- We have reworked the presentation of health care statistics, including basic math skills, measures of variance, and sample Excel formulas.

- All new content has been added to Chapter 11, "Quality and Uses of Health Information," to reflect the importance of process improvement, National Patient Safety Goals, and outcomes monitoring among managed care agencies, the Centers for Medicare and Medicaid Services (CMS), and accrediting bodies.

- Chapter 13 introduces the process of implementing and upgrading electronic health record systems from a management perspective.

- This edition contains more than 100 new vocabulary terms and definitions and more than 100 new illustrations.

One thing in particular that has not changed is the tone of the narrative. Our students have told us repeatedly that this is a very easy book to read and understand. As that was our original goal, we are pleased to maintain that aspect of the text.

For whatever reason you are reading this book, remember that it is the beginning of the journey. You will not have achieved understanding of health information management by the end of Chapter 14. You will need to obtain additional skills. You must acquire more knowledge from other sources in order to be a successful practicing professional in this field. Also, the industry and the profession are changing constantly. We have no doubt that elements in this book will be outdated the moment it goes to press. However, that is the challenge of lifelong learning.

We believe that health information management is an exciting and rewarding career choice for students, and we have tried our best to infuse the narrative with that enthusiasm. We hope you enjoy using this text and would welcome any comments that you may have to improve it for our next edition.

## Student Resources on Evolve

The Evolve companion Website offers additional resources to students using the text. Supplementary content details the ICD-9-CM coding system, including the structure and use of these codes as a legacy system, while the industry moves to adopt ICD-10-CM. Each of the sample paper forms shown in Appendix A of this textbook are also available on Evolve, enabling students to print blank copies of each form for practice.

## Instructor Resources on Evolve

The TEACH Instructor's Resource Manual provides detailed lesson plans, PowerPoints, and an Examview test bank. The lesson plans allow instructors to quickly familiarize themselves with the material in each chapter. Powerpoints are tailored to each lesson, highlighting the most important concepts from the text. The Examview test bank includes over 1000 questions. Each question is tied to a specific learning objective.

Instructors using this textbook also have access to a full suite of course management tools on Evolve. The Evolve Website may be used to publish the class syllabus, outlines, and lecture notes. Instructors can set up email communication and "virtual office hours," and engage the class using discussion boards and chat rooms. An online class calendar is available to share important dates and other information.

# ACKNOWLEDGMENTS

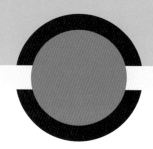

To John Tomedi, developmental editor extraordinaire, and all of the editorial and production staff who worked with us: thank you for your support, encouragement, and fabulous work.

To the reviewers: thank you for your encouragement and thoughtful comments.

Thanks to our contributors for helping to make this a more useful text.

I would like to thank the students and employees I have known, and those yet to come; it is a blessing to be motivated by your goals, expectations, and dreams!

To my family: you are my true motivation, inspiration, and love! I am Blessed!

To the contributors: Thank you for joining this team so that our students could benefit from your knowledge and expertise!

I am grateful to Nadinia Davis, and her relentless passion for writing for HIM students. You are courageous, knowledgeable, and tenacious! Your profound ability to convey all things HIM in ways that others may learn is beyond commendable. Thank you, Nadinia, for teaching me so much; I am so proud to be a part of this team!

Many thanks to my coauthor, Missy LaCour. You are an inspiration to all of us who believe that learning never ends and that we are limited only by our imagination.

To my family: thank you for your constant love and support.

Finally, thank you to all of our students, past, present, and future. We didn't write this book for ourselves, we wrote it for you. Thank you for making it a successful endeavor.

*Nadinia Davis*

John Tomedi, your unconditional support, motivation, and encouragement made this possible. I sincerely appreciate your tireless work along this journey—you are a wizard!

Likewise, a special thanks to the Elsevier team for all of the behind-the-scenes work that puts this edition into the hands of our students.

And finally, this edition began again with Susan Cole and her belief in us: Nadinia and me and the entire HIM community. She understood the need for this project to promote HIM to all students. Her support and enthusiasm for the HIM field made so many projects possible. Thank you, Susan, and God Bless!

*Missy LaCour*

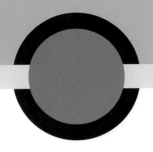

# ABOUT THE AUTHORS

## Nadinia Davis, MBA, CPA, RHIA, CHDA, FAHIMA

Nadinia Davis is the Program Coordinator for the Health Information Management Program at Delaware Technical and Community College in Delaware. She holds a Bachelor's degree in Political Science from Villanova University in Pennsylvania and an MBA with a concentration in accounting from Fairleigh Dickinson University in New Jersey. Nadinia worked for 12 years in the financial services industry before returning to school to obtain her postbaccalaureate certificate in health information management from Kean University in New Jersey. Nadinia has worked in a variety of capacities in acute care facilities and has been a coding consultant and a director of medical records in a rehabilitation facility. She taught health information management (HIM) at the associate degree level and then the baccalaureate level for a total of 12 years before returning to industry for nearly 4 years, as the Director of Health Records Services and subsequently the Executive Director of Revenue Cycle at Mountainside Hospital in New Jersey.

Nadinia is a past president of the New Jersey Health Information Management Association and received the New Jersey Health Information Management Association (NJHIMA) Distinguished Member Award in 1999. She served for 3 years on the Board of Directors of the American Health Information Management Association (AHIMA). In 2004 she was granted Fellowship in the AHIMA, and in 2007 she was inducted into the Honor Society of Phi Kappa Phi, Kean University Chapter.

## Melissa LaCour, MHIM, RHIA

Melissa (Missy) LaCour is the Dean of Distance Learning and Instructional Technology at Delgado Community College in New Orleans. She joined Delgado in August of 1996 as the Program Director of the Health Information Technology Department after holding a variety of positions in health information management, including Manager of Health Information Management at a rehabilitation center, Release of Information/Clerical Supervisor, Assistant Director, and Director of Health Information in acute care. Melissa earned a bachelor's of science in Medical Record Administration in 1990 and a Master's in Health Information Management in 2007 from Louisiana Tech University. Prior to becoming Dean she held the rank of Associate Professor.

She has volunteered her time with the Greater New Orleans Health Information Management Association, of which she is past president, and with the Louisiana Health Information Management Association (LHIMA), and she received the LHIMA Career Achievement Award in 2004.

In 2002 Nadinia and Melissa won the AHIMA Legacy award for the first edition of this book.

# ABOUT THE CONTRIBUTORS

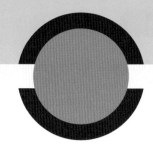

## Prerna Dua, PhD, HIT Pro

Prerna Dua is an Associate Professor in the Department of Health Informatics and Information Management at Louisiana Tech University. She obtained her PhD in Computational Analysis and Modeling in May 2006 from Louisiana Tech University. She majored in Computer Science, and her research was oriented toward finding high-performance computing solutions for health care informatics. She has published more than 20 research papers in leading journals and conferences in the area of health care data mining, knowledge discovery, and neuroinformatics. Her research has been funded by the National Institutes of Health (NIH), U.S. Department of Health and Human Services (DHHS), and Louisiana Board of Regents. She serves as an associate editor for the *Journal of Medical Imaging and Health Informatics* (*JMIHI*) and as a reviewer for the journal *Perspectives in Health Information Management*. She is an active member of AHIMA, the Health Information Management and Systems Society (HIMSS) and the Institute of Electrical and Electronics Engineers (IEEE).

## Kathleen A. Frawley, JD, MS, RHIA, FAHIMA

Kathleen Frawley, Professor and Chair of the Health Information Technology Program at DeVry University in North Brunswick, New Jersey, is the President of the AHIMA for 2013.

Kathleen has served in senior management positions in health care organizations for over 30 years. She is a past president of New Jersey Health Information Management Association (NJHIMA) and received the organization's Distinguished Member Award in 2011. She was the 2001 recipient of AHIMA's Distinguished Member Award.

In 1996 Kathleen was appointed by DHHS Secretary Donna Shalala to serve on the National Committee on Vital and Health Statistics. In November 2000 she was presented with the Secretary's Certificate of Appreciation for her time, effort, leadership, and counsel in the areas of computer-based patient records, standards, privacy, confidentiality, and security.

Kathleen participated in the landmark study "For the Record: Protecting Electronic Health Information," sponsored by the Computer Science and Telecommunications Board of the National Research Council. She has written numerous articles and chapters in textbooks on health information issues. She is a frequent speaker and has participated in audio seminars, teleseminars, and public radio and television broadcasts.

Kathleen received her Bachelor of Arts degree in English from the College of Mount Saint Vincent, her master of science degree in Health Services Administration from Wagner College, and her Juris Doctorate from New York Law School. She is certified as a Registered Health Information Administrator by the AHIMA and is a Fellow of AHIMA. She is also a member of the New York Bar.

## Marion Gentul, RHIA, CCS

Marion is an independent consultant, employing her 30 years of health information management experience to provide a variety of related services. Marion holds a Bachelor's Degree in Psychology from the University of Rhode Island and completed her Health Information Management education at the State University of New York Downstate Medical Center.

She has been an AHIMA-approved ICD-10 trainer since 2009, currently serving as an associate with the New Jersey Hospital Association for their ICD-10 educational programs. She is a subject matter expert for MC Strategies/Elsevier and assists with the writing and development of the company's online ICD-10 training programs.

She is coauthor of two chapters in AHIMA's publication *Effective Management of Coding Services* and has been a contributor to previous editions of Davis and LaCour's *Health Information Technology*.

Marion received AHIMA's Triumph Mentor Award, was named a Distinguished Alumna by SUNY Downstate Medical Center, and is also a recipient of the NJHIMA Distinguished Member Award.

She is a past president of the NJHIMA and past chair of the NJHIMA Scholarship Fund Board.

## Angela Kennedy, EdD, MBA, MEd, RHIA

Angela is an accomplished educator and leader who serves as the Chair of the Department of Health Informatics and Information Management at Louisiana Tech University. She has a rich history in association leadership. Angela served two terms as president of LHIMA. She most recently served as the Chair of the Commission on Accreditation for Health Informatics and Information Management Education (CAHIIM).

Angela served on the AHIMA Board of Directors in 2007 and is currently the 2013 AHIMA President-elect. She has served as President of the Louisiana Chapter of HIMSS and as a member of the National Association for HealthCare Quality (NAHQ) Leadership Council. Angela is an AHIMA Triumph Award winner, an LHIMA Distinguished Member, and an LHIMA Career Achievement recipient.

## Kim Theodos, JD, MS, RHIA

Kim is a tenured Associate Professor in the Health Informatics and Information Management Department at Louisiana Tech University in Ruston, Louisiana. She teaches undergraduate courses in the areas of legal and regulatory issues, quality and statistics, management, and the electronic health record. Kim holds a Bachelor of Science in Health Information Administration from Louisiana Tech University and a Master of Science in Healthcare Management from the University of

New Orleans. She has also earned a Juris Doctorate from Taft Law School. Kim has 8 years of teaching experience in both online and traditional on-campus formats. She is an active volunteer in the HIM industry, serving at local, state, and national levels. Kim served as President of the LHIMA and continues to volunteer in professional associations and on committees.

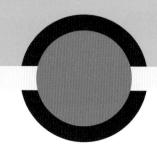

# EDITORIAL REVIEW BOARD

# CONTENTS

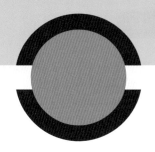

## UNIT II: Content, Structure, and Processing of Health Information 92

### CHAPTER 4 Acute Care Records 92

### CHAPTER 5 Health Information Management Processing 116

### CHAPTER 6 Code Sets 144

CHAPTER 7  **Reimbursement**                                           **163**

CHAPTER 8  **Health Information Management Issues in Other Care Settings    212**

## UNIT III: Maintenance and Analysis of Health Information 244

### CHAPTER 9 Managing Health Records 244

### CHAPTER 10 Statistics 289

## CHAPTER 11    Quality and Uses of Health Information                335

## UNIT IV: Legal and Supervisory Issues in Health Information    383

## CHAPTER 14  **Training and Development**                                        **459**

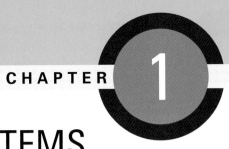

# HEALTH CARE DELIVERY SYSTEMS

Nadinia Davis

## CHAPTER OUTLINE

**HEALTH CARE PROFESSIONALS**
Physicians
Nurses
Allied Health Professionals
Professional Organizations
Health Information
  Management
Interdisciplinary
  Collaboration

**COMPARISON OF FACILITIES**
Types of Facilities
Facility Size
Ownership
Tax Status
Patient Population
Services
Continuity of Care
Modern Models

**LEGAL AND REGULATORY
ENVIRONMENT**
Federal
State
Local
Accreditation
Professional Standards

## VOCABULARY

accreditation
activities of daily living (ADL)
acute care facility
admission
allied health professionals
ambulatory care facility
American Health
  Information
  Management
  Association (AHIMA)
assisted living
bed count
behavioral health facility
Centers for Medicare and
  Medicaid Services
children's hospital
Commission on
  Accreditation for Health
  Informatics and
  Information
  Management (CAHIIM)

Conditions of Participation
  (COP)
consultation
continuity of care
continuum of care
credentials
deemed status
Department of Health
  and Human Services
  (DHHS)
diagnosis
discharge
dual governance
ethics
health information
  management (HIM)
health information
  technology (HIT)
home health care
hospice
hospital

hospitalist
inpatients
integrated delivery systems
  (IDS)
licensed beds
licensure
long-term care (LTC) facility
Medicaid
medical specialty
Medicare
medication
mental health facility
National Integrated
  Accreditation for
  Healthcare Organizations
  (NIAHO)
nurse
occupancy
outpatient
palliative care
patient care plan

physician
physician's orders
primary care physician (PCP)
procedure
psychiatrist
referral
rehabilitation facility
resident
The Joint Commission
  (TJC)

## CHAPTER OBJECTIVES

*By the end of this chapter, the student should be able to:*
1. Identify and describe the major medical specialties.
2. Distinguish among nursing occupations.
3. Identify and describe the major allied health
   professions and their principal occupational settings.
4. Distinguish between inpatients and outpatients.
5. Describe the differences among health care facilities.
6. Describe government involvement in health care.
7. Define *accreditation*.
8. Define *licensure*.
9. List four major accrediting organizations and the
   facilities they accredit.

The purpose of this chapter is to help you understand the basic structure and terminology of the health care industry. Most people have experienced the need for health care at one time, either at birth or for treatment of a particular illness or injury. In fact, some people know a lot about certain types of health care because of their own illness or the illness of a family member or friend. While reading this chapter, you may find it helpful to try to recall such personal experiences, to link what is presented here to your previous experiences and understanding of the health care industry.

## HEALTH CARE PROFESSIONALS

The health care industry includes professionals in many disciplines. These professionals vary from physicians and nurses to therapists and technicians to administrative and financial personnel. Each of these professionals plays a vital role in the delivery of health care. Physicians generally direct the delivery of care. They make decisions about the patient's condition and advise treatment. Physicians are vital to the health care team, because typically they are the individuals who direct the treatment plan, through physician orders. Nurses and therapists often work on teams with physicians, helping to make those decisions and carrying out the recommended treatments. Technical and administrative personnel support the teams by administering and evaluating tests, organizing data, and evaluating processes and procedures.

**physician's orders** The physician's directions regarding the patient's care. Also refers to the data collection device on which these elements are captured.

---

### HIT-bit

**PROFESSION**

What is a profession?

"An occupation whose core element is work based upon the mastery of a complex body of knowledge and skills. It is a vocation in which knowledge of some department of science or learning or the practice of an art founded upon it is used in the service of others. Its members are governed by codes of ethics and profess a commitment to competence, integrity and morality, altruism, and the promotion of the public good within their domain. These commitments form the basis of a social contract between a profession and society, which in return grants the profession a monopoly over the use of its knowledge base, the right to considerable autonomy in practice and the privilege of self-regulation. Professions and their members are accountable to those served and to society." (Cruess et al 2004)

---

**physician** A medical professional who has satisfied the academic, professional, and legal requirements to diagnose and treat patients at state-specified levels and within a declared specialty.

**treatment** A procedure, medication, or other measure designed to cure or alleviate the symptoms of disease.

**diagnosis** Literally, "complete knowledge"; refers to the name of the patient's condition or illness or the reason for the health care encounter.

**resident** A person who after attending college and medical school performs professional duties under the supervision of a fully qualified physician.

**MD** doctor of medicine
**DO** doctor of osteopathy

### Physicians

A **physician** is a person who is licensed to practice medicine. The practice of medicine is regulated by the individual state, which issues the license. To become licensed, a physician attends college and medical school and then serves a residency in his or her specialty. A physician earns a degree as a Doctor of Medicine (MD) or a Doctor of Osteopathy (DO). The schools that train MDs and DOs focus on different philosophies of medical **treatment** and **diagnosis**. A **resident** performs professional duties under the supervision of a fully qualified physician. Residency can last from 4 to 8 years, depending on the specialty. The medical licensing examination can be taken after the first year of residency. MDs take the United States Medical Licensing Examination (USMLE), which is developed and administered by the Federation of State Medical Boards (FSMB) in collaboration with the National Board of Medical Examiners (NBME). The USMLE is a three-step examination process that tests both the knowledge of the candidate and the ability of the candidate to apply that knowledge in the clinical setting. Examination results are provided to the individual state medical boards for licensing purposes (United States Medical Licensing Examination, 2012).

Historically, DOs relied on physical manipulation of the patient, particularly the spine, to alleviate symptoms of disease. MDs, on the other hand, used drugs and surgery, also

## TABLE 1-1

### COMMON MEDICAL SPECIALTIES

| PHYSICIAN SPECIALTY | DESCRIPTION |
| --- | --- |
| Allergist | Diagnoses and treats patients who have strong reactions to pollen, insect bites, food, medication, and other irritants |
| Anesthesiologist | Administers substances that cause loss of sensation, particularly during surgery |
| Cardiologist | Diagnoses and treats patients with diseases of the heart and blood vessels |
| Dermatologist | Diagnoses and treats patients with diseases of the skin |
| Family practitioner | Delivers primary health care for patients of all ages |
| Gastroenterologist | Diagnoses and treats patients with diseases of the digestive system |
| Gynecologist | Diagnoses and treats disorders of, and provides well care related to, the female reproductive system |
| Hospitalist | Employed by a hospital; medical practice focuses on patient care situations specific to acute care settings |
| Neonatologist | Diagnoses and treats diseases and abnormal conditions of newborns |
| Obstetrician | Cares for women before, during, and after delivery |
| Oncologist | Diagnoses and treats patients with cancer |
| Ophthalmologist | Diagnoses and treats patients with diseases of the eye |
| Orthopedist | Diagnoses and treats patients with diseases of the muscles and bones |
| Pathologist | Studies changes in cells, tissue, and organs in order to diagnose diseases and/or to determine possible treatments |
| Pediatrician | Delivers primary health care to children |
| Psychiatrist | Diagnoses and treats patients with disorders of the mind |
| Radiologist | Uses radiography and other tools to diagnose and treat a variety of diseases |

called *conventional medicine*, to treat patients. The term allopathic is sometimes used in reference to the conventional approach. In the United States, DOs take a whole-body approach and are likely to use both manipulation (osteopathic manipulative treatment) and conventional methods. However, in other countries, the historical differences remain. All states in the United States license both MDs and DOs (American Osteopathic Association, 2012).

Physicians are generally categorized by **medical specialty**. They can treat patients according to the area of the body, according to specific diseases, or by assisting with diagnosis. For example, an oncologist is a physician who diagnoses and treats cancers. A gastroenterologist specializes in diseases of the digestive system. Treatments range from diet and exercise, to oral **medications**, to **procedures**, such as surgical removal of diseased tissue. Some specialties may focus more narrowly on the patient's age group; a pediatric oncologist deals with children's cancers. Table 1-1 lists some common medical specialties.

Several of the tasks that physicians perform are considered specialties, even though many physicians may perform those tasks to a certain extent. For instance, a radiologist is a specialist who interprets radiographs and images from other types of examinations of internal organs. A gastroenterologist knows how to read a radiograph, but it is not his or her specialty. A growing practice is physicians who specialize in treating hospitalized patients. So, although many physicians admit patients into hospitals and care for them there, **hospitalists** care only for patients in that environment.

Medicine typically requires a minimum 10 years of study after high school. A physician who intends to specialize in family practice attends college for 4 years and medical school for another 3 years. He or she then applies for a residency of 3 years in family practice, studying internal medicine, pediatrics, obstetrics and gynecology, psychiatry, and geriatrics. An additional year of residency is required if the physician wants to further specialize in geriatrics, adolescent, or sports medicine (American Association of Medical Colleges, 2011).

**medical specialty** The focus of a physician's practice, such as pediatrics or oncology. Specialties are represented by Boards, which certify physicians in the specialty.

**medication** Chemical substance used to treat disease.

**procedure** A medical or surgical treatment.

**hospitalist** A physician employed by a hospital, whose medical practice is focused primarily on patient care situations specific to the acute care setting.

## HIT-bit ··········································································

### MEDICAL TERMINOLOGY

If you have not yet studied medical terminology, here is a brief lesson. Medical terms consist of combining forms, prefixes, and suffixes. These parts are assembled to form words, which can easily be deciphered when you know the definitions of the parts. For example, we just used the word oncologist. This word is assembled from the following parts:

onc/o = cancer
-logy = process of study
-ist = one who specializes

Therefore an oncologist is one who specializes in the study of cancer. The following are the word parts of some of the other specialties we mentioned:

gastr/o = stomach
enter/o = intestine
ped/i = children
iatr/o = treatment
-ic = pertaining to
oste/o = bone
-pathy = process of disease

Can you decipher the words in Table 1-1 now that you know their parts?

---

**referral** The act or documentation of one physician's request for an opinion or services from another health care professional, often another physician, for a specific patient regarding specific signs, symptoms, or diagnosis.

**consultation** The formal request by a physician for the professional opinion or services of another health care professional, usually another physician, in caring for a patient. Also refers to the opinion or services themselves as well as the activity of rendering the opinion or services.

**primary care physician (PCP)** In insurance, the physician who has been designated by the insured to deliver routine care to the insured and to evaluate the need for referral to a specialist, if applicable. Colloquial use is synonymous with "family doctor."

**PCP** primary care physician

**nurse** A medical professional who has satisfied the academic, professional, and legal requirements to care for patients at state-specified levels. Although usually delivering patient care at the direction of physicians, nurse practitioners may also deliver care independently.

Beyond licensing and completing the residency, physicians pursue additional training and take an examination to become board certified. Board certification is developed and administered by the specialty board that sets standards of education for the physician's specialty. The American Board of Medical Specialties is an umbrella group representing the 24 medical specialty boards (American Board of Medical Specialties, 2011). Among the 24 medical specialties, there are additional subspecialties. As noted previously, geriatrics is a subspecialty of family medicine. A board-certified family practitioner is referred to as a Diplomate of the American Board of Family Medicine. See Box 1-1 for a list of medical specialty boards.

Most individuals have a relationship with a family practitioner. This physician is trained to identify and treat a wide variety of conditions. However, the family practitioner also seeks guidance from other specialists as needed. For example, the family practitioner may identify a suspicious skin problem and send the patient to a dermatologist for evaluation. The process of sending a patient to another physician in this manner is called a **referral**. Alternatively, the family practitioner may ask the dermatologist to evaluate the patient's condition and confirm the family practitioner's ideas or give recommendations for treating the patient. The latter process is further called a **consultation**. A physician who coordinates the care of a patient, through referrals and consultations, is called a **primary care physician** (**PCP**). A family practitioner is most often the PCP for his or her patients. However, not all PCPs are family practitioners. For example, some women choose to use their gynecologists as their PCPs. A pediatrician is frequently the PCP for a child.

## Nurses

A **nurse** is a clinical professional who has received post-secondary school training in caring for patients in a variety of health care settings. There are several levels of nursing education, each qualifying the nurse for different positions. Historically, most nurses graduated from a hospital-based certificate program. Another large percentage received their training through associate degree programs. A growing number of nurses have a bachelor's or master's of science degree in nursing, and today, almost all nurses are college educated at some level. Nurses, like doctors, take licensing examinations. Table 1-2 lists the various levels of nursing and their educational requirements.

<table>
<tr><td>BOX 1-1</td><td>MEDICAL SPECIALTY BOARDS: AMERICAN BOARD OF MEDICAL SPECIALTIES MEMBER BOARDS</td></tr>
</table>

American Board of Allergy and Immunology
American Board of Anesthesiology
American Board of Colon and Rectal Surgery
American Board of Dermatology
American Board of Emergency Medicine
American Board of Family Medicine
American Board of Internal Medicine
American Board of Medical Genetics
American Board of Neurological Surgery
American Board of Nuclear Medicine
American Board of Obstetrics and Gynecology
American Board of Ophthalmology
American Board of Orthopaedic Surgery
American Board of Otolaryngology
American Board of Pathology
American Board of Pediatrics
American Board of Physical Medicine and Rehabilitation
American Board of Plastic Surgery
American Board of Preventive Medicine
American Board of Psychiatry and Neurology
American Board of Radiology
American Board of Surgery
American Board of Thoracic Surgery
American Board of Urology

## TABLE 1-2

### LEVELS OF NURSING PRACTICE

| TITLE | GENERAL DESCRIPTION AND REQUIREMENTS |
|---|---|
| Licensed Vocational Nurse; Licensed Practical Nurse | High school graduate or equivalent; graduation from a 1- to 2-year state-approved Health Occupations Education practical/vocational nurse program; pass NCLEX-PN examination. Licensed by state of employment or by the National Federation of Licensed Practical Nurses. |
| Registered Nurse | Minimum high school graduation or equivalent; programs leading to registration are offered at the associate, bachelor's, and master's degree levels. Examination and licensure in state of practice. |
| Nurse Practitioner | Registered nurse; completion of an accredited course in nurse practitioner training. |
| Advanced Practice Nursing examples: Acute Care Nurse Practitioner Adult Nurse Practitioner Family Nurse Practitioner Gerontological Nurse Practitioner Pediatric Nurse Practitioner | Completion of practice requirements and examinations offered by the American Nurses Credentialing Center, a subsidiary of the American Nursing Association. |

From American Nurses Association: http://www.nursecredentialing.org/Certification.aspx; All Nursing Schools: http://www.allnursingschools.com/faqs/lpn.php. Published 2012. Accessed July 10, 2012.

## Licensed Practical Nurse

A licensed practical nurse (LPN), sometimes referred to as a *vocational nurse*, receives training at a hospital-based, technical, or vocational school. The training consists of learning to care for patients' personal needs and other types of routine care. LPNs work under the direction of physicians or registered nurses, or both. The extent of their practice depends on the rules of the state in which they are licensed. It may include providing treatments and administering medications.

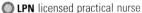 **LPN** licensed practical nurse

**medication administration** Clinical data including the name of the medication, dosage, date and time of administration, method of administration, and the nurse who administered it.

**○ RN** registered nurse

**○ APRN** advanced practice registered
   nurse

### Registered Nurse

In addition to caring for patients' personal needs, a registered nurse (RN) administers medication and renders other care at the order of a physician. RNs particularly focus on assessing and meeting the patients' need for education regarding their illness. RNs may specialize in caring for different types of patients. For example, a nurse may assist in the operating room or care for children or and older adult, each of which requires special skills and training. RNs who want to move into management-level or teaching positions generally pursue a master's degree, a doctoral degree, a specialty certification, or some combination of these qualifications.

### Advanced Practice Nursing Specialties

In response to physician shortages and nurses' desire for greater independence, several advanced specialties in nursing practice have developed under the general title advanced practice registered nurse (APRN). Examples of these specialties are nurse midwives and nurse anesthetists. A nurse midwife focuses on the care of women during the period surrounding childbirth: pregnancy, labor, delivery, and after delivery. A nurse anesthetist is trained to administer anesthesia and to care for patients during the delivery of anesthesia and recovery from the process. APRNs have a minimum of a master's degree and additional training and certification beyond the RN certification.

The American Nurses Credentialing Center, a subsidiary of the American Nursing Association, offers a variety of advanced practice certifications in subspecialties such as diabetes management and pediatrics (American Nurses Credentialing Center, 2006).

---

### HIT-bit

#### ALPHABET SOUP

The decoding of professional credentials is simplified by familiarity with a few guidelines:

**R**—generally stands for Registered. Individuals who are registered have complied with the standards of the registering organization. Standards may include passing an examination, completing academic requirements, and demonstrating experience in the field.

**C**—means the individual is Certified. This term is synonymous with Registered.

**F**—signifies a Fellow. A Fellow has generally demonstrated long-term, significant contribution to his or her discipline or a specific high level of competence. Fellowship is granted in a professional organization. For physicians, board certification is expressed as a fellowship.

**L**—refers to a License. Separate from other designations, licensure denotes compliance with state regulations. Individuals may be licensed. Facilities may also be licensed. In some disciplines, licensure is a prerequisite to practice.

These guidelines refer to the acronyms of the credential. Some credentials imply dual meanings. For example, registered nurses (RNs) are so designated when they are licensed to practice.

---

**○ allied health professionals** Health
   care professionals who support
   patient care in a variety of
   disciplines, including
   occupational therapy and
   physical therapy.
**radiology** Literally, the study of
   x-rays. In a health care facility,
   the department responsible for
   maintaining x-ray and other
   types of diagnostic and
   therapeutic equipment as well
   as analyzing diagnostic films.

## Allied Health Professionals

**Allied health** (or health-related) **professionals** can include both clinical and nonclinical professionals who provide a variety of services to patients. A clinical professional is one who provides health care services to a patient, generally pursuant to orders from a physician or APRN. Clinical professionals include radiology technicians and a variety of therapists. Nonclinical professionals support the clinical staff and provide other types of services to a patient. Nonclinical allied health staff includes health information management professionals. Table 1-3 provides examples of clinical allied health professions, their principal work environments, and their basic educational requirements.

## TABLE 1-3

### EXAMPLES OF CLINICAL HEALTH-RELATED PROFESSIONS

| TITLE | DESCRIPTION | REQUIREMENTS |
|---|---|---|
| Occupational Therapist | Focuses on returning patient to maximal functioning in activities of daily living. Primarily employed in rehabilitation facilities but may work in virtually any health care environment. | Bachelor's degree; licensure required in most states; certification (registration) can be obtained from the American Occupational Therapy Association. |
| Phlebotomist | Draws blood for donation and testing. Primarily employed in health care facilities and community blood banks. | High school graduate or equivalent. Completion of 10- to 20-hour certification program in a hospital, physician's office, or laboratory. Completion of a vocational education program as a phlebotomist. |
| Physical Therapist | Focuses on strength, gait, and range-of-motion training to return patients to maximal functioning in activities of daily living. Primarily employed in rehabilitation facilities but may work in virtually any health care environment. | Master's or doctoral degree; licensure by state of practice. All accredited programs will be required to offer the doctoral degree by 2015. |
| Registered Dietitian | Manages food services; evaluates nutritional needs, including planning menus and special diets and educating patients and family. Primarily employed in health care facilities. | Bachelor's degree; registration can be obtained from American Dietetic Association; licensure, certification, or registration required in many states. |
| Respiratory Therapist | Delivers therapies related to breathing. Employed primarily in health care facilities. | Associate or bachelor's degree; licensure or certification required in most states; registration can be obtained from the National Board for Respiratory Care. |

## Professional Organizations

Increasing demand for health care workers and the special emphasis on particular groups of patients has led to a proliferation of professional associations and credentials. One of the primary roles of a professional association is to improve the practice of the profession. Therefore professional associations play a critical role in the development of professional standards and improvement in health care delivery.

One of the standards of professional practice that can improve health care is mandatory education, both formal education and continuing education. Formal education in the discipline supports consistency of education, research, and growth of the knowledge base of the profession. The outcome of this formal education process is often the qualification to sit for an examination. That examination is designed to measure the competence of the individual. The specific level of competence varies from entry-level (basic) competence to advanced or specialty practice. Satisfaction of the profession's requirements for competence entitles the individual to certain **credentials**. Maintenance of a professional credential generally requires continuing education (CE). Continuing professional education supports the currency of professional knowledge among practitioners.

The credentialing requirements of professions vary widely. In some cases, no formal education is required. In other cases, no actual professional experience is required. In general, the professional associations themselves, or their credentialing affiliates, dictate the levels of expertise and evidence of competence required for the granting of credentials. For some professionals, such as nurses and physicians, licensure granted by the state or professional association is required in addition to competency examinations. *Health information management (HIM)* is an example of a category of professionals with multiple professional associations and a variety of credentials.

The **American Health Information Management Association (AHIMA)** supports the health care industry by promoting high-quality information standards through a variety of activities, including but not limited to accreditation of schools, continuing education, professional development and educational publications, and legislative and regulatory advocacy. The American Academy of Professional Coders (AAPC) promotes the accuracy of coding and billing in all health care settings, but particularly outpatient. AAPC offers multiple credentials in coding as well as auditing and training. Coding is discussed in Chapters 5 through 7 as it is an important HIM function.

**credentials** An individual's specific professional qualifications. Also refers to the letters that a professionally qualified person is entitled to list after his or her name.

**continuing education (CE)** Education required after a person has attained a position, credential, or degree, intended to keep the person knowledgeable in his/her profession.

**HIM** health information management

**American Health Information Management Association (AHIMA)** A professional organization supporting the health care industry by promoting high-quality information standards through a variety of activities, including but not limited to accreditation of schools, continuing education, professional development and educational publications, and legislative and regulatory advocacy.

**coding** The assignment of alphanumerical values to a word, phrase, or other non numerical expression. In health care, coding is the assignment of numerical values to diagnosis and procedure descriptions.

**AAPC** American Academy of Professional Coders

## Health Information Management

**health information management (HIM)** The profession that manages the sources and uses of health information, including the collection, storage, retrieval, and reporting of health information.

**electronic health records (EHRs)** A computer-based information resource allowing access to patient information when and where needed.

**Health information management (HIM)** encompasses all the tasks, jobs, titles, and organizations involved in the administration of health information, including collection, storage, retrieval, and reporting of that information. HIM professionals perform or oversee the functions that support these activities and frequently expand their practice to related activities, encompassing the financial and technical operations of a health care practitioner or organization. For example, HIM professionals may assist in the development and implementation of electronic health records (EHRs), oversee the maintenance of those databases, provide support services such as patient registration, retrieve data for reporting and continuing patient care, and participate in the billing process.

Literally hundreds of different jobs with many different titles are performed by HIM professionals throughout the world. This text presents specific job descriptions and job titles that can assist in planning a career in HIM. (See Table 1-4.)

### TABLE 1-4

#### EXAMPLES OF HEALTH INFORMATION MANAGEMENT PROFESSIONALS

| TITLE | DESCRIPTION | REQUIREMENTS |
|---|---|---|
| Certified Coding Specialist (CCS) or Certified Coding Specialist/ Physician-based (CCS-P) or Certified Coding Associate (CCA) | Assigns, collects, and reports codes representing clinical data. Primarily employed in health care facilities. | Certification by examination from the American Health Information Management Association. |
| Certified in Healthcare Privacy and Security (CHPS) | Specializes in privacy and security aspects of HIM practice. | A combination of education or credentials and health care data experience, ranging from an associate degree and 6 years of experience to a master's degree and 2 years of experience. |
| Certified Health Data Analyst (CHDA) | Analyzes health care data | A combination of education or credentials and health care data experience, ranging from an associate degree and 5 years of experience to an advanced degree and 1 year of experience. |
| Clinical Documentation Improvement Professional (CDIP) | Supports the collection of clinical documentation | An RHIA, RHIT, CCS, CCS-P, RN, MD, or DO and 2 years of experience in clinical documentation improvement, or an associate's degree or higher and 3 years of experience in the clinical documentation setting. |
| Health Unit Coordinator | Transcribes physician's orders, prepares and compiles records during patient hospitalization. Primarily employed in acute care facilities, long-term care facilities, and clinics. | High school graduate or equivalent; community college; hospital training program; completion of a vocational education program in the area of ward clerk, unit secretary, or health unit coordinator. Certification available from the National Association of Health Unit Coordinators. |
| Registered Health Information Technician | Provides administrative support targeting the collection, retention, and reporting of health information. Employed primarily in health care facilities but may work in a variety of settings, including insurance and pharmaceutical companies. | Associate degree from accredited Health Information Technology program; registration by examination from the American Health Information Management Association. |
| Registered Health Information Administrator | Provides administrative support targeting the collection, retention, and reporting of health information, including strategic planning, research, and systems analysis and acquisition. Employed primarily in health care facilities but may work in a variety of settings, including insurance and pharmaceutical companies. | Bachelor's degree from accredited Health Information Administration program; registration by examination from the American Health Information Management Association. |

HIM professionals work in virtually every area of the health care delivery system, from physician offices and hospitals to insurance companies and government agencies. They are also employed by suppliers, such as computer software vendors, and educational institutions as well as consulting firms. Throughout this text are discussions of historical roles, emerging roles, and the future of the HIM profession. As you review the many opportunities available to HIM professionals, it would be useful to check industry publications and Web sites for information about those specific jobs in your geographical area and around the world.

## Health Information Management Credentials
### *American Health Information Management Association*

The American Health Information Management Association (AHIMA) offers certification at progressively higher levels of education and experience. According to the AHIMA Web site, the organization offers the following (AHIMA, 2012):

Coding credentials (see Chapter 6 for a detailed discussion of coding issues):

- *Certified Coding Associate (CCA)*, the entry-level credential for coding. The credential is available by examination. No specific formal training is required; however, coding courses or on-the-job training is recommended. A high school education (or equivalent) is required.
- *Certified Coding Specialist (CCS)*, the mastery credential for coding. The credential is available by examination. No specific formal training is required; however, coding courses or on-the-job training is recommended. A high school education (or equivalent) is required.
- *Certified Coding Specialist/Physician-based (CCS-P)*, the mastery credential for coding in physician-based settings. The credential is available by examination. No specific formal training is required; however, the examination is designed to measure proficiency. Therefore significant study of coding or several years of experience (or both) are recommended. A high school education (or equivalency) is required.

General HIM credentials include the following:

- *Registered Health Information Technician (RHIT)*, the credential that demonstrates entry-level competency at the associate degree level. Graduation from an accredited HIT program is required to sit for the national examination.
- *Registered Health Information Administrator (RHIA)*, the credential that demonstrates entry-level competency at the baccalaureate or master's level. Graduation from an accredited Health Information Administration program or an approved master's program is required to sit for the national examination.

Advanced and specialty practice credentials include the following. Eligibility criteria and testing requirements are posted on the AHIMA Web site (AHIMA, 2012).

- *Certified in Healthcare Privacy and Security (CHPS)* is a specialty credential that demonstrates advanced competency in privacy and security aspects of HIM practice. Originally, individuals who were eligible for and who passed both the CHP and CHS examinations were designated CHPS. The CHP and CHS credentials are no longer offered separately. Individuals holding existing CHP or CHS designations may retain them.
- *Certified Health Data Analyst (CHDA)* is a specialty credential that demonstrates advanced competency in the analysis of health care data. Eligibility requirements include a combination of education or credentials and health care data experience, ranging from an associate degree and 5 years of experience to an advanced degree and 1 year of experience.
- *Clinical Documentation Improvement Professional (CDIP)* credential evidences competency in the skills necessary to support clinical documentation improvement activities, usually in the acute care setting.

The examinations for all of the previously mentioned credentials are offered through computer-based testing 6 days per week, year round, at locations nationwide. Additional information, including examination fees and continuing education requirements, may be found at http://www.ahima.org/certification/default.aspx.

**AHIMA** American Health Information Management Association

**CCA** Certified Coding Associate
**CCS** Certified Coding Specialist
**CCS-P** Certified Coding Specialist/Physician-based

**RHIT** Registered Health Information Technician
**RHIA** Registered Health Information Adimistrator

**CHPS** Certified in Healthcare Privacy and Security
**CHDA** Certified Health Data Analyst
**CDIP** Clinical Documentation Improvement Professional

● **AAPC** American Academy of Professional Coders

● **payer** The individual or organization that is primarily responsible for the reimbursement for a particular health care service. Usually refers to the insurance company or third party.

**outpatient** A patient whose health care services are intended to be delivered within 1 calendar day or, in some cases, a 24-hour period.

● **ONC** Office of the National Coordinator for Health Information Technology

● **health information technology (HIT)** The specialty in the field of health information management that focuses on the day-to-day activities of health information management that support the collection, storage, retrieval, and reporting of health information.

**workflow** The process of work flowing through a set of procedures to complete the health record.

● **diagnosis** The name of the patient's condition or illness, the reason for the health care encounter.

**patient care plan** The formal directions for treatment of the patient, which involves many different individuals, including the patient. It may be as simple as instructions to "take two aspirins and drink plenty of fluids," or it may be a multiple-page document with delegation of responsibilities. Care plans may also be developed by discipline, such as nursing.

**treatment** A procedure, medication, or other measure designed to cure or alleviate the symptoms of disease.

● **HIM** health information management

### American Academy of Professional Coders

The American Academy of Professional Coders (AAPC) offers a myriad of credentials, specifically for coders, with an emphasis on outpatient coding. The primary credentials are the CPC (Certified Professional Coder) and the CPC-H (Certified Professional Coder, hospital-based). There are also credentials for coding professionals in the payer community as well as 20 medical specialties. The AAPC also offers certification in auditing and compliance. The eligibility requirements for AAPC credentials consist of membership in AAPC and passing the exam.

### Office of the National Coordinator for Health Information Technology

Chapter 3 of this textbook discusses the impact of the landmark federal legislation passed in the United States in 2009 that set goals and provided funding for the implementation of technology in health care delivery. Some of the funding administered by the Office of the National Coordinator for Health Information Technology (ONC) is dedicated to educating and training the new workforce of **health information technology (HIT)** professionals that will support health care in the electronic age. As part of these efforts, the ONC has developed a series of competency examinations for an array of short, nondegree programs offered by community colleges across the country. Called *HIT PRO Exams*, these tests show competency for a number of specialties (Office of the National Coordinator for Health Information Technology, 2012):

- Practice workflow and information management redesign specialists
- Clinician/practitioner consultants
- Implementation support specialists
- Implementation managers
- Technical/software support
- Trainers

## Interdisciplinary Collaboration

Clinical professionals work together to care for the patient. Developing a diagnosis is generally the responsibility of the physician. The physician will also prescribe any medication or therapies. However, the care of the patient involves many different individuals, including the patient. The **patient care plan** may be as simple as instructions to "take two aspirin and drink plenty of fluids," or it may be a multiple-page document with delegation of responsibilities. Suppose a patient has been diagnosed with Type I diabetes mellitus, a disease characterized by chronic high blood glucose that can be controlled only with medication (i.e., insulin). The patient care plan might have the following parts:

- A nurse may be responsible for educating the patient about medication regimens.
- A psychologist can help the patient deal with the stress of chronic illness.
- An HIM professional can provide the patient with documentation of the diagnosis and treatment for continuing patient care.
- A social worker may help the patient's family learn about the disease and what to do in a crisis.

  If the patient is older and lives alone:

- A home health care worker may be brought in to check the patient's blood glucose level at home.
- A registered dietician may provide the patient with education about proper diet.
- A physical therapist may provide the patient with training for safe conditioning exercises.

    The patient, of course, must be involved every step of the way. A well-documented patient care plan helps all members of the interdisciplinary care team work together to deliver the best possible care to the patient.

## HIT-bit

### DIAGNOSIS AND PROCEDURE

Physicians identify and treat illnesses. They can also help prevent illnesses through patient education and various types of inoculations. Nurses and professionals in other health-related disciplines help physicians prevent, identify, and treat illnesses. Identification of the illness is the *diagnosis*. A *procedure* is performed to help in the identification (diagnostic) and treatment (therapeutic) processes.

|  | PROCEDURE | |
| --- | --- | --- |
| DIAGNOSIS | DIAGNOSTIC | THERAPEUTIC |
| A disease or abnormal condition | The evaluation or investigative steps taken to develop the diagnosis or monitor a disease or condition | The steps taken to alleviate or eliminate the cause or symptoms of a disease or condition |

*Examples*

| | | |
| --- | --- | --- |
| Appendicitis | Physical examination Blood test | Appendectomy |
| Cerebrovascular accident (stroke) | Physical examination Neurological examination Computed tomography scan | Medication Physical therapy Occupational therapy Speech therapy Psychological counseling |
| Myocardial infarction (heart attack) | Physical examination Blood test Electrocardiogram | Medication Coronary artery bypass graft |

## EXERCISE 1-1

### Health Care Professionals

1. List as many medical specialties as you can remember, and describe what they do. Refer to Table 1-1 in the text to see how well you did.
2. What is the difference between an RN and an LPN?
3. What is the purpose of advanced practice nursing credentials?
4. Physicians diagnose diseases and perform certain procedures, both diagnostic and therapeutic. Distinguish between diagnosis and procedure. Give examples of both.
5. Much of the care for patients is performed by various allied health professionals. List as many allied health professionals as you can remember, and describe what they do. Refer to Table 1-3 in the text to see how well you did.
6. List the health information management professional credentials and what they represent.
7. What is a patient care plan?

## COMPARISON OF FACILITIES

There are many different types of facilities, some of which are discussed in detail in Chapters 4 and 8. This section gives some general examples of how to distinguish between different types of facilities and how to compare and contrast similar facilities. Because no single characteristic separates one facility from another, the comparison of facilities requires consideration of their many characteristics to obtain a real understanding of the differences.

### Types of Facilities

Many facilities offer a variety of services, making it difficult to describe the facility as one particular type. In the following discussion, the distinctions are based primarily on the length of time during which the patient is treated and the services are provided.

## Acute Care Facilities

**hospital** An organization having permanent facilities that delivers inpatient health care services through 24-hour nursing care, an organized medical staff, and appropriate ancillary departments.

**acute care facility** A health care facility in which patients have an average length of stay less than 30 days and that has an emergency department, operating suite, and clinical departments to handle a broad range of diagnoses and treatments.

A **hospital** is a facility that offers 24-hour, a round-the-clock nursing, beds for patients who stay overnight, and an organized medical staff that directs the diagnosis and treatment of the patients. An **acute care** (or short stay) **facility** is a type of hospital. The word acute means sudden or severe. Applied to illnesses, it refers to a problem that generally arises swiftly or severely. An acute care facility treats patients who require a level of care that can be provided only in the acute care setting, such as serious injuries or illnesses and surgical procedures that require significant postoperative care. The typical patient in an acute care facility either is acutely ill or has some problem that requires the types of evaluation and treatment procedures that are available in the facility. In recent literature, the term short stay facility is being used synonymously with acute care. However, because the term short stay can also refer to the length of time a patient is in a facility and is occasionally used to describe facilities that are not also acute care, this text will continue to use the term acute care.

Typically, an acute care facility is distinguished by the presence of an emergency department and surgical (operating) facilities. The facility is also able to provide services for surgical procedures, such as appendectomies and hip replacements.

When people say that a patient is going to the hospital, they frequently mean that he or she is going to an acute care facility. However, the term hospital has a broader definition.

**dual governance** In hospitals, a shared organization structure consisting of the administration, headed by the CEO, and the medical staff, headed by the Chief of Medical Staff.

Hospitals are governed by a board of directors or a board of trustees, which is ultimately responsible for the facility and its activities. The board oversees strategic (long-term financial and operational) planning and approves administrative policies and procedures, budgets, and physician staff appointments. Hospitals typically have shared or **dual governance**. From the board of directors or trustees run two separate lines of authority: administration and medical staff. The administration, headed by the chief executive officer (CEO), is responsible for the day-to-day operations of the facility, such as ensuring adequate resources for patient care. The medical staff, which includes physicians and other practitioners, is responsible for the clinical care rendered in the hospital. Figure 1-1 shows an example of the organization of the upper management of a hospital and some of the departments that might report to those administrators.

**inpatient** An individual who is admitted to a hospital with the intention of staying overnight.

**physician's orders** The physician's directions regarding the patient's care. Also refers to the data collection device on which these elements are captured.

In an acute care facility, patients are cared for as **inpatients.** Inpatients typically remain in the facility at least overnight and are therefore patients whose evaluation and treatment result in admission to and discharge from the facility on different days. Exceptions can occur, such as if a patient dies or is transferred on the day of admission. However, these patients are still considered inpatients because the physician's order to admit the patient reveals the intention of the physician to keep the patient at least overnight. A physician's order is a verbal or written direction regarding the patient's care.

**Go To** Physician's orders are discussed in detail in Chapter 4.

**admission** The act of accepting a patient into care in a health care facility, including any nonambulatory care facility. Admission requires a physician's order.

**Admission** is the process that occurs when the patient is registered for evaluation or treatment in a facility upon the order of a physician. In most facilities, the admission process involves a variety of data collection activities. The admission date is defined as the actual calendar day that the order to admit was written. Whether the patient arrives at 1:05 AM or 11:59 PM on January 5, the admission date is the same: January 5.

**discharge** Discharge occurs when the patient leaves the care of the facility to go home, for transfer to another health care facility, or by death.

**Discharge** is the process that occurs when the patient leaves the facility. Discharge implies that the patient has already been admitted to the facility. The day of discharge is defined as the actual calendar day that the patient leaves the facility. Note that a physician's order for a patient to leave the facility is required for a normal discharge. However, as mentioned earlier, certain events might also cause a discharge. A patient may die, leave against medical advice, or be transferred to another facility. All of these events are discharges as of the calendar day on which they occur.

**Go To** Chapter 4 for information about the data collection that takes place during admission.

**Go To** Chapter 10 for a detailed explanation of (patient) average length of stay (ALOS).

By definition, in state licensure standards, the average time that patients stay in an acute care facility is less than 30 days. Exceptions can and do occur; greater lengths of stay are not uncommon and do not have an impact on the facility's acute care designation. Actually, the average number of days that a patient spends in a given acute care facility depends on what types of patients are treated in the facility. Many acute care facilities have an average patient stay between 3 and 6 days; significantly less than 30 days.

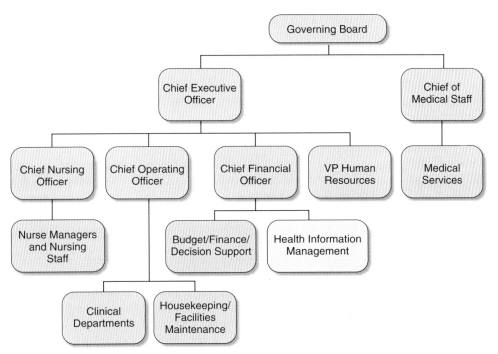

**Figure 1-1** Hospital organization chart. This is a very simple example of the possible organization of a hospital. There are many more possible departments than those depicted here and many different organizational structures. For example, a Health Information Management (HIM) department may report to any of the administrative chiefs even the Chief Nursing Officer.

Historically, acute care facilities have been stand-alone hospitals. Although they may have provided a variety of different services to the community, they did not have a formal business affiliation with other hospitals. In recent years, as a result of economic pressures, hospitals are consolidating. Sometimes they merge, which means that two or more hospitals combine their resources. Other times, one hospital acquires (purchases) the other. In recent years, looser "partnerships" or "affiliations" have been formed in order to take advantage of individual strengths and perhaps to leverage buying power. Also in recent years, partly as a cost-cutting measure and partly for improved customer service, acute care facilities have expanded into ambulatory care and other services.

---

**HIT-bit** ·······································································

**MERGERS AND ACQUISITIONS**

Although this is not a strict rule, two hospitals that have combined often get a new name. If two hospitals combine and their group name is different from either of the original names, a merger has usually occurred. If the group name is the same as one of the original hospitals, the hospital with the retained name may have acquired the one whose name has changed. For example, if Community Hospital and Spencer Hospital combine to form Star Health System, the two hospitals probably merged. If they combine to form Spencer Health System, then Spencer Hospital probably acquired Community Hospital.

---

## Ambulatory Care

In an **ambulatory care facility**, patients are admitted and discharged on the same day. A patient whose evaluation or treatment is intended to occur within 1 calendar day is an ambulatory care patient, also known as an **outpatient.** Diagnostic laboratory and radiology

**ambulatory care facility** An outpatient facility, such as an emergency department or physician's office, in which treatment is intended to occur within 1 calendar day.

**outpatient** A patient whose health care services are intended to be delivered within 1 calendar day or, in some cases, a 24-hour period.

visits are done on an outpatient basis. Many therapies are also classified as outpatient. The concepts of admission and discharge have little relevance in an ambulatory care facility because both processes typically are intended to take place on the same day. An ambulatory care admission, then, is referred to as a visit or an encounter. In general, outpatient services are rendered in a matter of minutes or hours and the patient returns home quickly. However, some hospital-based outpatient services blur the lines between outpatient and inpatient, either in duration or appearance.

The emergency department is one example of an ambulatory care service. An emergency department patient is always an outpatient, even if the visit extends from one calendar day to the next, as is often the case late at night. A patient who is experiencing excessive nausea and vomiting may remain in the hospital overnight; however, the visit is still classified as outpatient. If the patient needs to be admitted, the order to admit results in an inpatient admission, which is no longer classified as an ED visit. Ambulatory surgery is another example of an outpatient service that occasionally extends from one calendar day to the next.

Finally, an observation patient is also an outpatient. These patients are experiencing signs or symptoms that may indicate a serious condition; however, the definitive etiology has not been determined. Chest pain, for example, may be acid reflux or it might signal an impending myocardial infarction. Shortness of breath and syncope (fainting) are other symptoms that often require additional study but not necessarily an inpatient admission. For these patients, a period of observation may be appropriate. Patients in observation status may remain in the hospital for 24 to 48 hours, during which time they are considered outpatients—regardless of their actual location in the hospital or what specific bed they occupy. The underlying purpose of observation status is to give the physician an extended period in which to decide whether to admit the patient for inpatient treatment or to discharge the patient.

### Physician's Offices

A physician's office is one type of ambulatory care facility. Most physicians maintain an office where patients can visit. There are many different types of physicians, as discussed earlier. Some physicians have offices attached to their homes; others have space in office buildings; still others are employed by the organizations for which they work, such as an acute care hospital.

### Ancillary Services

Some facilities offer a broad range of evaluation services, such as radiology and laboratory services. The radiology department performs and reviews radiographs and other types of imaging. The laboratory analyzes tissue and body fluids, such as blood. These evaluation services are called *ancillary*, or *adjunct*, services. Many of these services are offered in freestanding (not hospital-based) facilities. Some freestanding services lease space in other health care facilities, such as acute care hospitals, so that it is not always obvious that the service is not part of the hospital. Whether hospital-based or freestanding, most ancillary services require a physician's order to perform.

### Long-Term Care Facilities

Historically referred to as "nursing homes," **long-term care (LTC) facilities** primarily cared for older patients who were ill or whose families could no longer care for them at home. Patients often moved into a nursing home and lived there until they died. Today, an LTC facility treats a wide variety of patients who need more care than they would be able to get at home, but who do not generally need the intensity of care provided by an acute care facility. In addition, the philosophy of these facilities has changed so that the focus is less on making a home for the patient and more on maintaining the patient's health and preparing him or her to go home, if possible. In long-term care, patients are termed residents. By definition, an LTC facility has an average length of stay (ALOS) in excess of 30 days. This is an important difference between acute care and long-term care.

---

**ED** emergency department

**ambulatory surgery** Surgical procedures performed on an outpatient basis; the patient returns home after the procedure is performed. Also called same day surgery.

**etiology** The cause or source of the patient's condition or disease.

---

**Go To** Chapter 8 for more information about health care delivery in non-acute settings.

---

**long-term care (LTC) facility** A hospital that provides services to patients over an extended period; an average length of stay is in excess of 30 days. Facilities are characterized by the extent to which nursing care is provided.

**LTC** long term care
**ALOS** average length of stay

### Behavioral Health Facilities

Behavioral health facilities are defined by their patient population. Patients in a **behavioral health facility** either have or are being evaluated for psychiatric illnesses. Such a facility may also be referred to as a **mental health facility** or psychiatric facility. These facilities can be inpatient, outpatient, or both. Large behavioral health facilities may be administered by the state or county government. In addition, there are many small, private facilities. There is no standard in terms of ALOS. Outpatient services may be provided in stand-alone clinics or as part of an inpatient facility.

### Rehabilitation Facilities

The focus of physical medicine and rehabilitation is to return the patient to the maximal possible level of function in terms of **activities of daily living (ADLs).** ADLs include self-care functions such as bathing and toileting as well as practical concerns such as ironing and cooking. This type of rehabilitation is referred to as physical medicine and rehabilitation. These facilities may be inpatient, outpatient, or both.

A **rehabilitation facility** treats patients who have suffered a debilitating illness or trauma or who are recovering from certain types of surgery. One typical patient may have survived a car accident but has suffered a head trauma and other injuries that require extensive therapy. Another patient may have had knee replacement surgery and needs therapy to learn to function with the prosthetic joint.

### Hospice

A **hospice** provides palliative care for the terminally ill. **Palliative care** involves making the patient comfortable by easing his or her pain and other discomforts. Hospice care can be delivered to the patient in an inpatient, residential setting or in the home. A hospice also provides support groups and counseling for both the patient and his or her family and friends. Hospice services may provide follow-up services for the survivors for up to a year after the patient's death.

### Home Health Care

As the name implies, **home health care** involves a variety of services provided to patients in the home. Services range from assistance with ADLs to physical therapy and intravenous drug therapy. Personnel providing these services also vary, from aides to therapists, nurses, and doctors.

## Facility Size

Another way of distinguishing one facility from another is by size. Frequently, not only is a facility described as being *acute care* or *long-term care* or *ambulatory care* or *rehabilitation*, but it also is differentiated by number of beds or number of discharges. The size of an ambulatory care facility is defined by the number of encounters or the number of visits. These concepts are detailed in the following sections. Table 1-5 summarizes some comparisons of different types of facilities.

### Number of Beds

In an inpatient facility, beds are set up for patients to occupy. There are two basic ways to view beds: licensed beds and bed count. **Licensed beds** are the number of beds that the state has approved for the hospital. One can think of licensed beds as the maximum number of beds allowed to the facility under normal circumstances.

Facilities do not always need all of their licensed beds. For example, a facility may not have enough patients to fill all of its beds. It is very expensive to maintain the equipment and staff members for an empty room. If the number of occupied beds is low over a long period, then administrators may decide to close some of the beds. To be economical, a facility may equip and staff only as many beds as it needs for the foreseeable future. A hospital may choose to offer private rooms as a courtesy or a marketing strategy, thereby reducing the number of available beds. This number of available beds, which can be less than the number of licensed beds but not more, is called the *bed count*. **Bed count** is the

---

**behavioral health facility** An inpatient or outpatient health care facility that focuses on the treatment of psychiatric conditions. Also called a **mental health** or **psychiatric facility**.

**activities of daily living (ADLs)** Refers to self-care, such as bathing, as well as cooking, shopping, and other routines requiring thought, planning, and physical motion.

**rehabilitation facility** A health care facility that delivers services to patients whose activities of daily living are impaired by their illness or condition. May be inpatient, outpatient, or both.

**hospice** Palliative health care services rendered to the terminally ill, their families, and their friends.
**palliative care** Health care services that are intended to soothe, comfort, or reduce symptoms but are not intended to cure.

**home health care** Health care services rendered in the patient's home; or an agency that provides such services.

**ADLs** activities of daily living

**discharge** Discharge occurs when the patient leaves the care of the facility to go home, for transfer to another health care facility, or by death. Also refers to the status of a patient.

**licensed beds** The maximum number of beds that a facility is legally permitted to have, as approved by state licensure.
**bed count** The actual number of beds that a hospital has staffed, equipped, and otherwise made available for occupancy by patients for each specific operating day.

**TABLE 1-5**

**HEALTH CARE FACILITIES COMPARED BY LENGTH OF STAY OR MEDICAL SPECIALTY**

| FACILITIES | LENGTH OF STAY |
|---|---|
| Ambulatory care facility | Patients are admitted and discharged on the same day |
| Acute care facility | Patients remain at least overnight and, on average, stay less than 30 days |
| Long-term care facility | Patients remain at least overnight (inpatient) and, on average, stay longer than 30 days |

| FACILITIES | MEDICAL SPECIALTY |
|---|---|
| Rehabilitation facility | Physical medicine, physical therapy, and occupational therapy; may be inpatient or outpatient |
| Behavioral health facility | Psychiatric diagnosis; may be inpatient or outpatient |
| Children's hospital | Treats only children, usually 16 years old and younger; may be inpatient or outpatient |

number of beds that the facility actually has set up, equipped, and staffed—in other words, the beds that are ready to treat patients.

In a comparison of facilities, the size of the facility is often referred to in terms of its licensed beds. It is also useful to analyze a facility's licensed beds versus bed count over time. A seasonal or otherwise short-term closing of beds is not automatically a matter of concern and may, in fact, indicate sound administration. Long-term low bed count (as compared with licensed beds), on the other hand, may indicate serious problems. Over the last 10 years, many hospitals have been forced to close beds partly as a result of the health care industry shift from acute care to ambulatory care and partly because there were too many hospitals concentrated in areas that did not necessarily need them. Because licensed beds are granted on the basis of the needs of the community, long-term reduction of bed count may signal that the facility is no longer needed in its community. As some facilities close, patients will use other facilities in the surrounding area. In this way, the number of available beds in an area adjusts to changes in the industry and in the environment.

**Discharges**

Another measure of the size of a facility is the number of discharges in a period, usually expressed monthly or annually. Number of discharges is a measure of activity, as opposed to a measure of physical size. Although two acute care facilities may each have 250 beds, one of them may discharge 15,000 patients per year while the other discharges 25,000 patients per year. Higher numbers of discharges require larger numbers of administrative and other support staff.

**Occupancy,** the percentage of available beds that have been used over a certain period, is one explanation for the difference in the number of discharges. To calculate occupancy, divide the number of days that patients used hospital beds by the number of beds available. For example, if there are 100 licensed beds in the facility and there are 75 patients currently in those beds, then the day's occupancy is 75% (Figure 1-2). The number of beds available can be based on either bed count or licensed beds. A facility may use bed count internally to monitor the rate at which available beds are being used, but it may use licensed beds to compare use over time because licensed beds are less likely to change.

Length of stay is another explanation for different discharge numbers. The longer a patient stays in the hospital, the fewer individual patients can be treated in the bed being used by the patient. Therefore if a hospital has an ALOS of 6 days, it can treat half as many patients as a hospital of the same size with an ALOS of 3 days (Figure 1-3).

For example, to calculate the ALOS of a 200-bed hospital in the month of June, multiply 200 beds by 30 days in June to equal 6000 "beds" or "days" available to treat patients. If the ALOS is 6 days, then the hospital is able to treat an estimated 1000 patients for 6 days (6000

**ambulatory care facility** An outpatient facility, such as an emergency department or physician's office, in which treatment is intended to occur within 1 calendar day.

**occupancy** In a hospital, the percentage of available beds that have been used over time.

**ALOS** average length of stay

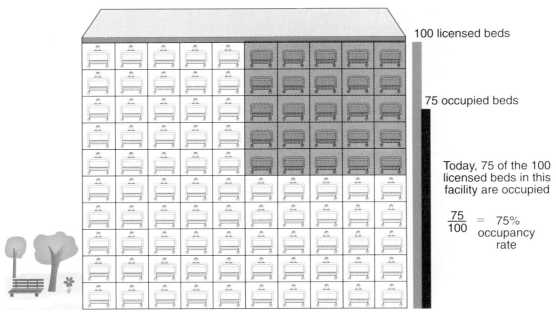

100 licensed beds

75 occupied beds

Today, 75 of the 100 licensed beds in this facility are occupied

$$\frac{75}{100} = 75\% \text{ occupancy rate}$$

**Figure 1-2** Calculating occupancy. ALOS, average length of stay.

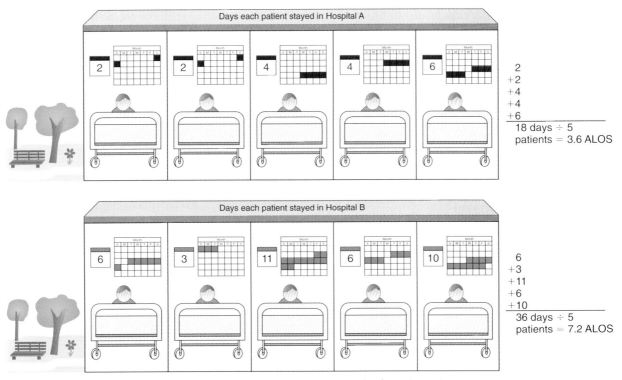

Days each patient stayed in Hospital A

2
+2
+4
+4
+6
_____
18 days ÷ 5 patients = 3.6 ALOS

Days each patient stayed in Hospital B

6
+3
+11
+6
+10
_____
36 days ÷ 5 patients = 7.2 ALOS

**Figure 1-3** The calculation of average length of stay (ALOS).

divided by 6 equals 1000). If the ALOS is 3 days, then the hospital is able to treat an estimated 2000 patients—twice as many as the hospital with an ALOS of 6 days (see Figure 1-4). That means twice as many admissions, twice as many discharges, and twice as much work for many of the administrative support staff who process these activities.

**Go To** Chapter 5 for a description of post-discharge processing; Chapter 10 contains more hospital statistics.

## Ownership

Health care facilities may exist under many different types of ownership. Some facilities, such as physician group practices and radiology centers, are owned by individuals or groups

Hospital A has 100 licensed beds

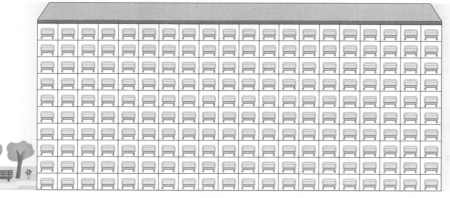

Since there are 30 days in June, Hospital A has 3000 bed days this month. If the ALOS at this facility is 3.6:

$$\frac{3000 \text{ days}}{3.6 \text{ ALOS}} = 833 \text{ patients}$$

It is estimated that Hospital A can treat 833 patients in the month of June, if each patient stays about 3 days

Hospital B has 200 licensed beds

Hospital B has twice as many licensed beds, and therefore twice as many bed days in June:

200 beds x 30 days in June = 6000 days

But since Hospital B's patients average a stay that is twice as long, an ALOS of 7.2 days, it is estimated that it will treat the same amount of patients in June (833). Maybe Hospital B's patients were more severely ill or maybe Hospital A is just more efficient.

Because Hospital A has a shorter ALOS it can treat about the same amount of patients in June as Hospital B, even though Hospital B is twice the size.

$$\frac{6000 \text{ days}}{7.2 \text{ ALOS}} = 833 \text{ patients}$$

**Figure 1-4** The comparison of average length of stay (ALOS) in two facilities.

of individuals. Facilities may also be owned by corporations, government entities, or religious groups. Hospital Corporation of America (HCA) is a corporation that owns many facilities. The Veterans Administration facilities are examples of government-owned facilities. The Catholic Church operates many hospitals throughout the country. Frequently, the ownership of the organization has an impact on both the operations and the services provided by the facility. For example, a facility owned by a religious organization may not allow abortions to be performed by their physicians. A government-owned facility may require supplies to be purchased from government-approved vendors.

## Tax Status

Another way to distinguish institutions from one another is by their tax status: for-profit or not-for-profit. A for-profit, or proprietary, organization has owners. It can have few or many owners (or shareholders). HCA is an example of a for-profit organization with many shareholders. A not-for-profit institution operates solely for the good of the community and is considered to be owned by the community. It has no shareholders who have a vested interest in the economic viability of the organization. Not-for-profit institutions enjoy certain tax benefits, including exemption from property and certain corporate income taxes. Most community hospitals are not-for-profit.

The tax status of an organization should have little or no impact on the day-to-day operations of the organization. The fundamental impact is on the distribution of net income. Net income is the excess of revenue (mostly income from patient services) over expenses (the resources used to provide the services) over a specified period. In a not-for-profit organization, net income (called surplus) must be used for charitable purposes. In a for-profit organization, net income belongs to the shareholders and may, at the discretion of the board of directors, be distributed in whole or in part to these owners of the organization. Because board members are elected by the shareholders, the board is answerable to them.

## Patient Population

As previously discussed, facilities may differ in terms of the types of patients that they treat. Many facilities specialize in treating only certain types of diseases. For example, Deborah Heart and Lung Center in New Jersey specializes in treating cardiac and respiratory problems. It would not accept a patient whose only problem is a broken leg. Behavioral health facilities treat patients with different types of psychiatric problems. Another common type of specialty hospital is a **children's hospital**. The medical treatment of children requires smaller equipment as well as specialized training. A children's hospital would not normally accept a 35-year-old patient.

**children's hospital** A specialty facility that focuses on the treatment of children.

## Services

Depending on the type of patients that they treat, facilities offer a variety of services. These services are often organized into departments. For example, an acute care facility has an emergency department and a surgery department. It also offers radiology, laboratory, and pathology services. If an acute care facility offers physical therapy, the physical therapy department may be small. Often, therapy is provided at the patient's bedside. A rehabilitation facility does not have an emergency department, but it may have a room set aside for the performance of minor surgical procedures. It may have radiology and laboratory services, but it probably does not have a pathology department. Because physical therapy is a major component of rehabilitation, the physical therapy department is large. A large amount of space is available for treatment, including a variety of specialized equipment.

**acute care facility** A health care facility in which patients have an average length of stay less than 30 days and that has an emergency department, operating suite, and clinical departments to handle a broad range of diagnoses and treatments.

## Continuity of Care

With so many different caregivers working in such a variety of facilities, communication among them is essential. The coordination among caregivers to treat a patient is called the **continuity of care** or **continuum of care.** Continuity of care is a concept with two separate but related elements. First, it refers to communication among all the patient's care providers in a facility from his or her admission to discharge. As a patient moves from place to place in a facility, communication among all his or her caregivers ideally should be as smooth and coordinated as possible. This means that each individual rendering care should be aware of and responsive to all known, relevant data about the patient. For example:

- The nurses need to know about the orders: what has been completed, what is outstanding, and what critical results must be communicated to the physician.
- The physician needs to be aware of the results and whether the nursing staff has reported any issues since the previous visit.
- The radiology staff needs to know whether the patient has any drug allergies if they are doing a test that requires contrast dye.

Continuity of care also refers to all the patient's experiences from one facility to another, either throughout a particular illness or throughout the life of the patient. A PCP needs to know that her patient has been admitted to the hospital so that she can follow-up at discharge to ensure that the patient understands the diagnosis and the treatment plan. This follow up not only helps the patient manage the illness effectively but also helps prevent unnecessary re-admissions to the hospital.

The following is an example of the continuity of care needed to treat a particular female patient through her lifetime.

**continuity of care** The coordination among caregivers to provide, efficiently and effectively, the broad range of health care services required by a patient during an illness or for an entire lifetime. May also refer to the coordination of care provided among caregivers / services within a health care organization.
**continuum of care** The broad range of health care services required by a patient during an illness or for an entire lifetime. May also refer to the continuity of care provided by a health care organization.

### Childhood

The patient, Emily, is born in an acute care facility. As a child, Emily is treated by a pediatrician. The pediatrician is her primary care provider, or PCP. She receives extensive well-child care: preventive vaccinations, checkups, and developmental assessments.

**primary care physician (PCP)** In insurance, the physician who has been designated by the insured to deliver routine care to the insured and to evaluate the need for referral to a specialist, if applicable. Colloquial use is synonymous with "family doctor."

**PCP** primary care physician

**psychiatrist** A physician who specializes in the diagnosis and treatment of patients with conditions that affect the mind.

**ADLs** activities of daily living

**personal health record (PHR)** A patient's own copy of health information documenting the patient's health care history and providing information on continuing patient care.

**continuum of care** The broad range of health care services required by a patient during an illness or for an entire lifetime. May also refer to the continuity of care provided by a health care organization.

**acute care facility** A health care facility in which patients have an average length of stay less than 30 days and that has an emergency department, operating suite, and clinical departments to handle a broad range of diagnoses and treatments.

**rehabilitation facility** A health care facility that delivers services to patients whose activities of daily living are impaired by their illness or condition. May be inpatient, outpatient, or both.

**long-term care (LTC) facility** A hospital that provides services to patients over an extended period; an average length of stay is in excess of 30 days. Facilities are characterized by the extent to which nursing care is provided.

**integrated delivery system (IDS)** A health care organization that provides services through most or all of the continuum of care.

**ACO** Accountable Care Organization

## Adult Care

As Emily ages and grows into adulthood, she visits a family practitioner as her new PCP. The family practitioner would benefit from having information about all of the patient's childhood diseases, immunizations, and problems that she has experienced previously. Emily sees her PCP on a regular basis. As she becomes an adult, she also visits a gynecologist for regular examinations. Emily moves several times in her adult life, changing physicians each time. The new PCP and gynecologist would benefit from copies of her prior records.

## Special Health Issues

When Emily becomes pregnant, she is examined and followed by her obstetrician throughout the pregnancy and cesarean delivery. Later in life, as she becomes older, other illnesses arise. For example, in her late 30s, Emily develops diabetes. Her PCP refers her to an endocrinologist for treatment of the diabetes. After Emily discovers a lump in her breast, she undergoes a mammography and is referred to a surgeon for a diagnosis. Then she enters an acute care facility to have a lumpectomy. Note that at this point, Emily has had at least three admissions to an acute care facility and has visited at least three specialists in addition to her PCP. When she is seeing specialists concurrently, it is important for Emily to ask them to communicate with one another about her care. This communication helps avoid unnecessary duplication of tests and conflicting plans of care.

## Elder Care

Maturing past menopause, Emily falls and breaks her hip. She needs to have a hip replacement and is treated by an orthopedic surgeon in an acute care facility for hip replacement surgery, after which she is transferred to a rehabilitation facility for a couple of weeks of rehabilitation to enable her to resume her ADLs. Eventually, Emily becomes incapacitated and is unable to take care of herself. She is diagnosed with Alzheimer disease and is seen by a neurologist and a **psychiatrist**. Ultimately, she is admitted to a nursing home for 24-hour monitored nursing care.

Throughout these encounters with various facilities and specialists, the history of Emily's care should follow her smoothly. The orthopedic surgeon will want to know her experiences under anesthesia when she had breast surgery and her reaction to anesthesia when her baby was born. This information should be available to subsequent surgeons. Emily can maintain a personal health record (PHR): copies of important documents such as operative reports, discharge summaries, immunizations, and test results. Her PHR can be a folder with the paper documents or an electronic file. There are also Web sites on which Emily can maintain her data. Increasingly, physicians and some hospitals are providing patient access to certain elements of the patient's records for this purpose. As the technology evolves, the communication among caregivers, and hence the continuity of care, is facilitated.

Table 1-6 compares some of the onsite services provided by various types of facilities.

## Modern Models

As noted previously, hospital mergers have increased in recent years. Many health care organizations are consolidating along the continuum of care. In other words, they are not just buying multiple acute care facilities; they are buying physician's office practices, rehabilitation facilities, and LTC facilities as well as acute care facilities. Thus they are able to provide patients with seamless coordination of care along this continuum. Such enterprises are referred to as **integrated delivery systems (IDSs).** Many see this approach as an efficient delivery of health care throughout a patient's lifetime. Evolving relationships between PCPs and other providers, as well as the emphasis on alternatives to expensive inpatient care, have led to the development of Accountable Care Organizations (ACOs) and the Medical Home model.

The Medical Home model has its foundation in the concept that the PCP is the gatekeeper for services to patients and the coordinator of those services. In this model, the PCP does not just refer patients to specialists but also coordinates the follow-up and any

## TABLE 1-6

### COMPARISON OF ONSITE SERVICES PROVIDED IN HEALTH CARE FACILITIES

| SERVICE OR DEPARTMENT | PHYSICIAN'S OFFICE | ACUTE CARE | LONG-TERM CARE | REHABILITATION |
|---|---|---|---|---|
| Nursing | Maybe | Yes | Yes | Yes |
| Medical staff | One, two, or many | Many; visit many patients daily | Many; visit patients as needed or defined | Many; visit many patients daily |
| Patient registration | Yes | Yes | Yes | Yes |
| Dietary | Not usually | Yes | Yes | Yes |
| Health information management | Not a separate department in small facilities | Yes | Not always a separate department | Usually |
| Patient accounts | Yes | Yes | Yes | Yes |
| Volunteers | Only in large facilities | Yes | Yes | Yes |
| Radiology | Maybe | Yes | Limited, if any | Usually |
| Laboratory | Maybe | Yes | Limited | Limited |
| Physical therapy | May be associated within group practice | Small department | Varies; may have small department | Large department |
| Occupational therapy | May be associated within group practice | Small department | Varies; may have small department | Large department |
| Emergency Services | Urgent care | Yes | No | No |
| Surgery | Minor procedures | Yes | Minor procedures | Minor procedures |
| Pathology | No; physician usually uses a freestanding or hospital-based service | Yes | Limited | Limited |

subsequent required care. In this model, the PCP is the patient's "home" for all medical care, regardless of the actual provider rendering the service. Transitioning from one setting to another is a key component of the Medical Home model.

Normally, all providers are paid separately for care that is rendered to patients. Physicians who care for patients in acute care facilities are entitled to payment separate and apart from the hospital's facility charges. Because inpatient care is expensive, one way to incentivize hospitals and physicians to work together toward efficient and effective inpatient care is through ACOs. ACOs provide a mechanism in which payment for inpatient services flows through the hospital and out to other providers. In this manner, the hospital and the physicians have a vested interest in working together to ensure the necessity and efficiency of services rendered.

**inpatient** An individual who is admitted to a hospital with the intention of staying overnight.

**Go To** Reimbursement is discussed in more detail in Chapter 7.

## ▪ EXERCISE 1-2

### Comparison of Facilities

1. Patients whose care requires them to remain in the hospital overnight are called _____.
2. What are the characteristics of a hospital?
3. Define admission and discharge.
4. If a patient is admitted as an inpatient on Monday at 10 AM but dies on Monday at 3 PM, is that patient still considered an inpatient?
5. A hospital with an average length of stay of less than 30 days, an emergency department, operating suite, and clinical departments to handle a broad range of diagnoses and treatments is most likely a(n) _____.
6. A specialty inpatient facility that focuses on the treatment of individuals with psychiatric disorders is a(n) _____.
7. Care for the terminally ill is the focus of _____ care.
8. _____ focuses on treating patients where they reside.
9. Chapone Health Care is an organization that owns a number of different health care facilities: three acute care hospitals, two long-term care facilities, and a number of physician offices. Chapone also owns a rehabilitation hospital and an assisted living facility, which also delivers home care. This organization delivers care to patients at every point along the continuum of care. Chapone Health Care can be described as a(n) _____ _____.

10. The coordination among caregivers to provide services to a patient within a facility or among different providers is referred to as _____.

11. A(n) _____ provides care to patients at all or most points along the continuum of care.

12. The Community Care Center has 200 beds. It has an average length of stay of 2 years. Most of the patients are older, but there are some younger patients with serious chronic illnesses. Community Care Center is most likely a(n) _____.

**Health Insurance Portability and Accountability Act (HIPAA)** Public Law 104-191, a federal legislation passed in 1996 that outlines the guidelines of managing patient information in terms of privacy, security, and confidentiality. The legislation also outlines penalties for noncompliance.

**Department of Health and Human Services (DHHS)** The U.S. federal agency with regulatory oversight of American health care, which also provides health services to certain populations through several operating divisions.

**Centers for Medicare and Medicaid Services (CMS)** The division of the U.S. federal government's Department of Health and Human Services that administers Medicare and Medicaid.

## LEGAL AND REGULATORY ENVIRONMENT

Various facilities have different ways of operating, but the mandate under which activities are performed often arises from legislation, regulation, and accreditation issues. Federal, state, and local governments all have an impact in varying degrees on health care institutions and delivery. For example, a patient's right to privacy is mandated at the federal level by the privacy provisions of the Health Insurance Portability and Accountability Act (HIPAA) as well as at the state level through court actions, laws, and regulation, depending on the state. The legal and regulatory environment is discussed in greater detail in Chapter 12, but the following discussion is a general overview of how government affects health care. Table 1-7 summarizes the agencies of the federal government that impact health care.

### Federal

The federal government has a major impact on health care through regulatory activity. The federal legislature (the U.S. House of Representatives and the Senate) enacts laws, which the executive branch (the President) must then enforce. Enforcement arises from the delegation of executive responsibilities to various agencies. In terms of health care, the critical regulatory agency is the **Department of Health and Human Services (DHHS),** which includes the **Centers for Medicare and Medicaid Services (CMS).** This agency administers Medicare and part of Medicaid.

**Medicare** is an *entitlement* to health care benefits for persons of advanced age (older than 65 years) or those with certain chronic illnesses (e.g., end-stage renal disease). Health

## TABLE 1-7

### FEDERAL AGENCIES INVOLVED IN HEALTH CARE

| DEPARTMENT | AGENCY | HEALTH-RELATED FUNCTIONS |
|---|---|---|
| Department of Health and Human Services | Food and Drug Administration | Ensures safety of foods, cosmetics, pharmaceuticals, biological products, and medical devices |
| | Centers for Medicare and Medicaid Services | Oversees Medicare and the federal portion of Medicaid |
| | National Institutes of Health | Supports biomedical research |
| | Centers for Disease Control and Prevention | Provides a system of health surveillance to monitor and prevent outbreak of diseases |
| | Health Resources and Services Administration | Helps provide health resources for medically underserved populations |
| | Indian Health Service | Supports a network of health care facilities and providers to Native Americans, including Alaskans |
| | Office for Civil Rights | Protects patients from discrimination in health care |
| Department of Defense | Military Health Services System | Maintains a network of health care providers and facilities for service personnel and their dependents |
| Department of Veterans Affairs | Veterans Affairs facilities | Maintains a network of facilities and services for armed services veterans and sometimes their dependents |
| Department of Labor | Occupational Safety and Health Administration | Regulates workplace health and safety |

care facilities are not automatically eligible for full reimbursement from Medicare simply on the basis of treating a Medicare patient. To be eligible for full reimbursement from Medicare, a health care facility must comply with Medicare's **Conditions of Participation (COP)**. COP standards include the quality of providers, certain policies and procedures, and financial issues; these are updated in the *Code of Federal Regulations* (CFR) and published in the *Federal Register*. Another important area of federal regulation concerns the release of information pertaining to patients with drug and alcohol diagnoses.

---

## HIT-bit

### ABBREVIATIONS AND ACRONYMS

You may have noticed that many of the terms and phrases used in health care frequently are shortened to a few recognizable letters. An abbreviation made from the initial letters or parts of a term is called an *acronym*. Acronyms and other abbreviations shorten writing time and save space. However, acronyms can also cause confusion. AMA, for example, means "against medical advice." It is also the abbreviation for the American Medical Association and the American Management Association. There are also interdisciplinary issues with abbreviations. "Dr." means doctor to a health care professional. To an accountant, it means debit. Therefore abbreviations should be used carefully. Health care facilities must define acceptable abbreviations and should restrict the use of abbreviations to only those that have been approved.

---

## State

The impact of state government on health care organizations varies from state to state and consists primarily of licensure and reporting. States also share in the administration of the **Medicaid** program.

### Licensure

For operation of any health care facility, a license must be obtained from the state in which the facility will operate. The process of **licensure** varies among states. Often, the state's legislature passes a hospital licensing act or a similar law that requires hospitals to be licensed and delegates the authority to regulate that process to a state agency, possibly the state's Department of Health. The delegated agency then develops and administers the detailed regulations, which are part of the state's administrative code. The licensure regulations contain a great deal of useful information pertaining to the operations of a health care facility, including the minimum requirements for maintaining patient records. Some states' regulations are very detailed and specific as to the organization and structure of a facility, including such items as services to be provided, medical staff requirements, nursing requirements, committees, and sanitation. Licensure is specific to the type of health care facility being operated. The regulations governing acute care facilities differ somewhat from those for long-term care facilities, which are in turn different from those for rehabilitation facilities.

It is fundamentally the responsibility of the board of directors or board of trustees of a facility to ensure compliance with each of the requirements of the license. The board delegates the day-to-day operations of the facility to management, through the chief executive officer or administrator of the hospital.

Many state agencies visit hospitals regularly and review the hospital operations and the documentation for compliance with the license of the facility. Of particular note are long-term care facilities, which tend to be scrutinized very closely. State surveyors may visit a facility as part of a general audit plan or in response to patient complaints. CMS may also delegate to state surveyors the task of conducting COP reviews.

### Reporting

A tremendous amount of reporting occurs among health care facilities and state agencies. Typically, reporting includes information about general patient data, cancer, trauma, birth

---

**Medicare** Federally funded health care entitlement program for older adults and for certain categories of chronically ill patients.

**entitlement program** In health care, government-sponsored program that pay for certain services on the basis of an individual's age, condition, employment status, or other circumstances.

**reimbursement** The amount of money that the health care facility receives from the party responsible for paying the bill.

**Conditions of Participation (COP)** The terms under which a facility is eligible to receive reimbursement from Medicare.

**Federal Register** The publication of the proceedings of the United States Congress.

**Go To** The release of information function is discussed in Chapter 5, and issues of privacy are detailed in Chapter 12.

**Medicaid** A federally mandated, state-funded program providing access to health care for the poor and the medically indigent.

**licensure** The mandatory government approval required for performing specified activities. In health care, the state approval required for providing health care services.

**CMS** Centers for Medicare and Medicaid Services
**COP** Conditions of Participation

defects, and infectious disease. Additional reporting may result from health care workers' observation of inappropriate activities, such as child abuse; health care workers have an obligation to report certain types of suspected abuses to the authorities.

One of the key reporting relationships between health care facilities and the state is the reporting of service activity. States typically require the transmission of specific data about patients that are discussed in Chapter 2. For example, the New Jersey Department of Health and Senior Services requires acute care facilities to upload all acute, ambulatory surgical, and emergency department discharges electronically to the New Jersey Discharge Data Collection System.

### Medicaid and Uncompensated Care

ESRD end-stage renal disease

Unlike eligibility for the Medicare program, which is based on age, disability, or ESRD, eligibility for Medicaid is based primarily on economic circumstances. Individuals with limited resources may be eligible for Medicaid, including some children whose parents may not personally be eligible. The eligibility rules and application process vary by state. Funding for Medicaid is shared between the federal government and the state.

In addition to Medicaid, states also provide funding for a variety of programs supporting the health care needs of individuals who do not have the resources to pay for care. For example, all hospitals that maintain an emergency department are required to evaluate patients prior to obtaining information about the patient's ability to pay for care. If the patient has an emergency, such as stroke, the hospital could admit and treat the patient without knowing whether the patient could pay for the services rendered. If the patient has no resources with which to pay for the services, and is not eligible for other government programs, the hospital may obtain some reimbursement from the state's uncompensated care program.

**admission** The act of accepting a patient into care in a health care facility, including any nonambulatory care facility. Admission requires a physician's order.

*Uncompensated care,* also called "charity care," refers to the value of services rendered to patients who have no ability to pay for those services. Patients may be eligible for Medicaid or some other state-funded program, for which they must apply and from which the hospital may obtain some level of payment. The state may also provide to hospitals payments that are not specifically tied to individual patients but are based on the quantity of uncompensated care rendered as a percentage of total care provided. So, a state may determine that a hospital rendering 20% of its total dollar value of care to indigent patients will be reimbursed by the state for 10% of that dollar value. If the value of care to indigent patients is 60 million dollars, then the hospital would receive 6 million dollars from the state.

## Local

Local government may also become involved in health care organizations, particularly in the aspect of zoning regulations. For example, a health care organization is a business, and zoning regulations may require that businesses be located only in certain areas of a town. If a health care organization is not-for-profit, it is likely exempt from property taxes. A facility that is not taxable is an economic burden to the local government. Therefore health care organizations often become deeply intertwined with the interests of the communities in which they are located. Current Internal Revenue Service regulations require that not-for-profit organizations, including hospitals, measure and report the benefit that they provide to their communities.

## Accreditation

Another issue that has a visible impact on the operation of a health care facility is voluntary accreditation. Whereas licensure is mandatory to operate a health care facility within a given state, accreditation is voluntary.

**accreditation** Voluntary compliance with a set of standards developed by an independent agent, who periodically performs audits to ensure compliance.

**Accreditation** begins with voluntary compliance with a set of standards that are developed by an independent organization. That organization then audits the facility to ensure compliance. Examples of accreditation standards include the existence and enforcement of policies and procedures regarding activities surrounding medical staff, environment of

## TABLE 1-8

## ACCREDITING ORGANIZATIONS IN HEALTH CARE

| ACCREDITING ORGANIZATION | FACILITIES/ORGANIZATIONS ACCREDITED |
| --- | --- |
| **Health Care Facilities** | |
| Accreditation Association for Ambulatory Health Care (AAAHC) | Ambulatory care facilities |
| American Osteopathic Association (AOA) | Osteopathic hospitals |
| The Joint Commission (TJC) | Acute care, ambulatory care, behavioral health long-term care, and rehabilitation facilities |
| National Integrated Accreditation for Healthcare Organizations (NIAHO) | Acute care facilities |
| Commission on Accreditation of Rehabilitation Facilities (CARF) | Rehabilitation facilities |
| National Committee for Quality Assurance (NCQA) | Managed care organizations |
| Healthcare Facilities Accreditation Program (HFAP) | Acute care, ambulatory care, behavioral health long-term care, and rehabilitation facilities |
| Community Health Accreditation Program (CHAP) (National League for Nursing) | Home- and community-based health care organizations |
| **Educational Programs** | |
| Accreditation Council for Occupational Therapy Education | Occupational therapist and occupational therapy assistant programs |
| American Physical Therapy Association | Physical therapist and physical therapist assistant programs |
| Committee on the Accreditation of Allied Health Education Programs | Education programs for multiple allied health specialties, including anesthesiologist assistant, cardiovascular technologist, blood bank technologist, medical assistant, exercise science, and respiratory therapist |
| Commission on Accreditation of Health Informatics and Information Management Education | Health information and informatics programs |
| Commission on Accreditation/Approval for Dietetics Education of the American Dietetic Association | Dietitian/nutritionist and dietetic technician programs |
| Liaison Committee of the Association of American Medical Colleges and the American Medical Association | Medical schools |
| National League for Nursing Accrediting Commission | Nursing schools |

care, information management, and provision of care. Numerous accrediting bodies exist for different industries. Table 1-8 lists some health care accrediting bodies and the subjects of their activities.

## The Joint Commission

Within the health care industry, the most important accrediting body is **The Joint Commission (TJC).** TJC is an organization located in Chicago that sets standards for acute care facilities, ambulatory care networks, long-term care facilities, and rehabilitation facilities as well as certain specialty facilities, such as hospice and home care agencies.

The standards set by TJC reflect best practices and in many ways define how a health care facility should operate in terms of patient care, the clinical flow of data, and documentation standards. Much of TJC's activity stems from the original 1913 American College of Surgeons (ACS) medical documentation standardization project. For many years after that project, ACS not only maintained the development of the standards of documentation for hospitals but also conducted the approval proceedings. In 1951, the ACS, along with the American Hospital Association, the American Medical Association, and the Canadian Medical Association, formed the Joint Commission on Accreditation of Hospitals, which took over that accrediting function. In 1987, the organization changed its name (Joint Commission on Accreditation of Healthcare Organizations) to reflect the variety of organizations that were seeking accreditation. In 2009, the current name, The Joint Commission, was adopted.

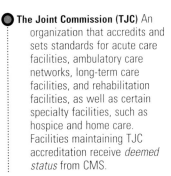

**The Joint Commission (TJC)** An organization that accredits and sets standards for acute care facilities, ambulatory care networks, long-term care facilities, and rehabilitation facilities, as well as certain specialty facilities, such as hospice and home care. Facilities maintaining TJC accreditation receive *deemed status* from CMS.

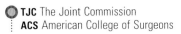

**TJC** The Joint Commission
**ACS** American College of Surgeons

**Medicare** Federally funded health care insurance plan for the older adult and for certain categories of chronically ill patients.

**reimbursement** The amount of money that the health care facility receives from the party responsible for paying the bill.

**deemed status** The Medicare provision that an approved accreditation is sufficient to satisfy the compliance audit element of the Conditions of Participation.

**CMS** Centers for Medicare and Medicaid Services

**COP** Conditions of Participation

**National Integrated Accreditation for Healthcare Organizations (NIAHO)** A compliance and accreditation entity partnered with CMS to ensure quality and standards in acute care settings. Facilities maintaining NIAHO accreditation receive *deemed status* from CMS.

**NIAHO** National Integrated Accreditation of Healthcare Organizations

**assisted living** A type of long-term care in which the resident is significantly independent in activities of daily living and does not need high levels of skilled nursing.

**acute care facility** A healthcare facility in which patients have an average length of stay less than 30 days and that has an emergency department, operating suite, and clinical departments to handle a broad range of diagnoses and treatments.

**ambulatory care facility** An outpatient facility, such as an emergency department or physician's office, in which treatment is intended to occur within 1 calendar day.

**TJC** The Joint Commission

**CARF** Commission on Accreditation of Rehabilitation Facilities

**Commission on Accreditation for Health Informatics and Information Management (CAHIIM)** The organization that accredits and sets quality and educational standards for HIM higher education programs.

TJC has a tremendous impact on health care facilities for a number of reasons. First, on-site accrediting surveys take place on a scheduled 3-year (maximum) cycle. Therefore, at least every 3 years, the facility is subject to an intensive onsite review. The accreditation standards change to differing degrees annually, with interim changes as needed. So within the 3-year cycle of review, facilities are required to stay abreast of the changes and implement procedures to comply.

Second, whether a facility attains favorable accreditation status has an impact on its relationship with government entities. As previously discussed, the CMS, through Medicare, allows reimbursement from Medicare to those facilities that comply with Medicare's COP. This ordinarily entails a survey to ensure that the facility complies with COP. However, a facility that is accredited by TJC is typically not subjected to the COP review; this situation is called **deemed status** because the facility is deemed to have complied with the COP because of its TJC accreditation. In addition, in some states TJC accreditation reduces the incidence of state licensure surveys. So in some cases, the voluntary accreditation by the TJC can alleviate two additional surveys, for the state department of health and Medicare COP. Many health insurance companies also require TJC or other accreditation before they will reimburse the organization.

Finally, accreditation is also desirable as a symbol of quality for marketing purposes.

### National Integrated Accreditation for Healthcare Organizations

Until 2008, TJC was the only accreditation option for acute care facilities that wanted to achieve deemed status. In 2008, CMS approved accreditation by the **National Integrated Accreditation for Healthcare Organizations (NIAHO)**. NIAHO is a subsidiary of Det Norske Veritas (DNV), a Norwegian foundation that specializes in risk management. DNV focuses on the maritime, energy, food and beverage, and health care industries.

NIAHO hospital accreditation is based on International Standards Organization (ISO) 9001 quality compliance and the CMS Conditions of Participation. Surveys are conducted annually and are focused on education and performance improvement. At the time of this writing, 211 hospitals had achieved NIAHO accreditation.

### Commission on Accreditation of Rehabilitation Facilities

Another important accrediting body is the Commission on Accreditation of Rehabilitation Facilities (CARF), also known as the Rehabilitation Accreditation Commission, which focuses on facilities that provide physical, mental, and occupational rehabilitation services. Accreditation of adult day care, **assisted living**, and employment and community services are also available. TJC also accredits rehabilitation facilities, but it has slightly different requirements and standards, adapting acute care and ambulatory care requirements. In fact, many rehabilitation facilities may be accredited by both TJC and CARF. The focus of the two reviews is slightly different, and rehabilitation facilities that are accredited by TJC find themselves in something of a dilemma in complying with both sets of requirements. CARF requirements tend to be more prescriptive, and surveyors focus beyond physician/ nurse documentation to emphasize documentation of occupational, physical, and other therapies. In recent years, TJC and CARF have collaborated to offer joint survey options to facilities. In this way, the surveys can be simultaneous and partially coordinated to reduce duplication of effort.

Many organizations accredit health care facilities and health care professional education programs. A partial list of these organizations and the facilities and institutions that they accredit is provided in Table 1-8.

### Commission on Accreditation for Health Informatics and Information Management

If you are studying health information management in a college that has an accredited health information management program, your program is accredited by the **Commission on Accreditation for Health Informatics and Information Management (CAHIIM).**

CAHIIM serves the public interest by establishing quality standards for the educational preparation of future HIM professionals. When a program is accredited by CAHIIM, it has voluntarily undergone a rigorous review process and has been determined to meet or exceed the standards set by CAHIIM. CAHIIM is an independent affiliate of the American Health Information Management Association (AHIMA). CAHIIM accreditation is a way to recognize and publicize best practices for HIM Education Programs (Commission on Accreditation for Health Informatics and Information Management Education, 2012).

## Professional Standards

In addition to licensure and accreditation requirements, yet another level of requirements must be followed in a health care organization: professional standards. On the one hand, licensure and accrediting bodies take a general overview of the facility and tend not to specifically address the day-to-day activities of individual practitioners. On the other hand, professional standards are developed by the professional organizations that grant the credentials to the individuals performing health-related tasks.

In addition to professional standards that govern the behavior of a variety of health care professionals, many of those professionals are also licensed by the state in which they practice and come under those licensing regulations as well. Specifically, physicians are licensed to practice medicine in the same way that health care facilities are licensed to operate, and the requirements for licensure may vary from state to state.

Professional standards play an important role in determining the activities of health care professionals. Often, it is the professional standards of the individual practitioner that dictate the type and extent of documentation required in the performance of any type of therapy or evaluation of patients. Medical professions have a code of ethics that govern the conduct of their members.

In the field of HIM, professional standards tend to revolve around issues of **ethics** and best practices. They also tend to target data quality, confidentiality, and access to health information. It is important in the practice of HIM that practitioners know and adhere to these professional standards. Professional standards in HIM are developed by AHIMA and take the form of an ethics statement as well as practice briefs and position papers, which are routinely published in the *Journal of the American Health Information Management Association*. Box 1-2 shows the AHIMA Code of Ethics.

**licensure** The mandatory government approval required for performing specified activities. In health care, the state approval required for providing health care services.

**accreditation** Voluntary compliance with a set of standards developed by an independent agent, who periodically performs audits to ensure compliance.

**ethics** A system of beliefs about acceptable behavior; a standard of moral excellence that all health information management professionals must uphold while managing patient information.

**HIM** Health Information Management

**AHIMA** American Health Information Management Association

---

**BOX 1-2  AMERICAN HEALTH AND INFORMATION MANAGEMENT ASSOCIATION'S CODE OF ETHICS**

The following ethical principles are based on the core values of the AHIMA and apply to all health information management professionals:

Advocate, uphold, and defend the individual's right to privacy and the doctrine of confidentiality in the use and disclosure of information.

Put service and the health and welfare of persons before self-interest and conduct oneself in the practice of the profession so as to bring honor to oneself, peers, and to the health information management profession.

Preserve, protect, and secure personal health information in any form or medium and hold in the highest regard health information and other information of a confidential nature obtained in an official capacity, taking into account the applicable statutes and regulations.

Refuse to participate in or conceal unethical practices or procedures and report such practices.

Advance health information management knowledge and practice through continuing education, research, publications, and presentations.

Recruit and mentor students, staff, peers, and colleagues to develop and strengthen professional workforce.

Represent the profession to the public in a positive manner.

Perform honorably health information management association responsibilities, either appointed or elected, and preserve the confidentiality of any privileged information made known in any official capacity.

State truthfully and accurately one's credentials, professional education, and experiences.

Facilitate interdisciplinary collaboration in situations supporting health information practice.

Respect the inherent dignity and worth of every person.

*Revised and adopted by AHIMA House of Delegates—July 1, 2004.*

## EXERCISE 1-3

**Legal and Regulatory Environment**

1. List and describe the purposes of the agencies within the Department of Health and Human Services.
2. Medicare is administered by_____.
3. Medicare waives compliance audits for appropriately accredited facilities by granting them _____.
4. Voluntary compliance with a set of standards developed by an independent agency is part of the _____ process.
5. Health care professionals must adhere to their discipline's _____.

## WORKS CITED

American Association of Medical Colleges: Family practice: Careers in medicine: Specialty information: Family practice https://www.aamc.org/students/medstudents/cim/specialties/63820/cim_pub_fp.html. Published 2011. Accessed July 30, 2011.

American Board of Medical Specialties: About ABMS. http://www.abms.org/About_ABMS/member_boards.aspx. Published 2011. Accessed July 30, 2011.

American Health Information Management Association (AHIMA): AHIMA Code of Ethics. http://library.ahima.org/xpedio/groups/public/documents/ahima/bok1_024277.hcsp?dDocName=bok1_024277. Published 2004. Accessed September 4, 2012.

American Health Information Management Association: Certification. http://www.ahima.org/certification/default.aspx. Published 2012. Accessed July 10, 2012.

American Nurses Credentialing Center: Certified nursing excellence. http://www.nursecredentialing.org/Certification.aspx. Published 2006. Accessed August 13, 2012.

American Osteopathic Association (AOA): About osteopathic medicine. http://www.osteopathic.org/osteopathic-health/about-dos/Pages/default.aspx. Published 2012. Accessed July 10, 2012.

Commission on Accreditation for Health Informatics and Information Management Education (CAHIM): Welcome to CAHIIM. http://www.cahiim.org. Published 2012. Accessed July 10, 2012.

Cruess SR, Johnston S, Cruess RL: Profession: a working definition for medical educators. Teach Learn Med Winter;16:74-76, 2004.

Office of the National Coordinator for Health Information Technology: Preparing skilled professionals for a career in health IT. http://healthit.hhs.gov/portal/server.pt/community/healthit_hhs_gov__workforce_development_program/3659. Published 2012. Accessed April 25, 2012.

United States Medical Licensing Examination: Overview. USMLE Bulletin 2012. http://www.usmle.org/bulletin/overview. Accessed April 25, 2012.

## SUGGESTED READING

Peden AH: Comparative health information management, ed 2, Clifton Park, NY, 2005, Delmar.
Sultz H, Young K: Health care USA: understanding its organization and delivery, ed 2, Gaithersburg, MD, 1999, Aspen.

# CHAPTER ACTIVITIES

## CHAPTER SUMMARY

Health care is provided by a variety of different practitioners, including physicians, nurses, and therapists. Practitioners in multiple disciplines work together to care for the patient. Physicians may maintain their own offices as solo practitioners or work with other physicians in group practices. Physicians' offices are a type of ambulatory care facility. Other types of facilities are acute care, long-term care, and a variety of specialty facilities, including rehabilitation facilities, mental health facilities, and children's hospitals. Facilities can be classified by length of stay, inpatient versus outpatient services, and financial status (i.e., for-profit or not-for-profit).

Government plays a role in the health care industry. Federal and state governments enact laws and enforce them through regulations. Health care facilities are licensed through the state, and there are a number of very specific reporting requirements. Another aspect of facility organization is accreditation status. Accreditation is very important to ensure quality and efficient reimbursement. Last, professional standards play a role in determining the activities of a facility because each profession has its own standards of both care and documentation.

## REVIEW QUESTIONS

1. Match the diagnosis, activity, or patient group on the left with the name of the specialty on the right.

| | |
|---|---|
| _____ 1. Administers substances that cause loss of sensation | A. Allergist |
| _____ 2. Cares for patients with cancer | B. Anesthesiologist |
| _____ 3. Provides care related to the female reproductive system | C. Cardiologist |
| _____ 4. Cares for women before, during, and after delivery | D. Dermatologist |
| _____ 5. Delivers primary health care for children | E. Family practitioner |
| _____ 6. Delivers primary health care for patients of all ages | F. Gastroenterologist |
| _____ 7. Treats diseases and abnormal conditions of newborns | G. Gynecologist |
| _____ 8. Treats diseases of the digestive system | H. Neonatologist |
| _____ 9. Treats diseases of the heart and blood vessels | I. Obstetrician |
| _____ 10. Treats diseases of the muscles and bones | J. Oncologist |
| _____ 11. Treats diseases of the skin | K. Ophthalmologist |
| _____ 12. Deals with disorders of the mind | L. Orthopedist |
| _____ 13. Provides care related to eye diseases | M. Pathologist |
| _____ 14. Treats patients who have strong reactions to pollen and insect bites | N. Pediatrician |
| _____ 15. Studies changes in cells, tissue, and organs | O. Psychiatrist |

2. List six medical specialties, and describe what those professionals do. Research five medical specialties that were not listed in the text, and discover what those professionals do.
3. Log on to the AHIMA Web site (http://www.ahima.org). Explore the site. What does AHIMA say about careers in health information management? How many schools offer degrees in health information management? What courses are included in these programs?
4. The fundamental difference between ambulatory care and acute care is the patient's length of stay. Ambulatory patients are called outpatients, and acute care patients are called inpatients. In your own words, describe the differences between the two. What problems arise in an acute care facility in distinguishing between an outpatient and an inpatient? What are some other differences between ambulatory care and acute care?
5. Health care facilities can be compared in many ways other than length of stay. Organizational structure and ownership are two of those ways. List and describe in your own words how facilities can be different from one another.

6. Several types of health care settings were mentioned in this chapter. List as many different settings as you can remember. Identify and distinguish the various health care settings.

7. If you were just diagnosed with diabetes, how would you go about finding a physician to care for you?

8. Identify a facility in your area by looking on the Internet. Find out as much as you can about the facility, including the types of services that it offers. Describe the facility in terms of size, organization, types of patients, and average length of stay. What type of facility is it?

9. The lines between inpatients and outpatients may become blurred under certain circumstances. An emergency department patient who is treated and released is clearly an outpatient. However, if the patient entered the emergency department at 11 PM and left at 4 AM, the patient clearly arrived on one day and left on the next. Is this patient an inpatient or an outpatient? Why?

10. Some patients are kept in the hospital for observation. This is a special category of patients, neither outpatients nor inpatients, who may stay in the hospital for up to 24 hours without being admitted as inpatients. Can you think of a reason that this category of patients was created?

11. Describe government involvement in health care.

12. Health care facilities must be licensed to conduct business. However, they often choose to be accredited as well. What is licensure? What is accreditation? What is the difference between licensure and accreditation?

13. Many different organizations accredit health care facilities and educational programs. List as many accrediting bodies that you can remember and which facilities or programs they accredit.

14. Match accrediting bodies on the left with the type of organization on the right. Some accrediting bodies accredit more than one type of organization.

| | | | |
|---|---|---|---|
| ____ 1. AAAHC | A. Acute care |
| ____ 2. AOA | B. Ambulatory care facilities |
| ____ 3. CARF | C. Home health care |
| ____ 4. CHAP | D. Managed care organizations |
| ____ 5. TJC | E. Osteopathic hospitals |
| ____ 6. NCQA | F. Rehabilitation facilities |

⬤ **PROFESSIONAL PROFILE**

### Physician Office Liaison

My name is Melanie, and I have a very interesting position at a community hospital. I am a physician office liaison in the Medical Staff Office at Diamonte Hospital. I am responsible for helping the hospital maintain good relationships with the physicians on our staff. We are a small community hospital with 250 licensed beds. Our physicians are not employees of the hospital; they have privileges. This means that the hospital allows the physicians to admit their patients for treatment at the hospital.

These physicians have private practices with their own offices and staff. It's my job to know them, to help with any problems they may have communicating with the hospital, and to coordinate the filing of their professional documentation.

I like my job because I get to meet many really interesting people, and I learn about their jobs as well. Even though I'm learning something new every day, I had to know a lot to get this job in the first place.

To be able to help a physician's office staff member, I have to know the various professionals who might work in an office and what they might do. It really helps that I know the difference between a medical assistant and a nurse practitioner. It's important that I know how a group practice works so that I can help the hospital keep track of which physicians can cover for one another.

The hospital collects statistics on physicians: how many patients they admit, what diagnoses they are treating, what procedures they are performing, and other information. I collaborate with other hospital departments to collect these reports and help present them at medical staff meetings. To do this, I have to know all the departments in the hospital and how they are related. I also need to understand the reports.

One of my most important tasks is credentialing. When a physician applies for privileges, I do a background check, collect the licensing documentation, and prepare a presentation for the credentialing committee. Because privileges aren't permanent, I remind the physicians when they need to reapply and help gather the updated documentation. I need to understand the differences among the medical specialties and what board certification means.

Finally, I coordinate continuing education sessions for physicians and their office staff. My next project is to develop a newsletter of hospital and physician activities that I can e-mail to the physicians' offices.

How did I get this job? I'm a registered health information technician. I have an associate degree in health information technology (HIT) from my local community college. In the HIT program, I learned a lot about physicians, hospitals, and other health-related professions. The hospital administrators were very happy to find a candidate for the job who already understood the system.

## PATIENT CARE PERSPECTIVE

### Maria—Mother of Two

When my husband and I moved to town, we needed to find a pediatrician right away. We contacted Diamonte Hospital because they had a physician referral service. I had some follow-up questions, so I called the hospital and spoke with Melanie in the Medical Staff office to help me understand how the referral service worked. We were able to interview several physicians right away and establish a great relationship.

## APPLICATION

### An Ethical Dilemma

Vanessa is the supervisor of health information management at Community Hospital. She is a member of AHIMA and is studying to become a registered health information technician. Community Hospital has a new chief operating officer, Brad, who is new to the hospital and comes from another state. Brad is concerned that too many physicians are not completing their paperwork when patients are discharged. He would like Vanessa and her staff to send the paperwork out of the hospital to the physicians' offices for completion because he thinks that the physicians would be more likely to do the work if it were on their desks. Vanessa knows that the state licensure regulations prohibit the removal of the paperwork from the hospital under normal circumstances.

Should Vanessa comply with Brad's request? Is compliance with Brad's request a violation of the AHIMA Code of Ethics?

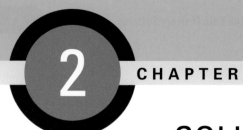

**CHAPTER**

# 2

# COLLECTING HEALTH CARE DATA

Nadinia Davis

## CHAPTER OUTLINE

BASIC CONCEPTS
  Health
  Data
  Information
  Health Data
  Health Information
KEY DATA CATEGORIES
  Demographic Data
  Socioeconomic Data
  Financial Data
  Clinical Data

MEDICAL DECISION MAKING
  Subjective
  Objective
  Assessment
  Plan
  Outcome
DESCRIBING DATA
  Building a Database
  Master Patient Index

ORGANIZATION OF DATA
ELEMENTS IN A HEALTH
RECORD
  Data Collection
  Paper
  Electronic Health Record
  Advantages and Disadvantages
DATA QUALITY
  Electronic Data Collection
  Quality Elements
DATA SETS
  Defined Data Sets

## VOCABULARY

aggregate data
assessment
authentication
Centers for Disease Control
  and Prevention (CDC)
character
clinical data
computerized physician
  order entry (CPOE)
data
data accessibility
data accuracy
data analytics
data collection devices
data consistency
data dictionary

data set
data validity
database
demographic data
electronic health record
electronic signature
epidemiology
field
file
financial data
guarantor
health data
health information
health record (medical
  record)
information

integrated record
master forms file
master patient index (MPI)
Minimum Data Set
  (MDS 3.0)
morbidity
mortality
National Center for Health
  Statistics (NCHS)
objective
outcome
Outcome and Assessment
  Information Set (OASIS)
payer
plan of treatment
problem list

problem-oriented record
record
rule out
SOAP format
socioeconomic data
source-oriented record
subjective
symptom
Uniform Bill (UB-04)
Uniform Hospital Discharge
  Data Set (UHDDS)
vital statistic

## CHAPTER OBJECTIVES

*By the end of this chapter, the student should be able to:*
1. Distinguish between data and information.
2. Define health and explain its relation to health data.
3. List and explain key data categories.
4. Distinguish among characters, fields, records, and files.

5. Describe how data are organized in a health record.
6. List and describe key data collection and quality issues.
7. Define the data sets used in health care and identify
   their applications and purposes.

● **assessment** An evaluation. In
  medical decision making, the
  physician's evaluation of the
  subjective and objective
  evidence. Also refers to the
  evaluation of a patient by any
  clinical discipline.
  **treatment** A procedure, medication,
   or other measure designed to
   cure or alleviate the symptoms
   of disease.

Chapter 1 contained a discussion of various health care professionals and the settings in which they work. While caring for patients, health care workers listen to the patients and make observations. They record those observations, along with their evaluations and plans for further assessment and treatment. All of the assessment and treatment activities are further documented along with the outcome of these activities. This chapter focuses on the ways that health care workers record what they observe and what they do.

It often surprises patients when health care workers record their observations on paper. Popular literature and cinema often present a futuristic view of health care delivery in which documentation is captured and saved in computers, which then magically analyze and diagnose the patient. Although the technology certainly exists and is used in some settings, its universal implementation has not arrived. Because the United States is making the transition from paper- to computer-based standards, both are addressed to the extent that is practical in this text.

## BASIC CONCEPTS

Some basic terminology will assist your understanding of the material in this chapter as well as the rest of the text. Although these terms may be meaningful in other ways, it is important to understand them in the context of health care.

### Health

Health begins with the absence of disease. For the purposes of this discussion, consider a disease to be an abnormality caused by organic, environmental, or congenital problems. Therefore a person with no diseases is considered "healthy." Suppose a person has no diseases but is very emotionally upset about events in his or her life: Is that person healthy? Not really. Long-term emotional upheaval can lead to a number of serious diseases. Consequently, emotional concerns detract from health. What about a child who does not get enough to eat but is currently free from disease? Won't that child eventually deteriorate and become unhealthy over time? Of course. A person who is healthy is free of disease and is also free of outside physical, social, and other problems that could lead to a disease condition. Our knowledge about health comes from information we have analyzed, based on health care data.

The primary purpose of this book is to discuss data in the health care setting; how data are organized, stored, and retrieved, and how one can create information from data. So it is important to understand that data are the building blocks of information that is used for many different purposes.

### Data

Health information starts with **data**. *Data* are items, observations, or raw facts. A person can collect data without actually understanding it. For example, say there are 100 patients in Community Hospital today. What does that mean? Is that a lot of patients? How many patients should there be? So the number of patients in the hospital is not meaningful without understanding the context of the data collection. Similarly, other characteristics of hospital patients must be identified before the data are useful. The gender of the patients (male or female), the ages of the patients, and the types of services the patients are receiving are all important characteristics that would help explain the 100 patients. Clearly, *information* is needed.

> **data** The smallest elements or units of facts or observations. Also refers to a collection of such elements.

### HIT-bit

#### DATA: PLURAL OR SINGULAR?

Is *data* a plural word or a singular word? *Datum* is the singular form of the Latin word, and it represents a single item, observation, or fact. However, we rarely refer to one item of knowledge. Generally, we discuss a group of similar items, such as the temperatures listed in Figure 2-2, and we call the group *data*. In this book, the plural form is used to refer to items of related data ("the data are significant").

| | April 15, 2012 |
|---|---|
| Total Inpatients | 100 |
| | |
| Service | |
| Medical | 42 |
| Surgical | 23 |
| Obstetrical | 7 |
| Psychiatric | 24 |
| Nursery | 4 |
| | |
| Length of Stay | |
| 1 day | 23 |
| 2 days | 22 |
| 3 days | 29 |
| 4 days | 14 |
| 5 days | 7 |
| 6 days | 3 |
| 7 or more days | 2 |

**Figure 2-1** Organized report of 100 patients.

**Data vs. Information**

| DATA | INFORMATION |
|---|---|
| Definition: Individual units of knowledge | Definition: Data with a frame of reference |
| Example: Maria Gomez | Example: Maria Gomez Temperature (oral) March 15, 2012 |

| DATA | INFORMATION | |
|---|---|---|
| 104 | | |
| 105 | | |
| 104 | 1 PM | 104° |
| 103 | 2 PM | 105° |
| 102 | 3 PM | 104° |
| 101 | 4 PM | 103° |
| 100 | 5 PM | 102° |
| 99 | 6 PM | 101° |
| | 7 PM | 100° |
| | 8 PM | 99° |

On the left, the data about Maria Gomez are not useful, because we do not have a frame of reference. Those same data, within the frame of reference of date and time, tell a story that is clinically significant.

**Figure 2-2** A list of data with a frame of reference becomes information.

## Information

To interpret data—to make sense of the facts and use them—the data must be organized. The goal of organizing the data is to provide **information**. The terms *data* and *information* are often used synonymously, but they are not the same. "Get me the data" usually really means "get me useful information." Data are the units of observation, and information is data that has been organized to make it useful. Figure 2-1 provides an organized report of the 100 patients that gives the user information.

On the left in Figure 2-2 is a list of data pertaining to Maria Gomez. The user cannot tell what the data on the left signify until it is determined that they are her oral temperatures, taken at 1-hour intervals. Only then do the data become useful.

**information** Processed data (i.e., data that are presented in an appropriate frame of reference).

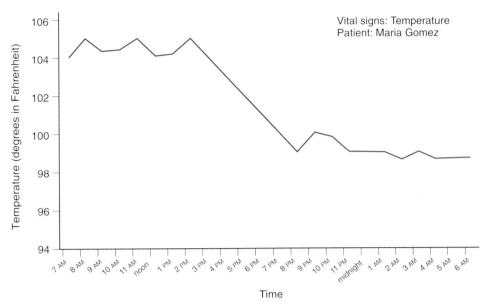

**Figure 2-3** The data presentation graph displays a large amount of data.

In Figure 2-2, the temperatures are listed in chronological order. On the basis of these few observations, it is easy to see that Maria's temperature is going down. If a nurse took Maria's temperature every hour for 5 days, there would be more than 100 items of data. But even listing them in order would not be helpful: there would be too many numbers to process visually. Therefore the most useful information is often data organized into a picture, such as the graph shown in Figure 2-3. Here, we can see that Maria's temperature was high in the morning, but returned to normal later in the evening and stayed there. The figure shows that the usefulness of data depends on their organization and presentation.

These two examples show that data becomes information when it is organized and when it is presented in the proper context. Sometimes, a list is enough; other times, pictures are more helpful.

**Go To** Chapter 10 for more information on vital statistics.

## Health Data

Many types of data can be collected. Figure 2-2 is an example of health data. **Health data** are items in reference to an individual patient or a group of patients. We can list all of the diseases that a patient has (for continuing patient care) or all of the patients who have a certain disease (to start an audit, for example). The series of temperatures collected and reported from Maria Gomez in Figures 2-2 and 2-3 is the health data from one patient.

Similarly, one can obtain vast quantities of data on individual patients or groups of patients. Imagine a list of 10,000 patients and their diseases. Are these useful data? What could be done with these data? Unless one is prepared to organize it, the list is not very informative. However, a list of the top 10 most common diseases of 10,000 residents in a particular location would be quite useful. This type of information is published frequently. For example, Figure 2-4 shows the top 10 causes of death in the United States in 1900 and 2007. Certainly, a list of the top 500 causes of death would not have been as useful.

**health data** Elements related to a patient's diagnosis and procedures as well as factors that may affect the patient's condition.

## Health Information

**Health information** is health data that have been organized. In Figure 2-3, the temperatures gathered become health information when the user understands that those temperatures are for one patient at certain times of the day. Health data related to 10,000 residents become health information when the data are organized in a way that is meaningful to the reader. Listing the top 10 diseases of a city's residents is useful health information. This is

**health information** Organized data that have been collected about a patient or a group of patients.

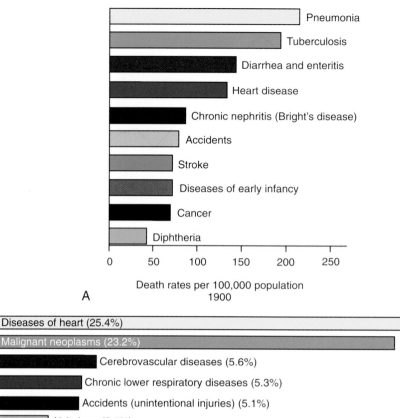

Figure 2-4 **A,** The top ten causes of death in the United States: 1900. **B,** The top ten causes of death in the United States: 2007. (**A,** Modified from Grove RD, Hetzel AM: Vital statistics rates of the United States, 1940-1960, Washington, DC, 1968, U.S. Government Printing Office; and Hoyert DL, Koehanek KD, Murphy SI: Deaths: Final data for 1997. National Vital Stat Report 47, No.19, 30 June 1999. **B,** Data from CDC/NCHS, National Vital Statistics System: Deaths, percent of total deaths, and death rates for the 15 leading causes of death: United States and each State, 2007. http://www.cdc.gov/nchs/data/dvs/LCWK9_2007.pdf. Published 2011. Accessed April 3, 2012.)

**mortality** Refers to death.
**vital statistic** Public health data collected through birth certificates, death certificates, and other data-gathering tools.
**morbidity** A disease or illness.
**epidemiology** The study of morbidity (disease) trends and occurrences.

**Go To** Chapter 10 for more information on vital statistics.

information that physicians can use to make decisions. In Figure 2-4, for example, tuberculosis and diarrhea/enteritis are no longer on the list of the top ten causes of death (mortality) in the United States. **Mortality** data are a **vital statistic** captured through the death certificate filing process, discussed in detail in Chapter 10. Births and marriages are also vital statistics. **Morbidity**, or disease process, data are captured through the reporting of patient-specific data from various types of facilities. Upon study, one finds that the development of antibiotics and vaccines and improvements in sanitation have significantly reduced the number of deaths caused by these conditions. The graphs in Figure 2-4 present interesting information that helps us ask questions that lead to more information. The study of these types of health trends or patterns is called **epidemiology**.

Health information is a broad category. It may refer to the organized data that have been collected about an individual patient, or it can be the summary of information about that patient's entire experience with his or her physician. Health information can also be summary information about all of the patients that a physician has seen (also called **aggregate data**). Furthermore, health information managers can take all of the available information about patients in a particular geographical area and make broad statements on the basis of this array of information (public health information). The process of examining the data and exploring them to create information is called **data analytics**.

Health information therefore encompasses the organization of a limitless array of possible data items and combinations of data items. It can range from data about the care of an individual patient to information about the health trends of an entire nation.

> **aggregate data** A group of like data elements compiled to provide information about the group.
> **data analytics** The process of analyzing data and exploring them to create information.

## EXERCISE 2-1
### Basic Concepts

1. Give two examples in your personal life of data and two examples of information. Think of two examples of ways that health data differ from health information.
2. How do data become information?
3. What is health information?

## KEY DATA CATEGORIES

The primary purpose of recording data is communication, which is necessary for a variety of reasons. For example, a medical assistant may take a patient's vital signs for the physician's reference. The physician records her observations so that she can measure the patient's progress at a later date. Thus recording health data is an important way for health care professionals to communicate and facilitate patient care.

Beyond patient care, there are many other uses of health data. Hospital administrators use health data in order to make decisions about what services to offer and how best to serve the communities in which they are located. Lawyers use health data to demonstrate the extent of injuries suffered by a client. **Payers,** such as insurance companies and Medicare, use health data to determine reimbursement to providers. Government agencies, such as the **Centers for Disease Control and Prevention (CDC)** use health data to monitor diseases. The CDC is a division of the U.S. Department of Health and Human Services (DHHS). Within the CDC is the **National Center for Health Statistics (NCHS)**, which collects and analyzes mortality and other vital statistics. Box 2-1 shows a complete list of the DHHS's Operating Divisions.

These government agencies are just two of the many users of data that are collected and reported by providers. Chapter 7 discusses the use of health data for reimbursement.

> **payer** The individual or organization that is primarily responsible for the reimbursement for a particular health care service. Usually refers to the insurance company or third party.
> **Medicare** Federally funded health care insurance plan for older adults and for certain categories of chronically ill patients.
> **Centers for Disease Control and Prevention (CDC)** A federal agency that collects health information to provide research for the improvement of public health.
> **National Center for Health Statistics (NCHS)** A division of the CDC that collects and analyzes vital statistics. Acts as one of the ICD-10-CM Cooperating Parties.

> **reimbursement** The amount of money that the health care facility receives from the party responsible for paying the bill; health care services are paid after services have been rendered.

| BOX 2-1 | OPERATING DIVISIONS OF THE U.S. DEPARTMENT OF HEALTH AND HUMAN SERVICES (DHHS) |
|---|---|

- Administration for Children and Families (ACF)
  - Administration for Children, Youth and Families (ACYF)
- Administration for Community Living (ACL)
- Agency for Healthcare Research and Quality (AHRQ)
- Centers for Disease Control and Prevention (CDC)
- Centers for Medicare and Medicaid Services
- Food and Drug Administration (FDA)
- Health Resources and Services Administration (HRSA)
- Indian Health Service (IHS)
- National Institutes of Health (NIH)
  - National Cancer Institute (NCI)
- Substance Abuse and Mental Health Services Administration (SAMHSA)

Chapter 10 discusses the statistical analysis of health data for many different purposes. Chapter 11 discusses some administrative uses of health data.

Health data that are collected in a consistent, systematic process are most easily organized into information. There are four broad categories into which health data are collected: demographic, socioeconomic, financial, and clinical.

## Demographic Data

**Demographic data** identify the patient. Name, address, age, and gender are examples of demographic data. The physician needs the patient's name and address to send the patient correspondence, follow-up notices, or a bill. Other necessary data include the home phone number, place of employment, work telephone number, race, ethnicity, and Social Security number. The physician needs these data both to contact the patient and to distinguish one patient from another. Figure 2-5 shows demographic data collected for a new patient.

Demographic data helps the physician answer questions such as: How old are my patients? Where do my patients live?

## Socioeconomic Data

Another type of data about a patient that a physician collects is **socioeconomic data**. These personal data include the patient's marital status, education, and personal habits. Many students ask why the patient's socioeconomic situation is relevant to health care. One of the reasons that such data are important is that the diagnosis of many illnesses, and sometimes their treatment, depends on the doctor's understanding of the patient's personal situation. A list of socioeconomic data is presented in Box 2-2.

A patient with asthma who smokes will likely be advised by his or her physician to quit smoking. This is an example of a personal habit that directly affects a disease

**health data** Elements related to a patient's diagnosis and procedures as well as factors that may affect the patient's condition.

**demographic data** Identification: those elements that distinguish one patient from another, such as name, address, and birth date.

**socioeconomic data** Elements that pertain to the patient's personal life and personal habits, such as marital status, religion, and culture.

**diagnosis** The process of identifying the patient's condition or illness.

**treatment** A procedure, medication, or other measure designed to cure or alleviate the symptoms of disease.

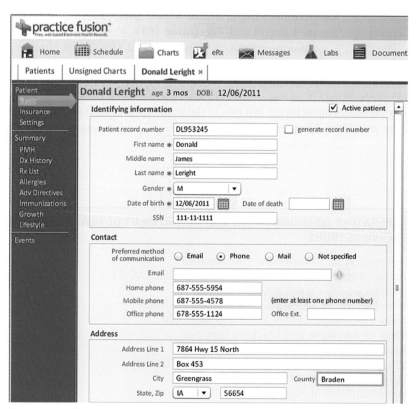

**Figure 2-5** Demographic data: data that help the user contact the patient or to distinguish one patient from another. (Courtesy Practice Fusion, Inc.)

condition. In addition, the socioeconomic situation or personal life of a patient sometimes dictates whether the patient will be compliant with a medication regimen or even whether he or she is able to obtain treatment. For example, if an older patient has just undergone a hip replacement, sending that patient home to a third-story walk-up apartment might be a problem. It will be very difficult for the patient to get in and out of the apartment and certainly very difficult for the patient to leave the apartment for therapy, particularly if there is no caregiver at home. Treatment at home might be needed as well as assistance with grocery shopping. Another possibility is to keep the patient in the hospital until the patient is comfortable with stairs. Therefore understanding a patient's personal life and living situation is important to the planning of how to care for the patient.

Sometimes the knowledge that a patient travels widely can lead a physician to suspect an illness that he or she would not consider if the patient never traveled. Travel in certain areas of the world could have caused exposure to diseases that are uncommon in his or her native area. Thus a patient's complaint of abdominal pain could lead the physician to suspect a parasite (an organism that may have been swallowed and is living in the intestines), whereas ordinarily the physician would consider only bacterial or viral causes.

## Financial Data

When requesting services from any health care provider, one expects at some point that payment of some sort will be required. The physician requests information about the party responsible for paying the bill. This information makes up the **financial data**. Financial data relate to the payment of the bill for services rendered.

The party (person or organization) from whom the provider is expecting payment for services rendered is called the payer. The payer is frequently an insurance company. It may also be a government agency, such as Medicare or Medicaid. Many patients have more than one payer. The primary payer is billed first for payment. A secondary payer is approached for any amount that the primary payer did not remit, and so on. For example, patients who are covered by Medicare may have supplemental or secondary insurance with a different payer. The physician first sends the bill to Medicare. Any amount that Medicare does not pay is then billed to the secondary payer. The patient may also have some responsibility for part of the payment.

Ultimately, the patient is financially responsible for payment of services that he or she has received. If the patient is a dependent, a person other than the patient may be ultimately responsible for the bill. The person who is ultimately responsible for paying the bill is called the **guarantor**. For example, if a child goes to the physician's office for treatment, the child, as a dependent, cannot be held responsible for the invoice. Therefore the parent or legal guardian is responsible for payment and is the guarantor. Figure 2-6 shows financial data required by a health care provider.

**financial data** Elements that describe the payer. For example, the name, address, telephone number, group number, and member number of the patient's insurance company.

**payer** The individual or organization that is primarily responsible for the reimbursement for a particular health care service. Usually refers to the insurance company or third party.

**Medicare** Federally funded health care insurance plan for older adults and for certain categories of chronically ill patients.

**guarantor** The individual or organization that promises to pay for the rendered health care services after all other sources (such as insurance) are exhausted.

**Go To** Financial data is typically collected at registration, which is discussed in greater detail in Chapter 4.

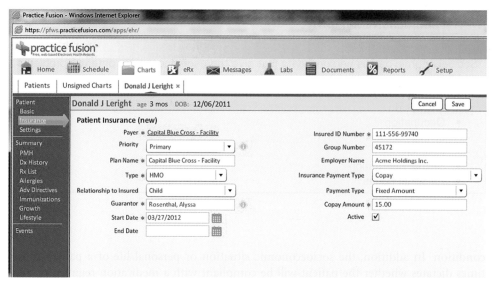

**Figure 2-6** Financial data include the identities of the parties responsible for paying the invoice. (Courtesy Practice Fusion, Inc.)

---

**BOX 2-3** | **CLINICAL DATA**

Clinical data is data that is specific to the patient's diagnosis and treatment; examples are as follows:

- Diagnosis
- Temperature
- Blood pressure
- Laboratory reports
- Radiographs and other types of imaging
- Medications
- Surgical procedures

---

## Clinical Data

Clinical data are probably the easiest to understand and relate to the health care field. **Clinical data** comprise all of the data that have been recorded about the patient's health, including the physician's conclusion about the patient's condition (diagnosis) and what plan or treatment (procedures) will be recommended. The following example illustrates clinical data.

The patient presents in the physician's office for pain in the abdomen. The physician knows that pain in the abdomen can be caused by a variety of conditions. The pain is merely a **symptom**, a description of what the patient feels or is experiencing. Other symptoms may include nausea, dizziness, and headache. The physician orders tests and performs a physical examination to determine which of those conditions is responsible for the abdominal pain. Some of these tests include radiographs and blood tests. Ultimately, the physician may conclude that the abdominal pain is caused by an inflamed appendix, or appendicitis. Appendicitis is the diagnosis, and the blood test and physical examination are the procedures. The physician records both the findings of the examination and the results of the tests in the patient's record. Clinical data constitute the bulk of any patient's record. All of the previous data that have been discussed—demographic, socioeconomic, and financial—can usually be contained in one or two pages in the front of a patient's health record. The rest of the record is the clinical data. Box 2-3 lists examples of clinical data.

**clinical data** All of the medical data that have been recorded about the patient's stay or visit, including diagnoses and procedures.

**symptom** The patient's report of physical or other complaints, such as dizziness, headache, and stomach pain.

## EXERCISE 2-2
### Key Data Categories

1. List and describe the four key data categories.
2. For each category of data, give four examples of data elements that would be contained in that category.

## MEDICAL DECISION MAKING

A logical thought process supports the medical evaluation process, or development of a medical diagnosis. Data are collected in one of four specific categories: the patient's *subjective* view, the physician's *objective* view, the physician's opinion or *assessment*, and the care *plan*. This method of recording observations or clinical evaluations is called the **SOAP format**: subjective, objective, assessment, and plan. Although physicians may not always follow this format exactly, they record their thoughts in this general manner. Table 2-1 lists the elements of a medical evaluation.

In conducting the evaluation, the physician collects data sufficient to develop a medical diagnosis. Initially, the data may support several different diagnoses. The physician continues to collect and analyze data until a specific diagnosis can be determined. For example, chest pain and shortness of breath can be symptoms of many conditions, including myocardial infarction (heart attack), congestive heart failure (a heart pumping problem that causes a buildup of fluid), and pneumonia (inflammation of the lungs). The physician examines the patient and orders enough tests to conclude which diagnosis (or diagnoses) applies in each individual case.

● **SOAP format** Subjective, Objective, Assessment, and Plan: the medical decision-making process used by physicians to assess the patient at various intervals.

● **diagnosis** The name of the patient's condition or illness.

### Subjective

The physician begins the medical evaluation process by asking the patient about the medical problem and the symptoms that he or she is experiencing. The patient's description of the problem, in his or her own words, is the **subjective** or history portion of the evaluation process. For example, the patient may have stomach pain. The patient may describe this as "abdominal pain," "pain in the belly," or "pain in the stomach." The physician's task is to narrow the patient's description through questioning. For instance, the patient can be assisted to identify the pain as a sharp, stabbing pain in the lower right portion of the abdomen. The physician also asks when the pain began, whether it is continuous or intermittent, and whether there are any other symptoms, such as nausea and vomiting. The physician will record the patient's description in the patient's own words.

● **subjective** In the SOAP format of medical decision making, the patient's description of the symptoms or other complaints.

### Objective

Once the physician has obtained and recorded the patient's subjective impressions about the medical problem, the physician must look at the patient objectively. The physician conducts a physical examination, exploring the places where the stomach pain may be located. The patient says his or her stomach hurts, but the physician records that the patient has "tenderness on palpation in the right lower quadrant." Tenderness on palpation in the right lower quadrant is a classic indication of appendicitis. Other possible diagnoses (also

| TABLE 2-1 | |
| --- | --- |
| **ELEMENTS OF MEDICAL EVALUATION (SOAP)** | |
| **DATA ELEMENT** | **EXPLANATION** |
| Subjective | The patient's report of symptoms or problems |
| Objective | The physician's observations, including evaluation of diagnostic test results |
| Assessment | The physician's opinion as to the diagnosis or possible diagnoses |
| Plan | Treatment or further diagnostic evaluation |

**objective** In the SOAP format for medical decision making, the physician's observations and review of diagnostic tests.

**rule out** The process of systematically eliminating potential diagnoses. Also refers to the list of potential diagnoses.

called differential diagnoses) are ovarian cyst and a variety of intestinal disorders, such as diverticulitis (inflammation of the intestines). The physician's **objective** notation is the specific anatomical location of the pain, vital signs, and the results of any laboratory tests that the physician ordered. The physician orders tests to confirm a likely diagnosis or to **rule out**, or eliminate, a possible diagnosis. In this example, the physician is looking for an elevation of the white blood cell (WBC) count, which indicates the presence of an infection. The physician may rule out differential diagnoses such as appendicitis if the WBC count is normal. Additional tests, such as an abdominal ultrasound, might be ordered if the blood test results are negative or inconclusive.

---

## HIT-bit

### RULE OUT

In recording the assessment of possible diagnoses, the physician often makes the following statement: "Rule Out." This phrase indicates that the listed diagnosis is still provisional—that it may prove to be the final diagnosis (or one of them). On the other hand, if the statement reads "Ruled Out," the diagnosis is no longer being considered. For example:

"Rule Out: CHF (congestive heart failure), pneumonia." This means that the patient may or may not have CHF and/or pneumonia.

"CHF, pneumonia ruled out." This means that the patient has CHF and does not have pneumonia.

---

## Assessment

**assessment** An evaluation. In medical decision making, the physician's evaluation of the subjective and objective evidence. Also refers to the evaluation of a patient by any clinical discipline.

Once the physician has obtained the patient's subjective view and has conducted an objective medical evaluation, he or she develops an *assessment*. The **assessment** is a description of what the physician thinks is wrong with the patient: the diagnosis or possible (provisional) diagnoses. If there are multiple possible diagnoses, the physician would record "possible appendicitis versus ovarian cyst" or "rule out appendicitis, rule out ovarian cyst." The phrase "rule out" means that the diagnosis is still under investigation. "Ruled out" means that the diagnosis has been eliminated as a possibility. In this abdominal pain example, if the physician has eliminated the possibility of an ovarian cyst and has concluded that the patient has appendicitis, the documentation would read: "appendicitis, ovarian cyst ruled out."

## Plan

**plan of treatment** In the SOAP format for medical decision making, the diagnostic, therapeutic, or palliative measures that are taken to investigate or treat the patient's condition or disease.

Once the physician has assessed what is wrong with the patient, he or she writes a **plan of treatment**. The plan may be for treatment or for further evaluation, particularly if the assessment includes several possible diagnoses. Figure 2-7 illustrates the pattern of data collection.

Other clinical personnel also record their observations but not necessarily in the SOAP format. Many nursing evaluations are recorded through the use of graphs or on preprinted forms. Graphs or preprinted forms are also used for clinical evaluations in physical therapy, respiratory therapy, and anesthesia records; also, some surgical records and many maternity and neonatal records use preprinted or graphical forms.

## Outcome

**outcome** The result of a patient's treatment.

**discharge** Discharge occurs when the patient leaves the care of the facility to go home, for transfer to another health care facility or by death. Also refers to the status of a patient.

It should be noted that an increasingly important component of the medical decision-making process is the **outcome**: the result of the plan. Insurance companies may use the history and trending of outcomes to determine which health care providers will be included in their networks.

In an acute care (hospital) record, the outcome of the admission is captured in several places: the diagnoses and procedures, the discharge disposition (e.g., home, nursing home, expired), and the physician's overall explanation of the stay in the discharge summary.

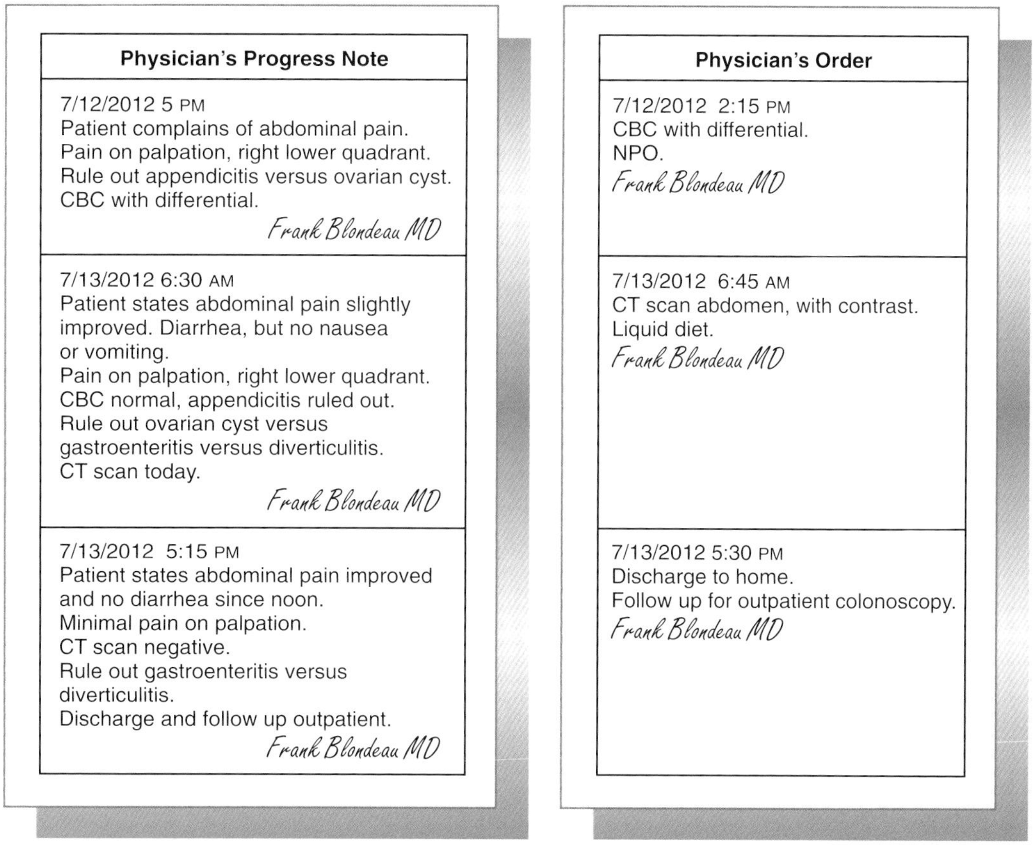

| Physician's Progress Note |
|---|
| 7/12/2012 5 PM<br>Patient complains of abdominal pain.<br>Pain on palpation, right lower quadrant.<br>Rule out appendicitis versus ovarian cyst.<br>CBC with differential.<br><br>*Frank Blondeau MD* |
| 7/13/2012 6:30 AM<br>Patient states abdominal pain slightly<br>improved. Diarrhea, but no nausea<br>or vomiting.<br>Pain on palpation, right lower quadrant.<br>CBC normal, appendicitis ruled out.<br>Rule out ovarian cyst versus<br>gastroenteritis versus diverticulitis.<br>CT scan today.<br><br>*Frank Blondeau MD* |
| 7/13/2012 5:15 PM<br>Patient states abdominal pain improved<br>and no diarrhea since noon.<br>Minimal pain on palpation.<br>CT scan negative.<br>Rule out gastroenteritis versus<br>diverticulitis.<br>Discharge and follow up outpatient.<br><br>*Frank Blondeau MD* |

| Physician's Order |
|---|
| 7/12/2012 2:15 PM<br>CBC with differential.<br>NPO.<br><br>*Frank Blondeau MD* |
| 7/13/2012 6:45 AM<br>CT scan abdomen, with contrast.<br>Liquid diet.<br><br>*Frank Blondeau MD* |
| 7/13/2012 5:30 PM<br>Discharge to home.<br>Follow up for outpatient colonoscopy.<br><br>*Frank Blondeau MD* |

**Figure 2-7** The link between physician's notes and physician's orders.

Often, the patient is not fully recovered when discharged, and additional follow-up is required. Therefore some outcomes are inferred. For example, if the patient is discharged on Monday and readmitted on Thursday for the same diagnosis, it could be inferred that the outcome of the plan during the first admission was not successful.

The reasons for unsuccessful outcomes are not necessarily the fault of the attending physician or the facility in which the patient was treated. The patient may not have complied with discharge instructions, for example. Nevertheless, the readmission is attributed to both the attending physician and the facility in the reporting of such data. One example of the shifting emphasis on outcomes and follow-up is the Medical Home model of primary care. Medical Home refers to the proactive coordination of patient care by the primary care physician. The Medical Home model requires coordination and collaboration among all caregivers in order to ensure that the patient's transition from one setting to another is seamless and is supported by the data collected in the prior settings. In this manner, the primary care physician would be informed concurrently of the patient's inpatient treatment and discharge instructions so that follow-up would occur promptly, ensuring that the patient understood and was following discharge instructions, potentially preventing unnecessary readmission.

**attending physician** The physician who is primarily responsible for coordinating the care of the patient in the hospital; it is usually the physician who ordered the patient's admission to the hospital.

**primary care physician (PCP)** In insurance, the physician who has been designated by the insured to deliver routine care to the insured and to evaluate the need for referral to a specialist, if applicable. Colloquial use is synonymous with *family doctor.*

## EXERCISE 2-3

### Medical Decision-Making Process

*Match the physician progress note entry on the left with the SOAP note component on the right.*

1. 60 mg pseudoephedrine every 4 hours; 100 mg Tylenol as needed for pain
2. Acute sinusitis with pharyngitis
3. Patient complains of headache
4. Patient's frontal sinuses sensitive to percussion; lungs clear; throat slightly inflamed

A. Subjective
B. Objective
C. Assessment
D. Plan

**demographic data** Identification: those elements that distinguish one patient from another, such as name, address, and birth date.

**financial data** Elements that describe the payer. For example, the name, address, telephone number, group number, and member number of the patient's insurance company.

**electronic health record (EHR)** A secure real-time, point-of-care, patient centric information resource for clinicians allowing access to patient information when and where needed and incorporating evidence-based decision support.

**clinical data** All of the medical data that have been recorded about the patient's stay or visit, including diagnoses and procedures.

**database** An organized collection of data.

**payer** The individual or organization that is primarily responsible for the reimbursement for a particular health care service. Usually refers to the insurance company or third party.

**character** A single letter, number, or symbol.

**field** A collection or series of related characters. A field may contain a word, a group of words, a number, or a code, for example.

## DESCRIBING DATA

Data are collected for a reason and stored for later use. The process is a little like grocery shopping. One buys food that is needed both now and in the future and stores it in the proper place for current and future use. Similarly, health care providers collect the data that are needed both now and in the future and store these data in the proper places for both current and future use.

The demographic and financial data collected for each patient are stored in a *database*. In an **electronic health record** (**EHR**), the clinical data are similarly captured and stored. This **database** is a collection of data elements organized in a manner that allows efficient retrieval of information. The data collection can occur on paper or in a software program. For this discussion, the database is the EHR; however, keep in mind that any collection of data elements can be considered a database if it is so organized.

Whether data are to be stored on paper or in a computer, they must be organized in such a way that they can be found quickly when they are needed. The first step in collecting the data is determining what data elements are needed. Demographic, socioeconomic, financial, and clinical data are needed, but the specific elements that are collected will vary depending on the health care provider, the patient's problem, the needs of the facility, and the requirements of other users such as the payer.

To take the analogy of grocery shopping further: Just as food comes in appropriate containers, data also come in packages. Data are collected and stored in logical segments. Individual data items are collected and packaged into useful bundles, according to the category of data. Think about the appendicitis example. What data did the physician need? How were the data obtained? Data are collected piece by piece in logical segments. The logical segments are called characters, fields, records, and files.

## Building a Database

### Characters

This chapter focuses on the way data are collected on paper or electronically. With regard to computers, the smallest segment of data is referred to as a *bit*. A bit is the computer's electronic differentiation between two choices: on and off. Small strings of bits in specific combinations of on/off patterns make bytes, which are represented on the computer screen as characters. A character is the smallest segment of written data.

A **character** is a letter, a single-digit number, or a symbol. "A" is a character, as are "3" and "&." A character is the smallest unit of data that is collected. Characters are the building blocks of data. Characters are strung together to make words, larger numbers, and other types of written communication.

### Fields

The individual recording the data needs to know what characters to combine to make the words that are the patient's name, for example. Placing the characters in the correct order is important so that the data collected are accurate (correct). For example: if a patient's name is Gomez, recording the name as Goemz is not accurate.

A **field** is a series of related characters that have a specific relationship to one another. Usually, a field is a word, a group of related words, or a specific type of number. In the demographic category, the patient's address in the United States contains a postal service zip code. The zip code for Linden, New Jersey is 07036. Therefore the field "zip code" contains five characters: 0, 7, 0, 3, and 6.

Fields are defined by the type of data that they contain. A field containing nothing but letters would be an alphabetical field. For example, a field for first name would be an alphabetical field (abbreviated as alpha). A field containing only numbers would be a numerical field. A field for dollars is an example of a numerical field. A field can also be a combination of alphabetical and numerical characters; this is called an *alphanumerical field*. A field for street address is an alphanumerical field.

| Name | Definition | Size | Type | Example |
|-------|-------------------------|---------------|--------------|--------------|
| FNAME | Patient's first name | 15 Characters | Alphabetic | Jane |
| LNAME | Patient's last name | 15 Characters | Alphabetic | Jones |
| TELE | Patient's phone number | 12 Characters | Alphanumeric | 973-555-3331 |
| TEMP | Patient's temperature | 5 Characters | Numeric | 98.6 |

**Figure 2-8** Common fields of data, including definitions.

## HIT-bit

### FORMATTING FIELDS

When creating fields in a computer, you may find it useful to tell the computer that a number is really alphanumerical. For example, if a zip code field is labeled "numerical," most computer systems drop the leading zeros. Zip code 07036 then becomes 7036 both on the screen and when printed out. This is not desirable if you are printing labels for mailing envelopes. Mail addressed this way would most certainly be delayed. Social Security numbers are another tricky field to define. Again, a field containing a Social Security number should be defined as alphabetical or text to preserve the zeros.

Fields are generally given logical names to identify them. Figure 2-8 illustrates data fields and definitions. The listing of fields is one component of creating a **data dictionary**. A data dictionary is a listing of all fields to be collected: their size, name, and description. Some fields, such as the month of the year, have a limited number of possible contents or values. The data dictionary describes the specific contents or values that can be contained in each field. For example, in the specific contents of the field for the month of the patient's admission, the whole numbers 1 through 12 are the only acceptable values.

Whether the data are collected on paper or in a computer, the size of the field must be considered to ensure uniformity in recording and retrieving the data (standardization).

### Records

In the same way that characters combine to make fields, fields combine to make **records**. A very simple example of fields that combine to make a record is an entry in a contact list in an electronic device such as a cell phone. First name, last name, street address, city, state, zip code, and multiple telephone numbers are listed. Similarly, a physician keeps track of patients using groups of fields that combine to make a record of the patient's demographic data. A simple example of how fields combine to make a record is shown in Figure 2-9.

### Files

The physician collects numerous records of different types of data, and this group of related records is called a **file**. In Figure 2-10, the entire contact list is a file made up of individual records.

Files can be large or small, depending on the number of records that they contain. A patient's entire health history can be contained in one file depending on how it is organized. An EHR or electronic patient record is developed by linking the data records collected for each patient. In common usage, the terms "file" and "record" are often used interchangeably, even though they have different technical meanings.

## Master Patient Index

The number of health records generated by a provider quickly becomes unmanageable with out a way to reference them. The **master patient index (MPI)** is the key to identifying patients and locating their records. Historically, an MPI was a manual system maintained

**data dictionary** A list of details that describe each field in a database.

**record** A collection of related fields. Also refers to all of the data collected about a patient's visit or all of the patient's visits.

**Go To** Chapter 3 discusses the development of an electronic health record.

**file** Numerous records of different types of related data. Files can be large or small, depending on the number of records they contain.

**master patient index (MPI)** A system containing a list of patients who have received care at the health care facility and their encounter information, often used to correlate the patient with the file identification.

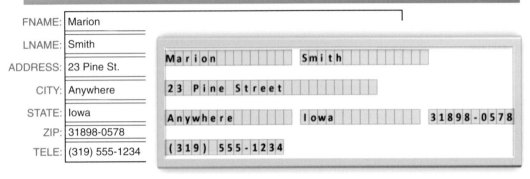

| Name | Definition | Size | Type | Example |
|------|-----------|------|------|---------|
| FNAME | Patient's first name | 15 Characters | Alphabetic | Marion |
| LNAME | Patient's last name | 15 Characters | Alphabetic | Smith |
| ADDRESS | Patient's home street address | 25 Characters | Alphanumeric | 23 Pine St |
| CITY | City associated with ADDRESS | 15 Characters | Alphabetic | Anywhere |
| STATE | State associated with ADDRESS | 14 Characters | Alphabetic | IOWA |
| ZIP | Postal zip code associated with ADDRESS | 10 Characters | Alphanumeric | 31898-0578 |
| TELE | Patient's primary contact number | 14 Characters | Alphanumeric | (319) 555-1234 |

FNAME: Marion
LNAME: Smith
ADDRESS: 23 Pine St.
CITY: Anywhere
STATE: Iowa
ZIP: 31898-0578
TELE: (319) 555-1234

Marion          Smith
23 Pine Street
Anywhere     Iowa          31898-0578
(319) 555-1234

Each field in the record above is blocked to illustrate the number of characters allowed, compared to the number this record required.

**Figure 2-9** An example of how fields combine to make a record in a contact list.

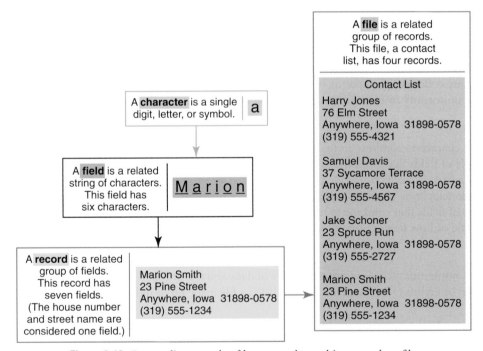

**Figure 2-10** Contact list example of how records combine to make a file.

**demographic data** Identification: those elements that distinguish one patient from another, such as name, address, and birth date.

on dual index cards organized in a file cabinet in alphabetical order (similar to the contact list example given previously) and numerical order (by identification number). Today, even providers with paper-based health records maintain an electronic MPI.

The data contained in the MPI is the demographic data collected during the patient registration process. These data are used to identify each patient within that health care facility and to locate the patient's health record.

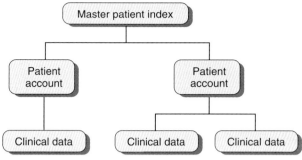

Figure 2-11  Building a database.

The first time a patient visits, a unique medical record number (MR#) is assigned. On subsequent visits, the registrar will be able to find the patient in the index and use the medical record number that already exists. For accounting purposes, each visit is also assigned a unique number, frequently called the **patient account number**, *patient number*, or *billing number*. The account number is linked to the MR# so that all visits can be identified and tracked. In a paper-based environment, the MPI is primarily a look-up for finding patients and their visits. However, more powerfully, this numbering and linking of patient identity and demographic data to visits and thus clinical data are the foundation for the database that becomes the EHR (Figure 2-11).

**patient account number** A numerical identifier assigned to a specific encounter or health care service received by a patient; a new number will be assigned to each encounter, but the patient will retain the same medical record number.

**medical record number (MR#)** A unique number assigned to each patient in a health care system; this code will be used for the rest of the patient's encounters with that specific health system.

**MPI** master patient index

## EXERCISE 2-4
### Describing Data

1. Create a file of five records that contain name, address, and telephone number. Begin by defining the fields in data dictionary format, and then show how you would represent these fields if you were trying to explain them to someone else.
2. Which of the following is the best example of a single character field?
   a. J
   b. NJ
   c. New Jersey
   d. All of the above

*Use the sample data dictionary below to answer Questions 3 through 5.*

| NAME | DEFINITION | SIZE | TYPE | EXAMPLE |
|------|-----------|------|------|---------|
| FNAME | Patient's first name | 15 Characters | Alphabetical | Jane |
| LNAME | Patient's last name | 15 Characters | Alphabetical | Jones |
| HTEL | Patient's home telephone number | 12 Characters | Alphanumerical | 973-555-3331 |
| TEMP | Patient's temperature | 5 Characters | Numerical | 98.6 |

3. Using 12 alphanumerical characters is one way to capture the patient's home telephone number. List at least one other way to capture that data.
4. List and describe two additional fields that would be needed to capture a patient's entire name.
5. Using the format above, define the fields that would be needed to capture a patient's diagnosis and a procedure.

## ORGANIZATION OF DATA ELEMENTS IN A HEALTH RECORD

All of the data that have been collected about an individual patient are called a **health record** or medical record. A health record may refer to the patient's record that is kept by a particular health care provider or to the patient's lifelong medical history. For the sake

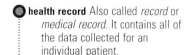

**health record** Also called *record* or *medical record*. It contains all of the data collected for an individual patient.

**Go To** Chapter 9 delves into the intricacies of storing health data in various formats.

of clarity, we refer to a patient's information as the health record, whether it refers to a single visit or the patient's collective experience.

The previous example of a contact list involved defining data in a certain useful format. Data collected in a health care environment can be similarly defined. When health care workers collect items of data, they record them so that they and other users can retrieve them later. Data can be recorded on paper, in an electronic format, or in both formats (hybrid record).

## Data Collection

Data collection is rarely the collection of a single data field but is more often a record of several data fields collected repeatedly over time. At this point, it is useful to consider the way in which the data are collected.

The primary difference between the data compiled in a physician's office record and the data collected in a hospital lies in the volume of data collected about a patient and the way it is organized in a record. In the physician's office, there are a limited number of individuals recording data in the record. The receptionist, a nurse, a medical assistant, and a doctor might contribute to collecting and recording of data. The categories of data are the same (demographic, socioeconomic, financial, and clinical) when a patient is receiving care in a facility, such as a hospital; however, the volume of data collected in a hospital is much greater. While the patient is in the hospital, an entire team of clinical personnel is collecting and recording data about everything that happens to the patient. Even a patient with multiple complications who visits a physician's office has a fairly brief record until he or she has visited many times. In a hospital, however, sometimes even the smallest procedures generate enormous volumes of data. Paper forms and computer hardware are the primary **data collection devices** for health data.

### Forms

In a paper-based record, most of the data are collected in a standard format that is devised by the individual facility. With some exceptions, notably the forms for newborns and women delivering babies, the forms in one hospital do not look exactly the same as those in another hospital. The purposes of the form are numerous, as follows:
* A form reminds the user of which data have to be collected.
* A form provides a structure for capturing that data so that the reader knows where to look for the desired data.
* The form ensures that complete data are collected according to the clinical guidelines of the facility and profession and according to regulation.

Paper forms are designed to meet documentation standards specific to the clinical discipline, the facility, facility guidelines, and regulatory considerations. They are frequently created by committees of the people who use them. Forms related to *medication administration*, for example, would be created by the nursing department in collaboration with the pharmacy and probably with physician input. Some facilities have an oversight committee, simply called the forms committee or documentation committee. This committee may be charged with ensuring that forms are created only when necessary, that duplicate forms are not created, and that the forms conform to hospital guidelines. The most important consideration in the development of a form is the needs of the users of the form. Those needs include: regulatory compliance, clear communication, ease of data entry, and ease of data retrieval.

Even facilities that collect the clinical data on paper tend to have computerized patient registration data. The key demographic data, financial data, and some of the socioeconomic data that are collected during the patient registration process can usually be printed out on one paper form, called the *admission record* or *face sheet*, although several computer screens may be necessary to capture these data.

### Content

Many considerations go into the development of a health data form. Consider the development of a *physician's order form* in the following example.

**data collection devices** Paper forms designed to capture data elements in a standardized format, or the physical computer hardware that facilitates the data collection process.

**medication administration** Clinical data including the name of the medication, dosage, date and time of administration, method of administration, and the nurse who administered it.

**face sheet** The first page in a paper record. Usually contains at least the demographic data and contains space for the physician to record and authenticate the discharge diagnoses and procedures. In many facilities, the admission record is also used as the face sheet.

**physician's order** The physician's directions regarding the patient's care. Also refers to the data collection device on which these elements are captured.

If a physician wants to administer penicillin to a patient, the nurse and the pharmacy need to know the following information:

- To which patient the medication is being dispensed
- The exact medication
- The exact dosage
- The specific route of administration (e.g., oral or intravenous [via a needle into the bloodstream])
- The ordered frequency of administration
- When the order was given
- Who gave the order

The needs of the users of the form is the most important consideration in its creation. In a hospital, the physician directs the care of the patient. The form for a physician's order has the very important function of communicating the patient's care to all members of the health care team. All lab tests, for example, must start with the physician's order. The form must satisfy every user's needs, not just the physician's. The form must be flexible enough to record the hundreds of different medications, therapies, and instructions that a physician might give and to communicate accurately the instructions needed by the recipient of the order, such as the radiology department. On a paper form, these data are recorded by the physician, who writes the orders in his or her own handwriting.

Generally, the patient's name and other identifying data are recorded in the top right-hand corner of every page of every form. Patient identification data must be on every page so that the data can be matched to the correct patient. The patient data usually go in the right-hand corner of the page because most records, particularly when the patient is still in the hospital, are kept in three-ring binders. Having the patient's name and MR# in the top right-hand corner makes the record easy to check and prevents misfiling. In fact, the patient's name and MR# should be on every page in order to ensure that only that patient's data are included in the record.

In addition to identifying the patient on the form, some information identifying the particular form is needed. Typically included are the name of the facility, the title of the form, and any special instructions about the form. The top left-hand corner of the page is a convenient place to put the name of the hospital and possibly its location (which is useful if the hospital has many facilities), along with the title of the form.

## Format

How many physician's orders can be put on one page of a paper record? Should there be separate blocks for each order or should the form be designed to have a lot of lines on which the physician may write as much as he or she desires for each order? This is a matter of facility preference. Forms with the orders in blocks, with each block containing only one set of orders, and forms that consist of a page of blank lines on which the physician may write free-form are both common. Some facilities may create separate forms for every type of order. Thus orders pertaining to newborns would be on one type of form; order forms for surgical patients would be different; orders for the general patient population would be on a third form.

A major consideration in constructing a form is the size of the fields that will be included. In the previous discussion about data dictionaries, the size of a field was illustrated. On a paper form, the size of the field in characters must be accommodated, as well as the space needed to hand-write the data.

The size of the printing on the page is a consideration. How close to the edge of the page can the form be printed? Will holes be punched in the form? If so, where will they be and how much space should be allowed? Figure 2-12 shows a forms design template. Table 2-2 summarizes forms design issues.

## Compliance

Compliance with licensure and accreditation standards is another consideration. Whether forms are maintained on paper or in an electronic medium, documentation standards for the record remain the same. If, for example, The Joint Commission (TJC) requires that physician's orders must be signed, then the form should facilitate that process. One problem

**radiology** Literally, the study of x-rays. In a health care facility, the department responsible for maintaining x-ray and other types of diagnostic and therapeutic equipment as well as analyzing diagnostic films.

**medical record number (MR#)** A unique number assigned to each patient in a health care system; this code will be used for the rest of the patient's encounters with that specific health system.

**field** A collection or series of related characters. A field may contain a word, a group of words, a number, or a code, for example.

**data dictionary** A list of details that describe each field in a database.

**compliance** Meeting standards. Also the development, implementation, and enforcement of policies and procedures that ensure that standards are met.

**licensure** The mandatory government approval required for performing specified activities. In health care, the state approval required for providing health care services.

**accreditation** Voluntary compliance with a set of standards developed by an independent agent, who periodically performs audits to ensure compliance.

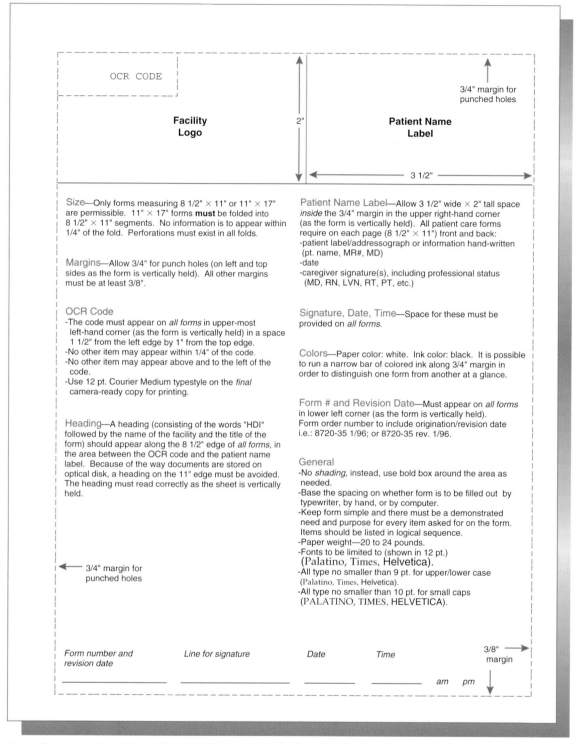

OCR CODE

Facility
Logo

2"

Patient Name
Label

3/4" margin for
punched holes

3 1/2"

Size—Only forms measuring 8 1/2" × 11" or 11" × 17" are permissible. 11" × 17" forms **must** be folded into 8 1/2" × 11" segments. No information is to appear within 1/4" of the fold. Perforations must exist in all folds.

Margins—Allow 3/4" for punch holes (on left and top sides as the form is vertically held). All other margins must be at least 3/8".

OCR Code
-The code must appear on *all forms* in upper-most left-hand corner (as the form is vertically held) in a space 1 1/2" from the left edge by 1" from the top edge.
-No other item may appear within 1/4" of the code.
-No other item may appear above and to the left of the code.
-Use 12 pt. Courier Medium typestyle on the *final* camera-ready copy for printing.

Heading—A heading (consisting of the words "HDI" followed by the name of the facility and the title of the form) should appear along the 8 1/2" edge of *all forms*, in the area between the OCR code and the patient name label. Because of the way documents are stored on optical disk, a heading on the 11" edge must be avoided. The heading must read correctly as the sheet is vertically held.

← 3/4" margin for punched holes

Patient Name Label—Allow 3 1/2" wide × 2" tall space *inside* the 3/4" margin in the upper right-hand corner (as the form is vertically held). All patient care forms require on each page (8 1/2" × 11") front and back:
-patient label/addressograph or information hand-written (pt. name, MR#, MD)
-date
-caregiver signature(s), including professional status (MD, RN, LVN, RT, PT, etc.)

Signature, Date, Time—Space for these must be provided on *all forms*.

Colors—Paper color: white. Ink color: black. It is possible to run a narrow bar of colored ink along 3/4" margin in order to distinguish one form from another at a glance.

Form # and Revision Date—Must appear on *all forms* in lower left corner (as the form is vertically held). Form order number to include origination/revision date i.e.: 8720-35 1/96; or 8720-35 rev. 1/96.

General
-No *shading*, instead, use bold box around the area as needed.
-Base the spacing on whether form is to be filled out by typewriter, by hand, or by computer.
-Keep form simple and there must be a demonstrated need and purpose for every item asked for on the form. Items should be listed in logical sequence.
-Paper weight—20 to 24 pounds.
-Fonts to be limited to (shown in 12 pt.) (Palatino, Times, Helvetica).
-All type no smaller than 9 pt. for upper/lower case (Palatino, Times, Helvetica).
-All type no smaller than 10 pt. for small caps (PALATINO, TIMES, HELVETICA).

Form number and revision date

Line for signature

Date

Time

am    pm

3/8" →
margin

Figure 2-12 Forms design template. (From Abdelhak M, Grostick S, Hanken MA, Jacobs E: Health information: management of a strategic resource, ed 4, Philadelphia, 2012, Saunders, p 122.)

**authenticate** To assume responsibility for data collection or the activities described by the data collection by signature, mark, code, password, or other means of identification.

with paper records is that clinicians may write an order but forget to sign it, meaning that the order is not *authenticated*. The "signature" is in ink on the paper form, but on the electronic form it will be a notation generated by the physician's acceptance of the order (Figure 2-13).

Two concepts are necessary to understand "signed." The first concept is authorship: the author of an order is the person who wrote it. The second concept is **authentication**: the

## TABLE 2-2

### DATA COLLECTION DEVICE DESIGN ISSUES

| ISSUE | CONSIDERATIONS |
| --- | --- |
| Identification of user needs | Not limited to the collectors of the data; it is also necessary to consider subsequent users of both the device and the data it contains |
| Purpose of the data collection device | Necessary to ensure both data collection and controls for quality |
| Selection of the appropriate data items and sequencing of data collection activities | Should fulfill the purpose of the device, without unnecessary fields; it is important to consider the order in which data is collected |
| Understanding the technology used | Not just paper versus computer (e.g., How is the paper used? How is the computer used? What input devices are available and how will they be used?) |
| Use of standard terminology and abbreviations as well as development of a standard format | Communication among users is improved by consistency in language and format |
| Appropriate instructions | Consistency improved by instructions on the form |
| Simplicity | The simpler the device, the easier it is to use |

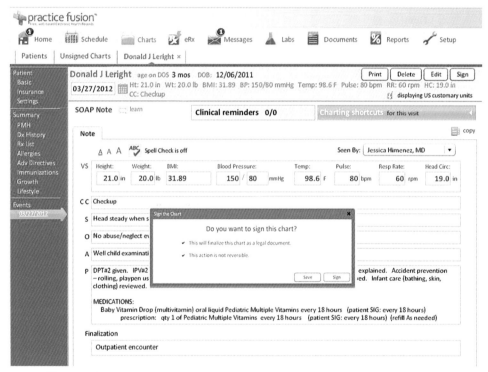

**Figure 2-13** Authentication in an electronic record. (Courtesy Practice Fusion, Inc.)

author's mark or signature. The distinction between author and authentication is important for compliance with rules regarding signing of clinical and other documentation. For example, a first-year resident may be the author of an order or progress note; however, that order or note probably must be countersigned by a supervising, licensed physician. The potential need (and space) for this second authentication must be taken into consideration in the design of forms. Another example of an authentication without authorship is the discharge instruction form. **Discharge** instructions are often prepared by nursing staff, then completed and authenticated by the discharging physician.

On a paper record, that mark or signature takes the form of the author's formal signature or his or her initials. Consequently, in the design of the form, places are provided for the author's authentication and a note of the date and time of the orders. This detail is

**countersigned** Evidence of supervision of subordinate personnel, such as physician residents.

**discharge** The occurrence of a patient leaving the care of the facility to go home, for transfer to another health care facility, or by death. Also refers to the status of a patient.

***Community Hospital***
***City, State***

***Frank Bright***
***ID #354792***

***DOCTOR'S ORDERS***

| | | | |
|---|---|---|---|
| *Date* | | *Date* | |
| *Time* | *Signature* ______ | *Time* | |
| *Date* | | *Date* | |
| *Time* | *Signature* ______ | *Time* | |
| *Date* | | *Date* | |
| *Time* | *Signature* ______ | *Time* | |
| *Date* | | *Date* | |
| *Time* | *Signature* ______ | *Time* | |

**Figure 2-14** Sample of a completed physician's order form.

important from a clinical perspective because the time between the writing of the order and the execution of the order is a compliance issue.

Next, the designers must consider what other information will be necessary on the form. The physician's orders are written to communicate instructions to other health care providers. In a paper record, the physician's orders are maintained in the nursing unit near the patient. The orders are not directly accessible to the radiology department, laboratory department, pharmacy, and so on. Someone has to communicate the orders to the correct party. Members of the nursing staff are usually charged with that responsibility. Therefore the form must contain an area for these staff members to indicate that they have read and executed the order. In the case of medication, the drug must be ordered from the pharmacy and then be administered to the patient. Figure 2-14 shows a completed physician's order on a form that leaves a separate blank for each order.

### Other Considerations

Creation of a form involves many other considerations. So far, the focus has been on the data that must be recorded on the form. In a paper record, a number of other issues must be considered:

- How heavy should the paper be? Should it be heavy cardstock or copy machine weight?
- Should the form be one part, two parts, or more?
- If it is a multipart form, should each part be a different color?
- On what color paper should the form be printed? White is best for photocopying, but would another color help the users of the form?

These are considerations that the forms committee reviews to ensure that the form conforms to the institution's guidelines. Designing forms was once a difficult and time-consuming process because they had to be developed with a pencil and paper, given to a printer, created, and then returned to the organization for editing—frequently multiple times. Today, it is possible to create forms using word-processing software and reproduce them on a photocopy machine. Nevertheless, the great volume of forms required and the unique characteristics of some of the forms often require the assistance of professional printers to this day.

## Forms Control

In a paper-based system, forms are used selectively depending on the type of patient record and the department using them. Someone in the hospital, frequently the director of the health information management (HIM) department, must keep track of all approved forms to ensure that documentation standards are met. In reality, forms get passed around, photocopied, and shuffled from department to department. If a form is not used frequently, it often becomes lost. When the form is needed but not readily available, the users may create a new form even though the old form still exists. Therefore a **master forms file** should be created and maintained by the director of the HIM department. The master forms file contains every form used by the hospital and can be organized in any way that the hospital finds useful.

One very efficient way to save a master forms file is to keep forms in categories corresponding to the departments that use them and then alphabetically by department name. Another way to maintain a master forms file is to give each form a numerical assignment and then save the forms in numerical order. In either case, the creation of an index and table of contents for the master forms file is necessary. The index is at the front of the file, and the title of each form and its individual number are listed in the table of contents. The responsibility for ensuring that forms are not duplicated and that each form conforms to the institution's needs usually lies with the forms committee, as previously mentioned.

The forms committee is an institution-wide committee that has the responsibility of reviewing and approving all forms. Therefore representatives of all the major clinical services must be included. The committee should include a representative from nursing, physician staff (probably several representatives if the facility offers numerous services), laboratory, and radiology. Because HIM personnel are frequently in charge of the master forms file, a representative from the HIM department should be included in the forms committee.

In a computer-based environment, the forms are created and displayed on computer screens. The development of or addition to a computer system should be under the direction of a systems development team. However, only the clinicians and other health practitioners are truly aware of the data that must be collected and how the data should be organized. The data dictionary then becomes critical in the development process. The data fields that are collected, the staff members who have access to them, and whether those with access can print, change, or view the data become increasingly important considerations. Existing institutional committees become involved in this development according to institution policies. In any event, HIM personnel should be directly involved in this process.

## Paper

Data are collected in an organized fashion. In a paper-based environment, the data collection device is a form. Forms are specific to their purpose, as discussed previously. As the forms are collected into the record, they must be put into some kind of order so that users will be able to locate and retrieve the data. Paper records are sorted in one or a combination of three ways: by date, source, or diagnosis.

### Integrated Record

Pages in the record can be organized by order of date. In a completely **integrated record**, the data themselves are also collected by date order (i.e., chronologically), regardless of the source of the data. The first piece of data is recorded with its date, and each subsequent piece of data is organized sequentially after the preceding piece of data. This method of maintaining data is particularly useful when we need to know when events happen in relation to one another. For practical purposes, different types of data are recorded on separate forms, but those forms are also placed in date order. Figure 2-15 illustrates the chronological organization of data.

This method of recording data in date order can also be called *date-oriented* or *sequential*. The organization of the data in date order is a fairly useful and efficient way to collect

**master forms file** A file containing blank copies of all current paper forms used in a facility.

**HIM** health information management

**Go To** Chapter 13 to explore the process of developing or upgrading health care information systems, called the Systems Development Life Cycle, or SDLC.

**data dictionary** A list of details that describe each field in a database.

**integrated record** A paper record in which the pages are organized sequentially, in the chronological order in which they were generated; also known as *date-oriented record* or *sequential record*.

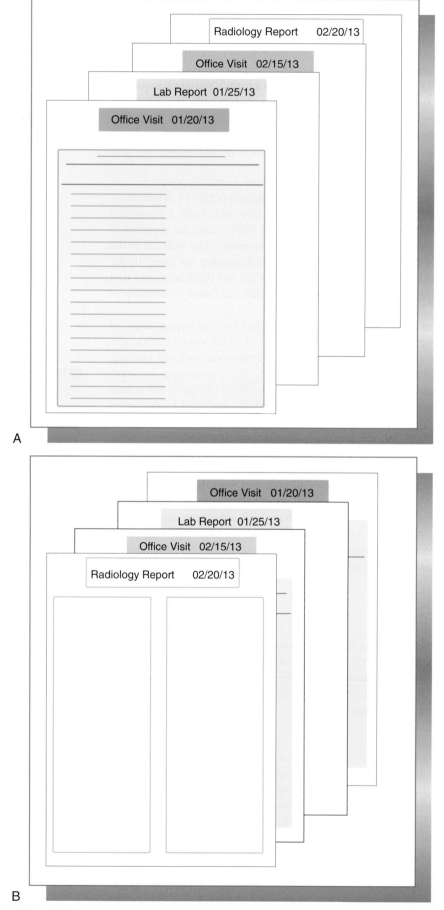

**Figure 2-15 A,** Integrated record. **B,** Integrated record in reverse chronological order.

data sequentially during each episode of care and from one episode to the next. In a paper record, it is easier to place the most recent pages on top; an integrated paper record organized in reverse chronological order is still considered an integrated record.

Because of the ease of filing and the chronological picture such records provide, many physicians and other ambulatory care providers use an integrated record.

### Source-Oriented Record

In addition to being organized by date, data may be organized by source. In other words, all of the data obtained from the physician can be grouped together, all of the data obtained from the nurse can be grouped together, and all of the laboratory data can be grouped together. This method of organizing data produces a **source-oriented record**.

Organizing data by source is useful when there are many items of data coming from different sources. For example, a patient who is in the hospital for several days may require numerous laboratory and blood tests, and many pages of physician and nursing notes are compiled. If all of these pieces of data are organized in date order, as an integrated record, one would have to know the exact date on which something occurred in order to find the desired data. Further, it would be very difficult to compare laboratory results from one date to the next. Consequently, in records that have numerous items from each type of source, the records tend to be organized in a source-oriented manner. Figure 2-16 illustrates a source-oriented record. Notice that within each source, the data are organized in chronological order so that specific items are more easily located and the record shows the patient's progress chronologically.

### Problem-Oriented Record

The data can also be organized by the patient's diagnosis, or problem. For instance, all of the data on a patient's appendicitis and appendectomy can be organized together. Similarly, all of the data that pertain to the patient's congestive heart failure can be organized together. Such a method greatly facilitates the monitoring of individual patient conditions. This method of organizing data produces a **problem-oriented record** and is useful when the

**ambulatory care facility** An outpatient facility, such as an emergency department or physician's office, in which treatment is intended to occur within 1 calendar day.

**source-oriented record** A paper record in which the pages are organized by discipline, department, and/or type of form.

**problem-oriented record** A paper record with pages organized by diagnosis.

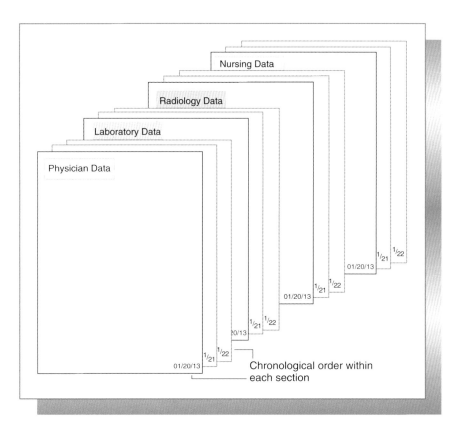

**Figure 2-16** Source-oriented record.

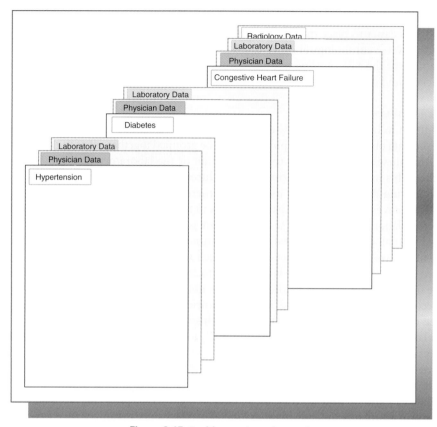

Figure 2-17  Problem-oriented record.

patient has several major chronic conditions that may be addressed at different times. For example, if a patient has congestive heart failure, diabetes, and hypertension, the patient might not be treated for all three simultaneously. Therefore the records for each of the conditions may be kept separately. Problems that have been resolved are easily flagged, and current problems are more easily referenced. Figure 2-17 illustrates a simple problem-oriented record. The problem-oriented record format is most often used by physician offices or clinics.

### Problem List

After several visits to an ambulatory care facility, a list of the patient's problems (diagnoses or complaints) is compiled. This **problem list** facilitates management of the patient's care and improves communication among caregivers. In a problem-oriented record, this list becomes an index to the record as well as a historical summary of patient care management. Therefore the problem list is an integral part of a problem-oriented record. However, a problem list is required regardless of the organization of the record. A simple problem list is shown in Figure 2-18. Maintaining a problem list is a requirement for TJC accreditation.

## Electronic Health Record

Computerization will continue to have an impact on HIM. The terminology of computerization is often confusing. The terms *electronic, computerized, computer-assisted*, and *computer-based* are sometimes used interchangeably. At the time of this writing, the generally accepted term for a computerized patient record EHR.

In an EHR, data are collected in fields and records that are linked together in such a manner that the data can be referenced, displayed, or reported in any of the ways previously mentioned. For instance, if a physician were reviewing the lab results in the EHR, the results

**problem list** A chronological summary of the patient's conditions and treatments.

**TJC** The Joint Commission

| Problem List | | | | | |
| --- | --- | --- | --- | --- | --- |
| Date | Problem # | Description | Date of Initial Diagnosis | Current Treatment | Comments |
| 01/20/12 | 1 | Hypertension | 11/27/09 | Diet | Follow-up 01/13 |
| 02/15/12 | 2 | Sprain/right ankle | 02/15/12 | Wrap and rest Tylenol 1000 mg as needed | |
| 03/15/12 | 2 | Sprain/right ankle | 02/15/12 | None | Resolved |
| | | | | | |
| | | | | | |
| | | | | | |

Figure 2-18  Problem list.

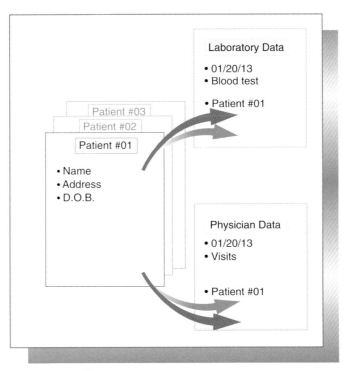

Figure 2-19  Electronic patient record.

could be displayed chronologically and by lab result, as in a source-oriented record. A user who wishes to print the entire record might have the option of printing all data in chronological order, by date recorded: the integrated format. This versatility is one of the major advantages of an EHR. The data are linked by reference numbers (e.g., medical record or billing number) so that all data about the patient are accessible. A complete discussion of a relational database is beyond the scope of this text, but Figure 2-19 shows one way in which computer records might be designed to link patient data together.

Another benefit of an EHR is the ability to capture authentications electronically: electronic signatures. An **electronic signature** may capture the practitioner's actual signature into the computer, similar to the electronic signing for a credit card charge. In other cases, it is the computer recognition of a unique code that only the author has in his or her possession. The computer can be programmed to reject orders that do not contain an appropriate authentication. The program would look for both the existence of the authentication (for data completeness) and the correct authentication (for data validity).

**EHR** electronic health record

**authenticate** To assume responsibility for data collection or the activities described by the data collection by signature, mark, code, password, or other means of identification.

**electronic signature** When the authenticator uses a password or PIN to electronically sign a document.

## Advantages and Disadvantages

Each of these methods of organizing patient records has its own advantages and disadvantages. The integrated record is simple to file, but subsequent retrieval and comparison of data are more difficult. The source-oriented record is more complicated to file, but this method facilitates the retrieval and comparison of source data. The problem-oriented record lends itself best to the long-term management of chronic illnesses; however, filing is complicated, and duplication of data may be necessary so that laboratory reports related to different problems are included in all relevant sections. All of these methods are essentially paper-based record organization systems. A well-designed computer-based system can solve filing and retrieval inefficiencies; however, until recently, cost and resistance to technology have slowed the universal implementation of electronic record systems.

It should be noted that the method of organizing a record is not patient specific. In other words, all patients' records are recorded in the same way. The method of organization is determined by its overall suitability to the particular environment and the needs that it satisfies.

## EXERCISE 2-5

### Organization of Data Elements in a Health Record

1. Think about a disease with which you are familiar, and create a list of all the data elements that you think a physician and allied health personnel in a physician's office would generate for this disease. You can make up the data, but make the list as complete as you can. This exercise will give you an idea of how complex health information is, even at the physician's office level.
2. The study of disease trends and occurrences is called _____.
3. Match the chart description on the left with the record order on the right:

    1. All of the information about the patient's congestive heart failure is together, the hypertension information is all together, and the appendicitis information is all together.

        A. Integrated

    2. Data are collected and recorded by different health care workers and linked to other data about the patient by common data elements.

        B. Source-oriented

    3. In the record, all of the physician's notes are together, the orders are together, the nursing notes are together, the medication sheets are together, and the laboratory reports are together.

        C. Problem-oriented

    4. The record is organized in chronological order only.

        D. Electronic health record

## DATA QUALITY

The expression "garbage in, garbage out" is appropriate in a discussion about data quality. In other words, if the data entered into the computer are wrong, then the data extracted from the computer will be wrong. Technicians responsible for entering data must exercise extreme care to ensure that the data are correct. The same rule applies to data collected on paper. If the data on the paper record are incorrectly recorded, then users will be presented with incorrect data upon review. High-quality data collection starts with an understanding of the data needs of the user. Data collection devices must be designed to capture the appropriate information with an emphasis on the quality of the data.

**data collection devices** Paper forms designed to capture data elements in a standardized format, or the physical computer hardware that facilitates the data collection process.

### Electronic Data Collection

Paper-based forms are the traditional way to record health data, and the skills for creating paper-based forms can be transferred to the creation of computer-based forms. Even entering data into a computer is still recording it on a form—the computer screen. It simply looks different. In the creation of a computer-based form, there must be a name for the form, which should be input at the top of the computer screen. The patient's name and

**health data** Elements related to a patient's diagnosis and procedures as well as factors that may affect the patient's condition.

MR# are carried forward onto every screen after the data have been entered. Computerized data capture facilitates the improvement of data quality. In a computer-based record, it is not necessary to "allow room" for variable handwriting; exactly enough room is allowed for the particular data field because the size of the field is defined in the data dictionary. The computer software may also be programmed to check the data for errors at the point of data entry. In other respects, many of the data collection considerations for a paper-based record are applicable to the development of a computer-based data record.

One consideration that is more important in computer data entry than in paper-record data collection is the sequence of data capture. Data can be recorded on a paper-based form in any order. Although the paper-based form may be designed to capture data in a logical sequence, as identified by the designers, recording items at the bottom of the form before recording items at the top does not pose a disadvantage if the data collector chooses to do it this way. With a computer-based data collection device, however, data collection may continue over several screens, or virtual pages. Flipping back and forth among the pages is confusing and time-consuming and may lead to errors and omissions. For example, a registrar collects patient demographic and financial data. The demographic data may be collected on one screen and the financial data on a subsequent screen. If the patient has multiple insurance plans, the financial data may flow into several screens. In designing the screens, one would take care to ensure that the logical sequence of data collection progresses through the screens and that each screen is completed before the data collector moves to the next. Although the computer may be programmed to check for incomplete data fields, this feature wastes time if the omission was caused by inefficient data capture.

In the context of a computer program, forms actually improve the data collection. As previously discussed, on a paper-based form the patient's name and MR# go in the top right-hand corner, which is added manually: Someone has to write it in, stamp it in, or affix a label in the corner. In an EHR, the patient's name is entered once, at the point of registration, and associated with the medical record number. Subsequent users who are recording data in that patient's record may select the patient from a directory of existing patients. Thus the patient name and medical record number are entered once and used many times.

Another example of improvement in data collection that results from EHR implementation is the **computerized physician order entry** (CPOE). For example, instead of the physician's actually typing or writing out the name of the drug, the dosage, and the route of administration, this information may be selected from drop-down menus. This method is particularly convenient because the only elements included in the menu are items that are definitely on the facility's approved drug list. In this particular instance, the use of a menu-driven computer-based data collection system significantly reduces the error that might occur if a physician ordered a nonapproved drug. Such a mistake might very well happen if the physician has privileges at a variety of different hospitals because approved drug lists in various hospitals are not necessarily identical. Moreover, the order entry can be linked to the pharmacy, which might generate the medication request without nursing intermediation. In addition, the order entry system can be linked to health data that have already been collected about the patient, such as sex, height, weight, age, and diagnosis. Then, if a physician ordered a drug at a dosage that exceeds the maximal amount that is considered safe for a newborn, for instance, a computer system could automatically generate a warning statement that the drug dosage was inappropriate, thereby alerting the physician of his or her error before any harm was done.

## Quality Elements

Spelling a patient's name correctly seems like an obvious goal for those collecting data. Recording accurate birth date, address, and vital signs (blood pressure, temperature, pulse) are also reasonable goals. Not quite as obvious is the need to record such data in a timely manner. Errors or delays in recording patient data can affect patient care and lead to poor health care delivery. Therefore the quality of data collection and recording has very specific elements that support efficient and effective patient care and organizational

**medical record number (MR#)** A unique number assigned to each patient in a health care system; this code will be used for the rest of the patient's encounters with that specific health system.

**EHR** electronic health record

**computerized physician order entry (CPOE)** A health information system in which physicians enter orders electronically. Includes decision support and alerts.

**Go To** Chapter 3 discusses electronic health records in more detail.

**American Health Information Management Association (AHIMA)** A professional organization supporting the health care industry by promoting high-quality information standards through a variety of activities, including but not limited to accreditation of schools, continuing education, professional development and educational publications, and legislative and regulatory advocacy.

**data accuracy** The quality that data are correct.

**data validity** The quality that data reflect the known or acceptable range of values for the specific data.

**data accessibility** Data can be obtained when needed by authorized individuals.

**data consistency** Data is the same wherever it appears.

administration. AHIMA has recently updated its Data Quality Management Model to reflect the issues in current data quality management. (AHIMA, 2012) The following discussion relates the characteristics of data quality to the topics discussed.

### Data Accuracy

To be useful, the data must be accurate. To understand the importance of **data accuracy**, think about how irritating it is to receive a telephone call from someone who has dialed the wrong number. Sometimes a person writes the wrong number in his or her telephone address book. In this case, the recorded data are inaccurate. Receiving misdirected telephone calls is merely an annoyance, whereas receiving someone else's medication could be fatal. If data are not accurate, wrong information is conveyed to the user of the data. Accuracy includes the concept of validity. **Data validity** ensures its usefulness. The term *validity* pertains to the data's conformity with an expected range of values. For example, "ABCDE" is not a valid U.S. Postal Service Zip Code, because Zip Codes in the United States contain only numbers. Similarly, 278° Fahrenheit is not a valid temperature for living human beings. Paper forms may contain instructions with valid ranges for specific data elements. A computer can be instructed to check specific fields for validity and alert the user to a potential data collection error (Figure 2-20).

### Data Accessibility

**Data accessibility** means that the data must be able to be obtained when needed from wherever it is being retained. From the discussion in this chapter as well as the discussion of electronic records in the previous chapter, it should be obvious that electronic data, if properly captured, is more easily retrieved than paper-based data. The concept of data security is part of accessibility. In other words, the ability to obtain the data must be restricted to authorized individuals.

### Data Consistency

**Data consistency** means that the data is the same, no matter where it appears. For example, the registrar records a patient's name in the hospital registration system as Martha Jackson. That same patient's name should appear as Martha Jackson in the radiology system and the laboratory system. In order to accomplish this efficiently and effectively, the data should flow from the hospital registration system to the laboratory and radiology systems electronically—without human intervention.

### Data Timeliness

During an episode of care, patient demographic, financial, socioeconomic, and clinical data are collected. Although it makes sense that demographic data are collected at the point of registration, if the patient is unconscious that might not be possible. Some financial data are collected at registration; however, in the emergency department, financial data are not

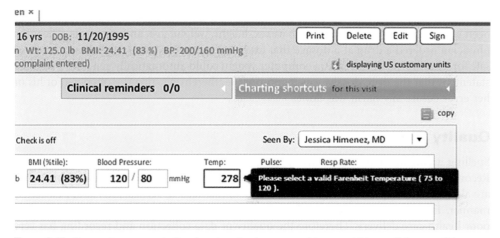

**Figure 2-20** Computer prompt indicating that the data entered is not within a valid range. (Courtesy Practice Fusion, Inc.)

collected until after the patient receives a medical screening. In both of these examples, the timeliness of data collection is relative to the situation in which the data are collected.

Other data collection requires specific guidelines. For example, the recording of a patient's vital signs must be done as soon as possible after collection of the readings because monitoring of vital signs is an important aspect of patient care. Similarly, physician documentation of observations and assessments is most useful when it is recorded concurrently with the activity of observing and assessing. The Joint Commission, Centers for Medicare and Medicaid Services (CMS), and state regulations are specific as to the timeliness required in many types of documentation. Failure to comply with timely documentation requirements is an indicator of lack of quality in the care of patients.

**Centers for Medicare and Medicaid Services (CMS)** The division of the U.S. Department of Health and Human Services that administers Medicare and Medicaid.

### Data Completeness

The data collected in a health record may be accurate and timely. However, if it is not complete, then quality is impaired. AHIMA refers to completeness as comprehensive. (AHIMA, 2012) For example, if a physician's progress note contains the subjective and objective descriptions but is missing the assessment and plan, then it is incomplete. The note may contain all of the SOAP elements, but if it is not signed, dated, and timed, it is incomplete.

**SOAP format** Subjective, Objective, Assessment, and Plan: the medical decision making process used by physicians to assess the patient at various intervals.

One of the many benefits of an electronic health record is that the data collection fields can be programmed to prompt the user to complete all of the fields in a form. So a nurse who records the beginning of an intravenous therapy could be prompted to note the site of the venous puncture and the time that the therapy began. Failure to complete the note with the time the therapy ended would leave the record incomplete. The system might then remind the nurse with each login or attempt to sign out that this element is outstanding.

### Data Definition

Earlier in this chapter, we discussed the need for a data dictionary in order to clearly define all of the fields to be collected in compiling a patient record. The creation of a data dictionary illustrates the concept of data definition. Every field must be clearly defined so that it can be collected consistently and accurately.

Additional data characteristics (currency, granularity, precision, and relevancy) (AHIMA, 2012) are discussed in subsequent chapters.

## ■ EXERCISE 2-6

### Data Quality

1. The nursing department in your facility has submitted a form to the forms committee for approval. The form is printed on dark gold paper so that it will stand out in the chart. You recommend a light yellow paper instead because it photocopies better than dark gold. This is an example of taking which of the following into consideration?
   a. The purpose of the data collection device
   b. The needs of all users of the device
   c. An understanding of the technology used
   d. Simplicity
2. Which of the following most closely describes the purpose of instructions on a data collection device?
   a. It ensures that the correct form is used.
   b. It helps users with complicated data collection.
   c. It helps ensure the consistency of data collection.
   d. It organizes the data in the correct sequence.

## DATA SETS

In addition to a basic understanding of the concept of data—where they come from, what types of things are collected, and why the data are necessary—the health information manager must know how the data will be used. Physicians use the data to improve the quality of their services and help treat individual patients. Health care consumers may use the data to select a physician or a treatment. Insurance companies and government agencies may also require health data to pay patients' bills or track health trends. Many of these

**data** The smallest elements or units of facts or observations. Also refers to a collection of such elements.

**health data** Elements related to a patient's diagnosis and procedures as well as factors that may affect the patient's condition.

| TABLE 2-3 | | |
|---|---|---|
| **COLLECTION AND REPORT OF GENDER DATA** | | |
| | **COLLECTED NUMERICAL** | **REPORTED ALPHA** |
| Female | 1 | F |
| Male | 2 | M |

**CMS** Centers for Medicare and Medicaid Services

**data set** A group of data elements collected for a specific purpose.

**aggregate data** A group of like data elements compiled to provide information about the group.

▌▌▌
**Go To** The analysis of data is explored in Chapter 10.

**field** A collection or series of related characters. A field may contain a word, a group of words, a number, or a code, for example.

**inpatient** An individual who is admitted to a hospital with the intention of staying overnight.

**Uniform Bill (UB-04)** The standardized form used by hospitals for inpatient and outpatient billing to CMS and other third-party payers.

users, particularly CMS, are very particular in their data needs and give health care providers specifications for the data sets that they require.

A **data set** is a defined group of fields that are required for a specified purpose. To efficiently mail a letter through the United States Postal Service, the data set is defined as: addressee, street address, apartment or unit number (if applicable), city, state, and Zip Code. Although the Zip Code could suffice to replace the city and state, the city and state help the post office validate the destination if there is an error in the Zip Code. Online shoppers are familiar with the dual data sets of "billing address" and "shipping address" as well as the "payment" data set, which includes the credit card, name on the card, card number, expiration date, and, recently, the security code.

The collection and reporting of defined data sets enables users to compare activities, volumes, patient care, and some outcomes among the reporting facilities. The detailed data can be aggregated and analyzed to make public health decisions and to study the spread of disease.

## Defined Data Sets

Throughout the course of the patient's care, data are collected by many health care professionals. Without a specific requirement for data collection, facilities might not include data elements that are helpful to users who wish to perform an analysis. For example, the patient's gender is a data element that is always helpful and therefore required. The patient's living arrangements, on the other hand, are not a required field in all settings.

Even for a required field, however, there are no specific rules governing the way in which the data are captured. So, even when the patient's gender is identified and recorded, facilities may choose to capture that data in the way that is most convenient or useful to itself. For example, without a specific rule to follow, the field that captures the patient's gender could read F, 1, or A, for female; and M, 2, or B, for male (Table 2-3).

If each health care facility determined its own method for collecting the patient's gender data and reported it that way, users would have to interpret each facility's method for classifying this information as they attempt to analyze the data. In fact, facilities may collect the data in any format that is useful to the facility. However, it must *convert* that data to the defined format at the time of reporting, depending on the needs of the user. For example, a hospital may decide to store patient admission and discharge dates as Microsoft Excel dates (January 1, 1900 = day "1"; October 3, 2014 = day "41915") in order to facilitate manipulation of downloaded data. But in order to report that data, the hospital must convert those dates into the format required by the user.

**HIT-bit** ··········································································

**GENDER CATEGORIES**

In rare cases, it is necessary to use the classification "unknown" for gender. Some health care applications have an "unknown" category for gender that may be recognized as U, 3, or C.

For billing hospital inpatients, the required format is the HIPAA 837I data set, which is represented on the **Uniform Bill (UB-04)**, a standardized billing form. By defining a specific data set and the method in which the information should be shared with payers on the UB-04 form, the government has mandated a data set for patients. Because of CMS's prevalence as a payer, this information is ultimately collected and reported on all patients in an acute care facility regardless of who is paying and therefore allows for the internal and external comparison of the information.

A data set is a group of elements collected for a specific purpose. A data set requires a standard method for reporting data elements so that they can be compared with similar data collected either in a different time or from a different facility. To compare data, everyone must collect the data in the same manner that can be readily converted into the same format. For example, certain data are collected on all patients regardless of the health care services needed—name, address, phone number, gender, and date of birth. This demographic data set is for the patient's personal identification. It allows the facility to distinguish one patient among other patients, and to distinguish between men and women, mothers and babies, and seniors and pediatric patients. Each facility must ensure that its data collection is designed to comply with regulatory and accreditation requirements as well as the internal needs of the facility. Table 2-3 illustrates data collection of "gender" as a numerical value that is converted to an alphabetical character upon reporting. The decision as to how to store particular data elements may depend on system capacity as well as data quality issues. For example, storing diagnosis data as the ICD-10-CM code rather than as free text saves computer storage space and prevents problems that may result from typing errors.

For most types of health care delivery, a minimum set of data must be collected and reported for each patient. Acute care hospitals, for example, report the **Uniform Hospital Discharge Data Set (UHDDS)**, which includes demographic, clinical, and financial data about individual patient visits. A summary of these elements is shown in Box 2-4. Skilled nursing facilities (SNF) use their **Minimum Data Set (MDS 3.0)** and home health organizations report the **Outcome and Assessment Information Set (OASIS)**. These setting-specific data sets are prescribed by CMS. Other data sets, such as that collected for disease-specific registries, are discussed in subsequent chapters in relation to the appropriate discussion of the health care setting or topic. Table 8-2 shows the data sets required by various types of facilities.

Collection of specific data, as required by the UHDDS for acute care, allows government entities, for example, to analyze patients, the health care provider, and services. Figure 2-21 shows the location of UHDDS data elements on the form locator (FL)

---

**CMS** Centers for Medicare and Medicaid Services

**payer** The individual or organization that is primarily responsible for the reimbursement for a particular health care service. Usually refers to the insurance company or third party.

**acute care facility** A healthcare facility in which patients have an average length of stay less than 30 days, and that has an emergency department, operating suite, and clinical departments to handle a broad range of diagnoses and treatments.

**Go To** Chapter 7 for more information on the Uniform Bill, UB-04.

**ICD-10-CM** International Classification of Diseases, Tenth Revision, Clinical Modification. A code set used for diagnosis of disease.

**Uniform Hospital Discharge Data Set (UHDDS)** The mandated data set for hospital inpatients.

**skilled nursing facility (SNF)** A long-term care facility providing a range of nursing and other health care services to patients who require continuous care, typically those with a chronic illness.

**home health** Health care services rendered in the patient's home; or an agency that provides such services.

**Minimum Data Set (MDS 3.0)** The detailed data collected about patients receiving long-term care.

**home health care** Health care services rendered in the patient's home; or, an agency that provides such services.

**Outcome and Assessment Information Set (OASIS)** Data set most associated with home health care. This data set monitors patient care by identifying markers over the course of patient care.

---

| BOX 2-4 | UNIFORM HOSPITAL DISCHARGE DATA SET (UHDDS) SUMMARY OF DATA ELEMENTS |
|---|---|

- Personal/unique identifier
- Date of birth
- Gender
- Race and ethnicity
- Residence
- Health care facility identification number
- Admission date
- Type of admission
- Discharge date
- Attending physician's identification number
- Surgeon's identification number
- Principal diagnosis
- Other diagnoses
- Qualifier for other diagnoses
- External cause of injury
- Birth weight of neonate
- Significant procedures and dates of procedures
- Disposition of the patient at discharge
- Expected source of payment
- Total charges

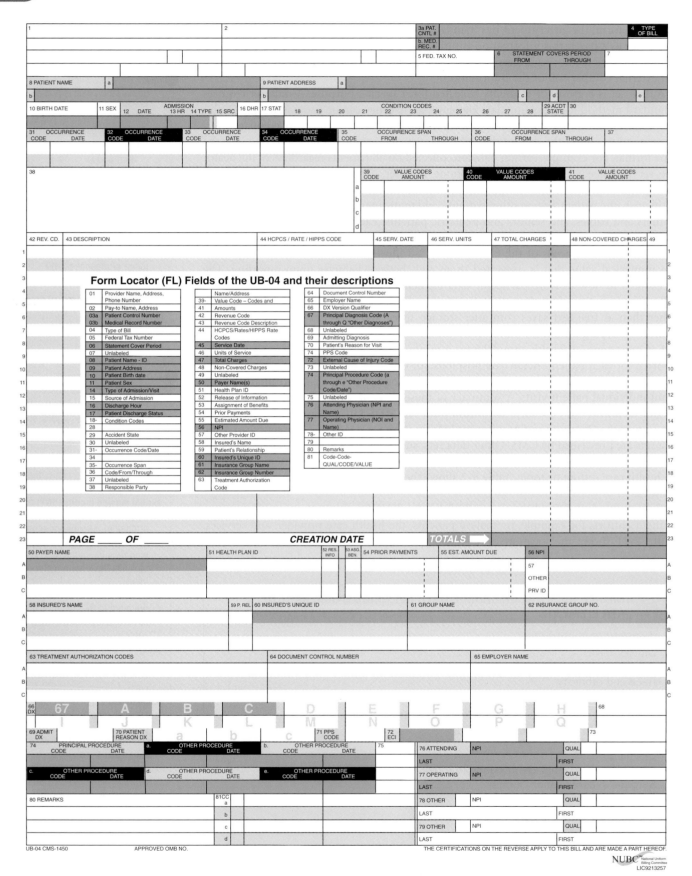

**Figure 2-21** UHDDS data elements on the UB-04. In this illustration, the fields highlighted in green represent data items required by the UHDDS which are also found here on the Universal Bill.

fields of the UB-04. The analysis is possible because each data element is being reported the same way for every inpatient receiving acute care in the United States. Health care entities provide UHDDS data to states through a defined reporting system. Within a specified time frame after discharge, the hospital must report all of the elements to the state Department of Health or other designated agency.

The specific manner in which billing is reported allows CMS, for example, to compare health care services received by Medicare patients regardless of where they receive those services. The definition provided for each data element specifies what should be captured for that data element (e.g., the principal diagnosis is defined by the UHDDS as the "condition established after study to be chiefly responsible for this admission") (CDC, ICD-9-CM Official Coding Guidelines).

Another source of defined data sets is the Health Insurance Portability and Accountability Act (HIPAA), federal legislation that specifies which code sets are to be used in transmitting clinical diagnoses and in what format. Because data are reported uniformly, the databases compiled through the collection of coded data can be extremely useful to users for research and other purposes. For example, a hospital considering the development of a breast cancer program may want to know how many cases of breast cancer were reported in its state. CMS uses this data not only for reimbursement but also to benchmark hospital activities.

**CMS** Centers for Medicare and Medicaid Services

**Health Insurance Portability and Accountability Act (HIPAA)** Public Law 104-191, a federal legislation passed in 1996 that outlines the guidelines of managing patient information in terms of privacy, security, and confidentiality. The legislation also outlines penalties for noncompliance.

**reimbursement** The amount of money that the health care facility receives from the party responsible for paying the bill; health care services are paid after services have been rendered.

**benchmarking** Comparing one facility's process with that of another facility that has been noted to have superior performance.

## WORKS CITED

American Health Information Management Association: Data Quality Management Model (Updated). Journal of AHIMA. 83:7:62-67, 2012.

Centers for Disease Control and Prevention, National Center for Health Statistics: ICD-9-CM Official Coding Guidelines. Section II. Selection of Principal Diagnosis. http://www.cdc.gov/nchs/data/icd9/icd9cm_guidelines_2011.pdf. Published 2011. Accessed August 19, 2012.

## SUGGESTED READING

Quinn J: An HL7 (Health Level Seven) overview, J AHIMA 70:32–34, 1999.

## CHAPTER ACTIVITIES

## CHAPTER SUMMARY

Data are collected about patients' health, then that data are organized to provide information. The key data categories are: demographic, socioeconomic, financial, and clinical. Data are collected during an encounter with a clinician that facilitates medical decision making; subjective, objective, assessment, and plan data are recorded in an organized manner. Outcomes are an increasingly important factor in reviewing the quality of health care. Health information management professionals are concerned with the collection, storage, retrieval, and documentation of health information.

Within the health record, data are organized into databases that are built from characters, fields, records, and files. The records and files are linked through the MPI index in an electronic health record. In a paper-based health record, data are collected on forms. The forms and other documents are gathered into the health record in a source-oriented, problem-oriented, or integrated order, depending on the needs of the clinical staff /facility. The general structure of a form is useful in designing electronic data capture screens. Health information technology is one area of the health information management profession.

The quality of data collected is important. Data must be accurate, accessible, consistent, timely, and complete. Many different data sets are collected about patients, including UHDDS and OASIS. Researchers and government entities are examples of users of these data.

## REVIEW QUESTIONS

1. Explain the difference between data and information.
2. Distinguish among fields, records, and files.
3. Compare and contrast the considerations in the development of paper-based versus computer-based data collection devices.
4. What are the characteristics of data quality introduced in this chapter?
5. For each of the elements of the Uniform Hospital Discharge Data Set, describe how you might define the field in a data dictionary.
6. How can uniform data sets be used to compare hospitals?

## ⬤ PROFESSIONAL PROFILE

### Patient Registration Specialist

My name is Michael, and I am a patient registration specialist at a large medical group practice. My primary responsibility is to register patients when they come into the facility to see a physician or a nurse practitioner. Because we keep all of our patient registration information in the computer, I don't have to pull any files to update patient information. We get a lot of walk-ins in addition to patients with appointments, so our office is very busy.

When a patient registers, I have to make sure that I enter the patient's demographic data correctly. I also must record the financial data so that the office can get paid! In addition to recording the data, I call the patient's insurance company to verify coverage. Every day, I call the patients who have appointments the next day to confirm their appointments. Sometimes they have forgotten, and they really appreciate the reminder.

I started out as a receptionist here when I graduated from high school. I liked the environment and the people, so I enrolled in college to study health information technology. I'm about halfway through the program now, and I was promoted to this position last month. I haven't decided what I want to do when I graduate, but there are a lot of opportunities here, working in the health information management department and in patient accounting.

## PATIENT CARE PERSPECTIVE

### Maria

I like using Dr. Lewis's medical group because all of the types of physicians we use on a regular basis are there. Our insurance changed last year, which I completely forgot about by the time I took Emma for her annual visit. Michael always asks to see our insurance card, even though he has known us for many years. So he caught the change right away and we had no problems with the insurance coverage for the visit.

## APPLICATION ⬤

### Creating a Data Dictionary

You are a health information professional working for Dr. Heath in his private practice. Dr. Heath has a large practice with several ancillary services attached. He and his partner see 50 patients a day in the practice, many of whom receive on-site diagnostic procedures. The diagnostic areas that Dr. Heath has are radiology, electrocardiography, and laboratory. He is concerned because a number of patients have complained that in each area of care, the health personnel seem to ask the same questions. The redundancy is annoying. He is considering computerizing his data collection to streamline the data collection process. Before he does, he wants to make sure that he understands the clinical flow of data in the facility. Dr. Heath seeks your advice and assistance in resolving his problem. What do you recommend? How would you go about implementing your recommendation?

## CHAPTER 3

# ELECTRONIC HEALTH RECORDS

Prerna Dua and Kim Theodos

## CHAPTER OUTLINE

## VOCABULARY

algorithm
American Recovery and
  Reinvestment Act
  (ARRA)
audit trail
bar code
Certification Commission
  for Health Information
  Technology (CCHIT)
clinical decision-making
  system (CDS)
clinical pathway
computerized physician
  order entry (CPOE)
data repository
data warehouse

Digital Imaging and
  Communication in
  Medicine (DICOM)
digital signature
document imaging
electronic document
  management system
  (EDMS)
electronic health record
  (EHR)
encryption
e-PHI
evidence-based decision
  support
evidence-based medicine

health information
  exchange (HIE)
Health Information
  Technology for
  Economic and Clinical
  Health Act (HITECH)
Health Level Seven (HL7)
hybrid record
indexing
infrastructure
integrity
interface
interoperability
longitudinal record
meaningful use

Nationwide Health
  Information Network
  (NHIN)
Office of the National
  Coordinator of Health
  Information Technology
  (ONC)
picture archiving and
  communication
  system (PACS)
point-of-care
  documentation
super user
workflow

## CHAPTER OBJECTIVES

*By the end of this chapter, the student should be able to:*
1. Define electronic health record.
2. Compare and contrast an electronic health record with a hybrid electronic health record.
3. Identify the advantages of the electronic health record.
4. Discuss government and private sector intervention in the development of an electronic health record.
5. Explain the history and future of the electronic health record.
6. Discuss meaningful use and its impact on the development of the electronic health record.
7. Identify the challenges and issues associated with implementing the electronic health record.
8. Explain the difference between the interoperable use and the longitudinal use of an electronic health record.
9. Discuss health information management career opportunities with reference to the electronic health record.

Modern health care requires modern technology. For health information professionals, this comes in the form of the **electronic health record (EHR)**. Although traditional paper records still exist in some organizations, significant progress is being made toward transitioning to a completely electronic record. Just as with any other type of major change, health care organizations can be found in many of the various steps and stages of transition. Although some facilities are operating in a fully functional EHR environment, others are in a hybrid phase, in which both paper and electronic mediums are utilized. Historically,

> ⬤ **electronic health record (EHR)** A secure real-time, point-of-care, patient centric information resource for clinicians allowing access to patient information when and where needed and incorporating evidence-based decision support.

**HIM** health information management

**medical record** Also called *record* or *health record*. It contains all of the data collected for an individual patient.

**admission** The act of accepting a patient into care in a health care facility, including any nonambulatory care facility. Admission requires a physician's order.

**encounter** A patient's health care experience; a unit of measure for the volume of ambulatory care services provided.

**treatment** A procedure, medication, or other measure designed to cure or alleviate the symptoms of disease.

**discharge** Discharge occurs when the patient leaves the care of the facility to go home, for transfer to another health care facility or by death. Also refers to the status of a patient.

**hybrid record** A record in which both electronic and paper media are used.

**clinical data** All of the medical data that have been recorded about the patient's stay or visit, including diagnoses and procedures.

**point-of-care documentation** Clinical data recorded at the time the treatment is delivered to the patient.

**report** The result of a query. A list from a database.

**interface** Computer configuration allowing information to pass from one system to another.

**master patient index (MPI)** A system containing a list of patients who have received care at the health care facility and their encounter information, often used to correlate the patient with the file identification.

this move was championed by health information management (HIM) professionals; however, it has become a focus of the federal government, several of its agencies, and many private consumer groups. This chapter is an introduction to the EHR in all its stages. HIM professionals are facing new responsibilities and new challenges, but their opportunities are greatly expanding. In addition to addressing those changes, this chapter discusses future trends for health care in the electronic exchange of information.

## THE EVOLUTION OF THE ELECTRONIC HEALTH RECORD

### The Paper Record

As discussed throughout this book, the medical record has been traditionally maintained in a paper format. Each department within a facility may develop a form to document treatment, tests, and other results pertinent to that department's functions. The paper record is generated at the time of the patient's admission or encounter and moves with the patient as he or she receives treatment throughout the health care facility. The paper record is assembled after discharge, analyzed, and then filed in the HIM department. A need for increased accessibility and a proven increase in quality of care have led to a trend away from paper records and toward the EHR.

One specific scenario highlighting the need for the EHRs occurred during Hurricane Katrina in 2005, when millions of health records were displaced and destroyed, leaving patients without access to their medical records. This made it difficult for the physicians working in disaster medical centers and community hospitals to deliver continued care based on established patient care plans. Responding in part to this disaster, more public and private efforts were initiated, and attention was focused on the development of an EHR system.

### The Hybrid Record

In a **hybrid record,** some departments of the hospital use computer information systems to document patient care, but other departments continue to use paper documentation. Recording of clinical data at the time treatment is delivered to the patient is called **point-of-care documentation.** Some clinical point-of-care documentation may be captured electronically through the system, making data collection into the patient's health record immediate. Physicians and other health care professionals may capture patient information directly into the health record using several different documentation systems, detailed throughout this chapter. The hybrid record represents a midpoint between the traditional paper record and the fully functional EHR, in which all the documentation surrounding patient care is captured and maintained electronically.

There are various degrees of computerization in the hybrid record, ranging from only one department generating electronic reports that make up the patient's health record to many departments generating electronic reports. Facilities may choose to transition to an EHR in stages by converting the various portions of the health record individually, and most facilities do use the hybrid stage as a step toward a completely EHR. This process may result in a hybrid record with some functions producing electronic data and others remaining paper-based.

Managing hybrid records presents unique challenges. Even with a complete electronic point-of-care system, there will still be paper that must be reconciled during downtime or from other organizations, often resulting in scanning or other electronic storage. It can be anticipated that health records will always be in some form of hybrid, and this probability should be acknowledged during development of the system.

As stated in Chapter 2, even facilities that rely on paper documentation for their clinical data tend to use computer systems for patient registration data. One example of a hybrid record can be seen during the **interfacing** (when two independent systems are configured to communicate with each other) between the financial department and the master patient index. The master patient index (MPI) is a major database stored in each facility that houses information about every patient, mostly consisting of demographic information. Although it contains a great deal of information about a patient, it is beneficial for the MPI to be able to gather information from other systems in the hospital as well. The financial system shares information with the MPI, enabling the facility to generate a computerized face sheet or admission record. Utilizing technology in this way is an efficient means of transmitting information between departments and creates an opportunity for further development and interfacing. Because information can be shared, communication between departments is faster, less redundant, and more accurate.

Practitioner documentation, consisting of clinical data, makes up a large portion of a traditional medical record. One form of documentation in the record is the transcribed reports, such as the history and physical (H&P), discharge summary, and operative reports. Traditionally, after these reports were dictated (read or spoken aloud and recorded) and transcribed (typed), the HIM department would print and file them in the patient's chart to be authenticated by the physician. In some hybrid records, these reports are integrated with the computer system and can be signed and stored electronically. In these systems, a **digital signature** can satisfy the authentication of the medical record, the process whereby the caregiver reads the content of the typed report and signs it, affirming that the content is accurate. Although traditionally done via a handwritten signature, this can be done electronically by clicking a button in the record that indicates "sign the record." Doing so adds a statement on the document or note indicating that it has been electronically signed by the user. That statement also includes the date and time that the user signed it. Hospitals may take another approach to digital signatures similar to those in retail establishments, where the user signs the name on an electronic signature pad that captures the handwritten signature and adds the image to the document.

Ancillary departments, such as laboratory, radiology, and pharmacy, may also use information systems to collect data and generate reports. Their data may be held in a separate database or interfaced with the HIM and/or financial systems. Collectively, these ancillary systems make up a great portion of the health record. Having this information available electronically to multiple users is a great advantage for caregivers, resulting in better quality of care.

Physician's orders are customarily handwritten, although the increased use of hybrid records has encouraged physicians to input this information electronically. A **computerized physician order entry (CPOE)** system is an application that allows a physician to enter orders for medications, tests, treatments, or procedures into a system. The traditional method of hand writing prescriptions and orders can be difficult, tedious, or even dangerous, and the electronic entry of physician's instructions for the treatment of the patients reduces potential medical errors. Information portals such as laptops, handheld electronic devices, and mobile computing terminals in the hospitals has made the input of point-of-care information convenient for physicians. The CPOE system provides the physician with a list of medications that can be used for the specific treatment of the patient's diagnosis. It offers a *clinical decision-making system* (including but not limited to generic drug ordering, drug interaction information, and laboratory information) that may be needed before the medication is prescribed. The CPOE system provides alerts to the physician based on the patient's drug list, allergies, interactions, or other potential contraindications. CPOEs are an important part of a fully EHR because they help improve the quality of clinical documentation, allow for more efficient delivery of medications, and reduce excessive and duplicate testing (Dixon, Zafar, 2009).

Maintenance of the complete medical record can be a challenge in hybrid records. Facilities with hybrid records may choose to retain part of the record electronically or to print out a paper copy of the computer-based portions, thus creating a paper record. Some facilities transfer or scan the paper-based portion into a digital format using a **document imaging** system, creating an electronic copy of that information. In document imaging, a scanner converts the paper document into a digital image, which is then stored on a document server, optical disk, or other storage medium. An example is illustrated in Figure 3-1. An **electronic document management system (EDMS)**, such as the one pictured, may be used as a storage and retrieval mechanism and allows for additional documents to be added

**face sheet** The first page in a paper record. Usually contains at least the demographic data and contains space for the physician to record and authenticate the discharge diagnoses and procedures. In many facilities, the admission record is also used as the face sheet.

**history and physical (H&P)** Heath record documentation comprising the patient's history and physical examination.

**discharge summary** The recap of an inpatient stay, usually dictated by the attending physician and transcribed into a formal report.

**authenticate** To assume responsibility for data collection or the activities described by the data collection by signature, mark, code, password, or other means of identification.

**digital signature** An electronic means to identify the authenticity and integrity of the user's identification.

**database** An organized collection of data.

**physician's order** The physician's directions regarding the patient's care. Also refers to the data collection device on which these elements are captured.

**hybrid record** A record in which both electronic and paper media are used.

**computerized physician order entry (CPOE)** A health information system in which physicians enter orders electronically. Includes decision support and alerts.

**point-of-care documentation** Clinical data recorded at the time the treatment is delivered to the patient.

**clinical decision-making system** A computer application that compares two or more items of patient data in order to advise clinicians on the treatment of that specific patient.

**CPOE** computerized physician order entry

**document imaging** Scanning or faxing of printed papers into a computer system. See also computer output to laser disk.

**electronic document management system (EDMS)** Computer software and hardware, typically scanners, that allow health record documents to be stored, retrieved, and shared.

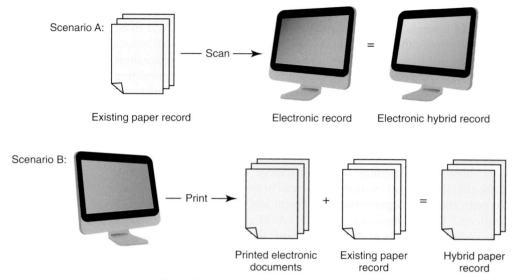

**Figure 3-1** Two kinds of hybrid records.

to an electronic record. For example, an EDMS may be used to scan records transferred from another facility to the EHR. Document imaging can be performed after discharge or at the point of care.

As the documents are scanned into the system, the different types of reports are then indexed. **Indexing** identifies the report by type and organizes them for easier retrieval when needed. It is similar to the plastic tab separators used in the paper records, in that it electronically divides the various sections and indicates in which section the information belongs. **Bar coding** is a type of automated indexing that is sometimes used to decrease errors and improve productivity in the indexing process. Document scanning and indexing are a solution that makes a paper record or paper portions of a record into electronic images. It proves to be useful especially in a hybrid environment or in an EHR, where it is used to add miscellaneous items and documents. It also allows various functions of the HIM department to be performed electronically, such as coding, analysis, and physician chart completion. In this hybrid record, each sheet of paper contained in the record can be viewed from the computer, but this method does not allow for more in-depth retrieval and use of the data contained in the scanned images. The computer simply recognizes the document as an image rather than recognizing the individual data elements contained in the document. Because individual data elements cannot be added or manipulated electronically, the use of document imaging is limited to storage and access.

The challenges associated with managing a hybrid record are substantial. Because portions of the record may be saved as scanned images, locating a specific data element in a document may be difficult. Controlling the various versions of the record is also important to ensure that the most up-to-date version of the record and documentation is stored in all parts of the patient's record. For example, if a patient changes her address and it is updated in the MPI, that change should be reflected in every system, including anything that has been scanned.

The goal is always to have a reliable and accessible patient record, in whichever way that record may be organized or stored. Many facilities have utilized hybrid records as a sensible, affordable solution to make progress toward an EHR.

## HIT-bit ········································································

**PERSONAL HEALTH RECORDS**

According to the American Health Information Management Association (AHIMA), the personal health record (PHR) is an individual's record of his or her own health information, which may be needed in making health decisions. The individual owns and manages the health information and decides who has access to it. It can be paper based, computer-based, Web-based, or some kind of composite thereof. The PHR is maintained separately from any legal record kept by health care providers (AHIMA e-HIM Personal Health Record Work Group, 2005). Beyond storing an individual's personal data, PHRs can interact with EHRs to obtain any relevant information about an ongoing disease in the family.

## EXERCISE 3-1

### Introduction

1. Describe a hybrid medical record.
2. _____uses scanners or fax machines to store records electronically.
3. _____ describes two independent systems configured to communicate with each other. Give an example.
4. An electronic means to identify the authenticity and integrity of the user's identification is a _____.
5. Describe the challenges of managing hybrid medical records.
6. Recording of clinical data at the time treatment is delivered is called _____.
7. The process of sorting a record by the different report types, making the viewing of the record uniform is called _____.
8. A _____ system is an application that allows a physician to enter orders for medications, tests, treatments, or procedures into a system.

## The Electronic Health Record

The Health Information Management Systems Society (HIMSS) Electronic Health Record Committee (2003) defines the EHR as follows:

"The Electronic Health Record (EHR) is a secure, real-time, point-of-care, patient-centric information resource for clinicians. The EHR aids clinicians' decision making by providing access to patient health record information where and when they need it and by incorporating **evidence-based decision support** (the best care results from the conscientious, explicit, and judicious use of current best evidence). The EHR automates and streamlines the clinician's workflow, closing loops in communication and response that result in delays or gaps in care. The EHR also supports the collection of data for uses other than direct clinical care, such as billing, quality management, outcomes reporting, resource planning, and public health disease surveillance and reporting."

To elaborate the preceding definition, a fully functional EHR incorporates the patient history, demographics, and patient problem lists, list of current medications, and patient's allergies, as well as physician clinical notes, which include patients' medical history and follow-up notes. In addition, prescriptions are sent to the pharmacy electronically before being verified for drug interaction, and contraindication warnings are provided. The laboratory and radiology tests are ordered and viewed electronically, with the results being incorporated into the EHR. Further, the out-of-range values for the laboratory tests are highlighted as they are included within the EHR.

An EHR results from computer-based data collection. Physicians and other clinicians capture data at the point of care, with the ability to retrieve the data later for reporting and use in research or administrative decision making. Health care workers document via various input ports on the various clinical units, using laptops, handheld computers, and bedside terminals, into templates. Very few, if any, paper reports are generated. The EHR allows all departments (e.g., nursing) to document care electronically using these templates. The electronic record should provide a CPOE. E-prescribing, which allows the electronic transmission of prescription information from physician's office to the pharmacy—shown in Figure 3-2—is a pronounced feature in EHRs. Other important

**point-of-care documentation** Clinical data recorded at the time the treatment is delivered to the patient.

**evidence-based decision support** Information systems that provide clinical best-knowledge practices to make decisions about patient care.

**workflow** The process of work flowing through a set of procedures to complete the health record.

**outcome** The result of a patient's treatment.

**EHR** electronic health record
**CPOE** computerized physician order entry

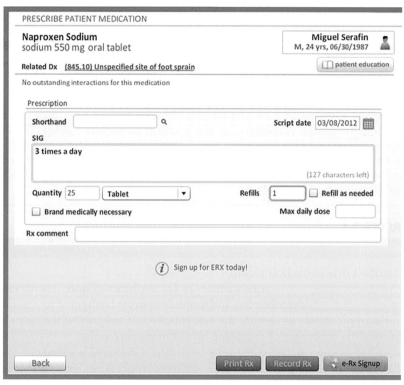

**Figure 3-2** A computerized physician order entry (CPOE) E-prescribing screen. (Courtesy Practice Fusion, Inc.)

features included in the EHRs are to send reminders to patients for patient preference or preventive follow-up care, to print out the diagnosis summary and current medication list, to provide patients with timely electronic access to their health information, and to apply evidence-based medicine. **Evidence-based medicine** (**EBM**) encompasses clinical expertise, patient values, and latest research available for making a decision in a patient's care. It helps the physicians understand that a certain treatment will be suitable for the patient and will do him or her more good than harm.

> **evidence-based medicine (EBM)** Health care delivery that uses clinical research to make decisions in patient care.

## HIT-bit

### EVIDENCE-BASED MEDICINE

Evidence-based medicine (EBM) is the integration of best research evidence with clinical expertise and patient values. It is the conscientious, explicit, and judicious use of current best evidence in making decisions about the care of individual patients and aims to apply the best available evidence gained from the scientific methods to medical decision making. The "best available external clinical evidence" means clinically relevant research, often from the basic sciences of medicine, but especially from patient-centered clinical research, into the accuracy and precision of diagnostic tests (including the clinical examination), the power of prognostic markers, and the efficacy and safety of therapeutic, rehabilitative, and preventive regimens. External clinical evidence both invalidates previously accepted diagnostic tests and treatments and replaces them with new ones that are more powerful, more accurate, more efficacious, and safer. The practice of evidence-based medicine means integrating individual clinical expertise with the best available external clinical evidence from systematic research (Sackett et al 1996).

> **algorithm** A procedure (set of instructions) for accomplishing a task.

The EHR can also provide clinical decision-making algorithms for physician and non-physician caregivers. An **algorithm** is a set of step-by-step instructions for solving a problem. An EHR can provide certain prompts or alerts specific to the physician's orders and provide drug-drug and drug-allergy interaction checks. As shown in Figure 3-3, the

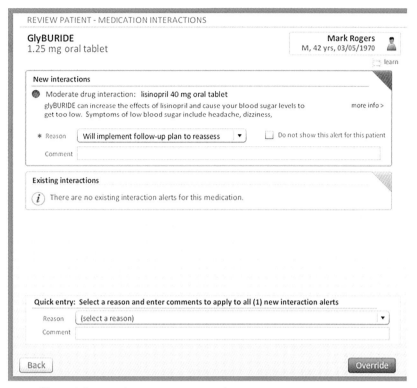

**Figure 3-3** Drug interaction prompt. (Courtesy Practice Fusion, Inc.)

EHR prompts the possibility of a moderate drug interaction between the previously pre-scribed drug, lisinopril, and the newly prescribed drug, glyburide. Wyatt et al (1991) pro-posed the formal definition of **clinical decision-making systems (CDSs)** as "active knowledge-making systems which use two or more items of patient data to generate case-specific advice." Care paths, or **clinical pathways**, are electronic aids (algorithms) that help caregivers make decisions about treatment. Reference material may be available for elec-tronic use when specific diagnoses are documented. Table 3-1 summarizes the functions of the EHR.

Since the data in a patient's EHR can come from many different facilities or sources, in many systems, a **data repository** is used. The data repository stores data from unrelated software programs. These software programs can be created by different vendors and have different applications. Health care organizations should be able to integrate the data and provide a multidisciplinary view of their elements. A data repository can store the data from these different systems and make them usable through the use of an interface without the need to run reports from each system. For example, data may be collected from three separate software programs and stored in the data repository. Consider a patient who has diabetes: The data repository would store data from the pharmacy software program extracted from the medication administration report indicating the amount of insulin the patient receives. The laboratory software program submits its findings, storing the patient's glucose levels, and the nursing notes would contain the glucose monitoring results obtained from the nursing flow sheets.

This repository data are then collected and reorganized in a **data warehouse.** Data warehousing facilitates the use of the data in the health records of many individuals by making all this information available for analysis. The data warehouse collects information from different databases and organizes it for use in ad hoc reports and analytical research. Data warehousing is used to make a variety of vital decisions in health care. Stakeholders in the health care industry use this information for analyzing revenue (e.g., to calculate the cost of treating a patient with diabetes) and for clinical management (e.g., to determine the average amount of insulin needed by a patient with diabetes in a specific age group). It has operational applications (e.g., to assess the staffing pattern for patients on a diabetic

**clinical decision-making system (CDS)** A computer application that compares two or more items of patient data in order to advise clinicians on the treatment of that specific patient.

**clinical pathway** A predetermined standard of treatment for a particular disease, diagnosis, or procedure designed to facilitate the patient's progress through the health care encounter.

**data repository** Where data is stored from different, unrelated software programs.

**medication administration** Clinical data including the name of the medication, dosage, date and time of administration, method of administration, and the nurse who administered it.

**data warehouse** Where information from different databases is collected and organized to be used for ad hoc reports and analytical research.

**TABLE 3-1**

**FUNCTIONS OF THE ELECTRONIC HEALTH RECORD**

| TOPIC | FUNCTION |
|---|---|
| Health information and data | Allows caregivers to have immediate access to key information such as allergies, medications, and lab test results |
| Result management | Allows caregivers to quickly access new and past test results, increasing patient safety and effectiveness of care |
| Order management | Allows caregivers to enter and store orders for prescriptions, tests, or services in a computer-based system that improves legibility, reduces duplication, and increases speed of executing the orders |
| Decision support | Allows the use of reminders, alerts, and prompts that will improve compliance with best clinical practices, ensure regular screening, and identify possible drug interactions |
| Electronic communication and connectivity | Allows for efficient, secure, and readily accessible communication among caregivers and patients that will improve the continuity of care, enhance timeliness of diagnoses and treatments, and reduce the frequency of adverse occurrences |
| Patient support | Provides tools that give patients access to their own health records, provides Internet education, and assists them carrying out home monitoring and self-teaching, which can help improve chronic conditions |
| Administrative processes | Allows for administrative tools such as scheduling, which would improve efficiency and provide more timely service |
| Reporting | Allows electronic data storage using uniform data standards that will enable organizations to respond to third-party regulatory agencies |

From Committee on Data Standards for Patient Safety: The National Academic News. http://www.iom.edu/Reports/2003/Key-Capabilities-of-an-Electronic-Health-Record-System.aspx. Accessed July 26, 2012.

**outcome** The result of a patient's treatment.

nursing unit) as well as use in outcome management (e.g., to estimate the percentage of patients who showed improvement after treatment). In a true EHR, data are collected, used, and shared with other all authorized hospital departments and users, as shown in Figure 3-4. The traditional HIM department functions can be performed electronically, either while the patient is still receiving treatment (concurrently) or after discharge (National Institutes of Health, 2006).

**HIT-bit**

**PATIENT PORTALS IN ELECTRONIC HEALTH RECORD**

Some web-based EHRs allow patients to actively participate in their records. Portions of an EHR may be made available to the patient to view or print. Patients are given a unique ID and password that grant them access to their own records. This is normally available through the health care organization's Web site. In some instances, patients can also message their physicians, make or change appointments, or add information such as allergies or new over-the-counter medications they are taking. Granting patients' access to their information is known as a *patient portal* and has become a popular function of Web-based EHRs.

**health information exchange (HIE)** The database of a network of health care providers (physicians, hospitals, laboratories, and public health organizations) allowing access to patient records within the network from approved points of care.

**Health information exchanges (HIEs)** allow health care providers (physicians, hospitals, laboratories, and public health organizations) to request and receive patients' records from other providers. For example, the HIEs facilitate sharing of electronic information that is requested by a physician at facility A for a patient from facility B (Figure 3-5). The rationale behind the establishment of HIEs and the way they are managed vary, as some are established by the state government and others by private organizations. Previous research indicates that most HIEs were formed to share and gather electronic information among health providers in a certain geographical areas such as a state, region, or nation. The HIEs benefit the health care providers by reducing costs through elimination of duplication of tests and increased staff efficiencies. Other benefits include:

- Easy access to a health record
- Better continuity of care for patients

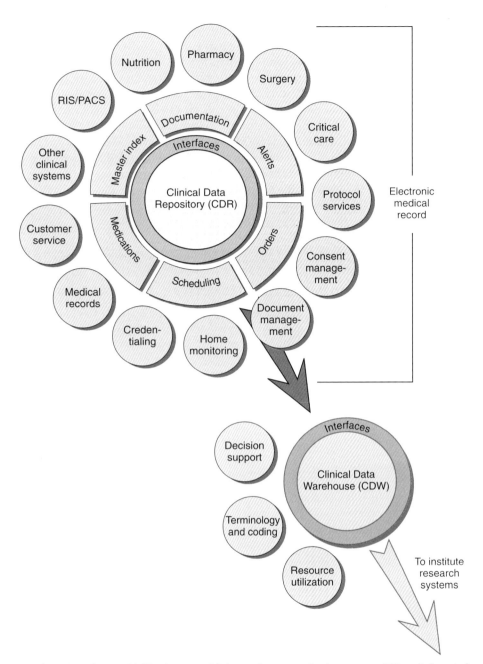

**Figure 3-4** Data repository/warehouse. PACS, picture archiving and communication system; RIS, radiology information system.

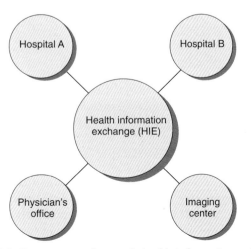

**Figure 3-5** Components of a sample health information exchange.

**outcome** The result of a patient's treatment.

**HIE** health information exchange

**Centers of Medicare and Medicaid Systems (CMS)** The division of the U.S. Department of Health and Human Services that administers Medicare and Medicaid.

**meaningful use** A set of measures to gauge the level of health information technology used by a provider, and required, in certain stages, in order to receive financial incentives from CMS.

- Decreased medical errors with ability to reconcile medications
- Improved patient outcomes and quality of care

In spite of the numerous benefits of HIEs, they face challenges in their long-term sustainability as they try to connect hundreds to thousands of participants in their networks. Each HIE usually receives seed grant money to establish itself, but as the money from the grant dries up it becomes difficult for the HIE to sustain itself financially.

Currently, the health care industry is undergoing drastic changes with greater use of EHRs. The United States federal government, through CMS, has provided financial incentives to the health care providers who use certified EHRs in a "meaningful" way, called **meaningful use**, to hasten the widespread use of the EHRs. These incentives provide a driving force for the adoption of EHRs to achieve the vision of a transformed health care that uses technology in the right way to save time and money, improve patient care, and ensure that each American can have a secure EHR.

## HIT-bit

### HEALTH INFORMATION EXCHANGES

Health information exchanges (HIEs) are being formed both regionally and locally by entities such as health care providers and health care businesses in an effort to share health information electronically. These providers and businesses may have been competitors in the past, but they are forming alliances in an effort to improve the quality and safety of health care in their city, state, or region.

## EXERCISE 3-2

### The Electronic Health Record

1. Explain why indexing of an EHR is important.
2. Explain how an algorithm can improve quality of care.
3. A medical record that contains computer-generated reports, collects data, and shares data with outside agencies is a(n) _____.
4. _____ collects information from different databases and organizes it to be used for ad hoc reports and analytical research.
5. Explain patient support as function of the EHR.
6. A set of measures used to measure the level of health information technology used by a provider, and required, in certain stages, to receive financial incentives from CMS is called: _____.
7. The database of a network of health care providers allowing access to patient records within the network from approved points of care is called a _____.
8. A(n) _____ is used to collect and organize data from different databases to be used for ad hoc reports and analytical research.
9. Information systems that provide clinical best-knowledge practices to make decisions about patient care are called _____.

## GOVERNMENT AND PRIVATE SECTOR INTERVENTION

**HIM** health information management

HIM professionals are not the only people interested in developing the EHR as a national standard for health care documentation. Although this technology promises improved health care delivery by making it easier to access patient data, obstacles such as the cost of implementation, agreement on standard technologies, and concerns about privacy have limited the adoption of fully functional EHRs. But both private consumer groups and government agencies have been working to speed up EHR implementation. The groups and agencies discussed here are working toward the goal of standardizing the technologies and content associated with EHRs to ensure confidentiality, accuracy, comprehensiveness, and the ability to share information among systems.

## Private Sector

Several private groups encourage and monitor the use of EHRs. Three notable private groups are the Markle Foundation, Health Level Seven (HL7), and the Certification Commission for Health Information Technology (CCHIT). These groups advocate the use of the EHR in an effort to improve patient care and safety. They have influence on governmental initiatives and play an important role in the adoption of new technologies.

The Markle Foundation was founded in 1927 by a husband and wife initially to encourage the progression of knowledge and the general good of mankind. One of its current goals is to eliminate barriers in the implementation of the EHR. Two of these barriers are lack of *interoperability* (the ability to exchange information) among computer systems and privacy issues. The Markle Foundation fosters collaboration in both private and public sectors through an initiative called Connecting to Health, which seeks to improve patient care by promoting standards for electronic medical information. In addition, the Markle Foundation has provided information and promoted meaningful use and the development of HIEs (http://www.markle.org).

**Health Level Seven (HL7)**, a nonprofit group composed of providers, vendors, payers, consultants, government groups, and others, is working to develop standards that will aid the interoperability of the exchange of electronic data in and among health care organizations. This group is one of many standards developing organizations (SDOs) producing standards for particular health care domains, such as pharmacy and radiology. HL7 works to provide standards for clinical and administrative domains, specifically the exchange, management, and integration of data supporting clinical patient care and the evaluation of health services. HL7 specifications allow for transfer of data between providers and health care organizations. These specifications ensure that data from one system or organization can be accepted and interpreted by HIE systems.

The **Certification Commission for Health Information Technology (CCHIT)**, a nonprofit organization, has taken a leadership role in the advancement of HIT by creating industry-approved certifications for EHRs (http://www.cchit.org). Although health care professionals have agreed that it is essential to move from paper-based or hybrid medical records to an electronic format, there had been little consensus on what components would constitute an EHR and how these systems would securely share data. The problem was made more complex by the large number of EHR products available (approximately 300) and the knowledge that many EHR implementations do not succeed.

CCHIT has taken on the task of defining the key functional components of an EHR, how it should communicate with other systems, and how it should protect patient information. The CCHIT criteria consist of a list of detailed product capabilities against which EHRs are evaluated. At the very least, CCHIT has created a functional requirements checklist for EHR buyers.

## Government Sector

The Institute of Medicine (IOM) and other health-related organizations have placed emphasis on the non-integrated nature of clinical information that is stored electronically, which affects the quality of care across the United States. One of the most important characteristics of an EHR while storing the clinical information is its ability to be **interoperable**: to share that information among other authorized users. If different information systems cannot communicate or interact with each other, then sharing is not possible. In order to achieve the objective to exchange clinical information, a secure, interoperable EHR is required that can share the information with other EHRs.

### Office of the National Coordinator for Health Information Technology

One of the noteworthy government interventions took place in April of 2004, when President George W. Bush issued Executive Order 13335. This executive order required the

**Health Level Seven (HL7)** A health information systems compliance organization whose goal is to standardize the collection of patient information in the electronic health care record.

**payer** The individual or organization that is primarily responsible for the reimbursement for a particular health care service. Usually refers to the insurance company or third party.

**health information exchange (HIE)** The database of a network of health care providers (physicians, hospitals, laboratories, and public health organizations) allowing access to patient records within the network from approved points of care.

**SDO** standards developing organizations

**Go To** the section titled "Standardization" for more information about how HL7 standards are used in the EHR.

**Certification Commission for Health Information Technology (CCHIT)** A nonprofit organization that seeks to advance health information technology by defining and certifying EHR technology.

**interoperability** The ability of different software and computer systems to communicate and share data.

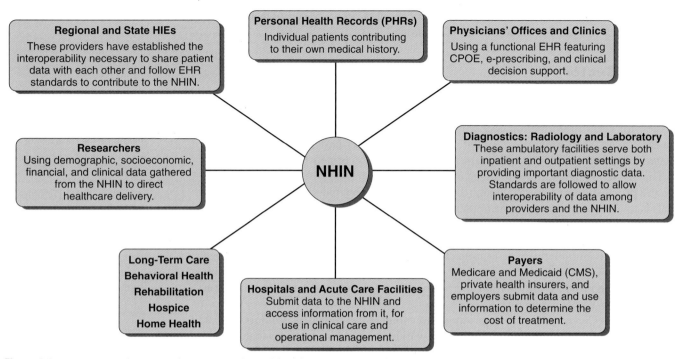

**Figure 3-6** Entities contributing to the Nationwide Health Information Network (NHIN). CMS, Centers for Medicare and Medicaid; CPOE, computerized physician order entry; EHR, electronic health record; HIE, health information exchange.

**Office of the National Coordinator of Health Information Technology (ONC)** An executive division of the U.S. Department of Health and Human Services that coordinates and promotes the national implementation of technology in health care.

**DHHS** U. S. Department of Health and Human Services

**Nationwide Health Information Network (NHIN)** A system of nationally shared health data, composed of a network of providers, consumers, and researchers, that aims to improve health care delivery through the secure exchange of information.

**clinical decision-making system (CDS)** A computer application that compares two or more items of patient data in order to advise clinicians on the treatment of that specific patient.

**HIE** health information exchange

widespread adoption of interoperable EHRs within 10 years. It also established the **Office of the National Coordinator for Health Information Technology (ONC)** within the DHHS. In addition, it directed the ONC to produce a report on the development and implementation of a strategic plan to guide the nationwide implementation of an interoperable EHR in both public and private sectors.

One of the initiatives taken by the ONC to move the entire nation from paper records to EHRs was to establish the **Nationwide Health Information Network (NHIN)**. The NHIN's goal is to provide an interoperable health information exchange among providers, consumers, and others involved in supporting health and health care that is secure and is capable of sharing information nationwide over the Internet. Conceptually, the NHIN is not a centrally located database. It aims to set common computer language requirements and secure messaging to allow regional and state-based networks of HIEs, laboratories, pharmacies, physicians' offices, and other entities involved in health care delivery to share information in a safe, efficient manner. (U.S. Department of Health and Human Services, 2011). The NHIN will make health data readily available for CDSs and use health care beyond direct patient care to improve public health. Because it will provide networks that would enable information sharing against geographical boundaries, the NHIN is a major component of the federal infrastructure. Figure 3-6 shows that the NHIN enables the secure exchange of health data among various entities.

Many other initiatives have been sponsored by the ONC, including one for meaningful use qualifications as well as one for privacy and security. Each of these areas is discussed in depth in this chapter. The ONC is a valuable resource for organizations seeking guidance and knowledge in these areas (Office of the National Coordinator for Health Information Technology, 2011a). Table 3-2 lists the goals of the ONC.

### ARRA/HITECH

In spite of the immense benefits of EHRs and the support of the federal government, there was little progress on their adoption except for a few large facilities and some smaller clinics.

**TABLE 3-2**

**GOALS OF THE OFFICE OF THE NATIONAL COORDINATOR FOR HEALTH INFORMATION TECHNOLOGY (ONC)**

| GOAL 1: Inform Clinical Practice | GOAL 2: Interconnect Physicians | GOAL 3: Personalize Care | GOAL 4: Improve Population Health |
|---|---|---|---|
| Provide incentives for electronic health record (EHR) adoption | Regional collaborations | Encourage use of personal health records | Unify public health surveillance architectures |
| Reduce risk of EHR investment | Develop a nationwide health information network | Enhance informed consumer choice | Streamline quality and health status monitoring |
| Promote EHR diffusion in rural and underserved areas | Coordinate federal health information systems | Promote use of telehealth systems | Accelerate research and dissemination of evidence |

From U.S. Department of Health and Human Services: Office of the National Coordinator for Health Information Technology: Executive summary. http://www.himss.org/handouts/executivesummary.pdf. Published 2004. Accessed October 13, 2012.

In order to break the barriers to the adoption of EHRs, President Barack Obama and his legislation provided a distinctive opportunity with the introduction of the **American Recovery and Reinvestment Act (ARRA)**, also commonly referred to as the stimulus bill or the recovery act, signed into law on Feb 17, 2009. ARRA was created to jumpstart and address the challenges in much-needed areas of the U.S. economy, providing many stimulus opportunities in different areas, one of them being health IT. This portion of the stimulus package was given the subtitle, the **Health Information Technology for Economic and Clinical Health Act (HITECH)**. This legislation further funded and set new mandates for the ONC, solidifying the office's existence.

Through HITECH, which focuses on various aspects of HIT, the federal government allotted a total of $27 billion over 10 years through the Center for Medicare and Medicaid Services (CMS) to clinicians and hospitals when they use the EHRs that meet certain guidelines, called meaningful use (Centers for Medicare and Medicaid Services, 2012). When they meet these requirements, physicians who utilize qualified technologies would receive an incentive or payment from the CMS. Payments are significant, from $18,000 in 2011 up to $44,000 for Medicare-assigned providers during the span of the program. Physicians can choose to be reimbursed as Medicaid-participating providers and receive payments up to $65,000 on the basis of state-defined guidelines. Hospital reimbursement for meeting meaningful use criteria can be significant and can provide substantial financial incentives in the millions of dollars.

Besides encouraging the implementation of EHRs through meaningful use, HITECH legislation promotes technological advancement in health care in other ways. Among them are (Office of the National Coordinator for Health Information Technology, 2011b):

- Support for the development of the NHIN through grants for states and local communities to build and support interoperable HIEs.
- Funding for research projects aimed at eliminating barriers to EHR adoption.
- Grants for colleges and universities to build academic programs for HIT and for Community Colleges to develop and expand HIT-specific nondegree training programs.
- A grant to establish a competency examination for graduates of nondegree HIT programs.

Another government entity, Consolidated Health Informatics, is composed of approximately 20 federal department or agencies, including the DHHS, the Department of Defense, and the Department of Veterans' Affairs. This group is working to establish uniform standards for the electronic exchange of clinical health information among federal health care agencies.

## Health Insurance Portability and Accountability Act

The security of health information has always been a large part of the discussion surrounding the large-scale adoption of EHR technologies, for both its proponents

**American Recovery and Reinvestment Act (ARRA)** Also called the "stimulus bill." 2009 federal legislation providing many stimulus opportunities in different areas. The portion of the law that finds and sets mandates for health information technology is called HITECH.

**Health Information Technology for Economic and Clinical Health Act (HITECH)** A subset of the American Recovery and Reinvestment Act (2009) legislation providing federal funding and mandates for the use of technology in health care.

**ONC** Office of the National Coordinator of Health Information Technology

**CMS** Centers for Medicare and Medicaid Services

**meaningful use** A set of measures to gauge the level of health information technology used by a provider, and required, in certain stages, in order to receive financial incentives from the CMS.

**Medicare** Federally funded health care insurance plan for older adults and for certain categories of chronically ill patients.

**NHIN** Nationwide Health Information Network

**HIE** health information exchange

**EHR** electronic health record

**HIT** health information technology

● **Health Insurance Portability and Accountability Act (HIPAA)** Public Law 104-191, federal legislation passed in 1996 that outlines the guidelines of managing patient information in terms of privacy, security, and confidentiality. The legislation also outlines penalties for noncompliance.

**Go To** A thorough discussion of this landmark legislation is provided in Chapter 12.

● **integrity** The data quality characteristic displayed when alteration of a finalized document is not permitted.
**e-PHI** Under HIPAA, protected health information in electronic format.

● **encryption** A security process that blocks unauthorized access to patient information.
**audit trail** Software that tracks and stores information related to the activity of users in the system.

● **HITECH** Health Information Technology for Economic and Clinical Health Act
**DHHS** The Department of Health and Human Services

and its detractors. The Health Insurance Portability and Accountability Act (HIPAA) of 1996 is best known for its dramatic effect on health care and protection of patient information, and several facets of the later HITECH regulations both strengthened and updated HIPAA provisions for application in a more computer-based health care environment.

One major component of HIPAA is known as the Security Rule. This portion of the regulation addresses how organizations protect information from unauthorized access while maintaining the *integrity* of the record. Record **integrity** refers to the idea that regardless of the format, the record is complete, reliable, and consistent. The Security Rule focuses on a subset of information known as **e-PHI** (electronic protected health information). It refers to "all individually identifiable health information a covered entity creates, receives, maintains or transmits in an electronic form" (Health Insurance Portability and Accountability Act of 1996). Unlike a simple paper document that contains protected health information (PHI), e-PHI encompasses any piece of data that identifies the patient and is considered electronic. If an e-mail is sent, for example, and it includes the patient's name or other identifying information, it is considered e-PHI. Organizations are required to conduct an overall security analysis reviewing potential risks to the security of the information, and to document measures put into place to minimize those risks (Health Insurance Portability and Accountability Act of 1996).

Specific security measures are required according to the HIPAA Security Rule. Administrative safeguards involve the organization's establishing personnel responsible for administering the security initiatives. This individual is named the Security Officer. Administrative safeguards also address training personnel on security regulations, including sanctions for violations and continuous evaluation of the security program.

Physical protection of e-PHI is also critical and part of the HIPAA Security Rule. This entails addressing the physical locations of workstations and servers and the management of storage devices. Although controlling the location of stationary workstations is easy, the use of laptop and handheld computers may pose a risk of unauthorized access. In addition, controlling the use of portable storage devices such as flash drives, compact disks (CDs), and cell phones is a critical aspect of this portion of the Security Rule.

Technical safeguards are the focus of another section that sets forth requirements to be implemented by health care providers that store e-PHI. These include controlling access through the use of user identification (user ID) and password creation and maintenance. Training employees in proper protection of their user IDs and passwords includes not sharing them with other employees or individuals, refraining from writing the information down, and proper techniques for changing and resetting passwords. **Encryption** (computerized scrambling of information to make it unrecognizable except to the intended recipient) and firewalls (electronic blocks) are preventive techniques that can help prevent unauthorized access as well. Finally, a technical safeguard that has proved to be beneficial is the **audit trail**. See Figure 3-7 for an example of an audit trail. This safeguard tracks the activity of users in the system and stores information related to what information the user accessed and when it was accessed, and some systems can even show what actions the user took (changed, deleted, printed information) while logged in. The audit trail can be a useful piece of evidence showing what a user did while logged in to the system. This process is an important reason why it is critical that users do not share their user IDs and passwords.

The remainder of the Security Rule requires the organization to create various policies and procedures that address storage, use, protection, and maintenance of e-PHI. If an unauthorized user gains access to e-PHI, the event is known as a *breach*. HITECH changed the Security Rule to require covered health care entities to report breaches. If a breach affects less than 500 patients, the organization must notify the individuals whose information was breached as well as the Secretary of the DHHS. In the instance that a breach affects more than 500 patients, the organization is required to notify the individuals, the Secretary, and the news media. All reported security breaches affecting more than 500 patients can be viewed on the DHHS Web site (Health Insurance Portability and Accountability Act of 1996).

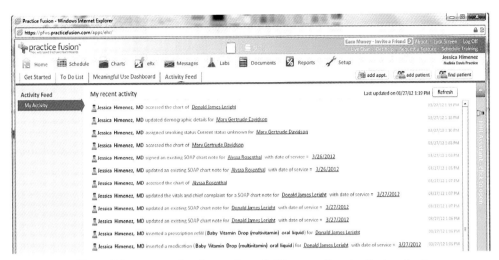

Figure 3-7 An example of an audit trail. (Courtesy Practice Fusion, Inc.)

The HIPAA Security Rule brought a new focus on the importance of securing electronic information. As the HIM industry transitions toward a fully electronic environment, the Security Rule is a critical factor in ensuring the security of health information.

## EXERCISE 3-3
### Government and Private Sector Intervention

1. Explain why HL7 is important.
2. Explain Executive Order 13335.
3. Which group is stressing the need for a national information infrastructure?
4. List the four goals of the ONC.
5. A security process that blocks unauthorized access to patient information _____.
6. A(n) _____ is a review of individual user access codes to determine who had access to patient health information and to ensure the access was deemed necessary for patient care.
7. What is ePHI?
8. Describe the data quality characteristic "integrity."

## IMPLEMENTING AN ELECTRONIC HEALTH RECORD

As discussed earlier in the chapter, many hospitals are already using some form of EHR. The process of implementing this technology has multiple facets that HIM professionals manage. Acknowledging and addressing challenges during the implementation process will result in successful adoption of new technology.

**Go To** Chapter 13 for more detail on the steps taken to implement or upgrade EHR technology.

### Standardization

Electronic health systems that share data will have to standardize the health record formats and language used within the various information systems in order for systems to integrate data. This interoperability between the systems is critical in order for users to gain maximum use of and efficiency from the EHR. When information is collected in different formats, it cannot be shared or exchanged with another organization without intervention by a user. For example, the data element, Date of Birth, can be collected numerous ways. Some systems may collect it in the format of: 2-digit date, 2-digit month, 4-digit year. Other systems may collect month first, then date, then year. Alternatively, some may collect the month as alphabetical characters (Oct instead of 10):

**interoperability** The ability of different software and computer systems to communicate and share data.

System 1: 09/10/1975
System 2: 10/09/1975
System 3: Oct/09/1975

Attempting to exchange or share information among these three systems will be difficult because of the lack of standardization in the Date of Birth field. Critical errors may result when systems cannot share information, such as misinterpreting treatment plans, medication strengths, or diagnoses.

Because standardization is a critical element to achieving seamless exchange of information, numerous standards have been issued, resulting in a need for coordination of these standards into one set. As discussed previously, HL7 has established standards specifically for the EHR and how it should be designed and formatted as well as the functions it should be capable of and the content it should contain. The standards are divided into three categories: *direct care, supportive,* and *information infrastructure* standards. Direct care standards relate to which EHR functions would relate to providing care to patients. The supportive standards section involves financial and administrative functions in a health care organization. Finally, the information infrastructure category is a more technical set of functions including security, user identification, and approved terminologies. For each standard, conformance criteria are listed that indicate how that standard is applied to the EHR system. HL7 has released various functional models describing these standards and how they should be incorporated into an EHR so that interoperability is ensured (Health Level Seven, 2004).

## Meaningful Use

The ARRA/HITECH legislation provides a financial incentive for the meaningful use of certified EHR technology to achieve quality health care and efficiency goals. By applying meaningful use, the health care providers not only reap financial benefits but also improve the quality of care by reducing medical errors and gaining CDS support and electronic prescribing—even though they might not be able to otherwise afford the technology. The ARRA has laid out three main components of meaningful use in the EHR incentive program, as follows (Centers for Medicare and Medicaid Services, 2012):

1. The use of a certified EHR in a meaningful manner, such as e-prescribing.
2. The use of certified EHR technology for electronic exchange of health information to improve quality of health care.
3. The use of certified EHR technology to submit clinical quality and other measures.

Because the widespread use of a fully functional and interoperable electronic health care documentation and delivery system represents tremendous investments of time and energy, meaningful use requirements have been set up in three stages over a period of 5 years, until the year 2015. Although physicians, hospitals, and other providers who meet meaningful use guidelines receive cash incentives from the CMS, those who do not embrace these technologies are slated to suffer a penalty in the payments they receive from Medicare, beginning with a 1% reduction in 2015.

There are 25 meaningful use objectives in Stage 1, 20 of which have to be met for a health care provider to qualify for the payment through the stimulus bill. The provider must choose 15 core objectives, and the remaining 5 objectives can be chosen from the set of 10 menu-set objectives. The objectives have been summarized in Boxes 3-1 and 3-2, which show the set of 15 core objectives and 10 menu objectives, respectively. Figure 3-8 shows the Stage 1 requirements being used at a sample physician's office.

Each of the three stages of meaningful use essentially builds upon the EHR. Stage 1, which started in 2011, requires the major functionality of a certified EHR, such as documenting visits, diagnosis, prescriptions, and other relevant health information, including reminders and alerts, and sharing patient information, reporting quality measures, and other public health information. Stage 2, which begins in 2013, includes all the functionality from Stage 1 in addition to sending and receiving laboratory orders and results. Stage 3 begins in 2015. It will incorporate the criteria from both Stage 1

**Health Level Seven (HL7)** A health information systems compliance organization whose goal is to standardize the collection of patient information in the electronic health care record.

**meaningful use** A set of measures to gauge the level of health information technology used by a provider and required, in certain stages, in order to receive financial incentives from the CMS.

**clinical decision-making system (CDS)** A computer application that compares two or more items of patient data in order to advise clinicians on the treatment of that specific patient.

**ARRA** American Recovery and Reinvestment Act
**EHR** electronic health record

**CMS** Centers for Medicare and Medicaid Services

**Medicare** Federally funded health care insurance plan for older adults and for certain categories of chronically ill patients.

---

**BOX 3-1  MEANINGFUL USE STAGE 1 CORE SET (ALL 15 MEASURES REQUIRED)**

Demographics (50%)
Vitals: BP and BMI (50%)
Problem list: ICD-9-CM or SNOMED (80%)
Active medication list (80%)
Medication allergies (80%)
Smoking status (50%)
Patient clinical visit summary (50% in 3 days)
Hospital discharge instructions (50%) *or* Patient with electronic copy (50% in 3 days)
CPOE (30% including a med)
Drug-drug and drug-allergy interactions (functionality enabled)
Exchange critical information (perform test)
Clinical decision support (one rule)
Security risk analysis
Report clinical quality (BP, BMI, Smoke, plus 3 others)
e-Prescribing (40%)

---

BMI, body mass index; BP, blood pressure; CPOE, computerized physician order entry; ICD-9-CM, International Classification of Diseases, 9th Revision—Clinical Modification; SNOMED, Systematized Nomenclature of Medicine; Smoke, smoking status.
Adapted from Practice Fusion, Inc: EHR Meaningful Use Criteria. http://www.practicefusion.com/pages/ehr-meaningful-use-criteria.html. Published 2012.

---

**BOX 3-2  MEANINGFUL USE STAGE 1 MENU SET (SELECT 5 OF 10)**

Drug-formulary checks (one report)
Structured laboratory results (40%)
Patients by conditions (one report)
Send patient-specific education (10%)
Medication reconciliation (50%)
Feed immunization registries (perform at least one test)
Hospital advance medical directives (50% >65 yrs)
Send reminders to patients for preventative and follow-up care (20% >65 yrs, <5 yrs)
Patient electronic access to laboratory results, problems, medications, and allergies
   (10% in 4 days)
Summary care record at transitions (50%)

---

Adapted from Practice Fusion, Inc: EHR Meaningful Use Criteria. http://www.practicefusion.com/pages/ehr-meaningful-use-criteria.html. Published 2012.

---

and Stage 2, adding on clinical decision support, access to comprehensive patient data, and improving patient health.

## Accessibility

A primary goal of the ONC is to allow authorized users to have access to medical information wherever and whenever it is needed, whether in a physician office, acute care facility, or home health agency. Rural facilities will be able to access the records from urban facilities where the specialists practice. Consumers will have personal health records (PHRs) that they can share with the caregivers at any facility.

One of the key advantages of a functional EHR linked to the NHIN is the accessibility of the patient's information by the caregivers regardless of the location of the patient. For example, consider a patient who enters a health care facility through the emergency department because of shortness of breath. The physician is able to retrieve the patient's previous

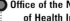 **Office of the National Coordinator of Health Information Technology (ONC)** An executive division of the U.S. Department of Health and Human Services that coordinates and promotes the national implementation of technology in health care.

**NHIN** Nationwide Health Information Network

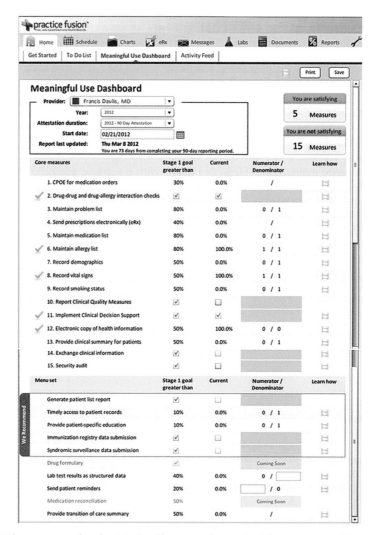

**Figure 3-8** The progress of a physician's office toward Meaningful Use Stage 1. (Courtesy Practice Fusion, Inc.)

**encounter** A patient's health care experience; a unit of measure for the volume of ambulatory care services provided.

**consultation** The formal request by a physician for the professional opinion or services of another health care professional, usually another physician, in caring for a patient. Also refers to the opinion or services themselves as well as the activity of rendering the opinion or services.

**discharge** Discharge occurs when the patient leaves the care of the facility to go home, for transfer to another health care facility or by death. Also refers to the status of a patient.

encounters, including test results and treatments that the patient received in the past from any facility. A surgery consultation is ordered for the patient. The surgeon is just finishing another patient's procedure and receives notice of the consultation. While in the surgery unit, he can access the patient's previous and current records and have some knowledge of the patient's health status before assessing the patient during this treatment encounter. The patient undergoes surgery during which an organ is removed. The organ is sent to the pathology laboratory for review. The pathologist may access the patient's record to review the clinical history and surgical findings before performing the pathological examination of the organ. The patient is discharged and has a follow-up appointment with the surgeon. The surgeon wants to review the pathology report again before discussing the findings with the patient. He can access the pathology report from his office rather than going to the HIM department to view the paper record.

When a paper record is used, the record is accessible wherever the patient is being treated because it goes where the patient goes; therefore only one health care provider at a time is usually able to see the record. The EHR allows the record to be viewed by several caregivers at the same time regardless of the location of the patient or the caregivers. In the HIM department, the EHR allows several staff members to use the record at the same time to support the many functions that occur. Having the ability to accomplish these tasks simultaneously leads to greater efficiency.

## EXERCISE 3-4
### Implementing an EHR

1. Why is standardization important for the widespread use of the EHR?
2. What are the stages of meaningful use?
3. How are providers encouraged to adopt technology through meaningful use?

## Challenges

It is because EHRs have been proven to enhance quality that the public and private organizations discussed previously, from the United States federal government to the Markle Foundation, have actively sought ways to defray the cost associated with implementing EHRs. From meaningful use to investments in education and technology, these entities are working to overcome the obstacles that stand in the way of large-scale implementation.

### Cost

The biggest deterrent to adoption of the EHR at this time is cost. Estimating the average cost of implementing an EHR is difficult because of the complex and various *infrastructures* of health care organizations. **Infrastructure** can be defined as the standard operating nomenclature, specifications, or protocols of a system. Modern health care delivery systems are diverse, and their structures and needs vary greatly from simple to complex. Logically, a more complex health system would require a more expensive EHR with greater functionality. Despite the variances in structure, a large portion of the costs relate to acquisition of both hardware and software. Organizations must also consider planning, design, reliable IT support, effective training, appropriate licenses, and maintenance fees.

**infrastructure** The interrelated components of a system.

### Training

Training users involves coordination among IT, HIM, all employees, and physicians. Even though computers are a part of our daily lives, many health care workers may not feel as comfortable managing electronic records, rather than paper records. Initially, productivity is expected to decrease as employees adjust to the new information management system. Good leadership practices should be utilized during the transition to help the organization meet established goals for the transition. Employees should be encouraged to learn the system properly, and managers should be patient during the transition phase. If delays are expected that would affect internal or external users, proper explanation and communication of the reason for delay should be offered.

**IT** information technology
**HIM** health information management

Training will cost an organization in development, time, personnel, and resources. Training methodology will vary according to the type, size, and complexity of the organization. Some organizations choose to train users in an electronic or online model with simulations in which users can learn at their own schedule. Other organizations use a traditional approach whereby users learn on site with hands-on practice. Organizations may customize training according to their users' comfort with technology.

However an organization chooses to train users, it is critical that training be carefully planned and executed. Training is essential to the success of any health information technology implementation. Failure to train or poor training can have catastrophic effects on the success of the EHR. The EHR is only as good as the individuals who use it. Identifying a super-user and making sure it is accessible to staff is one method of ensuring that users have adequate support during the migration and transition. A **superuser** is an individual that has been trained in all aspects of the system and can serve as an on-site help desk for users who may experience difficulties with the system. The super user can also be the main contact for the facility and may communicate technology issues with the software vendor. Many facilities train numerous super users to meet the needs of their staff.

**superuser** An individual trained in all aspects of a computer system who can offer on-site support to others.

**licensure** The mandatory government approval required for performing specified activities. In health care, the state approval required for providing health care services.

**certification** Approval by an outside agency, such as the federal or state government, indicating that the health care facility has met a set of predetermined standards.

**accreditation** Voluntary compliance with a set of standards developed by an independent agent, who periodically performs audits to ensure compliance.

**demographic data** Identification: those elements that distinguish one patient from another, such as name, address, and birth date.

**history** The physician's record of the patient's chief complaint, history of present illness, pertinent family and social history, and review of systems.

**progress notes** The physician's record of each interaction with the patient.

**longitudinal record** The compilation of information from all providers over the span of a patient's care, potentially from birth to death, which is facilitated by the electronic flow of information among providers.

**interoperable** The ability of different software and computer systems to communicate and share data.

## Privacy and Security

As discussed earlier in this chapter, security is a key issue in implementation of an EHR. In the transition from paper to electronic records, greater information accessibility poses higher risks to privacy and security. It is necessary to update policies, procedures, and sanctions to comply with federal and state regulations. The HIM department is responsible for establishing guidelines for privacy and security as well as conducting training to ensure that employees understand the policies and procedures. Special attention should also be paid to licensure, certification, and accreditation privacy and security requirements when applicable.

## Data Exchange and Interoperability

During a patient's lifetime, health care providers gather information in the form of demographic data, medical history, progress notes, vital signs, and clinical information such as laboratory, radiology, and pharmacy data. These data stored electronically in the form of an EHR are also referred as a **longitudinal record**, because they are collected over time and can provide a more complete picture of an individual's medical history. Because a patient may acquire this information from multiple clinical sources over the course of her life, the interoperability of information among the many stakeholders in health care, from hospitals and physician's offices to grocery store pharmacies, has been recognized as a key objective in utilizing the potential of an EHR (Figure 3-9).

Currently, most clinical information is stored in different locations across the health care community. Data about a given patient may be held in systems in physician's offices, laboratories, imaging systems, or other hospitals, and many times these systems do not "talk." In other words, these systems do not operate with one another to share information. Consider a scenario in which a patient who usually visits a physician's office has been transported to a nearby hospital because of an emergency. The attending physician may have difficulty obtaining patient's complete information. In some instances, the physician may have to repeat certain tests owing to lack of prior information about the patient. The lack of interoperability can be an enormous obstacle in advancing patient care. The

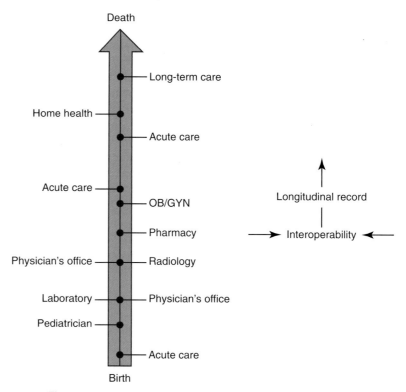

**Figure 3-9** Interoperable systems creating a longitudinal record.

interoperability between these organizations, the physician's office and the hospital, would reduce the need for redundant tests and would save the associated time and cost.

Moreover, without interoperable systems, the treatment the patient received at the hospital may not become part of the longitudinal record, possibly affecting the treatment decisions of the doctor directing the patient's care in the future.

---

**HIT-bit** ···········································································

### PICTURE ARCHIVING AND COMMUNICATION SYSTEMS AND THE DIGITAL IMAGING AND COMMUNICATION IN MEDICINE

Advances in medical imaging have ushered in a new era of noninvasive diagnostic tools in health care, but the way these images are captured and shared has evolved as well. Digital imaging has made the use of film increasingly rare in radiography, and it has also changed the way these data are stored. Rather than the development, filing, and retrieval of film jackets, modern medical imaging requires the storage and transmittal of very large digital pictures.

The technology that allows the effective use of these images is called a **picture archiving and communication system, or PACS**. A PACS allows many different kinds of diagnostic images (e.g., x-rays, magnetic images, ultrasound scans, computed tomography scans) obtained by many different kinds of machines to be archived and accessed from any computer terminal in the network, and even implemented into a patient's EHR.

Just as the data contained in an EHR require certain standards in order to be interoperable, images must follow a certain standard. Furthermore, some types of digital images generate so much data that their use is impractical without compression. The **Digital Imaging and Communication in Medicine (DICOM)** standard enables the management of these images—with regard to both storage and transmission over networks. Specifically, DICOM dictates the formats, protocols, the means of compression, and even the printing of images, making their exchange among physicians and other providers possible.

**Picture archiving and communication system (PACS)** A system that allows many different kinds of diagnostic images (e.g., radiographs, magnetic resonance images, ultrasound scans, computed tomography scans) produced by many different kinds of machines to be archived and accessed from any computer terminal in the network.

**Digital Imaging and Communications in Medicine (DICOM)** A standard that enables the storage and use of clinical digital imaging, making their exchange among physicians and other providers possible.

---

The Institute of Electrical and Electronics Engineers (IEEE, 1990) defines interoperability as the "ability of two or more components to exchange information and to use the information that has been exchanged." In simple terms, interoperability exists between two systems when both the systems can send and receive information and perform the necessary tasks in an appropriate manner without any intervention. Interoperability can be classified into three categories as follows (Garde et al 2007):

*Syntactic interoperability*—The two systems should be capable of exchanging *data*. In other words, the data should be accessible and in a machine-readable format. "Syntax" is the description of the rules by which the structure and the meaning are clearly defined.

*Structural interoperability/semantic interpretability*—The meaning of the information should be clear and understood by all users. An example of semantic interpretability is discrete code sets, such as in the International Classification of Diseases, 9th Revision—Clinical Modification (ICD-9-CM).

*Semantic interoperability*—The two or more systems that exchange information should be able to interpret the meaning of the information exchanged without any ambiguity. Semantic interoperability creates coherence among systems that do not speak the same language. In order to achieve semantic interoperability, the systems exchanging information should refer to a common information exchange reference model, such as HL7.

## The Future of the Electronic Health Record

In the current environment, in which approximately 27% of clinical research is conducted using electronic data capture, a significant number of these health care entities are also using EHRs for clinical research. A future vision is to collect patient data in the EHRs, which can be leveraged for clinical research in the same efficient and regulatory-compliant manner, thus benefitting the health care professionals, patients, and sponsors of clinical trials (eClinical Forum and PhRMA EDC task force, 2006). Increasing health care costs, patient safety, and its associated services make implementing the NHIN a priority. Managing and accounting for these needs now is critical to the future for the advancement of quality and cost-effective clinical research. This will enable clinical researchers to identify, attract, and manage patients and patient data and speed delivery of breakthrough medicines, therapies, and devices.

**workflow** The process of work flowing through a set of procedures to complete the health record.

---

## HIT-bit ······································

### ELECTRONIC HEALTH RECORD WORKFLOW

EHRs dramatically change the established *workflow* of the record. **Workflow** is the series of steps the record goes through from start to finish. Each process in the workflow is different, so training in each area is required. For example, the coding function changes when an EHR is implemented, so coders are trained specifically on the application that gathers, assigns, and/or edit codes (known as an encoder). Because this specialized training directly affects the potential success or failure of each person, careful consideration should be given to proper preparation for workflow changes. (eClinical Forum, 2006)

---

## Career Opportunities

**HIT** health information technology
**ONC** Office of the National Coordinator of Health Information Technology

As health care organizations transition to the EHR, a greater need exists for employees with HIT expertise. The ONC predicts that 51,000 additional Health Informatics workers will be needed during the next 4 years to satisfy EHR requirements and federal laws (Morton, 2011). The ONC has outlined 12 new roles, 6 of which require community college-based training; they are practice workflow and information management redesign specialists, clinician/practitioner consultants, implementation support specialists, implementation managers, technical/software support staff, and trainers. In addition, the health information technologist may find a variety of new careers concentrating on information management, including the following:

- Project management: act as a leader to teams in the process of developing or implementing EHR systems
- Design and development: test new systems, provide training on new systems
- Marketing and sales: sell products and services related to the EHR, provide support to new clients
- Implementation specialist: help facilities with the implementation of the EHR
- Technical support: provide support to the customers during and after system implementation, including access to facility records and development of a PHR
- Knowledge management: assist with database design and develop reports using databases
- Consumer affairs: educate members of the public about their rights and the appropriate uses of their health information

## ■ EXERCISE 3-5

### Advantages of and Barriers to Implementing an Electronic Health Record

1. Explain the difference between interoperable and longitudinal. Give an example of each.
2. List the barriers to implementing an EHR.
3. The framework that enables interoperability by using standard operating nomenclature, specifications, or protocols is called _____.
4. The electronic flow of information from one type of provider to another over the span of a patient's care is _____
5. The ability of different software and computer systems to communicate and share data is _____.
6. An individual who is trained on all aspects of a computer system, and who can help others on-site who are having difficulty is called a _____.

## WORKS CITED

AHIMA e-HIM Personal Health Record Work Group: The role of the personal health record in the EHR, J AHIMA 76:64A–64D, 2005.

Centers for Medicare and Medicaid Services: EHR Incentive Programs. Updated August, 2012. https://www.cms.gov/Regulations-and-Guidance/Legislation/EHRIncentivePrograms/index.html?redirect=/ehrincentiveprograms/. Accessed October 15, 2012.

Centers for Medicare and Medicaid Services: EHR Incentive Program. https://www.cms.gov/EHRIncentivePrograms/30_Meaningful_Use.asp. Accessed August 9, 2012.

Certification Commission for Health Information Technology: CCHIT: Home. http://www.cchit.org. Accessed August 1, 2011.

Dixon BE, Zafar A: Inpatient computerized provider order entry: findings from the AHRQ health IT portfolio (Prepared by the AHRQ National Resource Center for Health IT). AHRQ Publication No. 09-0031-EF, Rockville, Md, 2009, Agency for Healthcare Research and Quality.

The eClinical Forum and PhRMA EDC Task Group: The Future Vision of Electronic Health Records as eSource for Clinical Research. Draft Version 0.1. http://www.esi-bethesda.com/ncrrworkshops/clinicalResearch/pdf/CatherineCeligrantPaper.pdf Published March 2006. Accessed August 9, 2012.

Garde S, Knaup P, Hovenga EJS, Heard S: Towards semantic interoperability for electronic health records, Methods Inf Med 46:332–343, 2007.

Health Insurance Portability and Accountability Act of 1996. 45 CFR Part 160 and Subparts A and C of Part 164.

Health Level 7: HL7 EHR system functional model: A major development towards consensus on electronic health record system functionality. http://www.hl7.org/documentcenter/public_temp_0BD98B49-1C23-BA17-0C8B19C7ECF1ED5C/wg/ehr/EHR-SWhitePaper.pdf. Published 2004. Accessed August 12, 2012.

HIMSS Electronic Health Record Committee: HIMSS electronic health record definitional model version 1.0. http://www.himss.org/content/files/EHRAttributes.pdf. Published 2003. Accessed March 23, 2012.

Institute of Electrical and Electronics Engineers (IEEE): IEEE standard computer dictionary: a compilation of IEEE standard computer glossaries, New York, 1990, IEEE.

Morton A: UBT program: Preparing the health IT leaders of tomorrow, today. U.S. Department of Health & Human Services. http://www.healthit.gov/buzz-blog/university-based-training/ubt-program-preparing-health-leaders-tomorrow-today. HealthIt Buzz, Published May 12, 2011. Accessed August 28, 2012.

National Institutes of Health, Clinical Research Information System: The project: a clinical research information system for NIH. http://cris.cc.nih.gov/public/project.html. Accessed July 25, 2006.

Office of the National Coordinator for Health Information Technology: Health IT home. http://healthit.hhs.gov/portal/server/pt/comunit/healthit_hhs_gov Published 2011a. Accessed August 1, 2011.

Office of the National Coordinator for Health Information Technology: HITECH programs. http://healthit.hhs.gov/portal/server.pt/community/healthit_hhs_gov__hitech_programs/1487. Published 2011b. Accessed July 27, 2012.

Sackett DL, Rosenberg WM, Gray JA, et al: Evidence based medicine: what it is and what it isn't. BMJ 312:71–72, 1996.

U.S. Department of Health and Human Services: Nationwide Health Information Network (NHIN): Background and scope. http://www.hhs.gov/healthit/healthnetwork/background. Accessed August 6, 2011.

Wyatt JC, Spiegelhalter DJ: Field trials of medical decision-aids: potential problems and solutions. Proc Annu Symp Comput Appl Med Care 3-7, 1991.

## SUGGESTED READING

Amatayakul MK: Electronic health records: a practical guide for professionals and organizations, ed 2, Chicago, 2004, Clinical Research Information Management Association.

Downing K, Duncan M, Gustafson P, et al: The EHR's impact on HIM functions, J AHIMA 76: 56C–56H, 2005.

Ferris N: Regional health information network gains traction. Government Health IT. http://www.govhealthit.com/news/regional-health-information-networks-gain-traction. Published June 9, 2005. Accessed July 25, 2012.

# CHAPTER ACTIVITIES

## CHAPTER SUMMARY

The HITECH legislation under ARRA provides a huge government incentive for the meaningful use of EHRs. Many private and federal groups are working to make the EHR a reality. Many health care organizations are already using either hybrid or electronic health records. HIM employees who are using a hybrid record are already familiar with terms such as interfacing and document imaging. Health care organizations will standardize in order to enable interoperability, which is necessary for the creation and maintenance of longitudinal records, making health information more accessible to the users and thereby improving the quality of health care. The government has provided incentives to decrease the cost of EHR conversion. HIM departments making the transition to an EHR have to review and revise every function performed in the department. HIM professionals have to learn the information technology functions to manage the future HIM departments. As the interoperable EHR becomes a reality, there will be a growing need for professionals with HIM knowledge. In addition, the growth of data warehouses, clinical data repositories, and other large databases at the institutional, local, state, regional, and national levels requires professionals who are capable of understanding, retrieving, analyzing, and managing information. Job opportunities will be available for HIT personnel, project managers, privacy and security managers, vendor marketing and sales representatives, and database designers.

## REVIEW QUESTIONS

1. Explain the difference between the hybrid medical record and the EHR.
2. List the features of an EHR. Explain how these features are advantages for health care.
3. Identify government sector intervention designed to hasten the implementation of the widespread use of EHR technology.
4. Describe HIPAA protections governing the use of electronic health information.
5. Explain *meaningful use* and how it encourages providers to adopt EHR technologies.
6. List two barriers to the implementation of the EHR.
7. Explain the benefits of interoperable systems and the importance of a longitudinal record.
8. List three careers created by the widespread adoption of EHRs.
9. Describe the future of the electronic health record.

## ⬤ PROFESSIONAL PROFILE

My name is Ann, and I am a HIM implementation specialist in a 250-bed facility, Diamonte Hospital. This facility provides acute care, emergency services, ambulatory services, a cancer center, and two offsite rehabilitation centers. Our hospital is one of four hospitals in the city owned by the same corporation. We have approximately 500 physicians on the medical staff.

The four hospitals share a medical record database and use hybrid medical records. All four hospitals are currently in the process of implementing an EHR. Each hospital has hired an HIM implementation specialist who will work on different HIM applications in the electronic record. I was promoted from clerical supervisor to implementation specialist. This is a very exciting position. It has given me an opportunity to learn about the information systems throughout the facility as well as allowed me to work with many employees from other departments and from the other hospitals.

I am a member of the implementation team at our facility and provide input on HIM functions, forms, and communication. I am working with a joint forms committee with representatives from all four hospitals to revise the record forms to an electronic format. I am also working closely with the vendor and IT department to develop the workflow for the electronic record. I am spending many hours testing the HIM functions for my assigned applications as they are developed. I provide feedback on the results of the application testing to the vendor and implementation committee, who listen carefully to my suggestions for changes. Currently, we are working on the scanning and indexing application. I am developing training materials for the HIM employees at all four hospitals. Several of the file clerks will be performing the scanning and indexing functions. My next application will be working on the bar codes for the revised forms.

This position is allowing me the opportunity to use my computer skills, work with a team, and use my knowledge of HIM workflow and processes. Being part of the team developing the foundation for the EHR is very rewarding.

## PATIENT CARE PERSPECTIVE

**Dr. Lewis's partner, Dr. Boonton**

One thing we are trying very hard to accomplish is electronic communication between our practice and the hospitals at which we have privileges. Diamonte Hospital has negotiated a relationship with a software vendor who creates a connection among hospitals, physician offices, and patients. I send quite a few patients to Diamonte, although I don't admit them myself; the hospitalists care for them. So if one of my patients is admitted to Diamonte, key data elements flow automatically from the hospital to my office system. I am aware of the admission on a timely basis and can contact the hospitalist if necessary. For example, Maria's mother, Isabel, was admitted to Diamonte last week after a fall. I saw the notification the following morning, and the hospitalist called me to confirm her medications and discuss her condition and discharge plan. The day after she was discharged, we set up an appointment for follow-up.

## APPLICATION

### Current EHR Activities

Go to the ONC and HL7 Web sites and prepare a brief report on the current activities of these organizations relating to the implementation of the EHR. Prepare this report as if you were presenting it to the next monthly HIM department meeting at your hospital.

**4** CHAPTER

# ACUTE CARE RECORDS

Nadinia Davis

## CHAPTER OUTLINE

CLINICAL FLOW OF DATA
  The Order to Admit
  Initial Assessment
  Plan of Care
  Discharge

CLINICAL DATA
  Physicians
  Nurses
  Laboratory Data
  Radiology Data

Special Records
DISCHARGE DATA SET

## VOCABULARY

admission consent form
admission record
admitting diagnosis
admitting physician
advance directive
anesthesia report
attending physician
bar code
chief complaint

consultant
consultation
countersigned
direct admission
discharge summary
face sheet
general consent form
history
history and physical (H&P)

laboratory tests
medication administration
nosocomial infection
nursing assessment
nursing progress notes
operation
operative report
plan of treatment
physical examination

physician's order
progress notes
protocol (order set)
radiology examination
surgeon
telemedicine
treatment

## CHAPTER OBJECTIVES

*By the end of this chapter, the student should be able to:*
1. Describe the flow of clinical data through an acute care facility.
2. Given a specific clinical report, analyze the required data elements.
3. Given a data element, identify the appropriate original source of the data.
4. List the elements of the Uniform Hospital Discharge Data Set (UHDDS).

**data set** A group of data elements collected for a specific purpose.
**demographic data** Those elements that distinguish one patient from another, such as name, address, and birth date.
**financial data** Elements that describe the payer. For example, the name, address, and telephone of the patient's insurance company, as well as the group and member numbers the company has assigned to the patient.
**socioeconomic data** Elements that pertain to the patient's personal life and personal habits, such as marital status, religion, and culture.
**clinical data** All of the medical data that have been recorded about the patient's stay or visit, including diagnoses and procedures.

Data collection begins with building the hospital's data set for a given patient. Each type of facility has its own particular data set that must be considered in the planning of data collection strategies, inclusive of the discharge data set required for the U.S. Department of Health and Human Services (DHHS). Demographic, financial, socioeconomic, and clinical data constitute the health record. This chapter is about the clinical data that are collected throughout the patient's acute care (short stay) inpatient stay by various caregivers in the facility. Throughout the chapter, various paper forms or computer data collection screens are referenced, examples of which are located in Appendix A and Appendix B.

## CLINICAL FLOW OF DATA

In any health care delivery encounter, there is a pattern of activity and data collection that is characteristic of the facility and the type of care being rendered. Although there are unique differences, as will be seen in Chapter 8, most encounters have some basic points in common: patient registration, clinical data collection and evaluation, assessment, and treatment.

## The Order to Admit

All patients who seek treatment in any health care setting (e.g., emergency department, clinic, inpatient unit) within a hospital must be registered. Inpatient admissions usually correspond to one of the following four scenarios:

*Emergency*—Unexpected, in which case the patient is taken to the emergency department and admitted as an emergency admission. These patients have life-threatening conditions that require immediate medical care, such as myocardial infarction (heart attack).

*Urgent*—The patient may be admitted because of an exacerbation of a medical condition. The physician or someone from the physician's office calls in advance in much the same way that a patient calls a physician's office and makes an appointment. This type of admission is referred to as a **direct admission**. Other patients may be admitted directly as transfer patients from other hospitals or skilled nursing facilities (SNFs).

*Elective*—At other times, the patient's visit is expected, in which case the patient has an appointment (i.e., the patient's physician or someone in the physician's office arranges for, or schedules, the admission). For example, a woman may be coming in to give birth by elective caesarean section.

*Other*—Newborns are considered to be admitted at the time of birth and are registered soon thereafter.

A physician must write an order for a patient to be placed in a bed in the hospital. The patient's status is defined in the order: inpatient or outpatient. If the patient is to remain in the hospital for observation, the physician's order is to keep the patient on outpatient status so that the patient can be monitored by the clinical staff. Typically, chest pain and syncope are symptoms that might require close monitoring while laboratory tests and radiologic examinations are performed and their findings reviewed. Centers for Medicare and Medicaid Services (CMS) considers 48 hours to be the maximum amount of time that a patient would reasonably be held in observation status, at which point a decision to admit or to discharge should have been made. In exceptional circumstances, a patient might be held longer; however, the documentation should be very specific as to why the patient was held in observation for longer than 48 hours.

If the patient is to be an inpatient, the physician should write the order to say: admit to inpatient status. The status of the patient is very important, because the billing and coding are different for inpatients and outpatients. In order to ensure that the patient's status is clear, some hospitals use special forms for initial orders with the correct language embedded in the form. Similarly, in an electronic record, the patient status (inpatient vs. outpatient observation) would be a required field defined by menu.

In recent years, whether a patient is an inpatient or given outpatient observation status has become a problematic issue for hospitals. The reimbursement for outpatient observation is minimal in comparison with that for inpatient admission. Short-stay inpatient admissions (length of stay 1 or 2 days) are targets of CMS auditors, who look to deny the admission for lack of medical necessity. In order to change the patient status from outpatient observation to inpatient admission, the physician writes a new order to admit to inpatient status. However, if a patient is admitted to inpatient status first and is later (during the admission) changed to outpatient observation status, a specific order must be written and the patient bill must contain a condition code 44 to reflect this action. Many hospitals post case management personnel in the emergency department or patient registration department in order to facilitate the placement of patients in the correct status and to liaise with physicians in the event of uncertainty as to the nature of a physician's order.

### The Patient Registration Department

Hospitals often have an entire department whose function is similar to that of the registration or reception area of a physician's office. The patient registration department (also

**Go To** Chapter 8 explores the flow of data collection in non-acute health care settings.

**assessment** An evaluation. In medical decision making, the physician's evaluation of the subjective and objective evidence. Also refers to the evaluation of a patient by any clinical discipline.

**treatment** A procedure, medication, or other measure designed to cure or alleviate the symptoms of disease.

**inpatient** An individual who is admitted to a hospital with the intention of staying overnight.

**direct admission** An expedited inpatient admission arranged in advance by a physician's office or other entity due to a patient's urgent medical condition.

**skilled nursing facility (SNF)** A long-term care facility providing a range of nursing and other health care services to patients who require continous care, typically those with a chronic illness.

**physician's order** The physician's directions regarding the patient's care.

**outpatient** A patient whose health care services are intended to be delivered within 1 calendar day or, in some cases, a 24-hour period.

**CMS** Centers for Medicare and Medicaid Services

**Go To** Chapter 7 discusses this difference in more detail.

**billing** The process of submitting health insurance claims or rendering invoices.

**coding** The assignment of alphanumerical values to a word, phrase, or other nonnumerical expression. In health care, coding is the assignment of alpha numerical values to diagnosis and procedure descriptions.

**reimbursement** The amount of money that the health care facility receives from the party responsible for paying the bill.

**case management** The coordination of the patient's care and services, including reimbursement considerations.

**ambulatory surgery** Surgery performed on an outpatient basis; the patient returns home after the surgery is performed. Also called *same-day surgery*.

**attending physician** The physician who is primarily responsible for coordinating the care of the patient in the hospital; it is usually the physician who ordered the patient's admission to the hospital.

**admitting diagnosis** The reason given by the physician for initiating the order for the patient to be placed into care in a hospital.

**procedure** A medical or surgical treatment.

**master patient index (MPI)** A system containing a list of patients who have received care at the health care facility and their encounter information, often used to correlate the patient with the file identification.

**face sheet** The first page in a paper record. Usually contains at least the demographic data and contains space for the physician to record and authenticate the discharge diagnoses and procedures. In many facilities, the admission record is also used as the face sheet.

**admission record** The demographic, financial, socioeconomic, and clinical data collected about a patient at registration. Also refers to the document in a paper record that contains these data.

**advance directive** A written document, like a living will, that specifies a patient's wishes for his/her care and dictates power of attorney, for the purpose of providing clear instructions in the event the patient is unable to do so.

**primary care physician (PCP)** In insurance, the physician who has been designated by the insured to deliver routine care to the insured and to evaluate the need for referral to a specialist, if applicable. Colloquial use is synonymous with "family doctor."

**bar code** The representation of data using parallel lines or other patterns in a way readable to a machine, such as an optical bar code scanner or a smartphone.

called the admissions department or patient access department) is responsible for ensuring the timely and accurate registration of patients. Employees who perform the clerical function of completing the paperwork may be called admitting clerks, access clerks, registrars, or patient registration specialists. In a small hospital, the admissions department may consist of only one person; however, in a larger facility, dozens of health care professionals may be trained to register patients.

If there is one place in the hospital where all registration activities are performed, the registration function is said to be centralized. In some facilities, the registration function may be decentralized—that is, registrars are placed in locations throughout the facility. For example, dedicated registration areas may be located in the emergency department, clinics, and ambulatory (same-day) surgery area. However registration is organized, it is a function that must be staffed around the clock, every day of the week.

## Precertification

The patient registration staff must determine whether the patient has insurance and whether the insurance covers the care that the physician has requested. The attending physician must provide an **admitting diagnosis** to explain the reason for admission and a list of any planned procedures as part of the preapproval process. This preapproval, or precertification/insurance verification, process is extremely important to the hospital. Without the confirmation that the insurance company will pay for the patient's stay, the hospital is exposed to the risk of financial loss in the event that the patient is unable to pay for his or her treatment. When the patient's hospitalization is planned, the patient completes the initial registration process and possibly some preadmission testing (e.g., laboratory test and radiology procedures) before the actual hospitalization. This process gives the patient registration department time to obtain the necessary information.

The registration process can be complicated because the registrars must be able to handle any and all admission scenarios and must understand a variety of insurance rules. Because the registrar is often the first hospital staff member that patients and their families meet, providing excellent customer service is important for this professional. Many facilities require registrars to speak at least two languages, depending on the patient population served. In addition, facilities may subscribe to translation services or maintain a call list of employees who speak multiple languages. Many registration departments are staffed and managed by health information professionals. Registrars have their own professional association, the National Association of Healthcare Access Management (http://www.naham.org). The American Association of Healthcare Administrative Managers and the Healthcare Financial Management Association also serve patient registration constituents.

## Registration Process

After the patient arrives at the patient registration reception area, the registration clerk asks the patient for proof of identity and insurance, as well as demographic data, certain socioeconomic data, and financial data. These data are used to populate (or update) the master patient index. In a paper record, these data are printed together on a form known as a **face sheet** or an **admission record** (Table 4-1). In a paper record, it is important to file this form at the beginning of every health record so that the patient is clearly identified to everyone who uses it. Additional data collected at this point include whether the patient has an **advance directive** (a written document, like a living will, that specifies a patient's wishes for his/her care) and the name of the patient's primary care physician.

In addition to printing out the admission record, the admissions department also provides either an identification plate for stamping pages or labels to affix to the individual pages. Using the plate or labels, clinical personnel can identify every page in the record, front and back. If the hospital uses a bar code system, labels with the patient's bar code are also provided. **Bar codes** represent data in a way easily readable by a machine. Some systems allow the printing of forms with the patient's identification data and bar code preprinted on them.

## TABLE 4-1

### SAMPLE DATA INCLUDED IN AN ADMISSION RECORD OR FACE SHEET

| DATA ELEMENT | EXPLANATION |
|---|---|
| Patient's identification number | Number assigned by the facility to this patient |
| Patient's billing number | Number assigned by the facility to this visit |
| Admission date | Calendar day: month, day, and year |
| Discharge date | Calendar day: month, day, and year |
| Patient's name | Full name, including any titles (MD, PhD) |
| Patient's address | Address of usual residence |
| Gender | Male or female |
| Marital status | Married, single, divorced, separated |
| Race and ethnicity | Must choose from choices given on the admissions form |
| Religion | Optional |
| Occupation | General occupation (e.g., teacher, lawyer) |
| Current employment | Specific job (e.g., professor, district attorney) |
| Employer | Company name |
| Insurance | Insurance company name and address |
| Insurance identification numbers | Insurance company group and individual identification numbers |
| Additional insurance | Some patients are insured by multiple companies; all information must be collected |
| Guarantor | Individual or organization responsible for paying the bill if the insurance company declines payment |
| Attending physician | Name of the attending physician; may also include the physician's identification number |
| Admitting diagnosis | Reason the patient is being admitted |

These are typical items that are included in an admission record.

The patient is also asked to sign an **admission** or **general consent form**, with the patient's signature witnessed by the registration clerk. If the patient or the patient's representative is unable to sign this form, the registrar must make a note of this fact and follow up with an attempt to obtain a signature during the hospitalization. In some cases, if the patient is unconscious or not of legal age, an alternative signature is obtained from a parent, guardian, or spouse. The general consent form also contains several key permissions that the patient grants to the facility, as follows:

- Permission for caregivers in the hospital to provide general diagnostic and therapeutic care, such as laboratory tests, radiology examinations, most medications, and intravenous fluids
- Permission to release patient information to the patient's designated third party payer, if applicable, in order to obtain payment for the services rendered and to appeal denials of payment

Consent for invasive procedures, such as surgical procedures, requires additional consent, as discussed later in this chapter. The general consent form also contains acknowledgements that the patient has received certain notifications, such as the notice of patients' rights.

**admission consent form** A form signed by the patient in an inpatient facility granting permission to the hospital to provide general diagnostic and therapeutic care as well as to release patient information to a third party payer, if applicable. Also known as a **general consent form**.

**third party payer** An entity that pays a provider for part or all of a patient's health care services; often the patient's insurance company.

**consent** An agreement or permission to receive health care services.

## HIT-bit

### ADMISSION CONSENT FORMS

Depending on the patient population that the hospital serves, admission consent forms may be printed in various languages, such as Spanish, Polish, Chinese, and Arabic, as well as English. Great care must be taken when translating a form from English to other languages because this form becomes part of the legal patient record. Hospitals often send their forms to companies that specialize in such translations.

**Figure 4-1** The bar code on the patient's wristband contains the patient's medical record number, which links the patient to the patient's medical record. (Courtesy Zebra Technologies Corporation, Lincolnshire, IL.)

**medical record number (MR#)**
A unique number assigned to each patient in a health care system; this code will be used for the rest of the patient's encounters with that specific health system.
**encounter** A patient's interaction with a health care provider to receive services.

**Go To** See Chapter 12 for more information on patient privacy.

**ambulatory care** Care provided on an outpatient basis, in which the patient is not admitted; arriving at a facility, receiving treatment, and leaving within one day.

**admitting physician** The physician who gives the order to observe or admit a patient.
**attending physician** The physician who is primarily responsible for coordinating the care of the patient in the hospital; it is usually the physician who ordered the patient's admission to the hospital.

**SOAP format** Subjective, Objective, Assessment, and Plan: the medical decision-making process used by physicians to assess the patient at various intervals.

**assessment** An evaluation. In medical decision making, the physician's evaluation of the subjective and objective evidence. Also refers to the evaluation of a patient by any clinical discipline.
**plan of care (treatment)** In the SOAP format for medical decision making, the diagnostic, therapeutic, or palliative measures that are taken to investigate or treat the patient's condition or disease.

In addition to beginning the data collection process for the health record and labeling the documents (if required), the registrar must also properly label the patients themselves. Typically, facilities use wristbands to identify each patient. These bands might include the patient's name, birth date, admission date, medical record number (MR#), patient account number, account number, the bar code from admission, and the attending physician's name (Figure 4-1). Recent technology has enabled a picture of the patient to be included on the wristband as well. Once the wristband is donned, it is difficult to remove so that the patient can be clearly identified from it during the hospitalization or encounter at all times. Physicians and all hospital staff must check each patient's wristband before administering any treatments to confirm that they are performing the appropriate treatment for the right patient.

Occasionally, the facility requires that patients be photographed for the purpose of identification. If photographs are taken, care must be taken to comply with all applicable rules to ensure patient privacy.

As mentioned earlier, an acute care hospital has an emergency department. Patients arriving in the emergency department are initially treated as ambulatory care patients because they are expected to be treated and released. Sometimes, however, the condition of the patient warrants admission to the hospital or placement in observation. In this case, a member of the emergency department staff contacts the patient registration department to arrange for the change in status and for the patient to be transported from the emergency department to a bed on a patient unit. The patient registration department changes the patient's status in the registration system, and an inpatient or observation stay is initiated. Clinical information accompanies the patient to the patient unit. Seriously ill patients may not be able to walk to the patient registration area or to provide required data. Therefore additional data collection often takes place at the patient's bedside or with the assistance of family members.

Although it is often the emergency department physician who identifies the need to observe or admit the patient, that physician generally does not write the order to do so. The emergency department physician typically contacts a staff physician, an on-call physician, or the patient's primary care physician to discuss the patient's condition and to issue the order. The physician who issues the order to observe or admit the patient is termed the **admitting physician**. The physician who directs the care given to the patient while hospitalized is termed the **attending physician**. The admitting physician can be different from the attending physician. For example, an on-call or staff physician may admit a patient with chest pain. The patient's cardiologist may then take over the case and become the attending physician.

## Initial Assessment

After being formally admitted, the patient is taken to the appropriate treatment area. This area may be a patient unit, or sometimes it is the preoperative area, where the patient is prepared immediately for surgery. In the treatment area, the patient is assessed by nursing staff to determine the patient's needs during care and obtain vital signs. The physician also performs an assessment of the patient in the **SOAP** structure discussed in Chapter 2.

## Plan of Care

On the basis of the initial assessments, a plan of care is developed for the patient. Because the plan of care may involve many disciplines, often each patient is assigned to a patient care team that consists of various health care professionals in addition to physicians. The initial plan may consist of tests and other diagnostic procedures. A patient admitted for abdominal pain, etiology unknown, will undergo blood tests and possibly an ultrasound or computed tomography (CT) scan to determine the cause of the pain. Once a definitive diagnosis has been established, therapeutic procedures, such as surgery, may take place. For example, it may already have been determined that a patient has appendicitis and the patient has been admitted for an appendectomy. All procedures, whether diagnostic or therapeutic, are undertaken only on the direct order of the physician. Orders may also specify whether the patient has bathroom privileges, may ambulate independently, requires a special diet, or can have visitors.

Other disciplines involved in the care of the patient include nurses and may include but are not limited to: social workers, psychologists, nutritionists, physical and occupational therapists, and respiratory therapists. In the acute care setting, these health care professionals are directed by the physician. In other words, they collaborate in developing and implementing the plan of care but cannot independently direct patient care. Some clinical personnel, such as physicians assistants, midwives, and advanced practice registered nurses, may be licensed as independent practitioners and may, through the hospital's credentialing process, be approved to direct specific, limited types of patient care independently of a physician. In other cases, they may be dependent practitioners, directing patient care under the auspices of a particular physician.

Although physicians direct patient care and are responsible for the overall plan, they are not always present with the patient during the inpatient stay. They may have office hours elsewhere or admit patients to multiple facilities. Some exceptions to this situation are hospitalists, who spend most of their time on the hospital premises, and intensivists, who focus their efforts on patients in critical care units. In some cases, the physician is not present at all and care is directed long distance (called **telemedicine**). In such cases, the physicians rely on nursing staff to advise them of changes in the patient's status or problems that may arise. Nursing practice has evolved its own standards of practice, and nurses are diligent in documenting patient care and the events surrounding care. Because nurses spend far more time with a patient than the attending physician, nurse feedback is important to the physician's medical decision making.

## Discharge

Data continues to be collected and assessed throughout the patient's stay. The utilization review (UR) or case management personnel monitor the patient's care and facilitate the discharge of the patient to the appropriate setting. Discharge, like admission, is preceded by a physician's order.

### ▪ EXERCISE 4-1

#### Clinical Flow of Data

1. Upon admission, patient data are collected that help identify the patient and the payer for the services to be rendered. List as many data items (fields) as you can recall that would be included in an admission record.
2. Describe the patient registration process.
3. Who contributes to the collection of clinical data?

## CLINICAL DATA

Physicians, nurses, therapists, and numerous ancillary and administrative departments contribute a wide variety of notes, reports, and documentation of events. As discussed in Chapter 2, such documentation consists of collections of data organized in a logical manner into forms or data entry screens that build the health record. This section covers the major data elements that each of these professionals contributes and the traditionally named form into which the data are collected. Figure 4-2 shows the contributors of health data and the collections of data that they contribute.

---

**etiology** The cause or source of the patient's condition or disease.

**CT** computed tomography

**acute care facility** A health care facility in which patients have an average length of stay less than 30 days and that has an emergency department, operating suite, and clinical departments to handle a broad range of diagnoses and treatments.

**hospitalist** A physician employed by a hospital, whose medical practice is primarily focused on patient care situations specific to the acute care setting.
**telemedicine** Care provided through the use of mobile technology, which allows care providers to view and consult patient from satellite locations.

**utilization review (UR)** The process of evaluating medical interventions against established criteria, on the basis of the patient's known or tentative diagnosis. Evaluation may take place before, during, or after the episode of care for different purposes.
**case management** The coordination of the patient's care and services, including reimbursement considerations.

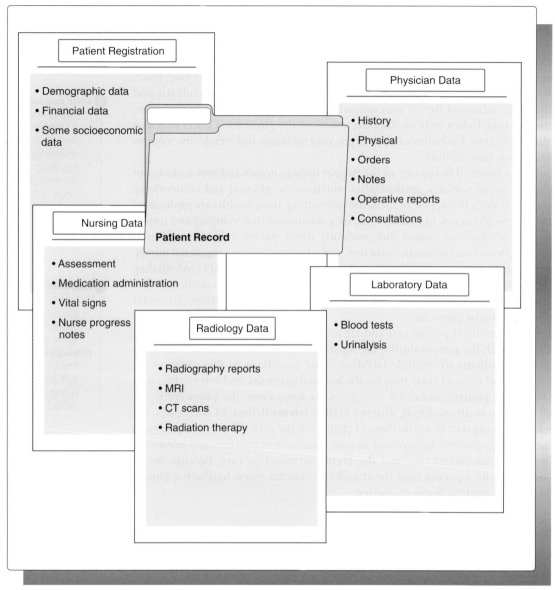

**Figure 4-2** Sample data elements in a health record by source. CT, computed tomography; MRI, magnetic resonance imaging.

The primary purpose of the clinical data is communication. The communication is certainly among clinicians before, during, and after the specific episode of care. It is also part of the business record of the hospital and therefore supports both the legal record of the care rendered as well as the documentation of the charges for that care. Therefore accurate, complete documentation is essential for multiple reasons.

## Physicians

When the patient is admitted, the attending physician conducts a medical evaluation. This SOAP-structured evaluation contains the subjective history, the objective physical examination, the assessment of a preliminary diagnosis or diagnoses, and a plan of care, for which orders are recorded. Medical decision making is a complex activity that depends on the number of possible diagnoses, the volume and complexity of diagnostic data that must be reviewed, and the severity of the patient's condition. This complexity is reflected in the physician's documentation. Figure 4-3 illustrates the components of medical decision making.

**attending physician** The physician who is primarily responsible for coordinating the care of the patient in the hospital; it is usually the physician who ordered the patient's admission to the hospital.

**SOAP format** Subjective, Objective, Assessment, and Plan: the medical decision-making process used by physicians to assess the patient at various intervals.

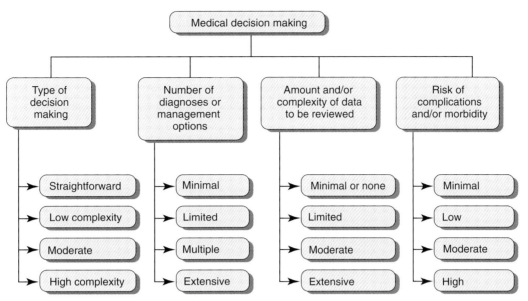

**Figure 4-3** Flowchart of medical decision making. (From Andress AA: Saunders' manual of medical office management, Philadelphia, 1996, Saunders, p 96.)

---

**BOX 4-1   THE PATIENT'S HISTORY**

If a patient visits the emergency department because of a splinter in a finger, a simple, or problem-focused, history is directed only toward the presenting problem (the splinter), and very little else is discussed or observed. The history would probably contain nothing more than the events surrounding the occurrence of the splinter and possibly an inquiry as to whether the patient had received a tetanus vaccination in the past 10 years.

The finger may appear to be infected, possibly leading to a blood test and thus an expanded review.

Perhaps the patient had fallen beforehand, prompting the physician to suspect possible head trauma or fracture, which would require review of the head and extremities as well as the abdomen and skin for possible soft tissue injury or injury to internal organs: a detailed review. The history becomes increasingly complex as the number of body systems involved and the potential threat to the patient's life become more evident.

A patient admitted to an acute care facility requires more substantive evaluation, particularly when the underlying illness is still under investigation. In that case, the physician collects a comprehensive history. The physician makes more detailed inquiries about the patient's entire medical history and asks questions about additional body systems.

---

**History**

A **history** is taken from the data that the patient reports to the physician regarding the patient's health. Table 4-2 lists the data elements that are collected in a history. This information may be written by hand, but it is preferably preserved in a dictated report that is later transcribed. In a fully electronic point-of-care documentation system, either the history could be dictated through the use of a speech recognition program or data could be collected by means of menu-driven prompts or templates. In an inpatient setting, the history is usually extensive and comprehensive. The history should consist of the **chief complaint** (the reason that the patient presented for evaluation and treatment), the history of the complaint, a description of relevant previous illnesses and procedures, and a review of body systems. The complexity of the history is directly related to the amount of data that the physician needs to evaluate the patient's problem, measured by the number of body systems that are reported. See Box 4-1 for an example.

**history** The physician's record of the patient's chief complaint, history of present illness, pertinent family and social history, and review of systems.

**point-of-care documentation** Clinical data recorded at the time the treatment is delivered to the patient.

**chief complaint** The main reason a patient has sought treatment.

## TABLE 4-2

### DATA ELEMENTS IN A HISTORY AND LEVEL OF HISTORY

| DATA ELEMENT | EXPLANATION | LEVEL OF HISTORY* | | | |
|---|---|---|---|---|---|
| | | PROBLEM-FOCUSED | EXPANDED PROBLEM-FOCUSED | DETAILED | COMPREHENSIVE |
| Chief complaint | The reason for the encounter, usually as expressed by the patient | — | — | — | — |
| History of present illness | The patient's report of the events, circumstances, and other details surrounding the chief complaint | Brief | Brief | Extended | Extended |
| Review of systems | The patient's responses to the physician's questions regarding pertinent body systems, including: Constitutional symptoms Eyes Ears, nose, mouth, and throat Cardiovascular Respiratory Gastrointestinal Genitourinary Musculoskeletal Integumentary Neurological Psychiatric Endocrine Hematological/lymphatic Allergic/immunological | N/A | Problem pertinent | Extended | Complete |
| Personal, family, and/or social history | Including the patient's prior illnesses and operations, socioeconomic concerns, and important family illnesses | N/A | N/A | Pertinent | Complete |

*All histories contain, at a minimum, the chief complaint and the history of present illness. The history can have four levels of complexity.
Modified from U.S. Department of Health and Human Services, Centers for Medicare and Medicaid Services: Evaluation and management services guide. http://www.cms.gov/Outreach-and-Education/Medicare-Learning-Network-MLN/MLNProducts/downloads/eval_mgmt_serv_guide-ICN006764.pdf. Published 2010. Accessed August 17, 2012.

**physical examination** The physician's record of examination of the patient.

**assessment** The physician's evaluation of the subjective and objective evidence.

**plan of treatment** In the SOAP format for medical decision making, the diagnostic, therapeutic, or palliative measures that are taken to investigate or treat the patient's condition or disease.

**history and physical (H&P)** Heath record documentation comprising the patient's history and physical examination; a formal, dictated copy must be included in the patient's health care record within 24 hours of admission for inpatient facilities.

### Physical Examination

After collecting the appropriate history data, the physician performs the objective portion of the evaluation: the **physical examination**. Like the history, the physical examination may be dictated and transcribed, dictated through speech recognition, entered through menus/templates, or handwritten. The physical examination (or more briefly, the physical) includes the physician's examination and observations of every pertinent body system. The term "pertinent" is used because the physical generally follows the same level of complexity as the history. For example, the patient with the splinter may require only an examination of the affected finger. In the absence of infection or other trauma, a problem-focused physical examination is appropriate. Moreover, it is not appropriate for the physician to perform a comprehensive physical examination of the patient with a splinter in the absence of a history indicating its necessity. In many cases, gynecological and rectal examinations are omitted, sometimes at the patient's request and certainly when no related abnormalities or disorders are suspected. The physical examination ends with the physician's assessment, also called the impression, and the initial plan of treatment. Table 4-3 lists data elements that are collected in a physical.

When the history and physical data are collected and reported together in a single, longer report, such a report is referred to as the **history and physical (H&P)**. Note that the H&P follows the medical evaluation process previously described. The subjective data (the patient's history) are followed by the objective data (the physical), and then the assessment and the plan of care are recorded.

**TABLE 4-3**

**DATA ELEMENTS IN A PHYSICAL EXAMINATION**

| LEVEL OF EXAMINATION | BODY AREA(S)/ORGAN SYSTEM(S) |
|---|---|
| Problem-focused | Affected body area (BA) and organ system (OS) |
| Expanded problem-focused | Affected BA and other BAs/OSs |
| Detailed | Extensive affected BAs/OSs |
| Comprehensive | Complete BAs and complete OSs |
| Area | Definition |
| Organ systems | Eyes |
| | Ears, nose, mouth, and throat |
| | Respiratory |
| | Cardiovascular |
| | Genitourinary |
| | Hematological/lymphatic immunological |
| | Musculoskeletal |
| | Skin |
| | Neurological |
| | Psychiatric |
| | Gastrointestinal |
| Body areas | Head |
| | Neck |
| | Chest |
| | Abdomen |
| | Genitalia, groin, buttocks |
| | Back |
| | Extremities |
| General | Constitutional (vital signs, general appearance) |

Modified from U.S. Department of Health and Human Services, Centers for Medicare and Medicaid Services: Evaluation and management services guide. http://www.cms.gov/Outreach-and-Education/Medicare-Learning-Network-MLN/MLNProducts/downloads/eval_mgmt_serv_guide-ICN006764.pdf. Published 2010. Accessed August 17, 2012.

The data collected in these two reports are critical for patient management; therefore specific rules direct the completion of this data collection activity. In an acute care facility, CMS (and consequently The Joint Commission [TJC]) requires that the history and physical be present in the record no more than 30 days before or 24 hours after admission or registration, but prior to surgery or a procedure requiring anesthesia services (Federal Register, 2012b; The Joint Commission, 2012). H&Ps performed more than 30 days prior to admission are not acceptable for the current admission, and a new H&P must be documented. H&Ps performed within 7 days of admission may be accepted as documented; however, H&Ps performed more than 7 days prior to admission must contain an interval note: a brief description by the physician regarding any changes in the patient's condition or the physician's assessment thereof.

The physician collecting and recording the H&P must authenticate those data. In teaching hospitals, the H&P may be performed by a resident physician. State law and medical staff bylaws or rules and regulations will specify to what extent an attending physician is required to cosign the documentation of a resident or medical student. Documentation by first-year residents (also known as interns) generally must be cosigned because these residents have not obtained their medical licenses.

Box 4-2 discusses the H&P in other health care settings.

## Orders

Only those authorized by the medical staff rules and regulations can write orders, and this authorization can be different for each organization. In some hospitals, physician assistants and midwives may be able to write physician's orders, but in other facilities only MD and DO clinicians may do so. While the patient is in the facility, the physician makes decisions

**CMS** Centers for Medicare and Medicaid Services
**TJC** The Joint Commission

**authenticate** To assume responsibility for data collection or the activities described by the data collection by signature, mark, code, password, or other means of identification.
**resident** A person who, after attending college and medical school, performs professional duties under the supervision of a fully qualified physician.

**H&P** history and physical

**MD** medical doctor
**DO** doctor of osteopathy

**treatment** A procedure, medication, or other measure designed to cure or alleviate the symptoms of disease.

**admitting diagnosis** The reason given by the physician for initiating the order for the patient to be placed into care in a hospital.

**plan of treatment** In the SOAP format for medical decision making, the diagnostic, therapeutic, or palliative measures that are taken to investigate or treat the patient's condition or disease.

**etiology** The cause or source of the patient's condition or disease.

**physician's order** The physician's directions regarding the patient's care. Also refers to the data collection device on which these elements are captured.

**clinical decision-making system (CDS)** A computer application that compares two or more items of patient data in order to advise clinicians on the treatment of that specific patient.

**CPOE** computerized physician order entry

**Go To** Review Chapter 3 for more information on clinical decision-making systems and CPOE.

**protocol** A predetermined plan of care that guides the health care professional toward best practices in diagnosing or treating the condition. Also called an **order set**.

**accreditation** Voluntary compliance with a set of standards developed by an independent agent, who periodically performs audits to ensure compliance.

**VO** verbal order
**TO** telephone order

about the patient's **treatment**, including those pertaining to any further diagnostic testing. For example, a patient who is scheduled for a hemicolectomy (excision of part of the colon) may have entered the hospital with an admitting diagnosis of chronic diverticulitis or colon cancer. The **plan of treatment** includes the removal of part of the colon. Other patients enter the hospital with vague or multiple symptoms, and the physician is not entirely sure which of several possible conditions the patient actually has. In the SOAP note example discussed in Chapter 2, the right lower quadrant abdominal pain could have a number of different etiologies, or causes, which are investigated while the patient is in the hospital. In an acute care facility, the physician must specifically order the diagnostic procedures that will help reveal the patient's diagnosis.

The physician's instructions for laboratory tests, radiological examinations, consultations, and medication are all contained in a separate data collection called **physician's orders**. Physician's orders may be recorded in a patient's record on an order form or by direct entry into a computer. Orders may be captured electronically at the point of care through a systematic process that includes interaction with the formulary (hospital's list of approved medications), the patient's information (such as height and weight), and clinical decision making systems (CDSs) (knowledge database that assists in the prescription of medications and the prevention of conflicting or erroneous orders). CPOE is the software that enables this electronic data capture. No tests or treatment can take place without the physician's order. Orders must be dated, timed, and authenticated by the physician.

Although each patient is treated individually on the basis of clinical presentation, many conditions call for a predetermined plan of care that guides the health care professional toward best practices in diagnosing or treating the condition. This predetermined plan may include a specific series of blood tests, radiographs, and urinalysis. It may also consist of a set of preoperative or pretherapeutic activities. Such predetermined plans are called **protocols** or **order sets**. Protocols arise from evidence-based, best practices as developed and documented by the relevant specialty. They may be applied voluntarily by the facility or they may be mandated for compliance with regulatory or accreditation standards. Protocols may be printed on a paper form or set up as a group of related orders in the CPOE. An example of a standard protocol or order set is that for venous thromboembolism (VTE) prophylaxis (Figure 4-4). Because virtually every patient admitted to the hospital is at risk for blood clots in the extremities, orders to assess and take preventive measures are an important factor in the quality of care. The order to put a set of protocols into effect comes from the physician, who is still required to authenticate, date, and time the orders.

Orders may be directly entered by the physician or dictated to a registered nurse, who then enters the orders. Orders that are dictated to a registered nurse are called verbal orders (VOs). VOs that are communicated over the telephone are called telephone orders (TOs). VOs and TOs are sometimes necessary in emergencies and in situations in which the physician is unable to be present at the hospital at the time the orders are required. VOs and TOs must be authenticated by the physician, although they can be executed immediately. The recipient of the order must record it, read it back for confirmation, and evidence the read-back. The recipient of the order must sign, date, and time the receipt and method of receiving the order. The CMS requires authentication of a VO or

| Low Risk | Moderate Risk | High Risk |
|---|---|---|
| Ambulatory patient without additional VTE risk factors or expected length of stay <2 days<br><br>Minor surgery in patient without additional VTE risk factors (same day surgery or operating room time <30 minutes).<br><br>*Early ambulation | Patients who aren't in either the low- or high-risk group (go to <u>VTE risk factor table</u>)<br><br>Select one pharmacologic* option:<br><br>• Enoxaparin† 40 mg SQ q 24 hours<br>• UFH 5,000 units SQ q 8 hours<br>• UFH 5,000 units SQ q 12 hours (use only if wt <50 kg or >75 years)<br>or<br>• No pharmacological prophylaxis because of contraindication<br><br>(go to <u>Contraindications table</u> below)<br><br>• No pharmacological prophylaxis because it is optional in this special population (GYN surgery).<br><br>Sequential compression device aka SCDs (Optional for these patients if they are on pharmacological prophylaxis, mandatory if not).<br><br>SCDs to<br>• Both lower extremities<br>• Right leg only<br>• Left leg only<br>• Patient intolerant or has skin lesions on both legs, do not use SCDs | Elective hip or knee arthroplasty<br>Acute spinal cord injury with paresis<br>Multiple major trauma<br>Abdominal or pelvic surgery for cancer<br><br>Select one pharmacologic† option:<br><br>• Enoxaparin* 40 mg SQ q 24 hours<br>• Enoxaparin* 30 mg SQ q 12 hours (knee replacement)<br>• Warfarin_____ mg PO daily, target INR 2-3; hold INR >3<br>or<br>• UFH 5,000 units SQ q 8 hours (only if creatinine clearance is <30, SCr >2, and warfarin is not an option)<br>• No pharmacological prophylaxis because of contraindication<br><br>(go to <u>Contraindications table</u> below)<br><br>and<br><br>SCDs to<br>• Both lower extremities<br>• Right leg only<br>• Left leg only<br>• Patient intolerant or has skin lesions on both legs, do not use SCDs |

* Go to <u>Contraindications table</u>.
† Enoxaparin should only be used in patients with CrCl>30 and SCr<2; do not use if epidural/spinal catheter is in place.
SCDs should be used in all patients for whom pharmacologic prophylaxis is contraindicated and in all high-risk patients unless patient is intolerant or with contraindications to SCDs.
Note: Enoxaparin is the USCD Medical Center formulary low molecular weight heparin (LMWH); other LMWHs are considered equivalent.
<u>Return to Contents</u>

| **Venous Thromboembolism Risk Factors** | | |
|---|---|---|
| Age >50 years<br>Myeloproliferative disorder<br>Dehydration<br>Congestive heart failure<br>Active malignancy<br>Hormonal replacement<br>Moderate to major surgery | Prior history of VTE<br>Impaired mobility<br>Inflammatory bowel disease<br>Active rheumatic disease<br>Sickle cell disease<br>Estrogen-based contraceptives<br>Central venous catheter | Acute or chronic lung disease<br>Obesity<br>Known thrombophilic state<br>Varicose veins/chronic stasis<br>Recent post-partum with immobility<br>Nephrotic syndrome<br>Myocardial infarction |

<u>Return to Contents</u>

| **Contraindications or Other Conditions to Consider with Pharmacological VTE Prophylaxis** | | |
|---|---|---|
| • Active hemorrhage<br>• Severe trauma to head or spinal cord with hemorrhage in the last 4 weeks<br>• Other _____ | • Intracranial hemorrhage within last year<br>• Craniotomy within 2 weeks<br>• Intraocular surgery within 2 weeks<br>• Gastrointestinal, genitourinary hemorrhage within the last month<br>• Thrombocytopenia (<50K) or coagulopathy (prothrombin time >18 seconds)<br>• End-stage liver disease<br>• Active intracranial lesions/neoplasms<br>• Hypertensive urgency/emergency<br>• Post-operative bleeding concerns†† | • Immune-mediated heparin-induced thrombocytopenia<br>• Epidural analgesia with spinal catheter (current or planned) |

†† Scheduled return to OR within the next 24 hours: major ortho: 24 hours leeway; spinal cord or ortho spine: 7 days leeway; general surgery, status post-transplant, status post-trauma admission: 48 hours leeway

**Figure 4-4** University of California, San Diego Medical Center VTE Risk Assessment and Prophylaxis Orders (paper version of computerized order set). CRCl, creatinine clearance, <30 mL/min.; GYN, gynecological; INR, international normalized ratio; OR, operating room; SCr, serum creatinine concentration, in mg/dL; SQ, subcutaneously; UFH, unfractionated heparin; VTE, venous thromboembolism. *Note:* Definition of thrombocytopenia (bottom table) is <50,000 platelets per mL of blood. (From U.S. Department of Health and Human Services, Agency for Healthcare Research and Quality: Preventing Hospital-Acquired Venous Thromboembolism. Appendix B: Sample Venous Thromboembolism Protocol Order/Set. http://www.ahrq.gov/qual/vtguide/vtguideapb.htm).

## TABLE 4-4

### DATA REQUIRED FOR AN ORDER PERSONALLY ENTERED BY THE PHYSICIAN

| DATA ELEMENT | EXPLANATION |
|---|---|
| Patient's name | Full name, including any titles (MD, PhD) |
| Patient's identification number | Number assigned by the facility to this patient |
| Order date | Date the order is rendered |
| Time | Time the order is rendered |
| Order | Medication, test, therapy, consultation, or other action directed by the physician |
| Physician's authentication | Physician's signature or password |
| Executor's authentication | Signature or password of party effecting the order |
| Execution date | Date the order was effected |
| Execution time | Time the order was effected |

An important element of a physician's order is the time that it is rendered. The interpretation of the requirement to authenticate verbal orders as soon as possible is often "within 24 hours." Implicitly, this requires a date and time attached to both the order and the authentication. If the physician personally makes the order, then the date and time of both are the same. If it is a verbal order, then the nurse taking the order must record the date and time, and the physician logs the appropriate date and time of the subsequent authentication. In a paper-based system, omitting the time of the order is a compliance issue. However, in a computer-based order entry system, the time can be automatically affixed by the computer.

## TABLE 4-5

### DATA REQUIRED FOR A VERBAL ORDER FROM THE PHYSICIAN

| DATA ELEMENT | EXPLANATION |
|---|---|
| Patient's name | Full name, including any titles (MD, PhD) |
| Patient's identification number | Number assigned to the patient by the facility |
| Order date | Date the order is received |
| Time | Time the order is received |
| Nurse's authentication | Signature or password of party receiving the order |
| Order | Medication, test, therapy, consultation, or other action directed by the physician |
| Verification | Note that the order was "read back" to the ordering physician |
| Physician's authentication | Physician's signature or password |
| Physician's authentication date | Date the order is authenticated |
| Physician's authentication time | Time the physician authenticated the order |
| Executor's authentication | Signature or password of party effecting the order |
| Execution date | Date the order was effected |
| Execution time | Time the order was effected |

**Centers for Medicare and Medicaid Services (CMS)** The division of the U.S. Department of Health and Human Services that administers Medicare and Medicaid.

**authenticate** To assume responsibility for data collection or the activities described by the data collection by signature, mark, code, password, or other means of identification.

**VO** verbal order
**TO** telephone order

TO within 48 hours of the communication of the order, or in a time frame specified by state law (Federal Register, 2012a). Individual facilities may have stricter requirements. All orders must be dated, timed, and authenticated. Compliance with authentication rules is measured from the time the order is communicated to the nurse to the date and time of the authentication.

The medical staff must clearly define who is eligible to accept a VO or TO and under what circumstances. Pharmacists, respiratory therapists, and radiology technicians, for example, may be permitted to accept a VO or TO specific to their discipline.

Tables 4-4 and 4-5 list the data contained in an order.

Nursing staff execute the orders, or put them into effect, by notifying the appropriate department or outside agency of the order. For example, medications may be requested from the hospital pharmacy, radiological examinations may be arranged, or a consultant may be contacted. The nurse who executes the order authenticates and dates the activity (see Figure 4-5).

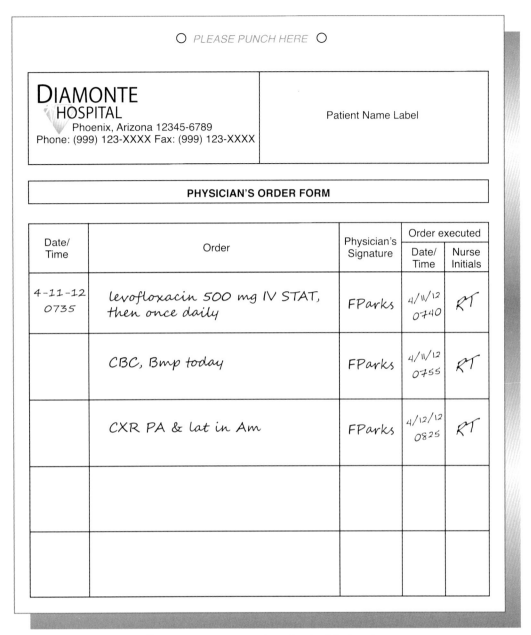

Figure 4-5 Nurse execution of a physician's orders.

Typically, the first order in the inpatient record is the order to admit. Not surprisingly, the last order is to discharge. Patients should not be released from the hospital without a discharge order. Patients who insist on leaving the hospital prior to a physician's order may be considered to have left against medical advice. Some orders are constrained by rules that are dictated by either the facility or a regulatory or accrediting body. DNR (do not resuscitate) and restraints are examples of special orders that require specific documentation.

### Progress Notes

While treating the patient, the physician continues to make observations and update the assessment and plan. These **progress notes** are important evidence of the care that the patient has received and serve to document the physician's activities and evaluation process. Progress notes are required as often as needed to document treatment provided to the patient and in acute care they must be written at least daily to validate the need for this level of care. Notes are often documented in the SOAP format; some physicians even write the SOAP acronym on the note. In an inpatient setting, progress notes become critical

**progress notes** The physician's record of each interaction with the patient.

**SOAP** subjective, objective, assessment, plan

**H&P** history and physical

**resident** A person who, after attending college and medical school, performs professional duties under the supervision of a fully qualified physician.

**countersigned** Evidence of supervision of subordinate personnel, such as physician residents.

**attending physician** The physician who is primarily responsible for coordinating the care of the patient in the hospital; it is usually the physician who ordered the patient's admission to the hospital.

**consultation** The formal request by a physician for the professional opinion or services of another health care professional, usually another physician, in caring for a patient. Also refers to the opinion or services themselves as well as the activity of rendering the opinion or services.

**consultant** A medical professional who provides clinical expertise in a specialty at the request of the attending physician.

**discharge summary** The recap of an inpatient stay, usually dictated by the attending physician and transcribed into a formal report.

because days, weeks, or months may elapse from the time of the H&P obtained at admission to the time of the patient's discharge. Notes must be dated, timed, and authenticated. In a facility in which physician residents are training, the resident may collect and record the data for the note. In many organizations, and always for unlicensed residents, the resident's note must also be authenticated, or **countersigned**, by the attending physician.

### Consultations

Physicians collaborate with one another through the **consultation** process. The attending physician, who is responsible for the patient's overall care, requests a consultation, citing the specific reason for the consultation. For example, a patient admitted for treatment of a heart condition may experience severe diarrhea. The attending physician may request a consultation from a gastrointestinal specialist or an infectious disease specialist. A patient undergoing a hemicolectomy may also have chronic obstructive pulmonary disease, emphysema, asthma, or other severe respiratory problem, in which case the attending physician may elect to call in a pulmonologist (a physician who specializes in diseases of the lung) to evaluate the patient's status before surgery. Some typical consultations that may be performed in an inpatient setting include an endocrinology consultation if the patient has diabetes mellitus; a podiatry consultation if the patient has hypertrophy of the nails (overgrown toenails) or onychomycosis (fungal infection of the toenail); a cardiology consultation if the patient has some sort of heart condition; and, as mentioned previously, a pulmonary specialist if the patient has respiratory concerns. Another typical type of consultation is a psychiatric consultation, which would be appropriate if the patient suffers from depression or other behavioral health issues. Table 4-6 lists the data required for a consultation document. The **consultant** evaluates the patient and responds to the request with specific diagnostic or therapeutic opinions and recommendations. The consultant's response is usually dictated and transcribed but may be handwritten if hospital policy permits.

### Discharge Summary

In an inpatient setting, a **discharge summary**, or case summary of the patient's care, is prepared by the attending physician or his or her designee. This summary should include a brief history of the presenting problem, the discharge diagnosis and other significant findings, a list of the treatments and procedures performed, the patient's condition at discharge, medications given during the stay and those prescribed for at-home administration, follow-up care or appointments, and any instructions given to the patient or patient's caregiver. As with other data, the discharge summary must be dated, timed, and authenticated. The recording of the discharge summary often takes the form of a dictated and transcribed report.

| TABLE 4-6 | |
|---|---|
| **DATA REQUIRED FOR A CONSULTATION** | |
| **DATA ELEMENT** | **EXPLANATION** |
| Patient's name | Full name, including any titles (MD, PhD) |
| Patient's identification number | Number assigned by the facility to this patient |
| Physician's order | Required before the consultation is performed (see Tables 4-4 and 4-5) |
| Date of request | Date that the attending physician requests the consultation |
| Specialty being consulted | Cardiology, podiatry, gastroenterology, etc. |
| Reason for consultation | Brief explanation of reason that the consultant's opinion is being sought |
| Authentication | Authentication of physician requesting consultation |
| Date of evaluation | When consultant saw patient |
| Consultant's opinion | Diagnosis or recommendations; may be an entire report, similar to an H&P (see Tables 4-2 and 4-3). The opinion will include relevant acknowledgements from the patient's record, such as mention of laboratory values or the attending physician's notes. |
| Report date | Date that consultant prepares report of the opinion |
| Authentication | Authentication of consultant |

Some inpatient stays do not require a discharge summary, such as that of a normal newborn. Generally, stays of less than 48 hours' duration do not require a detailed discharge summary; a form called a final progress note/record may be completed instead. An exception to this occurs when a patient who has been in a hospital for less than 48 hours expires. In such cases, a full discharge summary is required.

## Nurses

While the patient is in the hospital, the professionals who perform most of the patient's care, particularly in acute care and long-term care facilities, are the nurses and their ancillary staff. Nurses collect and record their own set of data for each patient. As with physician data, nursing data also require dates, times, and authentication.

### Nursing Assessment

Nurses perform an assessment of the patient when the patient first enters the facility. The purpose of the **nursing assessment** is not to diagnose the patient's illness—that is the responsibility of the physician—but to evaluate the patient's care needs. The assessment includes determining the patient's understanding of his or her condition and whether the patient has any particular concerns or needs that will affect nursing care. The nursing assessment includes an evaluation of the condition of the patient's skin, understanding of his or her condition, diagnosis or reason for admission, learning needs, and ability to perform self-care.

### Nursing Progress Notes

Nurses also must record **nursing progress notes**. During each shift, the nurse documents particular events or interactions with the patient. Patient complaints and any activities of the nursing staff to address those complaints are noted. The elements of a nursing progress note are given in Table 4-7. In a paper-based record, these notes typically take the form of free text. In an electronic health record (EHR), the documentation may be guided and at least partially menu-driven, using templates for required documentation. The organization of the notes may be chronological or by care plan.

### Vital Signs

Nurses are also responsible for observing and recording the patient's vital signs. Vital signs consist of temperature, blood pressure, pulse, and respiration. Frequently, vital signs are recorded in a graphic format, which can be referenced easily while the patient is in the facility. Chapter 2 demonstrates how displaying a patient's temperature in a graph or picture facilitates review of the data (see Figure 2-3). In an EHR the data are entered into

**long-term care (LTC) facility** A hospital that provides services to patients over an extended period; an average length of stay is in excess of 30 days. Facilities are characterized by the extent to which nursing care is provided.

**authenticate** To assume responsibility for data collection or the activities described by the data collection by signature, mark, code, password, or other means of identification.

**nursing assessment** The nurse's evaluation of the patient.

**nursing progress notes** Routine documentation of the nurse's interaction with a patient.

**EHR** electronic health record

| TABLE 4-7 | |
|---|---|
| **DATA REQUIRED FOR A NURSE'S PROGRESS NOTE** | |
| **DATA ELEMENT** | **EXPLANATION** |
| Patient's name | Full name, including any titles (MD, PhD) |
| Patient's identification number | Number assigned to the patient by the facility |
| Date | Date of the note |
| Time | Time of the note |
| Note | Nurse's comments, observations, and documentation of activities |
| Nurse's authentication | Nurse's signature or password |

Notes should be written as soon as possible after the activity has occurred. Thus the date and time of the note coincide with the date and time of the occurrence. If a note is written after the fact, the date and time of the occurrence must be separately noted.

In a paper-based system, the note field is generally a large alphanumerical field in which the nurse can comment freely. In a computer-based system, this field may be replaced with a series of fields from which the nurse can compose comments from predetermined menus, in addition to a free field for more specific remarks. The actual content of the note is governed by the patient's condition, nursing professional standards and facility requirements.

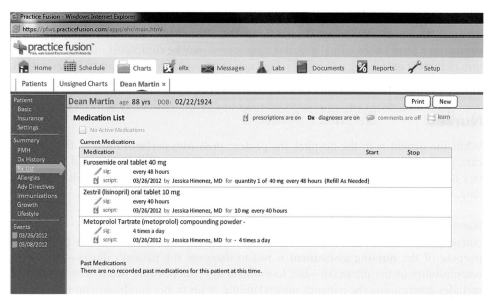

**Figure 4-6** Electronic report of medication administration. (Courtesy Practice Fusion, Inc., San Francisco, CA.)

a field that can then be linked to previous data collections to produce a report that is a graphic representation of the cumulative data over time. Electronic recording devices such as cardiac monitors may automatically record the data into the EHR for real-time data review. Other data that nurses collect that are frequently reported in graph format include fluid intake and output and mechanical ventilation readings.

### Medication Administration

One of the most important nursing data collections involves **medication administration**. The name of the medication, dosage, date and time of administration, method of administration, and the name of nurse who administered it are important data elements. Medication administration sheets traditionally take the form of a table, with the medication specifics down the left side and the administration dates across the top of the columns, with the times and nurse initials in the table cells. An example of a paper medication administration record is in Appendix A. In an electronic medication administration record, the data is captured at each administration, and a report of the administrations can then be printed, if necessary. See Figure 4-6.

Controls surrounding the administration of medications are focused on the prevention of medication errors. Personnel administering medications are required to identify the patient prior to administration by reviewing the data on the patient's wristband (name, medical record number) and comparing it with the data on the medication dispensed by the pharmacy. Ideally, a computer-generated bar code system used both on the wristband and by the pharmacy, linked to the electronic record, can facilitate this process. The nurse can scan the wristband, which brings up the medication order on the computer screen, then scan the dispensed medication, which matches the order with the drugs (Figure 4-7). If these elements match, the nurse can complete the administration. If not, the error can be identified and resolved.

## Laboratory Data

In an inpatient setting, the physician frequently orders routine **laboratory tests**, such as a complete blood count (CBC) and a urinalysis (UA). When these laboratory tests are performed at the time of the patient's admission, they help identify preexisting infectious conditions. Infections identified after 48 hours of hospitalization are attributed to the facility; these are called **nosocomial infections**. Laboratory tests are performed only when ordered by the physician. The results of the tests are included in the health record.

---

**medication administration** Clinical data including the name of the medication, dosage, date and time of administration, method of administration, and the nurse who administered it.

**bar code** The representation of data using parallel lines or other patterns in a way readable to a machine, such as an optical barcode scanner or a smartphone.

**laboratory tests** Procedures for analysis of body fluids.
**nosocomial infection** A hospital-acquired infection.

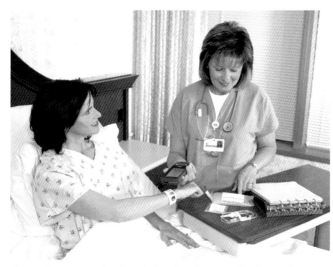

**Figure 4-7** Using bar codes on a patient's wristband and on medication to improve bedside medication verification (BMV). (Courtesy Zebra Technologies Corporation, Lincolnshire, IL.)

Laboratory results include both patient-specific data and data comparing the patient's test results with normative ranges of data. For example, the normal hemoglobin range is 12.0 to 15.0 g/dL for female adults. A female adult patient whose hemoglobin level is 14.3 g/dL is within normal limits. If a female adult patient's hemoglobin is 6.5 g/dL, the laboratory would flag these results as abnormal.

In an inpatient setting, the number of laboratory tests may be voluminous, depending on the extent to which a patient's condition needs to be monitored or the number of tests required to establish or validate a diagnosis. For some conditions, daily blood tests are appropriate. Other conditions may require hourly monitoring. Therefore multiple data fields, in which the results of multiple tests can be recorded, are necessary. As in other situations, the usefulness of an electronic record is evident. Once the test result data are collected, a computer can display them in whole or in part, as well as graphically.

## Radiology Data

**Radiology examinations** generate two sets of data: the original diagnostic image and the interpretation. The original diagnostic image is usually retained separately from the patient's record. For example, a radiology examination of the chest traditionally produces a large film, which is retained in a special envelope or file, usually in the radiology department. Facilities are increasingly relying on digital methods of radiographic imaging, recorded in a picture archiving computer system (PACS). These images are stored in the radiology imaging system, which may be linked to the EHR. Some electronic records can interface with the radiology system and display the radiographic image within the patient's electronic record. These digital images may be downloaded to a disk with the reading software and given to the patient for continuing patient care.

The radiologist's interpretation of the image, film or digital, which typically takes the form of a dictated and transcribed report, becomes part of the patient's record.

## Special Records

The previously discussed data elements are very common and occur in one form or another in almost all inpatient health records. The clinical flow of data is similar in every type of health care setting. Depending on the diagnosis and the clinical setting, many other data elements are collected.

However, even in an acute care facility, certain clinical situations require additional documentation or variations on the standard documentation described in the previous sections. For example, other types of documentation may include cardiology reports such

**radiology examination** The examination of internal body structures using radiographs and other imaging technologies.

**electronic health record (EHR)** A secure real-time, point-of-care, patient centric information resource for clinicians allowing access to patient information when and where needed and incorporating evidence-based decision support.

**interface** Computer configuration allowing information to pass from one system to another.

**Go To** Refer to Chapter 3 for an understanding of the way PACS works. Chapter 8 discusses data collection in radiology in more detail.

**Go To** Other types of health care facilities require special records, which are discussed in Chapter 8.

as electrocardiography (EKG) tracings, neurology reports such as electroencephalography (EEG) tracings, respiratory therapy diagnostic tests and treatment reports, physical/occupational therapy assessments and treatments, and dietary notes.

## Operative Records

Operative records require detailed data collection of the surgical procedure and the patient's condition before, during, and after the procedure. The record of the patient who undergoes a surgical procedure requires two sets of data: the operative data and the anesthesia data.

### Operative Data

⬤ **TJC** The Joint Commission

⬤ **operative report** The surgeon's formal report of surgical procedure(s) performed.
**surgeon** A physician who specializes in diagnosing and treating diseases with invasive procedures.
**operation** Surgery; an operation consists of one or more surgical procedures.

The **operative report** is recorded as a detailed, usually dictated and transcribed document. TJC standards call for the dictation to occur immediately following the procedure (The Joint Commission, 2012). Transcribed operative reports are not immediately available to users; therefore a brief operative note in the progress notes is usually written. The operative report lists the preoperative and postoperative diagnosis, the names of the **surgeon** and surgical assistants, the procedures performed, and a detailed description of the **operation**, operative findings, estimated blood loss, and specimens removed. As with all physician activities, the operative report is dated, timed, and authenticated. Additional data, such as preoperative checklists, implant information, transfusion record, and instrument counts, are collected and recorded by nursing staff in special forms. In an ERH this detailed perioperative documentation is collected and recorded with the use of templates. The surgical record system may be separate from the main electronic record system. The perioperative documentation may interface with or be scanned into the EHR.

### Anesthesia Data

⬤ **anesthesia report** An anesthesiologist's documentation of patient evaluations before, during, and after surgery, including the specifics of the administration of anesthesia.
**progress notes** The physician's record of each interaction with the patient.
**data collection devices** Paper forms designed to capture data elements in a standardized format, or the physical computer hardware that facilitates the data collection process.

The **anesthesia report** documents the evaluations and anesthesia administration of the anesthesiologist. The anesthesiologist performs preoperative and postoperative evaluations of the patient's condition in addition to the continuous recording of the patient's status during the procedure (the intraoperative anesthesia report). The anesthesiology preoperative evaluation is critical to the clearing of a patient for surgery. If the anesthesiologist has concerns about the patient's ability to undergo the administration of anesthesia, the surgery may be cancelled. The preoperative and postoperative evaluations may be documented in the progress notes or on a specially designed data collection device, either paper or electronic. The anesthesiologist is a specially trained physician. Anesthesia may also be administered by a certified registered nurse anesthetist.

## Same-Day Surgery Records

⬤ **ambulatory surgery** Surgery performed on an outpatient basis; the patient returns home after the surgery is performed. Also called *same-day surgery*.
**history and physical (H&P)** Heath record documentation comprising the patient's history and physical examination; a formal, dictated copy must be included in the patient's health care record within 24 hours of admission for inpatient facilities.

A patient can enter a hospital, have surgery, and leave on the same day; this process is called ambulatory surgery. In such cases, because of the short recovery time after the procedure, the data collection is frequently compressed so that the H&P, some anesthesia information, and some procedural information are included in shorter documents. For example, an otherwise healthy patient undergoing a screening colonoscopy might require only a brief H&P. The anesthesia and procedural notes might be uncomplicated and therefore quite brief compared with those for a more extensive procedure, such as a colon resection or a hip replacement. The patient recovery time after the colonoscopy might also be very short—perhaps less than an hour—so there is also less postprocedural nursing documentation. On the other hand, many complex surgical procedures, such as hysterectomy and medial meniscus repair can be performed on an outpatient basis, particularly if they are performed via laparoscope. These more complex procedures might require extensive documentation. In either event, the data collected and required documentation will be specified by the facility.

## Obstetrical Records

Obstetrical records differ from the ones already discussed because of the type of data that are collected. When a woman is pregnant and regularly visits a physician's office or clinic for prenatal care, data are collected on the progress of the fetus. Specific delivery data, such as the number of previous births, types of deliveries, and conditions of the newborns, are also collected. Shortly before the woman is due to give birth, the data are transferred to the hospital. The data are then incorporated into the inpatient record. Upon admission for childbirth, pregnant patients are monitored for contractions, fetal activity, and stress during labor. The prenatal record can be considered the history and physical for the admission for a normal, uncomplicated vaginal delivery.

### Neonatal Records

Neonatal records for healthy newborns are generally very short. Because these patients are in the hospital solely because of the mother's choice of delivery site, care is focused on promoting the infant's comfort and helping the mother learn how to care for the infant. The contents of a newborn record consist of an admission record, a brief physical examination that includes mention of any congenital anomalies, the birth record, nursing and pediatric progress notes, notes regarding medication administration, a note regarding the circumcision (if applicable), and a record of any testing done, such as a phenylketonuria (PKU) or hearing test. Newborns who exhibit signs of jaundice also have notes in their records pertaining to therapeutic interventions for jaundice, such as phototherapy.

Babies who are born with medical complications require more intensive care. Neonatal intensive care units (NICUs) feature more technological options, specialized caregivers, and specific documentation and data collection for their diagnosis and treatment plans.

### Intensive Care Unit Records

Sometimes, patients who are gravely ill when they enter the hospital are sent to special nursing care units called intensive care units (ICUs). A patient with a serious heart problem might be cared for in a coronary (or cardiac) care unit (CCU). Because of the intensity of nursing care in ICUs, nurses prefer to use graphic forms, which provide a great deal of visual data at a glance. In a paper record, such forms may consist of heavy-stock foldout graphs, which can be as large as 8 × 14 inches or 8 × 17 inches; they represent 24 hours of care. Vital signs are plotted on graphs that illustrate the patient's progress and the way the patient is being treated. Some of these forms are difficult to photocopy; however, they greatly facilitate the recording of patient data. In an ERH, vital signs and other data can be recorded either automatically, from the equipment that is capturing the data, or on data entry screens. Data captured electronically can be displayed in a variety of ways by the user: graphically or in table format, depending on the capabilities of the software.

Unlike standard progress notes, which are complete in the SOAP format, intensive care by physicians requires additional documentation, including details of the specific care given and the amount of time spent at the bedside (for physician billing purposes).

The following are some examples of special care units for close monitoring and care:

- Intensive care unit: for medical treatment
- Surgical intensive care unit: for postoperative treatment
- Cardiac care unit: for cardiac treatment and cardiac monitoring (telemetry)
- Neonatal intensive care unit: for newborns with medical problems

### Autopsy Reports

Occasionally, patients who expire are subject to autopsy. The *autopsy* is an examination of the deceased, usually for the purpose of determining the cause of death or other details surrounding the patient's illness at the time of death. The autopsy itself consists of an external and internal examination of the body or a particular organ. Additional testing, such as toxicology and histology (microscopic tissue evaluation), may be performed. The nature and extent of the autopsy are determined by the questions that need to be answered. In the case of an unexpected death from unknown causes in an otherwise healthy person, or if homicide is suspected, an extensive examination and many additional tests may be performed. However, if a confirmation of a suspected condition, such as Alzheimer's disease, is the only question to be answered, then the autopsy will focus on brain tissue.

Autopsies of hospitalized patients are performed according to the policies and procedures of the hospital, at the request of the family, or in compliance with the requirements of the medical examiner. The *medical examiner* is an official whose responsibility it is to

**admission record** The demographic, financial, socioeconomic, and clinical data collected about a patient at registration.

**medication administration** Clinical data including the name of the medication, dosage, date and time of administration, method of administration, and the nurse who administered it.

**NICU** neonatal intensive care unit
**ICU** intensive care unit
**CCU** coronary (or cardiac) care unit

**SOAP** subjective, objective, assessment, plan

investigate deaths that occur under specific circumstances. Suspected homicide, unexpected death of unknown cause of a person who is not under the care of a physician, and death from trauma are potential cases for a medical examiner.

Autopsies are performed by *pathologists*: physicians who are specially trained in this type of examination. The autopsy report is a detailed description of the extent of the examination and the findings. This report may take many weeks to prepare, particularly if extensive additional evaluations are required, but is usually available within 60 to 90 days of the autopsy. The report becomes a part of the permanent health record.

## ■ EXERCISE 4-2
### ■ Clinical Data

1. The first page in a paper record is usually the _____.
2. Describe the events that will occur when a patient is admitted to an acute care facility for an operation. What caregivers will be involved with the patient through this encounter?
3. In this chapter, we discuss some of the actual data collection devices that are used in acute care. Table 4-4 lists the key items in a physician's order. List those items as fields and describe them in data dictionary format, as discussed in Chapter 2.
4. At the end of a hospital stay, a _____ is usually required to be completed, as a dictated and transcribed report.
5. Routine documentation of the nurse's interaction with a patient is recorded in the _____.
6. Sometimes a physician needs to ask another physician for an opinion regarding the care of a patient. The physician asked is referred to as the _____.
7. Match the definition on the left with the vocabulary word(s) on the right.

   1. Acronym that describes the medical decision-making process. Also refers to the way physicians organize their progress notes
   2. Analysis of body fluids
   3. Examination of a patient using radiographs
   4. One or more surgical procedures performed at the same time
   5. Record of all drugs given to a patient during the hospitalization
   6. The diagnostic, therapeutic, or palliative measures that will be taken to investigate or treat the patient's condition or disease
   7. The nurse's evaluation of the patient
   8. The physician's directions regarding the patient's care. Also refers to the data collection device on which these elements are captured
   9. The physician's documentation of a surgical procedure, usually dictated and transcribed
   10. The physician's documentation of the examination of the patient, particularly at the initial visit
   11. The physician's record of each visit with the patient
   12. The predetermined, routine orders that have been designated to pertain to specific diagnoses or procedures. Must be ordered and authenticated by the appropriate physician
   13. The process of systematically eliminating potential diagnoses. Also refers to the list of potential diagnoses

   A. Laboratory tests
   B. Medication sheet
   C. Nursing assessment
   D. Operation
   E. Operative report
   F. Physical examination
   G. Physician's orders
   H. Plan of treatment
   I. Progress notes
   J. Radiology examinations
   K. Rule out
   L. SOAP format
   M. Order set

## ■ DISCHARGE DATA SET

**third party payer** An entity that pays a provider for part or all of a patient's health care services; often the patient's insurance company.

Throughout this chapter, specific data elements have been discussed. All of these data fall into one of the four main categories: demographic, financial, socioeconomic, and clinical. Many of these data are used to compile the bill that is sent to the third-party payer or the patient. Certain key data elements are also reported to various regulatory agencies, particularly the state's department of health or other agency that governs the

## TABLE 4-8

### UHDDS DATA ELEMENTS AND THEIR SOURCES

| UHDDS ELEMENT | TYPICAL RECORDER/SOURCE OF DATA |
|---|---|
| **Person/Enrollment Data** | |
| Personal/unique identifier | Patient registration |
| Date of birth | Patient registration |
| Gender | Patient registration |
| Race and ethnicity | Patient registration |
| Residence | Patient registration |
| **Encounter Data** | |
| Health care facility identification number | Maintained in system files |
| Admission date | Patient registration |
| Type of admission | Patient registration |
| Discharge date | Nursing or patient registration |
| Attending physician's identification number | Maintained in master physician data file |
| | Attending ID entered by patient registration or nursing; verified by HIM |
| Surgeon's identification number | Maintained in master physician data file |
| | Surgeon attributed by HIM in abstract |
| Principal diagnosis | HIM |
| Other diagnoses | HIM |
| Qualifier for other diagnoses | HIM |
| External cause of injury | HIM |
| Birth weight of neonate | Nursing in EHR; HIM abstracts if paper-based |
| Significant procedures and dates of procedures | HIM |
| Disposition of the patient at discharge | Nursing in EHR; HIM abstracts if paper-based |
| Expected source of payment | Patient registration |
| Total charges | Recorded by patient service areas; Total cumulated by system |

EHR, electronic health record; HIM, health information management.

licensure of hospitals. Although individual states may require additional data, the specific data elements that are required to be collected and reported by hospitals constitute the Uniform Hospital Discharge Data Set (UHDDS), which is the core data set required by most states (US DHHS, 2012). This data set was adopted in 1985 by the U.S. Department of Health & Human Services (DHHS) (US DHHS, 1996). Although many changes have been discussed, the data set has remained stable. Table 4-8 contains a summary of UHDDS data elements and each element's source in the acute care setting.

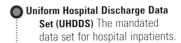 **Uniform Hospital Discharge Data Set (UHDDS)** The mandated data set for hospital inpatients.

## ▪ EXERCISE 4-3

### Discharge Data Set

1. Medicare requires a specific list of data elements to be collected about each patient who is discharged from an acute care facility. This list is called the Uniform Hospital Discharge Data Set (UHDDS). List as many items as you can remember from the UHDDS.

## WORKS CITED

Federal Register. Code of Federal Regulations, Title 42, Vol 5, Part 486.24 (c) 1.iii, 2012a.

Federal Register. Code of Federal Regulations, Title 42, Vol 5, Part 482.24 (c) 2.i.A, 2012b.

The Joint Commission: Hospital accreditation standards: record of care, treatment, and services, Chicago, 2012, The Joint Commission, RC.01.02.01 and RC.02.01.03.

U.S. Department of Health and Human Services (US DHHS), Centers for Disease Control and Prevention, National Center for Health Statistics (NCHS), Agency for Healthcare Research and Quality. Published 2012. http://www.ahrq.gov/data/infostd2.htm.

U.S. Department of Health and Human Services, National Committee on Vital and Health Statistics: Core Health Data Elements Report: Background. Published 1996. http://www.ncvhs.hhs.gov/ncvhsr1.htm#Background.

# CHAPTER ACTIVITIES

## CHAPTER SUMMARY

This chapter followed the clinical flow of data through an acute care visit. The clinical flow of a patient's data in an acute care facility starts with the initial assessments: history, physical, and nursing assessment. Various types of clinical data are collected from physicians and nurses as well as laboratory and radiology personnel. Most inpatient records contain the assessments as well as physician's orders, progress notes, and consultations. Nursing progress notes, medication administration, and vital signs are also universal. Some records contain additional information or the same data differently formatted. These records include surgical, obstetrical, neonatal, and medical intensive care cases. If the patient expires, an autopsy may be performed, which becomes a part of the patient's health record. Understanding the optimal point of data collection and the most appropriate source of needed data is important. Acute care facilities report the Uniform Hospital Discharge Data Set, containing key data elements of the inpatient stay.

## REVIEW QUESTIONS

1. List and explain the elements of an admission record.
2. Identify the appropriate source of the following data:
   a. Patient's name and address
   b. Patient's latest blood test results
   c. Patient's ability to explain his or her condition
   d. Patient/family education activities
   e. Plan of treatment on a specific day
   f. Whether the patient had a consultation during the inpatient stay
3. List and describe the data elements of the physician's order.
4. List and describe the elements of the Uniform Hospital Discharge Data Set and the source of the data elements.

### ● CAREER TIP

Transcription requires a level of speed and accuracy beyond that of the average typist. Transcriptionists need knowledge of medical terminology: not just diseases, but medical equipment, devices, and tools. They must be able to adapt to different styles of dictation and many different accents. Most transcriptionists take career school courses and progress from physician office or clinic dictation to specialized dictation such as radiology. Highly skilled transcriptionists may progress to inpatient dictation. Increasing computerization requires knowledge of computerized workflow distribution. Quality assurance and supervisory positions are logical career progressions.

## ● PROFESSIONAL PROFILE

### Transcriptionist

My name is Nicole, and I am a transcriptionist. I work for a large firm that performs transcription services for a lot of different facilities. I could work at home if I wanted to, but I like going into the office. My responsibility is to listen to what the physician dictated and to type exactly what the physician says. I learned transcription and took classes such as medical terminology and anatomy and physiology in the health-related professions program at my high school. I worked in a physician's office for a while and took some additional courses at my local community college.

My job isn't just typing. In order to transcribe accurately, I have to understand what the physician is saying and what it means. That means I need to understand and use medical terminology correctly. I need to know the requirements of the various medical reports, such as the H&P and the discharge summary, so that I transcribe them in the right format. I also need to know the regulatory requirements pertaining to the reports. For example, I know that the H&P is more urgent than the discharge summary, so I always transcribe the H&P report first.

Some people think that my job will go away when computers can understand and transcribe human language quickly and accurately. I certainly won't need to type as much, but my skills will become more important in reviewing the clinical reports for completeness, accuracy, and other data quality issues. I'm looking forward to that. To better prepare myself for that function, I am studying to become a registered health information technician.

## PATIENT CARE PERSPECTIVE

**Dr. Lewis**

Transcription is important to me, because the reports I dictate are often used by others for legal, billing, and patient care purposes. So, they have to be accurate. I can dictate an H&P in about 2 minutes. Within 4 hours, it's waiting in my queue in the hospital system for review and signature. The system allows me to make changes in the document before I sign it. Once I sign it, I cannot make any more changes, but I can dictate an addendum if I realize something is missing or needs to be corrected. Some of my patients like to keep personal health records and I find that a thorough discharge summary is one of their favorite tools to help keep track of inpatient admissions.

## APPLICATION

### Does Computerization Reduce the Use of Paper?

With increasing electronic health care documentation, *paperless environment* is commonly heard. The term is interesting and potentially misleading. Paperless implies that no paper is used at all. However, consider what happens when a patient's record transitions into the EHR. If admissions data are captured with a computer interface and the health record is still largely paper based, one must still print the admissions record on paper to include in the paper record. Many facilities that have an electronic admissions record still print out the record for the benefit of those using the paper record.

The physician reports a history and physical that can be dictated into a software application; the transcriptionist listens to the dictation and transcribes it into the computer using a word processing program. What happens to the history and physical then? It is printed out as a paper record. In an electronic environment, the report could be reviewed, corrected, authenticated, and stored electronically. What might be some legitimate reasons to print out an electronically stored report? One reason is for patient safety. If there is a disruption in service and the electronic record is unavailable, patient care could be affected. Therefore some facilities print out the history and physical as well as consultations and operative reports to keep in the nursing unit while the patient is still in the facility.

Think about the order entry system. The computerized physician order entry (CPOE) facilitates the entry of the order by the physician. However, when it is received in the pharmacy, the order is often printed out by the pharmacist while he or she is filling it. More paper may be generated when a prescription is transferred to the nursing station for the patient. Still more paper is generated if the order is printed so that it can be filed in the health record. This excessive generation of paper often occurs when a facility is in transition from a paper-based record system to a computer-based system. This example alone demonstrates that computerization of a patient record does not necessarily reduce paper, at least not immediately. How can an HIM department manager stop the excessive printing of data that can be viewed on the computer?

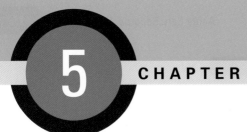

# HEALTH INFORMATION MANAGEMENT PROCESSING

Nadinia Davis

## CHAPTER OUTLINE

DATA QUALITY
  Timeliness
  Completeness
  Controls
POSTDISCHARGE PROCESSING
  Identification of Records to
    Process
  Assembly
  Quantitative Analysis
  Coding

Retrieval
Abstracting
Tracking Records While
  Processing
ELECTRONIC HEALTH RECORD
  MANAGEMENT
  Electronic Health Record
    Processing Issues
  Record Assembly
  Scanning and Indexing

Record Analysis
Coding
Abstracting
Storage and Retention
Transcription
Release of Information
Workflow
OTHER HEALTH INFORMATION
  MANAGEMENT ROLES

## VOCABULARY

abstract
abstracting
assembly
audit trail
batch control form
coding
completeness
concurrent analysis
concurrent coding

corrective controls
countersignature
data entry
deficiencies
deficiency system
  (incomplete system)
delinquent
detective controls

discharge register
  (discharge list)
exception report (error
  report)
indexing
nonrepudiation loose
  sheets (loose reports)
postdischarge processing
preventive controls

quantitative analysis
queue
release of information
  (ROI)
retention
revenue cycle
root cause analysis
timeliness
universal chart order

## CHAPTER OBJECTIVES

*By the end of this chapter, the student should be able to:*
1. List, explain, and give examples of the three types of controls.
2. Explain the flow of postdischarge processing of health information.
3. List and explain the major functions of a health information management department.
4. Explain the principles and process flow of an incomplete record system.
5. Compare and contrast paper-based versus electronic records processing.

**postdischarge processing** The procedures designed to prepare a health record for retention.

**retention** The procedures governing the storage of records, including duration, location, security, and access.

The previous several chapters have focused on the collection of data by clinical practitioners and the organization of that data. This chapter turns attention to the postdischarge processing of patient data, some data quality control measures, and the role of the health information management (HIM) professional in ensuring data quality, information access, and record retention.

This chapter discusses paper-based processing as well as electronic records processing. Ideally, electronic records replace paper-based records in their entirety. However, it is important to note that facilities must be prepared to conduct business as usual in the event of computer system "down time," interruptions in service that prevent use of the electronic health record (EHR). System down times can be planned, such as for system upgrades and other system maintenance. Unplanned down times, due to hardware failure, software crashes, and natural disasters, may also occur. Staff must be trained to continue to collect and record data for continuing patient care and patient safety, regardless of the availability of the electronic record. After down time, procedures must also be in place to either backload (enter later) the manually collected data or scan the paper collection into the computer.

## DATA QUALITY

Whether the data are recorded by hand or entered into an electronic record, the process of recording data into an information system is called **data entry.** In health care, a patient's life can depend on the accuracy and timeliness of the data entered. For example, if an incorrect blood type were recorded and a patient then received the wrong blood type during a blood transfusion, that patient might experience a life-threatening transfusion reaction. Consequently, the overall quality of the data that are recorded is critical. The data quality characteristics of timeliness and completeness defined in Chapter 2 are reinforced here.

### Timeliness

**Timeliness** refers to the recording of data within an appropriate time frame, preferably concurrent with its collection. Numerous regulations, both on the state licensure level and on the level of accreditation by voluntary agencies such as The Joint Commission (TJC), address the issue of when specific data must be recorded. The previous chapters discuss some of these regulations. For example, according to TJC rules, an operative report must be documented immediately after the operation (TJC, 2012). A history and physical (H&P) must be completed (dictated and present in the health record) within 24 hours of admission or before a surgical procedure (Federal Register, 2012; TJC, 2012). Timeliness applies to many other activities, as subsequent discussions demonstrate.

Timeliness is important, particularly from the health care facility's perspective, because the patient's health record is part of the normal business records of the facility. Therefore data that are being entered into the health record must be recorded as soon as possible after the events that the data describe. For example, if a nurse is monitoring a patient at 3:00 PM, then the note that he or she records in the patient's record must be written very shortly thereafter. Ideally, the note is written concurrently with the observation: point-of-care charting. Writing that same note at 9:00 PM, 6 hours after the actual observation, could impair the quality of the recorded note. Can the nurse really remember, 6 hours later, exactly what happened with the patient? Can a physician really remember, weeks later, exactly what happened during an operation well enough to dictate an accurate report?

After the patient has been discharged from an acute care facility, the record must be completed within a specified period of time, usually 30 days. State licensing regulations and medical staff bylaws, rules, and regulations will define the facility's standard for chart completion; however, the maximum is 30 days, by both TJC and Conditions of Participation (COP) standards. In the presence of conflicting standards, the most stringent takes precedence. So, if state licensing regulations require a record to be completed within 15 days of discharge, that shorter time frame takes precedence over 30-day standards. Because timeliness is so important, a significant amount of time and energy is spent facilitating the timely completion of health records.

### Completeness

**Completeness** refers to the collection or recording of data in their entirety. For example, a recording of vital signs that is missing the time and date is incomplete. A comprehensive

**data entry** The process of recording elements into a collection device.

**timeliness** The quality of data's being obtained, recorded, or reported within a predetermined time frame.

**The Joint Commission (TJC)** The largest and most comprehensive health care accrediting agency, focusing on improving patient safety and quality of care delivered.

**operative report** The surgeon's formal report of surgical procedure(s) performed.

**history and physical (H&P)** Health record documentation comprising the patient's history and physical examination; a formal, dictated copy must be included in the patient's health care record within 24 hours of admission for inpatient facilities.

**Go To** See the discussion of litigation in Chapter 12.

**health record** Also called *record* or *medical record.* It contains all of the data collected for an individual patient.

**acute care facility** A health care facility in which patients have an average length of stay less than 30 days and that has an emergency department, operating suite, and clinical departments to handle a broad range of diagnoses and treatments.

**Conditions of Participation (COP)** The terms under which a facility is eligible to receive reimbursement from Medicare.

**completeness** The data quality of existence. If a required data element is missing, the record is not complete.

**physical examination** The physician's record of examination of the patient.

**progress notes** The physician's record of each interaction with the patient.

**authenticate** To assume responsibility for data collection or the activities described by the data collection by signature, mark, code, password, or other means of identification.

**medication administration** Clinical data including the name of the medication, dosage, date and time of administration, method of administration, and the nurse who administered it.

**accreditation** Voluntary compliance with a set of standards developed by an independent agent, who periodically performs audits to ensure compliance.

**Go To** Reporting of data is discussed in Chapter 10.

physical examination that omits any mention of the condition of the patient's skin is incomplete. A progress note that is not authenticated is incomplete.

Complete data support the record of care of the patient. If a time is missing from a medication administration record, the hospital cannot provide evidence that the medication was administered on a timely basis. If the physician leaves out the condition of the patient's skin from a physical examination, the hospital may have difficulty claiming that a decubitus ulcer was present on admission.

In order to ensure that data collection and recording are timely and complete, health care organizations, such as hospitals and other providers of health care, must develop and implement data quality controls. Table 5-1 summarizes the data quality concepts that have been discussed in this text so far.

## Controls

There are many opportunities for errors to occur. Data entry errors may occur whether handwritten or electronically entered. The primary purpose of documentation is communication. For example, the documentation communicates among caregivers for continuing patient care as well as to payers, to justify and substantiate the care provided, and to regulatory or accrediting agencies to demonstrate the quality of patient care. If an individual's handwriting cannot be read by another health professional, how can those data elements be communicated? How can they be considered valid or accurate? If only the author of the data can decipher the writing, the data are useless to others. If a nurse records a temperature of 98.6° F without the decimal point (986° F), the temperature recorded is not valid. A physician's order that requests 100 mg of a medication instead of 10 mg could have fatal consequences if the larger dose is actually administered.

One way that data can be protected so that they are accurate, timely, and complete is through the development and implementation of controls over the collection, recording, and reporting of the data. This chapter focuses on the collection and recording of data. There are three basic types of controls over the collection and recording of data: preventive, detective, and corrective (Table 5-2).

---

| **TABLE 5-1** | | |
|---|---|---|
| **ELEMENTS OF DATA QUALITY** | | |
| **ELEMENT** | **DESCRIPTION** | **EXAMPLES OF ERRORS** |
| Accuracy | Data are correct. | The patient's pulse is 76 beats/min. The nurse recorded 67. That data entry was inaccurate. |
| Timeliness | Data are recorded within a predetermined period. | Operative reports not recorded immediately following surgery. |
| Completeness | Data exist in their entirety. | Date, time, or authentication missing from a record renders it incomplete. |

This is a partial list of the elements of data quality. Data quality elements are discussed throughout this book with regard to different aspects of health information management.

---

| **TABLE 5-2** | | |
|---|---|---|
| **PROCESSING CONTROLS** | | |
| **CONTROL** | **DESCRIPTION** | **EXAMPLE(S)** |
| Preventive | Helps ensure that an error does not occur | Computer-based validity check during data entry; examination of patient identification before medication administration |
| Detective | Helps in the discovery of errors that have been made | Quantitative analysis (e.g., error report) |
| Corrective | Correction of errors that have been discovered, including investigation of the source of the error for future prevention | Incomplete record processing |

## Preventive Controls

**Preventive controls** are designed to ensure that data errors do not occur in the first place. The best example of a preventive control is a software validity check. For example, suppose a user entered a date as July 45, 2012 (i.e., 07/45/2012). If the software is programmed to prevent one from entering invalid dates, it might send a message (an alert) saying, "You have entered an invalid date—please re-enter." It might even make a loud sound or block the character "4" from being typed in the first position of the day field.

Preventive controls are common, both in protocols surrounding clinical care and in paper-based data entry. For example, a nurse checks the patient's identification band before administering a medication to ensure that the medication is being given to the correct patient. In an electronic medication administration system, bar coding of both the patient wrist band and the medication itself (bar code medication administration) is a preventive control. The development of well-designed, preprinted forms to collect data also helps ensure that data collection is complete. Some facilities use a combination of paper and bar codes to collect data.

Preventive controls can be expensive and cumbersome to develop and implement. Health care providers might resist the implementation of preventive controls if they are burdensome and time consuming. Therefore the cost of a preventive control must always be balanced against its expected benefits. It is relatively easy to justify checking medications, orders, and patient identification because patient safety is of paramount concern. It is not quite as easy to justify developing a control to prevent the entry of an incorrect patient language or ethnicity.

One simple way to prevent invalid data entries is with the use of multiple-choice questions on a printed form or drop-down menu in an electronic record. All of the valid choices are listed so that the recorder merely chooses the correct one for the particular patient (Figure 5-1). This method also prompts the user to complete the form. However, this method does not prevent inaccurate or untimely entries because it is still possible to hit the wrong key without realizing it. For example, the staff member may enter the wrong sex

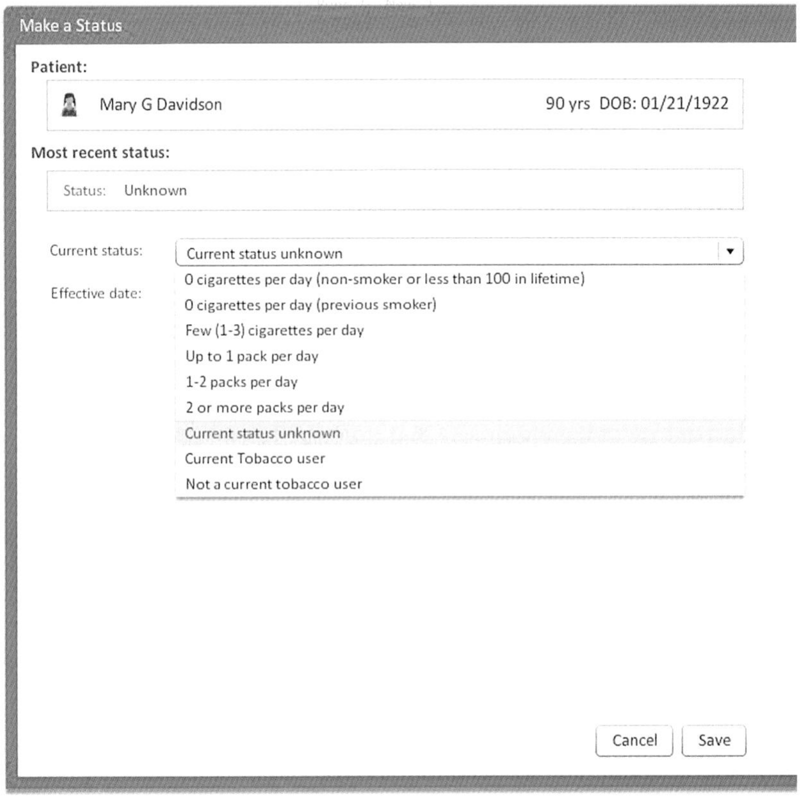

**preventive controls** Procedures, processes, or structures that are designed to minimize errors at the point of data collection.

**bar code** The representation of data using parallel lines or other patterns in a way readable to a machine, such as an optical bar code scanner or a smartphone.

**Figure 5-1** This drop-down list to enter a patient's tobacco habits limits the recorder to certain valid choices. (Courtesy Practice Fusion, Inc., San Francisco, CA.)

for a patient. Because the computer program has no way of "knowing" whether the patient is male or female, it does not prompt a correction. Thus comprehensive preventive controls are not always guaranteed.

### Detective Controls

**Detective controls** are developed and implemented to ensure that errors in data are discovered. Whereas a preventive control is designed to help prevent the person recording the data from making the mistake in the first place, a detective control is in place to find the data error after it is entered. In the previous date example (7/45/2012), a detective control might generate a list of entries that the software recognizes as problematic. Such a printout is called an **error report** or **exception report**. Error reports are also generated when the computer or other system encounters a problem with its normal processing. For example, a pharmacy system can be programmed to print an error report to alert the pharmacist that a medication order exceeds the normal dose. Omissions may also be highlighted in an error or exception report. For example, if the medication was ordered but not recorded as administered, this mistake could be detected on an exception report.

Detective controls are critical in a paper-based environment. Because there is no practical way to completely prevent erroneous data entry in a paper-based environment, the process of searching for errors is necessary. For example, nursing medication records may be reviewed regularly to ensure that medication administration notes are properly entered. Also, if a physician fails to dictate an operative report in a timely manner, a control must be in place to detect the missing report.

Detective controls are frequently the easiest and most cost-effective method to develop and implement, but as with preventive controls, they may be complex. The development of preventive and detective controls requires a thorough knowledge of the process being controlled as well as the potential negative impact of data errors in processing. For this reason a particular detective control may be performed either facility-wide, under the review of an overall quality improvement plan, or by a specific department.

### Corrective Controls

**Corrective controls** may be developed and implemented to fix an error once it has been detected. Corrective controls follow detective controls. In general, identifying an error wastes time and is ineffective if the facility does not correct the mistake. However, corrective controls, by their design, occur after the error has occurred. Thus if an error report identified an invalid date, such as July 45, the date would be corrected after the fact.

Nevertheless, some errors cannot be effectively corrected once they occur. In such cases, investigation of the error is necessary to determine whether sufficient controls are in place to prevent the error in the future. This is an important component of a *process improvement* or *quality improvement program*. For example, if a patient received an injection of an incorrect medication, the medication cannot subsequently be withdrawn. However, the events leading up to the administration of the drug can be thoroughly examined to determine why the error occurred. Did the physician order the wrong medication? Was the order transmitted incorrectly to the pharmacy? Did the health care provider check the patient's wristband before administering the medication? Once the source of the error is determined, the appropriate correction to the process can take place.

The process of determining the cause of an error is often referred to as a **root cause analysis**, or RCA. Facilities in which serious medical errors take place, such as an error that alters a patient's quality of life or results in death, may be required to report these errors with an RCA and a corrective action plan to the appropriate regulatory agencies. Employee education and disciplinary action are two examples of typical corrective actions that may take place if procedures were in place but not followed. Health care professionals, such as nurses and physicians, can lose their professional licenses if serious patient errors occur once or continue to occur even after the corrective action plan is in effect.

The HIM department plays a role in the detection and correction of certain documentation errors. Earlier in the chapter, an unsigned progress note was used as an example of

---

**detective controls** Procedures, processes, or structures that are designed to find errors after they have been made.

**error report** An electronically generated report that lists deficient or erroneous data. Also called an **exception report**.

**corrective controls** Procedures, processes, or structures that are designed to fix errors when they are detected. Because errors cannot always be fixed, corrective controls also include the initiation of investigation into future error prevention or detection.

**Go To** Chapter 11 explores process improvement programs in detail.

**root cause analysis (RCA)** The process of determining the cause of an error.

**HIM** health information management

incomplete data. In a paper-based environment, the HIM professional would have to obtain the record and read all of the progress notes in it to identify the incomplete note. In an electronic record environment, preventive control alerts, such as noises and verbal prompts, can be built into the program to encourage the authentication of the note at the time the note is originally recorded and also on subsequent access to the record. As a detective control, an exception report can identify incomplete notes. In both paper-based and electronic record environments, the corrective control consists of alerting the physician to the omission and giving him or her the opportunity to complete the note.

### Correction of Errors

The correction of errors is an important consideration in patient record keeping because nothing that is recorded should be deleted. Corrections must be made so that the error can be seen as clearly as the modified information. In a paper-based record, errors are corrected by drawing a line through the erroneous data and writing the correct data near it. It is important not to obscure the original entry because doing so may lead to the perception that someone attempted to cover up a mistake. The correction must be dated, timed, and authenticated. In addition, correction of errors cannot consist of destroying entire documents or pages of a record. All of the erroneous documents or pages must be clearly labeled as incorrect, authenticated, timed and dated, and kept with the correct portions of the record.

In electronic records, errors can be corrected in several ways depending on the type of error and the data that are being changed. For example, suppose that a patient admitted to a facility had been treated there before. A record of the previous visit exists. The patient registration specialist looks at the previous record and discovers that the patient has moved. The address and telephone number are now incorrect. Therefore the patient registration clerk may delete the old data and replace it in the patient's record with the new data. In doing so, the software should be programmed to create a historical file of the patient's previous addresses. On the other hand, a physician making a correction to a progress note must create an addendum to the record, identifying the error and entering the new note. In both cases, an audit trail should be created to indicate that the correction was made (Figure 5-2).

An **audit trail** is a list of all activities performed in a computer, including changes to the patient's record as well as viewings of the record. In addition to the date and time, medical record number (MR#), and patient account number, the audit trail contains a list of the activities, the workstation at which the activity took place, the user who performed the activity, and a description of the activity itself. In the case of changes, the audit trail also may be programmed to contain the precorrection and postcorrection data. Because the audit trail indicates the user, it can be used to determine whether errors are being made by certain staff members so that retraining can target the correct individuals. An audit trail may be generated automatically to review specific data elements, such as changing a patient's status from outpatient to inpatient. Other audit trails are designed to be generated on demand: for example, to review records for inappropriate access.

**authenticate** To assume responsibility for data collection or the activities described by the data collection by signature, mark, code, password, or other means of identification.

**audit trail** Software that tracks and stores information related to the activity of users in the system.

**medical record number (MR#)** A unique number assigned to each patient in a health care system; this code will be used for the rest of the patient's encounters with that specific health system.

**patient account number** A numerical identifier assigned to a specific encounter or health care service received by a patient; a new number will be assigned to each encounter, but the patient will retain the same medical record number.

**outpatient** A patient whose health care services are intended to be delivered within 1 calendar day or, in some cases, a 24-hour period.

**inpatient** An individual who is admitted to a hospital with the intention of staying overnight.

## EXERCISE 5-1

### Data Quality

1. When creating a paper form for new patients to complete at registration in a hospital, you should implement what preventive control to ensure that the patient lists all significant childhood illnesses?
2. Maintaining high standards of data quality is essential for patient care and effective use of health data. Data quality has a number of characteristics, many of which are discussed in this chapter and the preceding chapters. List and define as many characteristics as you can remember.
3. The development and implementation of internal controls aid in the protection of data quality and integrity. List and define three fundamental types of internal controls.

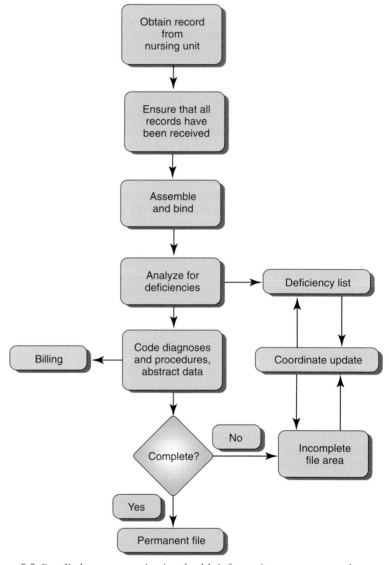

My recent activity     Last updated on 03/27/12 1:19 PM   Refresh

Jessica Himenez, MD accessed the chart of Donald James Leright    03/27/12 1:19 PM

Jessica Himenez, MD updated demographic details for Mary Gertrude Davidson    03/27/12 1:18 PM

Jessica Himenez, MD assigned smoking status Current status unknown for Mary Gertrude Davidson    03/27/12 1:10 PM

Jessica Himenez, MD accessed the chart of Mary Gertrude Davidson    03/27/12 1:08 PM

Jessica Himenez, MD signed an existing SOAP chart note for Alyssa Rosenthal with date of service = 3/26/2012    03/27/12 1:08 PM

**Figure 5-2** This activity feed or audit trail shows that Dr. Himenez changed the address (demographic details) for the patient Mary Davidson on March 27th at 1:18 PM. (Courtesy Practice Fusion, Inc., San Francisco, CA.)

**Figure 5-3** Postdischarge processing in a health information management department.

## POSTDISCHARGE PROCESSING

**postdischarge processing** The procedures designed to prepare a health record for retention.

**retention** The procedures governing the storage of records, including duration, location, security, and access.

The understanding of data concepts and control issues is critical for the development and implementation of postdischarge processing procedures (Figure 5-3). **Postdischarge processing** is what happens to a patient's record after the patient is discharged. In a paper-based environment, postdischarge processing is a series of procedures aimed at **retention**, or storage, of an accurate and complete record. In an electronic record environment, the record is already stored in the system; therefore postdischarge processing consists of

| TABLE 5-3 | |
|---|---|
| **COMPONENTS OF RECORD RETENTION** | |
| COMPONENT | DESCRIPTION |
| Storage | Compiling, indexing, or cataloging, and maintaining a physical or electronic location for data (see Chapter 9) |
| Security | Safety and confidentiality of data (see Chapters 9 and 12) |
| Access | Ability to retrieve data; release of data only to appropriate individuals or other entities (see Chapters 9 and 12) |

ensuring that the record is accurate and complete before being archived. With a hybrid record, both paper record and electronic record procedures may be necessary.

Key concepts to understand in the retention of records include the following:

*Retention*: Storing the record appropriately and for the necessary amount of time

*Security*: Preventing accidental destruction or inappropriate viewing or use of records

*Access*: Ensuring that the record is available timely should it be needed

Table 5-3 summarizes the components of record retention. Members of the HIM department and facility staff must adhere to requirements for record retention. These requirements vary from state to state.

Postdischarge processing is traditionally performed by the facility's HIM department. In a small physician's office or long-term care (LTC) facility, the entire process may be performed by one person. In a group practice or small inpatient facility, the process may be divided into functions and distributed among several individuals. In a large facility, many individuals may perform each of the separate functions of the process. The data concepts and control issues are relevant to many other health information environments. The following descriptions pertain to inpatient facilities. Although the principles are the same when applied to outpatient facilities, the application of the principles may vary.

## Identification of Records to Process

Postdischarge processing begins with the identification of discharged patients: what records need to be processed. This can be accomplished by reviewing a list of the patients who have been discharged: the **discharge register** or **discharge list.** As patients are discharged from the facility, their status is updated in the computer system. The discharge date and time are entered. This data entry may be performed by nursing or registration staff because they are the individuals most likely to know exactly when the patient has left. Bed control is notified, either manually or electronically, that the patient's bed is unoccupied. Housekeeping is notified that the room needs to be cleaned. All three tasks (discharge, notification, and cleaning) must take place in order to admit another patient to that bed. If the patient leaves but the discharge date is not recorded and bed control not notified, the number of patients in the facility (census) is incorrect and the discharge list is missing a patient. This detailed understanding of the discharge process and how it is performed in one's facility enables users of the discharge register to detect and correct errors. For example, if a record is received but the patient is not on the discharge register, the HIM department must determine what error has been made and notify the correct area to fix the problem.

**hybrid record** A record in which both electronic and paper media are used.

**long-term care (LTC) facility** A hospital that provides services to patients over an extended period; an average length of stay is in excess of 30 days. Facilities are characterized by the extent to which nursing care is provided.

**group practice** Multiple physicians who share facilities and resources and may also cooperate in rendering patient care.

**Go To** Chapter 10 for the calculation of census figures and other hospital statistics.

**discharge register** A list of all patients discharged on a specific date or during a specific period. Also called a **discharge list**.

**discharge** Discharge occurs when the patient leaves the care of the facility to go home, for transfer to another health care facility, or by death. Also refers to the status of a patient.

**bed control** The function of assigning beds in an acute care facility.

**census** The actual number of inpatients in a facility at a point in time, for comparative purposes, usually midnight.

## HIT-bit

### WHAT IS A DISCHARGE REGISTER?

In order to obtain control of the discharged records, the HIM professional first needs to know what patients have been discharged. A list of all patients who display a particular characteristic is a register. An admission register lists all patients who were admitted in a particular time frame. A discharge register lists all patients who were discharged. As patients are discharged, the discharge date is recorded in the master patient index (MPI). A discharge register is generated from the MPI.

| Admission Date | Patient Identification Number | Patient Name | | Attending Physician | Discharge Disposition | Room Number |
|---|---|---|---|---|---|---|
| | | Last | First | | | |
| 6/2/12 | 234675 | Johnson | Thomas | Bottoms | Transfer LTC | 313A |
| 6/4/12 | 234731 | Kudovski | Maria | Patel | Home | 303A |
| 6/4/12 | 234565 | Kudovski | Vladimir | Thomas | Home | Nursery |
| 5/31/12 | 156785 | Macey | Anna | Flint | Home | 213B |
| 6/3/12 | 234523 | Mattingly | Richard | Johnson | Home | 202A |
| 6/5/12 | 274568 | Ng | Charles | Kudro | Home | 224A |
| 5/15/12 | 234465 | Rodriguez | Francisco | Benet | Deceased | ICU-4 |
| 6/1/12 | 198543 | Rogers | Danielle | Patel | Home | 226B |
| 6/2/12 | 224678 | Young | Rebecca | Muniz | Home | 325B |

**Figure 5-4** A discharge register.

**master patient index (MPI)** A system containing a list of patients who have received care at the health care facility and their encounter information, often used to correlate the patient with the file identification.

**AMA** against medical advise

**point-of-care documentation** Clinical data recorded at the time the treatment is delivered to the patient.

**discharge summary** The recap of an inpatient stay, usually dictated by the attending physician and transcribed into a formal report.

A corrective control in this process may involve someone physically visiting all nursing units around midnight, essentially doing a bed check to verify whether all discharges have been recorded and that the census correctly identifies all of the patients and their locations. Nursing may perform this check comparing the patients in the beds with a computer printout of all inpatients. In paper-based facilities, the discharge would be a manual entry into a register, which could be photocopied or manually copied to a list for distribution to departments that use the discharge register, such as HIM. Manual census and discharge registers in a hospital are rare because the MPI has been computerized for decades. In a computer-based facility, flagging the patient status and entering the discharge date and time are performed through computer data entry. The discharge register is then a printed report of all patients discharged on a specific day or during a specified period. However it is compiled, the discharge register contains a list of the patients who have been discharged on a specific calendar day. A day is from 12:01 AM to 12 midnight, so discharges may include a patient who died at 11 PM and one who left against medical advice (AMA) at 5 PM. Figure 5-4 illustrates a discharge register.

In a paper-based acute care environment, patient records move from the point of care, or patient unit, to the HIM department after discharge. Once the patient has been discharged, documentation should be nearly complete and could theoretically be moved to the HIM department immediately upon discharge. Because the patient has already left the facility, the record is no longer needed for direct patient care. Usually, however, records remain on the patient unit until the morning of the day after discharge. This practice gives the physicians, who are not necessarily at the facility all day, time to sign off on orders and perhaps dictate the discharge summary. It also gives nursing and other clinicians time to complete their documentation.

## HIT-bit

### PNEUMATIC TUBE SYSTEMS

Pneumatic tube systems are widely used today at banks for drive-through customers. The customer drives up to a stand that holds a container. The checks or other documents are placed in the container, which is then transported at the press of a button, by forced air, to the teller inside the bank. Larger documents, such as health records, require larger containers. These systems are quick and generally efficient; however, the tendency of containers to get stuck in the tubes and the relatively short range of the system limit their appeal for this purpose. Nevertheless, they may be used for transporting physician's orders to the pharmacy, for example. Although theoretically not needed in an EHR, the systems may be retained for use when the electronic system is "down."

The process by which paper records move from the patient care unit to the HIM department varies by facility. Some of the considerations that determine what process is used include the distance from the patient units to the HIM department, the staffing levels on the patient unit, the staffing levels in the HIM department, and the availability of alternative personnel, such as volunteers. An example of a common practice is as follows: Patient unit personnel remove the records from their binders and leave them in a pile for pickup; the records are then picked up by any authorized person and delivered to the HIM department. Alternatively, the patient unit personnel may deliver the records. Some facilities use physical transportation systems such as pneumatic tube systems, elevators, and even transport robots.

The cost of moving paper records from one place to another is also a consideration. The cost is measured by the amount of time it takes to obtain the records times the hourly wage of the person performing the task. If it takes $1\frac{1}{2}$ hours for an HIM clerk to obtain the records daily and that clerk earns $12 per hour, then it costs $18 per day ($1\frac{1}{2} \times 12$) to pick up the records. However, it may take 6 unit clerks 5 minutes each (30 minutes per day) to drop off the records on their way to the time clock at shift change. If the unit personnel can drop off the records at shift change, the cost may be reduced to $6 per day—assuming that the unit personnel also earn $12 per hour. Thus the hospital could save 1 hour of staff time ($12) per day by making this process change. That is an annual savings of $4380 (365 days × $12/day).

Once the record arrives in the HIM department, postdischarge processing can begin. The first step is to ensure that all records have been received. This can be accomplished by checking the records received against the discharge register. If a patient was discharged but a record was not received, the patient unit staff should be contacted immediately so HIM can obtain the record. If a record was received but the patient is not listed on the discharge register, the record may have been sent in error (e.g., the patient may not actually have been discharged). Alternatively, the discharge register may be incorrect (e.g., the patient was discharged but not added to the discharge register). The patient unit staff should be contacted to verify the patient's status, and whatever error was made should be corrected immediately.

Other departments also rely on the accuracy of the discharge register. Members of the nutritional or dietary department would not want to deliver meals to patients who are no longer at the facility. The nursing department must know the exact bed occupancy statistics for every unit to ensure appropriate staffing levels. The admitting department must know which beds are open for new admissions. Therefore the facility must have a procedure in place, whether telephone, facsimile (fax), Internet communication, or computer-based system, to systematically notify the relevant departments. In an entirely electronic system, notifications among departments would be unnecessary, if the new status automatically "populates" into the department modules as the patient's status changed.

## Assembly

**Assembly** is the set of procedures by which a paper record is reorganized after discharge and prepared for further processing. The extent to which a record is reorganized varies among facilities. The need to reorganize the record arises from the differences between the order of the sections and documents of the record as filed on the patient unit and the order of the sections and documents of the record used in postdischarge processing. The patient care unit staff may place all sections pertaining to physician documentation in the beginning of the record so that the physicians do not have to search through other sections in order to find their section, which may be time consuming. In addition, the documentation is generally organized within sections in reverse chronological order, with the most recent date on top. Reverse chronological order makes sense while the record is on the patient unit, but after the patient is discharged, this method may actually hamper record review and understanding of the hospitalization because most people are used to reading events in chronological order. Similarly, sections that were considered sufficiently important to be placed up front for ease of documentation, such as physician's orders may be shifted after the patient is discharged so that the overall record may be more easily read.

**assembly** The reorganization of a paper record into a standard order.

**universal chart order** Pertaining to a paper health record, the maintenance of the same page organization both before and after discharge.

Reorganization of a paper record is done manually by HIM staff members, who are often called assemblers. Some administrators question the cost effectiveness of this function. Why take an organized record and reorganize it? The answer is that the needs of the users on the patient unit, while the patient is being treated, are different from the needs of the users after the patient has been discharged. Nevertheless, the cost of reorganizing the paper record may be prohibitive. So the paper record can be stored in the same order as it is kept on the patient unit. This approach is called **universal chart order.** In theory, universal chart order is a practical solution. However, it does require cooperation and coordination among the staff of the patient units and the HIM department. Further, the principal users of the record must agree on the universal order. Without such collaboration and agreement, universal chart order cannot be successfully implemented.

Once the paper record has been organized, it is bound. Binding consists of affixing the pages of the record within a permanent cover, usually a manila folder. The front of the folder usually contains the name of the facility. It may also contain warnings about the confidentiality of the record and other pertinent facility record policies. The front and tabs of the folder contain the patient's name and medical record number as well as the discharge date. Because health records are generally stored in open shelves, the tab is on the short side of the folder. This position enables the user to identify the contents of the folder when the folder is placed on a shelf.

**consent** An agreement or permission to receive health care services.

**advance directive** A written document, like a living will, that specifies a patient's wishes for his/her care and dictates power of attorney, for the purpose of providing clear instructions in the event the patient is unable to do so.

**electronic document management system (EDMS)** Computer software and hardware, typically scanners, that allow health record documents to be stored, retrieved, and shared.

It may seem obvious that an electronic record is not paper and therefore there is nothing to assemble. However, quite a bit of paper may be generated from an electronic record during the patient's stay, for a variety of reasons. Critical documents, such as dictated reports and laboratory results, may be printed on the nursing unit as a precaution in the event of down time. Also, a document may be generated or received during the patient stay that must be evaluated for inclusion in the record, such as copies of patient documents from other facilities, patient consent forms, and advance directives. The assembler must evaluate which documents received from the patient unit are original and which documents are printouts (i.e., copies or duplicates) that should be destroyed to prevent confusion. Original documents may contain signatures or indicate in other ways that they are originals. Printouts may need to be retained if they contain written documentation. For this reason, printing out documents from the computer-based record should be regulated by policy and procedure. Once assembled, these paper components are typically scanned into the computer system through the use of an electronic document management system (EDMS).

## Quantitative Analysis

**quantitative analysis** The process of reviewing a health record to ensure that the record is complete according to organization policies and procedures for a complete medical record.

Another important detective control that takes place in the HIM department is quantitative analysis. **Quantitative analysis** is the process of reviewing a health record to ensure that the record is complete according to organization policies and procedures for a complete medical record. As previously discussed, *completeness* refers to the entirety of data: Are all of the data elements present? The HIM professional who performs this function is frequently called a medical record analyst, medical record analysis specialist, health information specialist, or health information analyst. This person's responsibility is to review the patient's record and determine whether any reports, notes, or necessary signatures are missing. In many facilities, assembly and analysis are both performed by the same individual.

The extent of quantitative analysis performed in a facility depends on the type of facility and the rules of its licensure and accreditation. However, there are three guiding principles:

*Existence*: The record must contain all of the elements required by the licensure and accrediting bodies for the particular type of facility and all of the elements required by the clinical services pertaining to that patient's treatment as well as the elements common to all patients

*Completeness*: The existing documents must be complete and must not be missing data elements

*Authentication*: Each element of the record must be properly dated, timed, and authenticated in accordance with the rules and regulations of state or accrediting agencies that apply to the facility, with the authors clearly identified

## Elements of the Record

Different clinical services typically have special forms that pertain to those services. Physical therapy may have special assessment and progress forms that differ from those used by nursing. The analyst must know which forms are used in each service and must be able to identify any forms that are missing. Again, the complete absence of the data element is easier to identify than the partial absence. For example, an H&P must be documented on every inpatient record. Failure to perform an H&P is a serious error. If either the history portion or the physical portion of the transcribed report is missing, it may not have been performed. More often, however, the H&P was performed, noted in the record, and dictated, but the dictated report has not yet been matched with the chart. The same is true of operative reports and consultation reports. No rule or regulation states that reports must be dictated, so on some records, depending on hospital policy, a handwritten H&P is acceptable. The analyst must know the rules and must be able to identify noncompliance. The analyst must also be able to identify forms that are incomplete.

The absence of the author's authentication or of identification of authorship is easily recognized as long as the analyst is aware of when and where a signature must appear. However, the analyst must also know who should have authenticated the document. This knowledge becomes critical if a document has been signed but not by the correct individual. Perhaps a *countersignature* is required. A **countersignature** is authentication by an individual in addition to the author. For example, an unlicensed resident may write (author) a progress note, which the attending physician must then countersign to provide evidence that the resident was supervised.

> **H&P** history and physical
>
> **operative report** The surgeon's formal report of surgical procedure(s) performed.
>
> **consultation** The formal request by a physician for the professional opinion or services of another health care professional, usually another physician, in caring for a patient.
>
> **authenticate** To assume responsibility for data collection or the activities described by the data collection by signature, mark, code, password, or other means of identification.
>
> **countersignature** Evidence of supervision of subordinate personnel, such as physician residents.
>
> **progress notes** The physician's record of each interaction with the patient.

---

### HIT-bit

#### SIGNATURES SERVE DUAL PURPOSES

The author of a verbal order may be a registered nurse, who then authenticates the entry by initialing or signing it. The physician then authenticates the order to prove that it has been reviewed. Because both parties can be identified by their unique signatures, a signature can verify identity as well as represent an activity, such as review or approval.

---

Finally, the analyst ensures that the record is complete according to licensure and accreditation rules. For example, the H&P, discharge summary, and progress notes are required elements. Sometimes, this requirement overlaps with the requirement for authentication. Table 5-4 summarizes the major record elements for which quantitative analysis acts as a detective control.

> **licensure** The mandatory government approval required for performing specified activities. In health care, the state approval required for providing health care services.
>
> **accreditation** Voluntary compliance with a set of standards developed by an independent agent, who periodically performs audits to ensure compliance.
>
> **detective controls** Procedures, processes, or structures that are designed to find errors after they have been made.

### TABLE 5-4

#### ELEMENTS OF QUANTITATIVE ANALYSIS

| ELEMENT | ANALYSIS TO DETERMINE | COMMON DEFICIENCIES |
|---|---|---|
| Existence | Do the data exist? | Missing operative report<br>Missing discharge summary |
| Completeness | Are the data entirely present, or are there missing components? | Missing reason for consultation |
| Authentication | Is the author's or other appropriate signature/password present? | Unsigned H&P<br>Unsigned discharge summary<br>Unsigned order |

H&P, history and physical report.

**nursing progress notes** Routine documentation of the nurse's interaction with a patient.

**error report** An electronically generated report that lists deficient or erroneous data. Also called an exception report.

**abstracting** The recap of selected fields from a health record to create an informative summary. Also refers to the activity of identifying such fields and entering them into a computer system.

**deficiencies** Required elements that are missing from a record.

**concurrent analysis** Any type of record analysis performed during the patient's stay (i.e., after admission but before discharge).

As the analyst identifies missing elements, the pages are flagged and the missing elements are noted, along with the party responsible for correction. *Flagging* consists of affixing stickers to the pages of the record. The stickers come in multiple colors so that various clinicians can be identified, each with a different color, in a single record. In many facilities, the policy is to analyze only the physician portions of the record, such as orders, progress notes, and all dictated reports. In other facilities, the policy is to analyze many sections or all of the clinical documentation, which would include nursing progress notes.

In an electronic record, most of the quantitative analysis can be performed by the computer. For example, the analyst would receive a computer exception or error report for follow-up purposes. Analysts can then turn their attention to the analysis of other data quality issues, such as the correct assignment of physicians to specific cases. Assignment of physicians to cases occurs at several points during the inpatient stay and is verified and corrected by HIM staff during the abstracting process.

## Record Completion

Once the missing elements, or **deficiencies**, are identified, the responsible parties are then required to complete the record. The usefulness of requiring clinical staff to authenticate records after discharge is somewhat controversial because the lack of authentication has no clinical significance for patient care. For example, if a physician forgot to sign the progress note of a patient who has already been discharged, what possible impact could the addition of the signature have on the patient 30 days later? Any control function that would have been affected by the physician's signature has been lost. A small benefit may be obtained in the event that the entry is later questioned. These arguments, of course, are not relevant as long as licensure and accrediting agencies are still reviewing postdischarge records for compliance with such standards.

On the other hand, the argument has prompted some administrators to implement analysis procedures while the patient is still at the facility. This process is called **concurrent analysis** because it occurs concurrently with the patient's stay. Concurrent analysis facilitates compliance with the intent of authentication rules. For example, if verbal or telephone orders are required to be signed within 24 hours, this deficiency can be identified and corrected within the time frame by concurrent analysis but probably not by postdischarge analysis. In addition, concurrent analysis may speed postdischarge processing of the record. In an electronic record, concurrent flagging of incomplete entries should be automatic. For example, a physician's order entered by the physician will complete itself automatically when the physician finishes the entry. However, a telephone order entered by a nurse on behalf of the physician will be incomplete as to the physician's authentication of the order. In a well-designed system, that incomplete order will automatically be flagged and the physician will be alerted upon log-in that there is an order to be signed. Although this automatic flag does not guarantee that the physician will, in fact, review and sign the order on a timely basis, it does alleviate the need to manually review the orders.

It should be noted that an analyzer performing a concurrent analysis can look only for deficiencies that will have occurred up to that point. For example, if the chart is being reviewed 48 hours after admission, it should certainly contain an H&P, but there will not be a discharge summary because the patient is still in the facility. Review of the chart after the patient has gone home is called a retrospective or postdischarge analysis.

In some cases, there may have been a delay in obtaining a particular report. Suppose, for example, that the results of a radiology examination were communicated verbally to the physician but the transcribed report did not arrive at the nursing unit before the patient's discharge. Because the record is used primarily for communication and is a legal document, the lack of a report must be resolved. If an excessive amount of documentation is still being received by the HIM department after discharge, organizational issues may have to be resolved with the other departments involved. Filing this trailing documentation or "loose sheets" is not an effective use of HIM staff members' time if the reports should have been filed by patient unit personnel while the patient was still in house.

### Loose Sheets

In a paper-based record, some reports, test results, and other data have not been compiled with the record before the patient's discharge. While the patient is in the facility, it is the responsibility of the clinical staff, usually nursing or patient unit clerks, to compile these pages into the record. This is not an issue in a completely electronic record. Because many reports and other data are delivered to the area that requested them, a delay may occur in rerouting the data to the HIM department. These noncompiled pages are frequently called **loose sheets** or **loose reports**.

Loose sheets may arrive in the HIM department hours, days, or weeks after the patient has been discharged. By that time, the paper record has been processed and must be located. If the record is stored electronically, the loose sheets will be scanned into the record. Handling the volume of loose sheets arriving daily may be a full-time job in a large facility. Regular, systematic sorting and filing or scanning of loose sheets is necessary to ensure a complete record.

### Deficiency System

Once the patient's record has been reviewed and missing elements have been identified, the corrective control procedure is initiated. The responsible party—that is, the individual who was responsible for preparing the report or signing the note or report—is notified and asked to complete the record. The most common deficiencies that exist in inpatient records are absences of a discharge summary, an operative report, a formal consultation report, and signatures. This process of recording, reporting, and tracking missing elements in a record is called the **deficiency system** or, in some facilities, the **incomplete system.** This system applies to retrospective analysis. Concurrent analysis is not generally recorded and tracked because the clinician is expected to see the flag, whether it is manually inserted or computer generated, the next time he or she reviews the record.

Keeping track of "who did not do what" is a classic application for computerization and was one of the first HIM department functions to become computerized in many facilities. To track deficiencies, the name of the clinician and the type of the deficiency must be captured and recorded on the record and reported to the clinician. Figure 5-5 depicts a deficiency sheet.

When deficiencies are tracked in a computer, screens are generally organized by chart, with different lines or pages for each physician. In many cases, the deficiencies are first captured on a paper form and then transferred to the computerized tracking system. This is an example of a computer-assisted function. In either case, the analysis form or printout is kept with the chart, enabling clinicians to quickly reference their deficiencies and facilitating the distribution of the records to their colleagues.

Incomplete charts are routinely maintained in a special area of the department to allow clinicians easy access to complete the charts and correct deficiencies. The organization of this area depends on the extent to which the record has been computerized as well as the level of staffing available. If physicians are expected to retrieve their own charts, the area is typically organized alphabetically, by physician last name. An incomplete chart is shifted

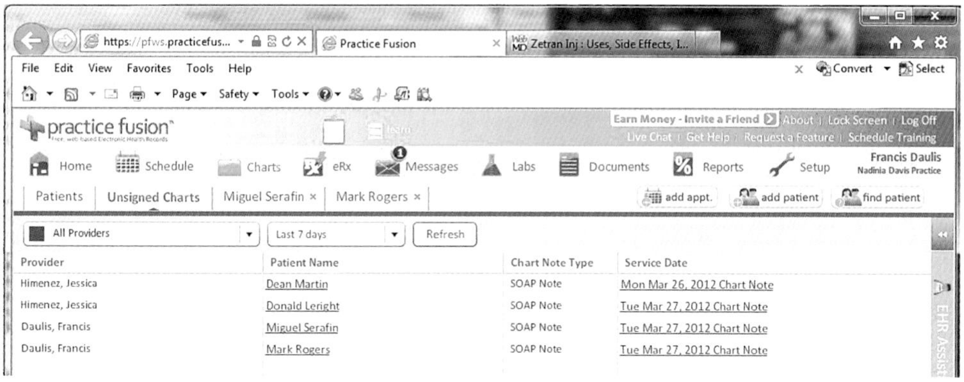

**loose sheets** In a paper health record, documents that are not present when the patient is discharged. These documents must be accumulated and filed with the record at a later date. Also called *loose reports*.

**deficiency system** The policies and procedures that form the corrective control of collecting the missing data identified in quantitative analysis. Includes the recording and reporting of deficiencies. Also called an **incomplete system**.

**Figure 5-5** A deficiency sheet. (Courtesy Practice Fusion, Inc., San Francisco, CA.)

from physician to physician until the chart is complete. If the HIM department is sufficiently well staffed that the charts can be gathered (pulled) for the physician on request, then all the charts are generally filed together by medical record number.

When a record appears to be complete, it is analyzed again to ensure that nothing was missed. When the record is complete, it is transferred to permanent storage. Incomplete records are returned to the incomplete chart area.

On a regular basis, typically weekly or biweekly, clinicians are reminded of their incomplete records. This report of incomplete records must be compiled at least quarterly for accreditation purposes. TJC-accredited facilities must comply with rules covering the maximum allowable number of incomplete records. Because acute care records must be completed within 30 days of discharge, all records incomplete after 30 days of discharge are considered **delinquent**. The maximum number of delinquent records that acute care facilities are permitted equals 50% of their average monthly discharges for the past 12 months (TJC, 2012). Therefore a facility with an average of 2000 discharges per month would be allowed to have 1000 delinquent records. Facilities can track deficiency rates to ensure compliance by using the Medical Record Statistics Form available online from TJC (http://www.jointcommission.org/Hospital_Medical_Record_Statistics_Form). Specific deficiencies, such as missing H&Ps and operative reports, are very serious. Some facilities track these deficiencies separately to ensure that the records are completed in a timely manner (e.g., within 24 hours of admission for H&Ps and immediately after surgery for operative reports).

Each facility has its own policies and procedures for ensuring that records are completed; these depend on the number of incomplete charts, the location of the HIM department, and the historical compliance of clinicians with policies governing record completion.

Electronic records can assist with the tracking of chart completion because the software can identify and report incomplete records. Because certain types of documentation are completed at the point of care, such as physician's orders, nurses' recordings of vital signs, and nursing assessments, authentication is typically effected concurrently with the documentation. Missing components of the documentation can be flagged by alert to the practitioner. Other documentation, such as dictated reports, may be incomplete until they are reviewed and authenticated. In this case, the physician would log in to the computer system using a personal identification number (PIN), review the document, and give approval for authentication. A report of unsigned documents would help HIM identify and track incomplete records. Other elements of the medical record, such as progress notes, are more difficult to capture electronically at the point of care. When these elements are still in paper form, some systems allow authentication after scanning; however, the procedure to identify whether the document is complete is manual.

## Coding

**Coding** is the representation of diagnoses and procedures as alphanumerical values in order to capture them in the database. Diagnosis and procedure codes are used for example to communicate data about patients among providers, to track and analyze diseases, for reimbursement, and to facilitate research. Standardizing pieces of information in this way allows communication of very specific diagnoses, procedures, and other kinds of clinical data with a better control over data quality. For example, an attending physician may request a consultation from a neurologist for evaluation of a patient with Lou Gehrig disease. The neurologist, upon examination, diagnoses the patient with amyotrophic lateral sclerosis. Although software can certainly evaluate and match the two names for the same disease, a misspelling of either term could lead to confusion. Assignment of the specific code (G12.21) clearly identifies the diagnosis.

### Inpatient Coding

There are three times during a patient's encounter with the facility that coding routinely occurs, all of which relate to the physician's development of the diagnosis: on admission, during the stay, and at discharge.

When a patient is being admitted, regardless of the inpatient setting, a physician must state the reason for the admission. The physician's statement of the reason for admission is expressed as a diagnosis—in this case, an admitting or provisional diagnosis. For example, the patient arrives in the emergency department with a complaint, is assessed by the emergency department physician, and is admitted by the attending physician. The emergency department form contains a section for a diagnosis, which is the reason for the emergency department encounter—for example, chest pain. The inpatient admitting diagnosis might also be chest pain, or it might be angina or myocardial infarction. The attending physician should state the reason for admission.

In another scenario, a physician sees a patient in his or her office and determines that the patient requires admission, contacts the hospital to make the arrangements for admission, and communicates an admitting diagnosis at that time. At the time of admission, a code should be assigned to the diagnosis so that computer-assisted tracking of the patient's stay can take place. If the admitting diagnosis is expressed only as free text, variations in the expression of the diagnosis impair the ability of the software to match and track the patient's diagnosis with known lengths of stay and clinical treatment plans. Further, if the patient registration staff member merely writes out the words, it is frequently left to the HIM department, after the patient is discharged, to assign a code to the admitting diagnosis.

Codes also may be assigned during the patient's stay in the facility. While the patient is in the facility, there are many reasons for HIM professionals to review the patient's record and assign codes to it. For example, computer matching and tracking of the patient's diagnosis is useful to help estimate the patient's length of hospital stay and thus can help control the delivery of health care. Coding that is done while the patient is still in the facility is called **concurrent coding**. In patients with long lengths of stay, concurrent coding, often called interim coding, must be completed for interim billing based on payer requirements.

The most common point at which patient charts are coded by HIM professionals is *retrospectively*, after the patient's discharge. Coders then read the entire record and assign the codes to identify the diagnoses and procedures appropriately. In acute care facilities, these postdischarge codes drive the reimbursement to the facility for many payers. Therefore the assignment of codes postdischarge have become a critical revenue cycle function. **Revenue cycle** is the groups of processes that identify, record, and report the financial transactions that result from the facility's clinical relationship with a patient (Davis, 2011). Figure 5-6 illustrates the revenue cycle as it relates to an inpatient stay.

The importance of coding cannot be overemphasized. The capture and reporting of accurate diagnosis and procedure codes enable facilities, payers, government agencies, researchers, and other users to analyze health data over populations and geographic areas. The coded data reported by health care facilities and other providers to payers, government, and regulatory agencies are used to determine reimbursement, monitor patient outcomes, maintain registries, and report quality of care—including adverse events. Knowledgeable individuals, including HIM professionals, who can manage data and can help health care providers identify risks and take preventive action to improve quality are valuable assets in all of those settings.

**admission** The act of accepting a patient into care in a health care facility, including any nonambulatory care facility. Admission requires a physician's order.

**admitting diagnosis** The reason given by the physician for initiating the order for the patient to be placed into care in a hospital.

**concurrent coding** Coding performed during the patient's stay (i.e., after admission but before discharge).

**reimbursement** The amount of money that the health care facility receives from the party responsible for paying the bill.
**payer** The individual or organization that is primarily responsible for the reimbursement for a particular health care service. Usually refers to the insurance company or third party.
**revenue cycle** The groups of processes that identify, record, and report the financial transactions that result from the facility's clinical relationship with a patient.

**outcome** The result of a patient's treatment.
**registry** A database of health information specific to disease, diagnosis, or implant used to improve the care provided to patients with that disease, diagnosis, or implant.

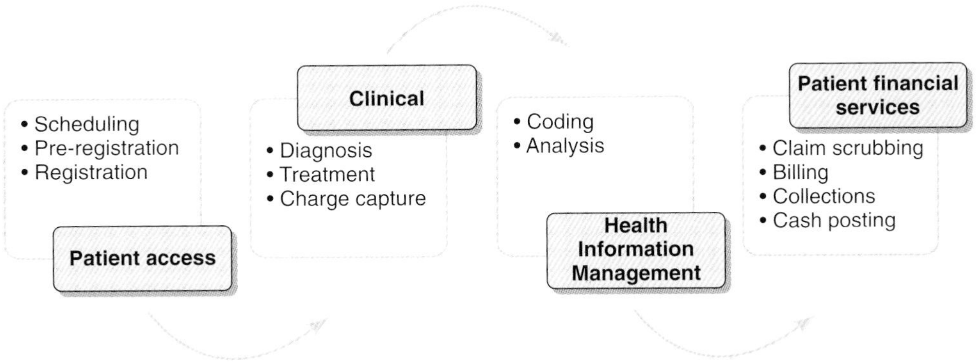

Figure 5-6  A revenue cycle.

**retention** The procedures governing the storage of records, including duration, location, security, and access.

**Go To** The function of releasing a record is discussed in Chapter 12, in the section concerned with confidentiality.

**release of information (ROI)** The term used to describe the HIM department function that provides disclosure of patient health information.

**abstracting** The recap of selected fields from a health record to create an informative summary. Also refers to the activity of identifying such fields and entering them into a computer system.

**database** An organized collection of data.

**postdischarge processing** The procedures designed to prepare a health record for retention.

**electronic health record (EHR)** A secure real-time, point-of-care, patient centric information resource for clinicians allowing access to patient information when and where needed and incorporating evidence-based decision support.

**abstract** A summary of the patient record.

**ICD-10-CM** International Classification of Diseases, Tenth Revision—Clinical Modification. The United States clinical modification of the WHO ICD-10 morbidity and mortality data set. ICD-10-CM is mandated by HIPAA for reporting diagnoses and reasons for healthcare encounters in all settings.

**ICD-10-PCS** International Classification of Diseases, Tenth Revision, Procedural Coding System. A unique classification system, developed in the U.S., for reporting procedures performed in inpatient settings. It is a HIPAA mandated code set.

**Current Procedural Terminology (CPT)** A nomenclature and coding system developed and maintained by the American Medical Association to facilitate billing for physicians and other services.

## Retrieval

It is appropriate to mention here that in a paper environment, storage is a very critical function in the facility. The storage and retention of health records, as well as the ability to retrieve those records efficiently, are traditionally the responsibility of HIM professionals.

Once the records are complete and filed, the need for retrieval is based on a number of factors. If no one would ever need to look at the record again after the patient has gone home, it would not need to be organized, analyzed, or stored. As previously mentioned, however, the health record is the business record that supports treatment and payment and is a critical communication tool; it will be reviewed many times after the patient leaves the facility.

The function of retrieving the health record and providing it, or parts of it, to individuals who need it is commonly called **release of information (ROI)**. It is extremely important that HIM professionals understand who is authorized to receive a record, who is authorized to receive a copy of a record, and how to prepare a record for review.

## Abstracting

HIM professionals are uniquely trained to perform functions that require identification of the best source of data. Coding is one such function. Abstracting is another. The term **abstracting** refers to a number of activities in which specific data are located in the record and transferred to another document or to a database. The necessity for abstracting arises for various reasons, including data transfer, volume reduction, discharge data sets, and analysis. Two activities are called abstracting. One occurs during postdischarge processing, after coding. The other occurs as a data retrieval activity.

### Abstracting as a Component of Postdischarge Processing

Patient health data are gathered at admission and throughout the course of the patient's care. In the paper environment, once the patient is discharged, the HIM employee must review key elements in the patient record to ensure that they are present and accurately recorded in the computer system. For example, the medical record number, account number, discharge disposition, and admitting diagnosis are typically reviewed and corrected as needed. In an EHR most of the data are already captured, and the HIM employee verifies the abstract. The **abstract** can be defined as a summary of the patient's encounter. Verification of the abstract is a detective control. Fixing any noted errors is a corrective control. It provides a brief synopsis of the patient's care that would otherwise require a thorough review of the entire patient record. The abstract typically contains the key demographic field, the physician data, diagnosis and procedure codes, dates of service, and discharge disposition.

The process of summarizing the patient's information in a database through the entry of specific data elements is called *abstracting*. To complete an abstract, the HIM clerk must review the health record. The review is necessary to determine the appropriate data element for each field. As previously discussed, the HIM coder must review the record to determine the accurate code (*ICD-10-CM/PCS* or *Current Procedural Terminology [CPT]*) to represent the patient's diagnosis and procedures. To make this determination, the coder relies on the documentation in the record and his or her knowledge of coding. Other information that is captured as part of the abstract is the patient's disposition: the place the patient goes after discharge from the facility—home, nursing home, or another acute care facility, for example. Discharge disposition is entered in the form of one of the codes listed in Table 5-5.

If the data in a paper-based record are to be transmitted electronically, the data must be transferred from the paper record to the electronic medium. The data are located in the record and copied into the system through data entry. An abstractor reviews the record and enters the desired data into fields on an abstracting form. Sometimes, an interim step is performed in which the data are transcribed to a form as they are located and then

## TABLE 5-5

### DISCHARGE DISPOSITION CODES

| CODE | DISCHARGE STATUS |
|------|------------------|
| 02 | Discharged/transferred to another short-term general hospital for inpatient care |
| 03 | Discharged/transferred to a Skilled Nursing Facility (SNF) with Medicare certification in anticipation of covered skilled care |
| 04 | Discharged/transferred to a facility that provides custodial or supportive care |
| 05 | Discharged/transferred to a designated cancer center or children's hospital |
| 06 | Discharged/transferred to home under care of organized home health service organization in anticipation of covered skilled care |
| 21 | Discharged/transferred to court/law enforcement |
| 43 | Discharged/transferred to a federal health care facility |
| 50 | Discharged/transferred to hospice—home (inpatient only) |
| 51 | Discharged/transferred to hospice—medical facility (inpatient only) |
| 61 | Discharged/transferred within this institution to a hospital-based Medicare-approved swing bed |
| 62 | Discharged/transferred to an inpatient rehabilitation facility, including distinct part units of a hospital |
| 63 | Discharged/transferred to a long-term care hospital (LTCH) |
| 64 | Discharged/transferred to a nursing facility certified under Medicaid but not certified under Medicare |
| 65 | Discharged/transferred to a psychiatric hospital or psychiatric distinct-part unit of a hospital |
| 66 | Discharged/transferred to a critical access hospital (CAH) |
| 70 | Discharged/transferred to another type of health care institution not defined elsewhere in the code list |

A swing bed hospital is a hospital or critical access hospital (CAH) participating in Medicare that has CMS approval to provide post-hospital SNF care and meets certain requirements. A swing bed is an acute bed used by such a hospital to provide this service. http://www.cms.gov/Medicare/Medicare-Fee-for-Service-Payment/SNFPPS/SwingBed.html

A long-term care hospital (LTCH) is defined by Medicare as a hospital having an average length of stay over 25 days. http://www.cms.gov/Outreach-and-Education/Medicare-Learning-Network-MLN/MLNProducts/downloads/LTCH-News.pdf

A critical access hospital (CAH) is a special designation to hospitals that provide necessary care in remote locations. http://www.cms.gov/Outreach-and-Education/Medicare-Learning-Network-MLN/MLNProducts/downloads/CritAccessHospfctsht.pdf

entered all at once into the computer. Diagnosis and procedure codes are often captured this way, as are surgical procedure dates and physician identification numbers.

Figure 5-7 is an example of patient abstract screens. Note the information required in the abstract: patient's name, address, admission and discharge dates, discharge disposition, diagnosis, procedure, procedure date, and physicians' names. The demographic and financial data are populated into the abstract at registration. Nursing personnel typically complete the discharge date, time, and status. HIM personnel enter the diagnostic and procedural data and validate the existing data before billing.

### Abstracting the Record for Data Retrieval

Another reason for abstracting is to reduce the volume of data. There are often far more data in a health record than are needed for a particular user. For example, a patient keeping a file of his or her health records at home (a personal health record) would not usually need an entire copy of the record. The patient may need only a copy of the discharge summary or the operative records. These data could be abstracted for the patient. In this process, rather than the addition of data to the record, selected parts of the data are copied—to either paper or an electronic file.

Finally, health data are frequently analyzed for other purposes, such as research. In this type of abstracting, patient records are reviewed for specific data elements, which are then recorded on a data collection sheet for subsequent analysis. For example, all patients with a diagnosis of acute cerebrovascular infarction should receive diagnostic and therapeutic care related to stroke care. The hospital reviewer would review records of all patients with stroke and identify whether the specific tests were performed and specific medications given. The effectiveness of such intervention would be reported to Centers for Medicare and Medicaid Services (CMS) for quality review purposes.

HIM professionals are well suited by their training to be involved in these abstracting functions. Although data abstracting and abstracting for ROI are traditional HIM functions, regulatory and research analysis activities are well within the scope of HIM

**demographic data** Data elements that distinguish one patient from another, such as name, address, and birth date.

**financial data** Elements that describe the payer. For example, the name, address, and telephone number of the patient's insurance company as well as the group and member numbers the company has assigned to the patient.

**CMS** Centers for Medicare and Medicaid Services

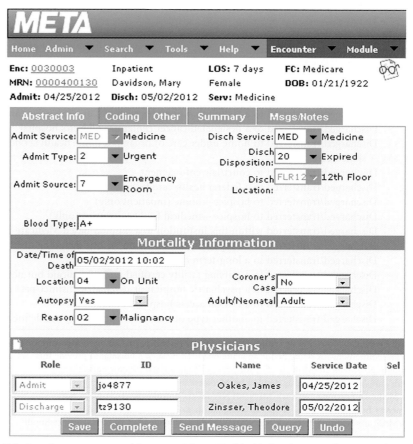

**Figure 5-7** An abstract screen. (Courtesy Meta Health Technology, a division of Streamline Health Solutions, Inc., Cincinnati, OH. Meta was acquired by Streamline Health Solutions, Inc. in August 2012.)

professional capabilities. Knowledge of the components of the record as well as an understanding of the clinical documentation content are core competencies for HIM professionals. Development of analytical skills sets, including clinical data analysis and regulatory reporting requirements, are useful for professionals who wish to move their careers in this direction.

## Tracking Records While Processing

While the patient is in the facility, the responsibility for maintaining his or her record rests with clinical staff members, particularly nursing and patient unit clerical staff members. Traditionally, in a paper-based environment, the HIM department assumes control once the patient is discharged. In an EHR environment, a number of departments may control aspects of the record. Because the record never actually moves from the computer, the physical location of the record is not in question. However, a paper-based record moves virtually every time an individual touches it. Therefore keeping track of it requires control procedures.

### Batch by Days

One way to keep track of paper records during postdischarge processing is to batch the records together by day. In this method, all records of discharges from April 15, for example, are gathered and kept together as they are moved as a group through assembly, analysis, and coding. At the end of the process, they are separated according to completion status. Completed charts are moved to the permanent file or scanning area for storage; incomplete charts are moved to the incomplete chart area. A **batch control form** lists the processing status of each record. This is particularly helpful if the record must be removed from the processing cycle for any reason.

**assembly** The reorganization of a paper record into a standard order.

**analysis** The review of a record to evaluate its completeness, accuracy, or compliance with predetermined standards or other criteria.

**coding** The assignment of alphanumerical values to a word, phrase, or other nonnumerical expression.

**batch control form** A listing of charts in process, postdischarge, that identifies which steps have been completed.

Records may be removed from the processing cycle for various reasons. The patient may have been readmitted, requiring review of the previous record. The record may need to be reviewed for quality assurance by another department, such as nursing. When the record is removed from the processing cycle, a batch control sheet clearly highlights the status of the record and facilitates its return to the appropriate processing step.

### Efficiency

To facilitate the many uses of the health record, related documents must be processed in a timely manner. It may make sense in some facilities that one must obtain the record in order to assemble it, assemble the record in order to analyze it, and analyze the record in order to code it. In some facilities, all personnel perform all of the steps. In other facilities, the chart is coded before analysis. All facilities process the health record in the way that best suits their particular workflow and their revenue cycle needs. For efficient processing, the paper record should be moved as little as possible, and each step should be performed in its entirety before the next step is attempted. In an EHR environment, some processes, such as analysis and coding, can take place concurrently. Many facilities maintain a central staging area, where paper records in process are kept between steps. This approach facilitates the location of records and the movement to the next processing step. Figure 5-3 illustrates the postdischarge processing flow.

> **workflow** The process of work flowing through a set of procedures to complete the health record.
>
> **revenue cycle** The groups of processes that identify, record, and report the financial transactions that result from the facility's clinical relationship with a patient.

### EXERCISE 5-2

#### Postdischarge Processing

1. What type of control is provided by the first processing step of receiving the records, as previously described?
2. Because physicians often are not actually employees of the facility at which they have privileges, what incentive do they have to complete their records?
3. The physician accidentally entered an order into the computer to request a cardiology consultation for the wrong patient. A staff nurse noticed the error. How should the correction be handled?
4. Health information management professionals perform a variety of internal control tasks within the context of postdischarge processing. List and describe one example of each type of control that is performed during this process.
5. In a paper environment, records must physically move from the patient care area to the HIM department for processing and storage. Give two examples of how that movement can occur.
6. Postdischarge processing follows a logical order. List the postdischarge processing steps in chronological order, beginning with obtaining control of the record.

## ELECTRONIC HEALTH RECORD MANAGEMENT

As discussed in Chapter 3, documentation of health records is moving to an electronic format. There have been changes in the postdischarge processing of patient records for the many facilities operating in a hybrid environment or fully functional EHR. This section discusses the issues that can arise and the changes in processing common to the conversion to electronic records.

### Electronic Health Record Processing Issues

Several issues and decisions must be made when a facility is converting from a paper record to an electronic record. Processing flow, staffing, and even department layout can change. Many facilities have made the decision to convert some data collection to electronic format and leave other in paper format, creating a hybrid record. Professionals must be well-versed in the nuances of processing, regardless of the data collection format.

> **hybrid record** A record in which both electronic and paper media are used.

### Record Assembly

An important consideration in the transition to EHR is how the health information is going to get into the EHR. Processing methods vary depending on what information is captured

**Go To** See Chapter 2 for information on forms control.

**point-of-care documentation** Clinical data recorded at the time the treatment is delivered to the patient.

**document imaging** Scanning or faxing of printed papers into a computer system or optical disk system. See also *Computer output to laser disk (COLD).*

**interface** Computer configuration allowing information to pass from one system to another.

**indexing** The process of sorting a record by the different report types, making the viewing of the record uniform.

electronically at the point of care or recorded first on paper. Will a paper record be generated first and then scanned in after discharge by the HIM department? Will some reports be scanned and combined with data that have already been captured at the point of care? Will clerks be needed to input data in the HIM department or at the points of care? Will it be a total electronic record in which each caregiver enters documents and orders directly into a computer system? Whatever the scenario, form control must be closely monitored and becomes more important with a document imaging system and the use of the EHR. Completely electronic data collection must be reviewed in the same way that paper data collection is reviewed so that all necessary data are captured in the correct format, in order to ensure data quality and satisfy the needs of the users.

If paper records are to be scanned, the use of bar codes for both the type of form and patient demographics is advantageous. Documents that have bar codes identifying the document and patient demographics may be scanned directly into the system. Documents without bar codes must be scanned with cover sheets to identify them to the system. The demographic bar code can be generated on labels and attached to each form. In some systems, the demographic bar code is automatically printed out on each report. The bar code indicating the form name is usually preprinted on the form. The bar codes allow for automatic indexing by patient record and report type. Indexing is discussed in more detail later in this chapter. Pages are scanned into the computer and linked to the patient's medical record number and admission (or encounter). If pages do not have machine-readable bar codes, the scanning operator must enter that data manually, a step that delays processing.

Chart order in a document management system is just as important as in the paper record. In the paper record, the order of the reports in the chart is standardized and the pages sorted to conform to that standard. Scanned documents are batched logically so that users can locate the portion of the record that is needed. For example, much like with a source-oriented paper record, scanned pages may be organized under tabs that indicate the type of documentation. Thus physician progress notes would be indexed so that they are accessible by clicking on a tab or menu for physician progress notes. Users of the EHR will rely on the indexes to find the reports that they need to read; if the format is standardized, they will become familiar with it more quickly.

Many reports are generated by systems that interface with the main electronic record system. Laboratory systems, radiology systems, and transcription systems are three examples of systems that generate data or reports and interface directly into the EHR. Just as scanned paper records are indexed, so are these data or reports indexed in the EHR for easy access.

As mentioned earlier, many reports may be printed while the patient is in the hospital. Thus the assembly process must also be continued in an electronic system, though it has been replaced by scanning. The assembler needs to analyze the disposition of these documents when they are obtained by the HIM department. Depending on how the documents are developed, they may be directly scanned or batch scanned.

## Scanning and Indexing

Scanning and *indexing* are necessary function with both the hybrid record and the EHR. With the hybrid record, the HIM department may be scanning the whole record or parts of a record. With the EHR, the HIM department may have only a few reports to scan because most data already reside in the EHR, either through direct data entry or by interface from another system. Scanning equipment must be purchased on the basis of the volume of reports (number of pages) to be scanned.

**Indexing** sorts the records by the different report types, making the viewing of the record uniform. Use of bar codes automates the indexing process. Indexing is important because users must be able to find the information that they need quickly in the computer system. The creation of an accurate index facilitates future retrieval of the images. With correct identification (i.e., indexing and naming) of the document for each patient, the computer system is able to locate the correct image when a search is performed.

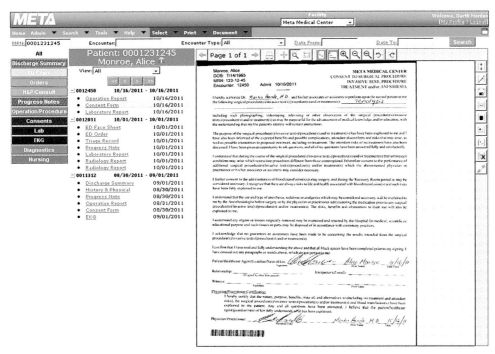

**Figure 5-8** An indexed electronic health record. (Courtesy Meta Health Technology, a division of Streamline Health Solutions, Inc., Cincinnati, OH. Meta was acquired by Streamline Health Solutions, Inc. in August 2012.)

What happens if the image is indexed by the wrong patient's name? How does one find the missing images of a record in the computer? All computer systems use various search methods to aid in the retrieval of the images. Additional methods to locate missing files require searching the discharge register or list to identify other patient records indexed on the same day. When records are scanned into a computer system, they are typically scanned in groups or batches. A typical group or batch of records would consist of 1 day of discharges. Therefore looking through the images of all the patients' records scanned on the same day may produce the missing image. Once the missing image is identified, it is renamed or indexed appropriately. Figure 5-8 is an example of an indexed EHR.

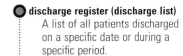

**discharge register (discharge list)** A list of all patients discharged on a specific date or during a specific period.

## Record Analysis

As discussed in previous chapters, analysis using a paper record is performed by HIM personnel, who review each page of the record to determine whether all the reports are present and any authentication is missing. A tally of what must be completed on the record can be maintained with use of a paper notification system or system-generated notification. For a hybrid or electronic record, it must be decided how and when the record will be analyzed. When using a hybrid record, an analysis clerk may still need to review the record and provide the physician with the chart deficiencies electronically. In the EHR, an automated deficiency analysis program may be included with the electronic record system; this program allows the record to be completed at the time of ordering or documenting. Policies and procedures must be established to define what constitutes a deficiency, and what a complete record.

**deficiencies** Required elements that are missing from a record.

The physicians can complete the records electronically using their passwords and can, in most cases, actually correct their own transcribed documents before signing them. The system can notify the physician that dictation, signatures, and even text are missing. In some facilities, the physician can complete the record remotely: from the private office or even from home. This arrangement removes the necessity for a physician visit to the HIM department. However, it also removes the opportunity for HIM personnel to interact with physicians when they visit. When the physician completes the records in the HIM department, procedures are set up to notify the physician of any coding queries or questions that HIM personnel may have about record completion. Because the physician can complete the EHR from areas other than the HIM department, procedures must be established to notify the physician in some other way about such matters. For example, instead of leaving a query on the record, the coder might send a fax to the physician's office. The temptation to send emails or text messages is strong; however, patient confidentiality must be preserved, eliminating unsecure methods of communication.

Authentication in a hybrid or electronic record must be carefully considered. A digitized signature is an original signature on a report that is then scanned into an electronic document. A digital signature occurs when the authenticator uses a password or personal identification number (PIN) to electronically sign a document. In some facilities, the authenticator must use both a password and a PIN to sign. The authentication method must provide a means to identify the user, **nonrepudiation** (a process that provides a positive identification of the user), and integrity of the signature (i.e., the document cannot be altered after the signature has been applied).

## Coding

In most facilities, the coding function is being assisted with a computer application called an encoder to help assign diagnosis and procedure codes more efficiently and accurately. In order to avoid duplication of effort, such as entering the codes on both the encoder and the abstracting screens, the encoder should interface directly with the abstracting system. The timing of coding is also an issue. In the case of a hybrid record, the coder must use both paper components and electronic record components to identify all of the diagnoses and procedures. If the paper component will be scanned, it might be more efficient for the coding personnel to wait until the record is scanned before attempting to code. However, if scanning delays coding beyond the facility's needs, the coders cannot wait for scanning. A fully electronic record eliminates the inefficiency of accommodating paper components and also permits the coding process to migrate to a remote location, as is common with transcription.

When the electronic record is used for coding, the facility may opt to provide large monitors or dual monitors to the coders that give them better visualization of the record and allow them to use two windows at once.

With the availability of electronically captured data, some coding can be automated. As clinicians select diagnoses from drop-down menus, these diagnoses can be captured for billing purposes. Although there is technically no reason for a coder to have to intervene in such a scenario, the reality is that clinicians do not always understand sequencing of codes and billing rules. Therefore review of charts by coders, periodic audits of coded data, and careful attention to billing errors are essential.

For more complex records, computer-assisted coding (CAC) applications can "read" transcribed documents and assign codes to meaningful phrases. Radiology transcriptions lend themselves to this process, as do operative reports. In a complex inpatient record, a CAC report of coded phrases could facilitate coding by reducing the amount of time a coder has to spend reading detailed reports.

## Abstracting

Even though all the data in a patient's health record have already been captured digitally in a fully functional EHR, the process of abstracting is no less important. Just as in a paper environment, the data elements listed in Figure 5-7 must be isolated and entered into a separate abstract database. Sophisticated software programs are able to abstract minimum data elements from the health record of each patient, although the job of HIM professionals remains critical. Because the abstract database is a central source of data for a variety of users, each patient's abstract must be carefully reviewed for accuracy. As discussed earlier, verification of the abstract is a detective control. Fixing any noted errors is a corrective control.

Most HIM departments use a computer program to abstract data electronically and generate reports from that system. When a facility is converting to a hybrid or fully electronic record, HIM staff must address how abstracting will occur—in a freestanding

---

**digitized signature** An original signature on a report that is then scanned into an electronic document.

**digital signature** An electronic means to identify the authenticity and integrity of the user's identification.

**nonrepudiation** A process that provides a positive identification of the user.

**abstracting** The recap of selected fields from a health record to create an informative summary. Also refers to the activity of identifying such fields and entering them into a computer system.

**billing** The process of submitting health insurance claims or rendering invoices.

**CAC** computer-assisted coding

program, with an interface, or through a vendor's product that includes report-writing capabilities. It must be determined whether data will be captured at the point of care or abstracted retrospectively. In the EHR, the abstracting function could be automated, with data captured at the time of documentation (see Figure 5-7). Certainly, discharge date and discharge disposition (e.g., home, transfer to rehabilitation, expired) can be captured by point-of-care staff. Some billing and patient insurance benefits depend on accurate discharge disposition data. Therefore data quality audits still must be performed to ensure that the data are accurate.

**point of care** Clinical data recorded at the time the treatment is delivered to the patient.

## Storage and Retention

During conversion to a hybrid or an electronic record, policies and procedures must be established to define what constitutes the legal health record. In a hybrid system this definition should be specified by hospital policy. In the hybrid record in which a paper chart is generated and then scanned into the electronic record, policies must specify what will happen to the paper record. The policy must address whether the paper record will be destroyed or maintained in offsite storage. Retention issues must be addressed in the policy. How long will the paper record be maintained in storage before it is destroyed? Will computer-based data be available online or archived over time?

**retention** The procedures governing the storage of records, including duration, location, security, and access.

## Transcription

The way in which the transcribed report moves to the EHR is an important issue to consider. The hybrid or electronic record will have the transcribed reports available for viewing on the health record as soon as the report is released by the transcriptionist. In some cases, signature deficiencies can be assigned automatically when the document moves from the transcription system to the electronic record system. Additionally, with a speech recognition interface at the point of dictation (front-end), the dictator can view the transcribed document while dictating and make changes concurrently.

Another issue to consider is whether the physicians can correct the transcribed reports electronically. If electronic corrections are allowed, do the different versions of the report need to be saved? Can corrections be made after a digital signature is applied or only before? If such corrections are not allowed, how will corrections be made? For documents with different versions, what type of an audit trail will the system maintain in order to keep track of which version was available at a particular point in time? What about transcribed reports generated from different systems, such as radiology and cardiology? How will these reports be interfaced with the main system? If front-end speech recognition is used, what quality controls will be implemented to ensure complete, properly formatted reports?

**audit trail** Software that tracks and stores information related to the activity of users in the system.

Clearly, there are many questions to be answered when dealing with transcribed documents. One key issue when paper-based records are still in use is: Will physicians be required to dictate certain reports or will they still have the option to write out their reports by hand, if desired? For most dictated reports, the cost of transcription is not the issue. The clarity achieved by having a typed document is generally worth the cost. The author must review the typed document for accuracy, thereby providing an audit of the reports—an important detective and corrective control. However, in a teaching facility where residents are also preparing reports, the cost may become prohibitive. Templates and menu-driven reports may be alternatives to free-form dictations in some cases.

## Release of Information

The Health Insurance Portability and Accountability Act (HIPAA) Privacy and Security Rules require health care facilities to have administrative, technical, and physical safeguards in place to ensure privacy and safeguard information whether it is on paper or in an electronic format.

Administrative safeguards include policies and procedures regarding confidentiality and security agreements signed by each staff member as well as by any non–staff member users of the medical record. The Security Rule requires that facilities identify all systems that

**Health Insurance Portability and Accountability Act (HIPAA)** Public Law 104-191, federal legislation passed in 1996 that outlines the guidelines of managing patient information in terms of privacy, security, and confidentiality. The legislation also outlines penalties for noncompliance.

contain electronic personal health information and perform a risk assessment to identify areas that may pose a security risk. Staff training is an integral part of the Privacy and Security Rules. The following topics are important and should be included in training:

- How to guard against threats of computer viruses or hackers and where to report suspicious activity
- Routine performance of audits to ensure that employees are using protected health information (PHI) on a need-to-know basis and that actions have been taken if inappropriate viewing or use of PHI is found
- Education on how to dispose of PHI on paper or electronic media such as optical disks
- Management of passwords: how often they will change and sanctions for sharing passwords

Technical safeguards are addressed in detail in HIPAA's Security Rule. An example of a technical safeguard is a procedure to deny system access immediately upon employee termination. Another example is automatic log-offs: If a computer idles for more than a specific number of minutes, it will automatically log the user off. Some facilities may also use encryption of data as a technical safeguard. Encryption is an effective way to support data security. To read an encrypted file, you must have access to a secret key or password that enables you to read it.

Physical safeguards must be established to protect unauthorized access to areas or systems containing PHI. If a paper-generated record is used, locked doors are used as barriers to protect the information. The following are examples of physical safeguards in an electronic context:

- Placing sensors on portable devices such as laptops and handheld devices that sound an alarm if the devices are taken off the premises
- Placing computer monitors in areas that minimize the chance that a stranger could view confidential information
- Using a dark screen monitor cover to prevent passersby from seeing data on the screen

## Workflow

In the paper context, workflow referred to the way in which the paper record was processed from one HIM function to another or moved from one desk to another. In the electronic context, workflow describes how the electronic record moves from one electronic component to another. Once a function is completed, the electronic record may automatically be sent to the appropriate work areas. These electronic work areas are called **queues.** An example of an HIM queue would be the coding queue or the analysis queue. Queues can be further defined (e.g., a coding queue may be called an outpatient coding queue). Individual coders may be assigned records automatically on the basis of predetermined criteria, such as type of record, may select records from the queue, or may be assigned records manually by the supervisor. These queues are an important workflow distribution tool. Supervisors can manage the workflow among coders, for example, and track the time items spend in queue. Queues are common in coding, transcription, and billing activities.

When an action is completed in a queue, the workflow software sends the electronic record to the next work area or queue. For example, when the coder has completed the abstract, the record may be routed to the coding supervisor for review. If the supervisor identifies an error, the record may then be routed back to the coder for correction. Other possible routing includes postdischarge review by documentation improvement specialists, pending query to physician, or finalize for billing.

Note that the record does not actually move in a completely electronic system. Workflow distribution in this context is a communication tool that alerts a specific user that there is a task to be performed. Once it is performed, the next user is notified. Some users may be able to work concurrently. For example, incomplete chart analysts may be able to work with the record at the same time the record is being coded. Physicians can certainly be reviewing and signing documents while the record is in process. In other cases, tasks may be sequential, such as scanning being followed by coding (particularly if the coder is working remotely).

---

**protected health information (PHI)** Individually identifiable health information that is transmitted or maintained in any form or medium by covered entities or their business associates.

**encryption** A security process that blocks unauthorized access to patient information.

**workflow** The process of work flowing through a set of procedures to complete the health record.

**queue** Electronic work area.

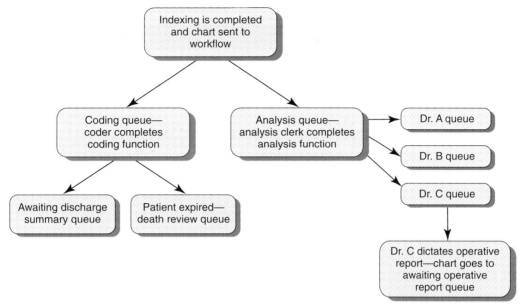

**Figure 5-9** A simple example of workflow in an electronic health record.

Workflow issues are complex and must be carefully planned. It must be decided what queues will be included and, more important, which staff members will be responsible for working the numerous queues. Error or pending queues, for example, are an important control function. A transcribed report goes to the queue when the HIM interface cannot identify the physician's name. HIM personnel review the report and route the report to the correct patient record.

A simple example of workflow in an electronic record is shown in Figure 5-9.

## OTHER HEALTH INFORMATION MANAGEMENT ROLES

This chapter discusses the traditional roles that HIM professionals play in the postdischarge processing of a health record. However, HIM professionals are employed in various roles and settings in the health care industry. As some of the traditional paper-based activities are replaced by electronic activities, exciting new opportunities arise for well-trained professionals with an eye to the future and a willingness to learn new skills. Entry-level positions in assembly and analysis now require increased technology skills. The focus on data quality and customer service points entry-level HIM professionals toward patient access. Billing is another area in which HIM professionals, because of their knowledge of coding and documentation requirements, may find opportunities to advance their careers. The move toward an electronic record opens new roles in training and technology implementation, not just in hospitals but in virtually all health care settings, including pharmaceuticals, insurance, and research. Students are encouraged to explore traditional as well as new avenues in planning their careers in HIM.

## WORKS CITED

Davis N: Revenue cycle management best practices, Chicago, 2011, American Health Information Management Association.

Federal Register. Code of Federal Regulations, Title 42, Vol 5, Part 482.24 (c) 2.i.A, 2012.

The Joint Commission: Hospital accreditation standards: record of care, treatment, and services, Chicago, 2012, The Joint Commission, RC.01.02.01, RC.02.01.03, and RC.01.04.01.

## SUGGESTED READING

Andress AA: Manual of medical office management, Philadelphia, 1996, Saunders.

Buck CJ: Step-by-step medical coding, ed 3, Philadelphia, 2000, Saunders.

## CHAPTER ACTIVITIES

### CHAPTER SUMMARY

Accuracy, validity, timeliness, and completeness are important data qualities. Prevention, detection, and correction of errors promote data of the best quality. HIM professionals are traditionally responsible for the postdischarge processing of health data. The focus of postdischarge processing of a health record is the preparation of health data for billing and retention (storage, security, and access).

After the patient's discharge, records must be obtained, assembled or scanned, analyzed, coded, and completed. Once control over the health record has been obtained, the record must be tracked and controlled throughout the postdischarge processing cycle. Ultimately, the record passes to the permanent file area or is finalized electronically. The HIM department is generally responsible for the release of patient information to authorized users. HIM professionals are employed in these traditional functions and also in many other functions throughout the health care industry.

### REVIEW QUESTIONS

1. List and explain the elements of data quality discussed in this chapter.
2. List, explain, and give examples of the three types of internal controls.
3. Explain the flow of postdischarge processing of health information.
4. List and explain the major functions of postdischarge processing in a health information management department.
5. Explain the principles and process flow of an incomplete record system.

### ● CAREER TIP

There are many opportunities for coders from physician offices to hospitals to consulting firms and even software developers. Knowledge of medical terminology, anatomy and physiology, pathology, and coding is essential. On the physician-based side, the American Academy of Professional Coders (AAPC) offers focused courses that lead directly to specific coding credentials. This training can lead to opportunities in physician offices or hospital outpatient settings. For inpatient coding, courses from a certificate program approved by the American Health Information Management Association (AHIMA) or from AHIMA itself are optimum. A degree in HIM is helpful for individuals who want to progress to supervisory or management roles.

### ● PROFESSIONAL PROFILE

#### Coder

My name is Olga, and I am a coder in the health information management department at Diamonte Hospital. There are six coders in our department: four inpatient coders and two outpatient coders. In addition, there is a coding supervisor, who trains us and checks our work.

I started out as an assembler in the department. I assembled records for a year. I had to learn the postdischarge order of the record and how to file loose sheets. When an opening came up in the analysis section, I applied for it and was promoted. I enjoyed analysis, but I also began to understand the importance of the data contained in the records. I was really interested in the clinical data and decided to go to school to learn about coding, because coders work with the data.

Our local community college has a health information management department, and I enrolled in their coding certificate program. I studied medical terminology, health record development and retention, anatomy and physiology, and disease pathology. I took several coding courses, learning ICD-10-CM and CPT. While I was a student, the coding supervisor allowed me to study completed records so that I could practice coding. When I finished the program, I was promoted to outpatient coder. I kept practicing inpatient coding with the completed records, and I asked a lot of questions. Now I code inpatient records most of the time and help out with the outpatient records.

After 2 years as an inpatient coder, I sat for and passed the Certified Coding Specialist (CCS) examination that is offered by the American Health Information Management Association. I am now a CCS! I really enjoy coding. It's challenging and interesting, and there are a lot of opportunities for me as I learn more about clinical data and how to manage health information.

## PATIENT CARE PERSPECTIVE

### Dr. Lewis

The hospital uses codes for data analysis and billing purposes, and so do I. Recently, I sent my patient, Isabel, to the hospital for a blood test. I was surprised to get a call from patient registration that I had used an invalid code on the request (script). So, I called Shamees right away to help me find the right code. Without the right code to explain the medical necessity of the test, Isabel's insurance would not have paid for the test. Isabel was very happy to get that problem resolved on the spot.

## APPLICATION

### Merging Expectations

You are the director of HIM at Community Hospital, a small hospital that has just merged with another hospital in your area. The facilities are roughly the same size. Approximately half of the physicians at your facility also have privileges at the other facility. With some exceptions, the two facilities have similar departments and services. Both facilities have some EHR capabilities and are able to interface because they use the same software vendor. Full computerization will not take place for at least 5 years. The administration of the two facilities would like to standardize the data collection with the goal of reducing the cost of forms and facilitating communication between the two facilities. As the senior director, you have been asked to coordinate this effort. What issues do you think should be addressed first? Who will you ask to assist in the project? What impact does this standardization project have on the HIM department?

**CHAPTER**

# CODE SETS

Marion Gentul

## VOCABULARY

American Medical
Association (AMA)
American Psychiatric
Association (APA)
case mix
classification
Cooperating Parties
Current Procedural
Terminology (CPT)
*Diagnostic and Statistical
Manual of Mental
Disorders, Fourth Edition
(DSM-IV)*

electronic data interchange
(EDI)
*Federal Register*
Healthcare Common
Procedure Coding
System (HCPCS)
*HIPAA Official Guidelines
for Coding and
Reporting*
ICD-10-CM
ICD-10-PCS
ICD-9-CM
ICD-O

Interactive Map-Assisted
Generation of ICD-
10-CM Codes (I-MAGIC)
algorithm
International Health
Terminology Standards
Development
Organisation (IHTSDO)
multi-axial
National Cancer Institute's
Surveillance,
Epidemiology and End
Results (SEER)

National Drug Codes (NDC)
National Library of
Medicine (NLM)
nomenclature
SNOMED-CT
standards for code sets
Standards of Ethical Coding
transaction code sets
World Health Organization
(WHO)

## CHAPTER OBJECTIVES

*By the end of this chapter, the student should be able to:*
1. Describe the general purpose of coded data in relation to its various uses.
2. Name the transaction code sets required under HIPAA.
3. Describe the format of ICD-10-CM.
4. Describe the format of ICD-10-PCS.
5. Describe different coding and classification systems and their uses.
6. Identify unethical coding practices.

---

**coding** The assignment of alphanumerical values to a word, phrase, or other nonnumerical expression. In health care, coding is the assignment of numerical values to diagnosis and procedure descriptions.

**postdischarge processing** The procedures designed to prepare a health record for retention.

**reimbursement** The amount of money that the health care facility receives from the party responsible for paying the bill.

## CODING

Coding is discussed in Chapter 5 as an element of postdischarge processing. This chapter focuses on several of the most commonly used coding systems and on how and when codes are used for health care reimbursement.

Although the coding function is most often associated with payment and reimbursement, coded data are used for other, equally important purposes. For example, coding professionals are key players in ensuring providers' compliance with official coding guidelines and government regulations. The statistical data collected from complete and accurate coding are necessary to provide a facility or health care provider with the following:

- Resource utilization information: volume and disease data
- Databases for maintaining indices and registries: lists of diagnosis, procedure, and physician data (see Chapter 10)
- Physician practice profiling information: physician volume data
- Information to assist in financial and strategic planning: volumes, services, and severity of illness
- Research and clinical trials
- Evaluation of the safety and quality of care
- Quality and outcomes measurements
- Prevention of health care fraud and abuse
- Other administrative initiatives and activities, such as audits and productivity analysis

On the patient level, the codes assigned to diagnoses and procedures for an individual patient's encounter or hospital stay may follow that patient throughout the health care delivery system and have an impact on future treatments and insurability. In the quest for fast billing turnaround time and payment, it is sometimes easy to forget that the patient record is a highly personal document, one that often describes a person's last days, and therefore must be treated respectfully with regard to the coded data assigned. The American Health Information Management Association (AHIMA) has issued "**Standards of Ethical Coding**," guidelines that all coders, regardless of setting, should be aware of and follow (Figure 6-1).

**AHIMA** American Health Information Management Association

**Standards of Ethical Coding** Guidelines from the AHIMA to guide professional coders toward ethical decisions.

Coding professionals should:

1. Apply accurate, complete, and consistent coding practices for the production of high-quality healthcare data.

AHIMA

2. Report all healthcare data elements (e.g. diagnosis and procedure codes, present on admission indicator, discharge status) required for external reporting purposes (e.g. reimbursement and other administrative uses, population health, quality and patient safety measurement, and research) completely and accurately, in accordance with regulatory and documentation standards and requirements and applicable official coding conventions, rules, and guidelines.
3. Assign and report only the codes and data that are clearly and consistently supported by health record documentation in accordance with applicable code set and abstraction conventions, rules, and guidelines.
4. Query provider (physician or other qualified healthcare practitioner) for clarification and additional documentation prior to code assignment when there is conflicting, incomplete, or ambiguous information in the health record regarding a significant reportable condition or procedure or other reportable data element dependent on health record documentation (e.g. present on admission indicator).
5. Refuse to change reported codes or the narratives of codes so that meanings are misrepresented.
6. Refuse to participate in or support coding or documentation practices intended to inappropriately increase payment, qualify for insurance policy coverage, or skew data by means that do not comply with federal and state statutes, regulations and official rules and guidelines.
7. Facilitate interdisciplinary collaboration in situations supporting proper coding practices.
8. Advance coding knowledge and practice through continuing education.
9. Refuse to participate in or conceal unethical coding or abstraction practices or procedures.
10. Protect the confidentiality of the health record at all times and refuse to access protected health information not required for coding-related activities ( examples of coding-related activities include completion of code assignment, other health record data abstraction, coding audits, and educational purposes).
11. Demonstrate behavior that reflects integrity, shows a commitment to ethical and legal coding practices, and fosters trust in professional activities.

Revised and approved by the House of Delegates 09/08

**Figure 6-1** The American Health Information Management Association (AHIMA) standards of ethical coding. (AHIMA Standards of Ethical Coding. http://library.ahima.org/xpedio/groups/public/documents/ahima/bok2_001166.hcsp?dDocName=bok2_001166. Revised September 2008. Accessed July 20, 2011. Adapted and Reprinted with permission from the American Health Information Management Association. Copyright © 2012 by the American Health Information Management Association. All rights reserved. No part of this may be reproduced, reprinted, stored in a retrieval system, or transmitted, in any form or by any means, electronic, photocopying, recording, or otherwise, without the prior written permission of the association.)

**Go To** HIPAA is discussed in greater detail in Chapter 12.

**standards for code sets** Standards that must be used under HIPAA for the electronic exchange of data for certain transactions, namely encounter and payment data.

**Health Insurance Portability and Accountability Act (HIPAA)** Public Law 104-191, federal legislation passed in 1996 that outlines the guidelines of managing patient information in terms of privacy, security, and confidentiality.

**transaction code set** A code set, established by HIPAA guidelines, to be used in electronic data transfer to ensure that the information transmitted is complete, private, and secure.

**electronic data interchange (EDI)** A standard in which data can be transmitted, communicated, and understood by the sending and receiving computer systems, allowing the exchange of information.

**ICD-10-CM** International Classification of Diseases, Tenth Revision—Clinical Modification. The United States clinical modification of the WHO ICD-10 morbidity and mortality data set. ICD-10-CM is mandated by HIPAA for reporting diagnoses and reasons for healthcare encounters in all settings.

**ICD-10-PCS** International Classification of Diseases, Tenth Revision, Procedural Coding System. A unique classification system, developed in the U.S., for reporting procedures performed in inpatient settings. It is a HIPAA mandated code set.

**inpatient** An individual who is admitted to a hospital with the intention of staying overnight.

Coding is essentially the translation of documented descriptions of diagnoses (e.g., diseases, injuries, circumstances, and reasons for encounters) into a numerical or alpha-numerical code. Thus the diagnosis *hypertension* is translated to the code I10. The same can be said of translating documented descriptions of procedures, services, or treatments. Coding standardizes the communication of clinical data between users and facilitates electronic transmission of clinical data.

Of interest to coders today are the **standards for code sets** under the Health Insurance Portability and Accountability Act (HIPAA) of 1996, which names standards for exchanging information through the use of codes. Under HIPAA, **transaction code sets** are sets of codes used to communicate the diagnosis and procedure codes, data elements, and medical concepts used in electronic health care transactions transferred through an **electronic data interchange (EDI).** The code sets used in the EDI were mandatory for use in reporting and reimbursement using electronic transaction format version 5010, effective January 1, 2012. The electronic version of a Uniform Bill (UB-04), for example, is the 837I, which is sent in 5010 format. Transaction code sets prior to October 1, 2014, are as follows:

- *ICD-9-CM, Volumes I and II; ICD-9-CM, Volume III,* for transmitting diagnoses and inpatient procedures
- *National Drug Codes (NDCs),* used for defining drugs by name, manufacturer, and dosage
- *Current Dental Terminology (CDT),* for dental terms
- *Healthcare Common Procedure Coding System (HCPCS)*; and *Current Procedural Terminology, 4th edition (CPT-4),* for transmitting outpatient procedures and defining inpatient charges

Effective October 1, 2014, **ICD-10-CM** and **ICD-10-PCS** replace ICD-9-CM Volumes I, II and III.

Coded data are also retained in electronic format within a facility, such as a hospital, or for a provider, such as a physician office. This coded data can also be shared within a network. Imagine attempting to share information about hundreds or thousands of patients without translating the written descriptions of diagnoses and procedures into codes, and one begins to appreciate the complexity of coded data and the importance of those who perform the coding function.

Many coding systems are in use today throughout the United States and the world. The United Kingdom, for example, uses the *Office of Population Censuses and Surveys (OPCS-4) Classification of Interventions and Procedures,* a coding system comparable to the ICD-10; Canada developed an adaptation to the ICD-10, ICD-10-CA. The word in*ternatio*nal can be found in the titles of many of these different coding systems. For example, the *International Medical Terminology,* for the reporting of regulatory activities, was developed under the auspices of the *International Conference on Harmonization of Technical Requirements for Registration of Pharmaceuticals for Human Use (ICH)* (National Center for Biomedical Ontology, 2012). Some systems are sponsored and maintained by governmental agencies and others by various medical or health associations in the United States and internationally. In the United States, the coding system used depends on the applicable HIPAA transaction code set used in the provider setting. For example, inpatient hospital-based coders use transaction code sets ICD-10-CM and ICD-10-PCS effective October 1, 2014.

## HIT-bit

### ICDs USED IN CANADA

Canada has used ICD-10-CA since 2002 for diagnosis coding. ICD-10-CA is very similar to ICD-10-CM but was adapted from ICD for use in Canada. For procedure coding, Canada uses the Canadian Classification of Interventions (CCI). CCI resembles ICD-10-PCS in some ways but differs significantly in other ways.

This chapter focuses on HIPAA transaction code sets, including ICD-10-CM and ICD-10-PCS, and HCPCS/CPT-4. Other important coding systems, including SNOMED-CT, are also discussed.

## Nomenclature and Classification

There are two basic types of coding systems: *nomenclature* and *classification*. A **nomenclature** is a system of naming things. Scientific and technical professions typically have their own nomenclatures. A number of different nomenclatures are used in medicine. A common nomenclature is found in the **Healthcare Common Procedure Coding System (HCPCS)** and **Current Procedural Terminology (CPT).** Nomenclatures facilitate communication because the users have available the specific definition of the codes. For example, HCPCS code G0010 represents the *administration of Hepatitis B vaccine*, and HCPCS code G0027 (the next G code) represents *semen analysis; presence and/or motility of sperm excluding Huhner*. Although many HCPCS codes are related to the next sequential code, there is no global relationship from one code to the next, and the purpose of the assignment of codes is primarily to enable users to communicate efficiently and effectively via computer data entry.

**nomenclature** A formal method of naming used by a scientific or technical profession; in medical coding, users of the nomenclature determine the definition of each code.

**Healthcare Common Procedure Coding System (HCPCS)** The CMS coding system, of which CPT-4 is level one. Used for drugs, equipment, supplies, and other auxiliary health care services rendered.

**Current Procedural Terminology (CPT)** A nomenclature and coding system developed and maintained by the American Medical Association to facilitate billing for physicians and other services.

### HIT-bit

#### WILLIAM FARR—MEDICAL STATISTICIAN

William Farr (1807-1883) was the first medical statistician in the General Registrar Office of England and Wales. In 1839, at the first Annual Report of the Registrar General, he discussed the principles, still relevant, that should govern a statistical classification of disease and urged the adoption of a uniform classification system, as follows:

> The advantages of a uniform statistical nomenclature, however imperfect, are so obvious, that it is surprising no attention has been paid to its enforcement in Bills of Mortality. Each disease has, in many instances, been denoted by three or four terms, and each term has been applied to as many different diseases: vague, inconvenient names have been employed, or complications have been registered instead of primary diseases. The nomenclature is of as much importance in this department of inquiry as weights and measures in the physical sciences, and should be settled without delay.

Farr proposed a classification system that included the principle of classifying diseases by anatomical site, a concept that was incorporated into early classification systems and that has survived to this day.

In addition to nomenclatures, **classification** systems are very important in health care. The primary disease classification system used in health care delivery systems is the International Classification of Diseases (ICD). ICD is used worldwide and is in its tenth revision (ICD-10). In the United States, it has been modified to increase its level of detail and to add procedural coding. Classification systems group codes so that coding sequences have logical relationships. For example, ICD-10 groups diagnoses by body system and sequences related conditions together. I21 is the ICD-10 category for acute myocardial infarctions, and I25 is the category for coronary artery disease. Subcategories describe the location, episode, or extent of the condition.

**classification** Systematic organization of elements into categories. ICD-10-CM is a classification system that organizes diagnoses into categories, primarily by body system.

Health information management (HIM) professionals must be knowledgeable about the coding systems used in the setting in which they are employed. Many HIM professionals are coders; however, a great deal of data analysis and reporting also occurs in health care, much of it in coded format. Therefore students of HIM should pay particular attention to developing sufficient coding skills to enhance their career opportunities.

## EXERCISE 6-1

**Coding**

1. Provide three examples for which coded data might be used in a facility.
2. What transaction format is used to transfer electronic data?
3. Name three coding systems used for reimbursement.

**morbidity** A disease or illness.

**mortality** The frequency of death.

**vital statistics** Public health data collected through birth certificates, death certificates, and other data gathering tools.

**World Health Organization (WHO)** An agency under the United Nations establishing focus areas for international public health policy.

**ICD-10** International Classification of Diseases, Tenth Revision

**ICD-9-CM** International Classification of Diseases, Ninth Revision—Clinical Modification. The United States version of the ICD-9.

**reimbursement** The amount of money that the health care facility receives from the party responsible for paying the bill.

**diagnosis-related groups (DRGs)** A collection of health care descriptions organized into statistically similar categories.

**prospective payment system (PPS)** A system used by payers, primarily the CMS, for reimbursing acute care facilities on the basis of statistical analysis of health care data.

**longitudinal** The electronic flow of information from one type of provider to another over the span of a patient's care.

**ICD-10-CM** International Classification of Diseases, Tenth Revision—Clinical Modification. The United States clinical modification of the World Health Organization ICD-10 morbidity and mortality data set. ICD-10-CM is mandated by HIPAA for reporting diagnoses and reasons for healthcare encounters in all settings.

**ICD-10-CM Examples**
- **E10.641**—Type 1 diabetes mellitus with hypoglycemia with coma
- **O11.3**—Pre-existing hypertension with pre-eclampsia, third trimester

## GENERAL PURPOSE CODE SETS

### ICD-9-CM

Coding for disease nomenclature purposes began in the 18th century with the attempt to name diseases. The first classification system, the Bertillon Classification of Causes of Death, was adopted by the International Statistics Institute (ISI) in 1893. Named after Jacques Bertillon, the chair of the ISI committee that developed the system, the Bertillon Classification of Causes of Death was adopted in the United States in 1899. Although some morbidity classifications were being developed at this time as well, it was not until 1948 that the adoption of classifications for disease took root and the sixth revision of the Bertillon Classification was incorporated into the *Manual of the International Statistical Classification of Diseases, Injuries, and Causes of Death* under the auspices of the World Health Congress. This also marked the beginning of the formal international effort to coordinate mortality reporting from national committees of vital and health statistics to the **World Health Organization (WHO)**. The WHO continued to revise the morbidity and mortality classification system, currently called the International Statistical Classification of Diseases and Related Health Problems, 10th Revision (ICD-10) (World Health Organization, 2011).

The United States lags behind the rest of the world in adopting ICD-10 for general use. WHO member nations began implementation of ICD-10 in 1994; however, the United States used it only for mortality reporting. The United States has continued to use ICD-9 as the basis for its clinical modification of the ICD-9 code set (**ICD-9-CM**) while it evaluated and eventually developed ICD-10-CM.

When ICD-9-CM was mandated for use in 1979, it really had no special purpose other than to ensure an updated and unified coding system in the United States. Coding became directly linked to reimbursement in 1983 with the implementation of the diagnosis-related group (DRG)–based hospital prospective payment system (PPS).

Although ICD-9-CM is scheduled to be replaced by ICD-10-CM/PCS, it is still important for HIM professionals to have at least a basic understanding of it. It is unlikely that organizations will convert their databases to ICD-10-CM/PCS, so historical data will continue to be displayed and used in ICD-9-CM format. Further, historical data will be subject to audits and used for research purposes and for longitudinal studies of coded data.

### ICD-10-CM

ICD-10-CM is published by the United States Government. The foundation of ICD-10-CM is the International Statistical Classification of Diseases and Related Health Problems, Tenth Revision, or ICD-10, published by the World Health Organization. With some variations, ICD-10 is also used in approximately 100 countries. ICD-10-CM is scheduled to replace ICD-9-CM Volumes I and II effective October 1, 2014.

ICD-10-CM contains characteristics that were not available in previous versions of the clinical modification of ICD. ICD-10-CM's structure is such that considerable expansion is possible, enabling the addition of new, specific codes as needed without compromising the general code structure.

ICD-10-CM consists of two main parts, the Index to Diseases and Injuries (the main index), and the Tabular List of Diseases and Injuries (the main tabular list). The Index consists of an alphabetical listing of terms followed by their corresponding complete or partial (incomplete) codes. The incomplete codes found in the Index must be completed, on the basis of additional information and instruction in the Tabular, to become valid

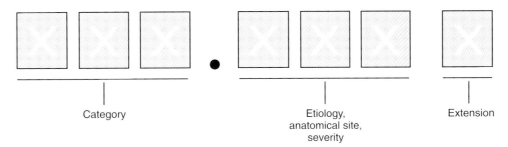

Figure 6-2 ICD-10-CM (International Classification of Diseases, Tenth Revision—Clinical Modification) code format.

codes. The Tabular is the complete list of codes, in numerical order. It is essential to use both the Index and Tabular for code assignment, because instruction notes and other elements such as punctuation in both the Index and Tabular must be followed. These instruction notes, called conventions and guidelines, are found in the **HIPAA Official Guidelines for Coding and Reporting.** The *Official Guidelines* are updated each October. They can be located in the CDC Web site; for example, the link to the *2011 Official Guidelines* is http://www.cdc.gov/nchs/data/icd9/10cmguidelines2011_FINAL.pdf.

ICD-10-CM codes are alphanumerical; a letter is always the first character in each code. The first three characters represent the code category. Characters four, five, and six represent etiology, anatomical site, and severity, respectively. Valid codes range from three to six characters in length. Certain code categories have applicable seventh characters, or code extensions, the meaning of which depends on the code and chapter where it is required. In the event that a code requiring a seventh character extension is less than six characters in length, a placeholder character, "x," is used to ensure that the seventh character extension is in the seventh character data field. See Figure 6-2 for an illustration.

Other unique features of ICD-10-CM include expanded injury codes, more codes relevant to ambulatory and outpatient encounters, combination codes, and classifications specific to laterality.

The main index also contains the Index to External Causes of Injury, the Neoplasm Table, and the Table of Drugs and Chemicals, all with corresponding codes in the main tabular.

ICD-10-CM can be downloaded in either PDF (printer-downloadable format) or XML (Extensible Markup Language) format from the CDC's Web site; the draft of the 2013 ICD-10-CM can be found here: http://www.cdc.gov/nchs/icd/icd10cm.htm#10update.

In the United States, the *Cooperating Parties* are responsible for ICD-10-CM. The **Cooperating Parties** consist of representatives of the American Hospital Association (AHA), AHIMA, the Centers for Medicare and Medicaid Services (CMS), and NCHS. The Cooperating Parties meet twice yearly, usually in April and October, to hear and discuss proposed code changes or revisions. Anyone can attend these meetings. Notices and agendas can be found on the CMS Web site in the *Federal Register* section at http://www.gpoaccess.gov/fr. If and when a proposed code change meets final approval, it can be accessed in the *Federal Register* section as a Final Rule. Coding changes may be approved and issued for use twice yearly, in April and October, although most major changes are effective in October.

**ICD-10-CM Examples—cont'd**
- **O32.1XX2**—Maternal care for breech presentation, fetus 2
- **S42.201A**—Unspecified fracture of upper end of right humerus, initial encounter for closed fracture
- **T43.8X6D**—Underdosing of other psychotropic drugs, subsequent encounter

● **HIPAA Official Guidelines for Coding and Reporting** Annually updated instructions for the use of ICD-10 codes.

● **character** A single letter, number, or symbol.

● **outpatient** A patient whose health care services are intended to be delivered within 1 calendar day or, in some cases, a 24-hour period.

◉ **CDC** U.S. Centers for Disease Control and Prevention

● **Cooperating Parties** The four organizations responsible for maintaining the ICD-10-CM: CMS, NCHS, AHA, and AHIMA. **Federal Register** The publication of the proceedings of the United States Congress.

◉ **AHIMA** American Health Information Management Association
**NCHS** National Center for Health Statistics

**HIT-bit**

**GRANULARITY**

The level of detail that a system provides is referred to as its *granularity*. A system with a high level of granularity is able to capture more specific, detailed information than a system with a lower level of granularity. Think of an ocean beach: If examined closely, one can see millions of grains of sand. Viewed from a distance, it may appear as more of a solitary object. In coding, granularity applies to the specificity of the coding system. ICD-10-CM, for example, has a higher level of granularity than the WHO's ICD-10. With regard to choosing a code system, the level of granularity required will be determined by the reason that a code system is being used.

**0DJ**

| Section | 0 | Medical and surgical |
|---|---|---|
| Body system | D | Gastrointestinal system |
| Operation | J | Inspection: Visually and/or manually exploring a body part |

| Body part | Approach | Device | Qualifier |
|---|---|---|---|
| **0** Upper intestinal tract<br>**6** Stomach<br>**D** Lower intestinal tract | **0** Open<br>**3** Percutaneous<br>**4** Percutaneous endoscopic<br>**7** Via natural or artificial opening<br>**8** Via natural or artificial opening endoscopic<br>**X** External | **Z** No device | **Z** No qualifier |
| **U** Omentum<br>**V** Mesentery<br>**W** Peritoneum | **0** Open<br>**3** Percutaneous<br>**4** Percutaneous endoscopic<br>**X** External | **Z** No device | **Z** No qualifier |

**Figure 6-3** Example of table used to build ICD-10-PCS codes.

## ICD-10-PCS

**ICD-10-PCS** International Classification of Diseases, Tenth Revision, Procedure Classification System

**CMS** Centers for Medicare and Medicaid Services.

ICD-10-PCS was developed by 3M under contract from the CMS to replace ICD-9-CM Vol. III, used for inpatient procedures. ICD-10-PCS will become effective for use at the same time as ICD-10-CM, October 1, 2014. The CMS is responsible for maintaining ICD-10-PCS, which currently comprises more than 70,000 codes. Information, including guidelines can be found at the CMS Web site: http://www.cms.gov/ICD10/01_Overview.asp#TopOfPage.

All ICD-10-PCS codes are composed of seven characters, either letters or digits. Each character has a character value, and each character value represents a specific option for the general character definition. Although there is an alphabetical index in ICD-10-PCS, codes are "built" from tables by selection of the specific character values for each of the seven characters on the basis of the details of the procedure that was performed (Figure 6-3). Because each character in the code has specific meaning, depending on its position in the sequence, ICD-10-PCS is a **multi-axial** code structure. Each position is an axis, so a 4 in the second position means something different from a 4 in the fifth position.

**multi-axial** A code structure in which the position of a character has a specific meaning.

Each ICD-10-PCS Code has a character or digit from each of seven different categories in the following order: Section, Body System, Root Operation, Body Part, Approach, Device, Qualifier. Sometimes it is easy to use a mnemonic to help remember this order, such as "Sally buys root beer at Dairy Queen." Note that ICD-10-PCS is alphanumerical, so there will potentially be numbers and letters in a code.

For example, Section 1 of ICD-10-PCS contains the tables for Medical/Surgical procedure codes, as follows:

- The first character represents the Section. In the medical/surgical section, the first character has a character value of 0. All codes in the medical surgical section will begin with the character 0.
- The second character indicates the Body System. Each body system has its own character value, such as 2 for Heart and Great Vessels, and D for Gastrointestinal System.
- The third character indicates the Root Operation. Assigning the correct root operation to the procedure that was performed is critical to building the correct code. There are 31 different root operations in the Med/Surg section, each with its own character value. The coder must understand and apply the definitions of each root operation and assign the correct character value. Some Root Operations are as follows:

*Excision:* Cutting out of or off, without replacement, a portion of a body part, character value B

### ICD-10-PCS Examples

*Note:* The first description after the code is the abbreviated or short description that is used in abstracting systems: the second description in brackets is the expanded form.

- **021V09P**—Bypass Sup Vena Cava to Pulm Trunk w Autol Vn, Open [Bypass Superior Vena Cava to Pulmonary Trunk with Autologous Venous Tissue, Open Approach]
- **0D5N4ZZ**—Destruction of Sigmoid Colon, Perc Endo Approach [Destruction of Sigmoid Colon, Percutaneous Endoscopic Approach]

*Resection:* Cutting out of or off, without replacement, all of a body part, character value T
*Inspection:* Visually and/or manually exploring a body part, character value J

- The fourth character indicates the Body Part, the site on which the procedure was performed. These are numerous and may be found in each table.
- The fifth character indicates the Approach, the technique used to reach the site of the procedure. There are seven types of approaches, each with its own character value. For example, an Open approach has a character value of 0.
- The sixth character indicates the Device, of which there are four different types, each with its own character value. The specific types of devices are found in the applicable tables. For example, a Monitoring Device has a character value of 2. If there is no device, character Z is assigned.
- The seventh character is called the Qualifier and contains unique values for certain individual procedures. For example, assigning character value X to certain procedures in the Qualifier position indicates a biopsy. If there is no qualifier, character Z is assigned (Centers for Medicare and Medicaid Services, 2012).

For example, a colonoscopy is coded in ICD-10-PCS as 0DJD8ZZ. Using the Table in Figure 6-3, one builds the PCS code for colonoscopy by assigning the character values for each character in the Table, as follows:

0—Section: Medical Surgical, character value 0
D—Body System: Gastrointestinal, character value D
J—Root Operation: Inspection
D—Body Part: Lower intestinal tract, character value D
8—Approach: Via natural or artificial opening, endoscopic
Z—No device (no device left inside the body after completion of the procedure)
Z—No qualifier (no unique information specific to the procedure)

The ICD-10-PCS Tables and Index can be downloaded from the CMS Web site: http://www.cms.gov/ICD10/Downloads/2011_Code_Tables_and_Index.pdf.

## HCPCS/CPT-4

HCPCS stands for Health Care Common Procedure Coding System. HCPCS was developed as a standard coding system for claims processing and is therefore extremely important to physicians and other providers for billing. HCPCS consists of two levels.

### HCPCS Level I

Level I is CPT, which stands for Current Procedural Terminology, currently in its fourth version (CPT-4). CPT is copyrighted, developed, and maintained by the **American Medical Association (AMA)**. CPT codes are composed of five numerical characters. They are used to report procedures and services performed by physicians and other health care professionals and in facilities or institutions for services performed in the outpatient setting (e.g., ambulatory surgery centers, emergency departments, clinics, rehabilitation facilities). There are CPT-4 codes that describe office visits, surgical procedures, radiology procedures, and laboratory tests, for example. CPT-4 codes are updated and published yearly by the AMA and become effective for use each January 1. The code changes and new codes must be purchased from the AMA.

Additions, deletions, and revisions to CPT-4 are determined by the AMA's editorial panel. The editorial panel consists of physicians representing the AMA, the Blue Cross and Blue Shield Association (BCBSA), the Health Insurance Association of America (HIAA), the AHA, and the CMS. Providing input to the panel are two Advisory Committees. The CPT Advisory Committee consists solely of physicians. The Health Care Professionals Advisory Committee is composed of allied health professionals, including health information management (HIM) professionals. AMA staff reviews and evaluates requests from the industry for suggestions for new codes. When appropriate, these suggestions are forwarded to the Advisory Committee for consideration. If the Advisory Committee is in agreement that a new code should be added, or if the Advisory Committee cannot reach an agreement, the issue is referred to the CPT Editorial Panel for resolution. Details of the process may be found on the AMA's Web site: http://www.ama-assn.org/ama/pub/physician-resources/solutions-managing-your-practice/coding-billing-insurance/cpt/cpt-process-faq/code-becomes-cpt.page.

---

**ICD-10-PCS Examples—cont'd**

- **0QS646Z**—Reposition R Up Femur with Intramed Fix, Perc Endo Approach [Reposition Right Upper Femur with Intramedullary Internal Fixation Device, Percutaneous Endoscopic Approach]
- **10D00Z1**—Extraction of POC, Low Cervical, Open Approach [Extraction of Products of Conception, Low Cervical, Open Approach]

**Healthcare Common Procedure Coding System (HCPCS)** A coding system, of which CPT-4 is level one, used for drugs, equipment, supplies, and other auxiliary health care services rendered.

**Current Procedural Terminology (CPT)** A nomenclature and coding system developed and maintained by the American Medical Association in order to facilitate billing for physicians and other services.

**American Medical Association (AMA)** National professional organization involved in supporting all medical decision makers; the AMA also owns and maintains the Current Procedural Terminology (CPT) code set.

**CPT (HCPCS Level I) Examples**

- **43251**—EGDc̄ polypectomy snared
- **49320**—Laparoscopy, diagnostic (separate procedure)
- **21320**—Closed treatment, nasal bone fracture; with stabilization

**HCPCS Examples**
- **C1715**—Brachytherapy needle
- **J0897**—Injection, denosumab, 1 mg
- **T1015**—Clinic visit/encounter, all-inclusive

**HCPCS** Healthcare Common Procedure Coding System
**BCBSA** Blue Cross and Blue Shield Association
**CMS** Centers for Medicare and Medicaid Services

### HCPCS Level II

Level II codes are generally called HCPCS codes. HCPCS Level II codes are reported by regulation that the CMS published on August 17, 2000 (45 CFR 162.10002). They consist of codes used by providers and institutions to report products, supplies, and services not included in CPT. For example, HCPCS Level II codes would be used to submit claims for durable medical equipment and ambulance services. Every HCPCS code is alphanumerical, consisting of a letter followed by four numerical characters. HCPCS Level II codes are maintained jointly by America's Health Insurance Plans (AHIP), the BCBSA, and the CMS. These same groups also serve on an HCPCS national panel, the functions of which include maintaining national permanent HCPCS Level II codes as well as additions, revisions, and deletions. According to the CMS, the purpose of the permanent national codes is to provide a "standardized coding system that is managed jointly by private and public insurers. It supplies a predictable set of uniform codes that provides a stable environment for claims submission and processing" (Centers for Medicare and Medicaid Services, 2011). HCPCS Level II codes are updated as needed, usually every quarter, and become effective once announced. Updates can be found on the CMS Web site.

## EXERCISE 6-2

### General Purpose Code Sets

1. What is the purpose of the Cooperating Parties?
2. What entity is responsible for ICD-10-CM?
3. What entity is responsible for ICD-10-PCS?
4. HIM professionals contribute to addition, deletions, and revisions to CPT through what committee?

**Go To** Chapter 3 discusses the EHR and interoperability.

**interoperability** The ability of different software and computer systems to communicate and share data.
**nomenclature** In medical coding, a systematic assignment of a name to a diagnosis or procedure and associating that name with a numeric or alphanumeric value.
**classification** Systematic organization of elements into categories. ICD-10-CM is a classification system that organizes diagnoses into categories, primarily by body system.

**International Health Terminology Standards Development Organisation (IHTSDO)** A multinational organization the supports the standardized exchange of health information through the development of clinical terminologies, notably SNOMED-CT.

## SPECIAL PURPOSE CODE SETS

### SNOMED-CT

*SNOMED-CT* provides the standardized core general terminology for an electronic health record (EHR), enabling better communication and interoperability of the EHR exchange. It is a nomenclature system consisting of more than 1 million medical concepts and attributes arranged in complex hierarchies. SNOMED-CT contains codes for diseases and procedures as well as relational terms that enable the translation of natural language into a classification system, such as ICD-10.

SNOMED-CT stands for Systemized Nomenclature of Medicine—Clinical Terms. This system was created by the College of American Pathologists (CAP) and the National Health Service (NHS) in England. Since 2007, SNOMED-CT has been owned, maintained, and distributed by the **International Health Terminology Standards Development Organisation (IHTSDO),** a not-for-profit association in Denmark composed of

---

### HIT-bit

#### INTERNATIONAL HEALTH TERMINOLOGY STANDARDS DEVELOPMENT ORGANISATION

The purpose of IHTSDO is to develop, maintain, promote, and enable the uptake and correct use of its terminology products in health systems, services, and products around the world and to undertake any or all activities incidental and conducive to achieving the purpose of the association for the benefits of the members.

The IHTSDO seeks to improve the health of humankind by fostering the development and use of suitable standardized clinical terminologies, notably SNOMED-CT, in order to support safe, accurate, and effective exchange of clinical and related health information. The focus is on enabling the implementation of semantically accurate health records that are interoperable. Support of Association Members and Licensees is provided on a global basis, allowing the pooling of resources to achieve shared benefits (International Health Terminology Standards Development Organisation, 2012).

representatives from many countries. According to the IHTSDO, SNOMED-CT is considered the most comprehensive multilingual clinical health care terminology in the world.

The United States representative to the IHTSDO is the **National Library of Medicine (NLM)**. Canada's representative is Canada Health Infoway. Both countries use SNOMED-CT to facilitate the exchange of clinical data through electronic health record (EHR) systems. Canada Health Infoway's goal is that, by 2016, all Canadians will have their electronic health records available to the authorized professionals who provide their health care services.

SNOMED-CT differs from classification systems such as ICD-10-CM, which are designed to assign codes to patient encounters according to diseases. The "output" of the coding process is an ICD-10-CM code that is not generally used during the course of, or directly for, patient care. Data generated from ICD-10-CM codes are most useful when aggregated after the encounter and are necessary for reimbursement. Classification systems such as ICD-10-CM are not designed to capture all of the available data and clinical information in a health record that is used by clinicians *during the course* of patient care. SNOMED-CT, however, can be applied to free text and, by translating the text or natural language, describe in coded format the diagnosis or activity, such as a procedure. The SNOMED-CT code is then mapped to the ICD-10-CM/PCS or HCPCS code for further processing. Therefore it is a critical link in connecting the data collected in an EHR with the classification or nomenclature system that describes the encounter.

Table 6-1 shows the SNOMED-CT codes, ICD-10-CM code, ICD-10-PCS code, and CPT-4 code assigned to the diagnosis "acute lower gastrointestinal hemorrhage" and to the procedure "flexible fiberoptic diagnostic colonoscopy." More SNOMED-CT diagnoses and procedure codes can be viewed at http://www.snomedct.nu/SNOMEDbrowser.

Because SNOMED-CT codes are assigned during the course of patient care, they can be linked with other software programs that can facilitate current patient care. For example, a SNOMED-CT code may be assigned with the use of input from a complex set of data extracted from various sections of the EHR. This SNOMED-CT code may be programmed to link to a software system to alert the clinician to a life-threatening condition.

Because classification systems and nomenclature systems are designed for different purposes and uses, one type of system cannot entirely replace the other. SNOMED-CT is designed to use very specific data, including gender and age, in order to assign a SNOMED-CT code called a "concept." For example, the SNOMED-CT concept, using SNOMED-CT terminology, for "a female with a herniated urinary bladder" is 410070006, Herniated urinary bladder (disorder) + gender = Female. This SNOMED-CT concept can be mapped to ICD-10-CM code N81.10, Cystocele, unspecified.

**Systemized Nomenclature of Medicine—Clinical Terms (SNOMED-CT)** Systematized nomenclature of human and veterinary medicine clinical terms; a reference terminology that, among other things, links common or input medical terminology and codes with the output reporting systems in an electronic health record.

**International Health Terminology Standards Development Organisation (IHTSDO)** A multinational organization the supports the standardized exchange of health information through the development of clinical terminologies, notably SNOMED-CT.

**National Library of Medicine (NLM)** The medical library operated by the U.S. government under the National Institutes of Health. Serves as representative for the United States in the international standards organization IHTSDO.

**SNOMED-CT Examples**
- **4557003**—Preinfarction syndrome
- **63650001**—Cholera
- **387712008**—Neonatal jaundice

**reimbursement** The amount of money that the health care facility receives from the party responsible for paying the bill.

**Healthcare Common Procedure Coding System (HCPCS)** A coding system, of which CPT-4 is Level I, used for drugs, equipment, supplies, and other auxiliary health care services rendered.

### TABLE 6-1

**COMPARISON OF CODES FOR THE DIAGNOSIS ACUTE LOWER GASTROINTESTINAL HEMORRHAGE AND THE PROCEDURE FLEXIBLE FIBEROPTIC DIAGNOSTIC COLONOSCOPY**

| CODE SET | CODE | MEANING |
|---|---|---|
| SNOMED-CT | 123688018 | Gastrointestinal hemorrhage |
| | 492675019 | Fiberoptic colonoscopy |
| ICD-10-CM | K92.2 | Gastrointestinal hemorrhage, unspecified |
| ICD-10-PCS | 0DJD8ZZ | Inspection, lower intestinal tract via natural or artificial opening, endoscopic |
| CPT-4 | 45378 | Colonoscopy, flexible, proximal to splenic flexure; diagnostic, with or without collection of specimen(s) by brushing or washing, with or without colon decompression (separate procedure) |

**Interactive Map-Assisted Generation of ICD-10-CM Codes (I-MAGIC) algorithm** An algorithm used to map EHR-generated SNOMED-CT codes to the more specific ICD-10-CM code set, seeking input from a coder to supply missing information as necessary.

**encounter** Unit of measure for the volume of ambulatory care services provided.

**aggregate data** A group of like data elements compiled to provide information about the group.

**ICD-O** International Classification of Diseases—Oncology The coding system used to record and track the occurrence of neoplasms (i.e., malignant tumors, cancer).

**multi-axial** A code structure in which the position of a character has a specific meaning.

**transaction code set** A code set, established by HIPAA guidelines, to be used in electronic data transfer to ensure that the information transmitted is complete, private, and secure.

**WHO** World Health Organization
**HIPAA** Health Insurance Portability and Accountability Act (1996)

In many instances, there is no direct map from a SNOMED-CT concept to an ICD-10-CM code, because the ICD-10-CM code includes information not captured in SNOMED-CT. For example, SNOMED-CT concept 58149017 (Antepartum hemorrhage) maps to the ICD-10-CM code O46.90, Antepartum hemorrhage, unspecified, unspecified trimester, by default. The coder would have to insert the trimester as specified in ICD-10-CM, but the SNOMED-CT concept does not include trimester.

The **Interactive Map-Assisted Generation of ICD-10-CM Codes (I-MAGIC) algorithm** was developed to encode ICD-10-CM codes from computer-generated SNOMED-CT codes of clinical problems. I-MAGIC works in real time to decide what user input is needed to assign the correct, detailed ICD-10 code from the SNOMED-CT code. Figure 6-4 illustrates the I-MAGIC algorithm.

The transition to the EHR and SNOMED-CT will not eliminate the need for coders in the foreseeable future. The accuracy of the coded data still must be reviewed and verified as they pertain to each specific patient encounter. Although no electronic system is infallible, the extent to which we can depend on such systems will probably increase with time. Even if the coding function were somehow entirely eliminated in the future, health information professionals with that knowledge base would assume more complex and advanced roles in, for example, development and maintenance of the code mapping (matching SNOMED-CT codes to the correct target code set), quality control of individual patient and aggregate data (making sure coded data are correct and complete), and sophisticated data analysis (including reporting and data presentation).

## ICD-O-3

**ICD-O** stands for International Classification of Diseases for Oncology, currently in its third revision as of January 1, 2001 (ICD-O-3). The WHO is responsible for this multi-axial classification system. Its purpose is to be the standard tool for coding neoplasm diagnoses. In a hospital setting, ICD-O-3 is used in the pathology department and in tumor (cancer) registries to code the site (topography axis) and the histology (morphology axis) of neoplasms. A *tumor registry* is a central repository of data about cancer, collected from the providers who identified the cancer cases. As an international coding system, it is available in several languages. The codes are the same; only the descriptions and instructional notes are translated where appropriate. ICD-O-3 is not used for reimbursement purposes and is not a transaction code set under HIPAA.

The topography axis uses as its foundation the ICD-10 classification of malignant neoplasms for all types of tumors. For nonmalignant tumors, ICD-O-3 is more detailed than ICD-10. ICD-O also adds topography for sites of certain tumors.

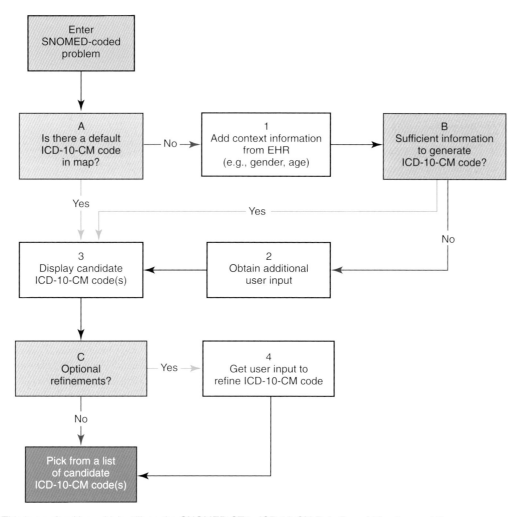

This is an algorithm which utilizes the SNOMED CT to ICD-10-CM Rule Based Map in a real-time, interactive manner to generate ICD-10-CM codes from SNOMED CT encoded clinical problems.

**Figure 6-4** The I-MAGIC algorithm (Interactive Map-Assisted Generation of ICD Codes). EHR, electronic health record; ICD-10-CM, International Classification of Diseases, 10th Revision—Clinical Modification; SNOMED-CT, Systematized Nomenclature of Medicine–Clinical Terms. (From National Library of Medicine: Mapping SNOMED CT to ICD-10-CM: Technical Specifications. http://www.nlm.nih.gov/research/umls/mapping_projects/snomedct_to_icd10cm_tech_spec_20120208.pdf.)

The morphology axis consists of five-digit codes ranging from M-8000/0 to M-9989/3. The first four digits indicate the specific histological term. The fifth digit after the slash (/) is the behavior code, which indicates whether a tumor is malignant, benign, in situ, or uncertain (whether benign or malignant). A separate one-digit code is also provided for histologic grading (differentiation) (World Health Organization, 2011).

For example, the diagnosis "neoplasm of the lung and bronchus, small cell carcinoma, fusiform cell" is assigned a code from C34.0 to C34.3 to indicate site (identical to the ICD-10-CM code equivalent) and also 8043/3 to indicate histology. Figure 6-5 shows the 33 to 34.3 site codes on a drawing of lung anatomy.

In the United States, the **National Cancer Institute's Surveillance, Epidemiology and End Results (SEER) Program** collects and compiles cancer statistics, including mortality data, for the United States using ICD-O-3. SEER provides information on incidence, prevalence, and survival from geographical areas in the United States. Tumor registrars use the *SEER Program Coding and Staging Manual* for coding and reporting cancer cases.

**Go To** Chapter 10 for a detailed discussion of registries.

● **National Cancer Institute's Surveillance, Epidemiology and End Results (SEER)** The National Cancer Institute's program that collects cancer statistics using the ICD-O-3 code set.

**mortality rate** The frequency of death.

**incidence** Number of occurrences of a particular event, disease, or diagnosis or the number of new cases of a disease.

**prevalence** Rate of incidence of an occurrence, disease, or diagnosis or the number of existing cases.

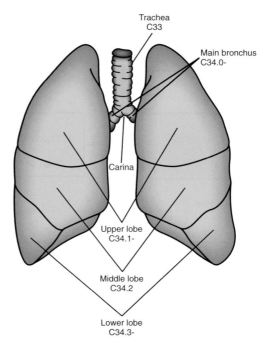

Figure 6-5 Lung anatomy with ICD-O-3 (International Classification of Diseases—Oncology, third edition) site codes. (From SEER Training Modules, *Module Name.* U. S. National Institutes of Health, National Cancer Institute. http://training.seer.cancer.gov/. Accessed July 15, 2011.)

---

## HIT-bit

### CERTIFIED TUMOR REGISTRAR

Many health information professionals choose to specialize in cancer coding and cancer registries and obtain the credential Certified Tumor Registrar (CTR). Those professionals working in Tumor Registries use ICD-O-3 to code cancer cases similar to the way inpatient coders use ICD-10-CM. Depending on the facility, in an inpatient setting, a patient with cancer will have been coded using both ICD-O-3 and ICD-10-CM, usually by different professionals in different departments, with each distinct case and code set reported electronically to entirely separate databases.

---

## DSM-IV, DSM-IV-TR, and DSM-5

**DSM-IV** stands for *Diagnostic and Statistical Manual of Mental Disorders,* Fourth Edition. It is a system used to classify mental disorders in a structured format. DSM-IV was first published in 1994, and DSM-5 is scheduled for final approval May 2013. In the interim, DSM-IV-TR was published in 2000 "to maintain the currency of the *DSM-IV* text, which reflected the empirical literature up to 1992" (http://www.psych.org/practice/dsm/dsm-iv-tr). DSM-IV-TR stands for *Diagnostic and Statistical Manual of Mental Disorders,* Fourth Edition, Text Revision. DSM-5 stands for *Diagnostic and Statistical Manual of Mental Disorders,* Fifth Edition. (Note that the Roman numeral is replaced by an arabic numeral for this edition.)

Its sponsoring organization is the **American Psychiatric Association (APA)**. Although DSM-IV and DSM-IV-TR codes are similar in appearance to ICD-9-CM codes, DSM-5 codes resemble ICD-10-CM codes. DSM is used only for data analysis of patients with psychiatric disorders, not for reimbursement purposes. DSM is a multi-axial system, in which each axis relates to a different aspect of the patient's mental disorder, as follows:

*Axis I:* Specific major mental, clinical, learning, or substance abuse disorders

*Axis II:* Personality disorders and intellectual disabilities

*Axis III:* Acute medical conditions and physical disorders

---

**Diagnostic and Statistical Manual of Mental Disorders, Fourth Edition (DSM-IV)** Used for coding behavior and mental health care encounters in a structured format.

**American Psychiatric Association (APA)** National professional organization involved in supporting licensed psychiatrists; maintains the DSM-IV Behavioral Health code set.

**ICD-9-CM** (International Classification of Diseases, Ninth Revision—Clinical Modification) The United States version of the ICD-9, maintained and updated by the Cooperating Parties.

**reimbursement** The amount of money that the health care facility receives from the party responsible for paying the bill.

*Axis IV:* Psychosocial and environmental factors contributing to the above disorders
*Axis V:* Functional assessment

Taken as a whole, DSM is a clinical assessment tool with its own set of definitions and criteria for each axis. Not all axis terms are coded; for example, there is no code assigned for axis V.

## National Drug Codes

**National Drug Codes (NDCs)** are found in the National Drug Code Directory and serve as universal product identifiers for human drugs. The U.S. Food and Drug Administration (FDA) maintains a list of these identifiers, or codes, on its Web site, which is updated at the beginning and middle of each month. NDCs are a transaction code set under HIPAA. They are important for commercial purposes, in selling and purchasing pharmaceuticals. They are also tied to a facility's pharmaceutical system and can therefore be traced to dispensing of medication at the patient level. Consequently, NDCs are critical in the event of a recall of pharmaceuticals.

Medicaid requires NDCs for reimbursement, as do some managed care providers. The NDC is appended to the Uniform Bill and gives the payer specific information regarding the cost of certain drugs.

NDCs contain three segments: labeler, product, and packaging codes. The individual segments are assigned partly by the FDA, which assigns the labeler code, and partly by the labeler, which assigns the product and packaging codes. The labeler may be the manufacturer of the drug or the distributor. For example, a drug manufactured by a pharmaceutical company and sold under that company's name as well as a retail drug store's name would have two different NDCs. The product code describes the strength, dosage, and formulation of the drug. The packaging code defines the packaging size and type.

Examples from the National Drug Code Directory in Table 6-2 show two labelers of acetaminophen: McNeil, which distributes it under the proprietary name Tylenol, and CVS Pharmacy, which distributes a nonproprietary version. Because acetaminophen is not restricted by patent at this time, a search of the NDC Directory yields more than 2900 entries for acetaminophen (U.S. Food and Drug Administration, 2011). In Table 6-2, 50580 is the FDAs labeler code for McNeil Consumer Healthcare Div. McNeil-PPC, Inc., 112 is McNeil's product code for Tylenol, and 02, 06, 10, and 12 are the various package codes for the configurations listed. The CVS Pharmacy version of acetaminophen is available in different strengths and packaging compared to the McNeil example.

**National Drug Codes (NDCs)** A transaction code set used to identify drugs by the firm, labeler, and batch.
**transaction code set** A code set, established by HIPAA guidelines, to be used in electronic data transfer to ensure the information transmitted is complete, private, and secure.

**HIPAA** Health Insurance Portability and Accountability Act (1996)

**Medicaid** A federally mandated, state-funded program providing access to health care for the poor and the medically indigent.
**Uniform Bill (UB-04)** The standardized form used by hospitals for inpatient and outpatient billing to CMS and other third party payers.

**Go To** Chapter 7 for a full discussion of reimbursement and explanation of the Uniform Bill.

## Current Dental Terminology Codes

The *Code on Dental Procedures and Nomenclature (Code)* (CDT) uses descriptive terms for procedures and treatments unique to dentistry. The American Dental Association (ADA) owns and holds the copyright to CDT. The CDT Code is used for reporting dental services and procedures to payers. The CDT Code is reviewed and revised as needed on the basis of changes in dentistry practice. Revisions to the CDT Code are published and effective biennially, at the start of odd-numbered years (e.g., 2011, 2013). The CDT Code is a transaction code set under HIPAA. Prior to 2011, CDT codes were incorporated into the HCPCS code list; however, they are currently available only through the ADA.

**CDT Examples**
- **D0120**—periodic oral evaluation—established patient
- **D2710**—crown—resin-based composite (indirect)
- **D5410**—adjust complete denture—maxillary

**HCPCS** Healthcare Common Procedure Coding System
**ADA** American Dental Association

## USES FOR CODED CLINICAL DATA

Coded clinical data are used for a variety of purposes by many different users. Therefore, the quality of the data is critical to ensure that all users are able to rely on the data. Some common uses of coded data are: case mix analysis, reporting, comparative analysis, and reimbursement. Table 6-3 lists the code sets discussed in this chapter and their applications.

**clinical data** All of the medical data that have been recorded about the patient's stay or visit, including diagnoses and procedures.

**TABLE 6-2**

## NATIONAL DRUG CODES (NDC) DIRECTORY FOR ACETAMINOPHEN

| PRODUCT NDC | PRODUCT TYPE NAME | PROPRIETARY NAME | NON-PROPRIETARY NAME | DOSAGE | ROUTE | LABELER | STRENGTH | PACKAGE CODE | PACKAGE DESCRIPTION |
|---|---|---|---|---|---|---|---|---|---|
| 50580-112 | Human OTC drug | Tylenol Arthritis Pain | Acetaminophen | Tablet, film coated, extended release | Oral | McNeil Consumer Healthcare Div. McNeil-PPC, Inc | 650 mg/L | 50580-112-02 | 34 pouch in 1 carton/2 tablet, film-coated, extended-release in 1 pouch |
| 50580-112 | Human OTC drug | Tylenol Arthritis Pain | Acetaminophen | Tablet, film coated, extended release | Oral | McNeil Consumer Healthcare Div. McNeil-PPC, Inc | 650 mg/L | 50580-112-06 | 3 pouch in 1 carton/2 tablet, film-coated, extended-release in 1 pouch |
| 50580-112 | Human OTC drug | Tylenol Arthritis Pain | Acetaminophen | Tablet, film coated, extended release | Oral | McNeil Consumer Healthcare Div. McNeil-PPC, Inc | 650 mg/L | 50580-112-10 | 1 bottle in 1 carton/100 tablet, film-coated, extended-release in 1 bottle |
| 50580-112 | Human OTC drug | Tylenol Arthritis Pain | Acetaminophen | Tablet, film coated, extended release | Oral | McNeil Consumer Healthcare Div. McNeil-PPC, Inc | 650 mg/L | 50580-112-12 | 1 bottle in 1 carton/120 tablet, film-coated, extended |
| 59779-484 | Human OTC drug | Pain relief (extra strength) | Acetaminophen | Tablet | Oral | CVS Pharmacy | 500 mg/L | 59779-484-62 | 1 bottle in 1 carton/24 tablet in 1 bottle |
| 59779-484 | Human OTC drug | Pain relief (extra strength) | Acetaminophen | Tablet | Oral | CVS Pharmacy | 500 mg/L | 59779-484-71 | 1 bottle in 1 carton/50 tablet in 1 bottle |
| 59779-484 | Human OTC drug | Pain relief (extra strength) | Acetaminophen | Tablet | Oral | CVS Pharmacy | 500 mg/L | 59779-484-76 | 1 bottle in 1 carton/120 tablet in 1 bottle |

## TABLE 6-3

## COMPARISON OF CURRENT CODING SYSTEMS

| ACRONYM | FULL NAME | USE |
|---|---|---|
| SNOMED-CT* | Systemized Nomenclature of Medical Clinical Terms | Extensive clinical vocabulary, machine-readable terminology for potential use in an electronic health record (EHR) |
| ICD-O-3 | International Classification of Diseases for Oncology, 3rd Revision | Coding of neoplasm/cancer diagnoses for tumor reporting |
| DSM-5 | *Diagnostic and Statistical Manual of Mental Disorders,* 5th edition | Coding of psychiatric disorders for psychiatric patients |
| ICD-9-CM* | International Classification of Diseases, 9th Revision—Clinical Modification | Coding and reporting diagnoses for patient encounters. Used for reimbursement. Scheduled to be replaced by ICD-10-CM in Oct 2014. |
| ICD-10-CM* | International Classification of Diseases, 10th Revision—Clinical Modification | Coding and reporting diagnoses for patient encounters. Used for reimbursement |
| ICD-10-PCS* | International Classification of Diseases, 10th Revision—Procedure Coding System | Coding and reporting procedures for inpatient encounters. Used with ICD-10-CM for reimbursement |
| HCPCS/CPT-4* | Healthcare Common Procedure Coding System and Current Procedural Terminology, 4th Version | Coding and reporting for reimbursement for outpatient and physician office procedures |
| CDT* | Current Dental Terminology | Used to report dental services and procedures to dental plans for reimbursement |
| NDC* | National Drug Codes | U.S. Food and Drug Administration (FDA) list of drugs used by humans |

*HIPAA Transaction Code Set.

## Case Mix Analysis

**Case mix** analysis looks at groups of patient data to determine what types of patients are treated in a particular setting. For example, some hospitals treat a large number of maternity and newborn cases; other hospitals treat a large number of trauma patients. Even within a particular facility, a hospital may see that there is a trend over time: less cataract surgery being performed this year than last year or more complicated cases treated in the first half of the year than the last.

Case mix analysis can be used to identify coding errors. If there is a sudden change in the number of complicated cases, the coders (or one coder) may be missing complicating diagnoses. Hospitals often pay close attention to case mix and perform routine audits to ensure accurate coding, which produces coded data that accurately reflect the case mix. The CMS also looks at case mix within the Medicare population and may initiate an audit of a hospital whose case mix shows an inexplicably high number of complications over time.

**case mix** Statistical distribution of patients according to their utilization of resources. Also refers to the grouping of patients by clinical department or other meaningful distribution, such as health insurance type.

**CMS** Centers for Medicare and Medicaid

**Medicare** Federally funded health care insurance plan for older adults and for certain categories of chronically ill patients.

## Reporting

As discussed in previous chapters, coded data are used for reporting purposes. Hospitals report the UHDDS, for example, which provides the states and subsequently the federal government with details of inpatient stays. Coded data are also provided to accrediting agencies and the CDC (to report infectious diseases).

Internally, coded data may be used to identify quantities of procedures performed for physician credentialing purposes and service area volume analysis. Many reports that are generated internally from the hospital system pull the data on the basis of the desired coded data element, such as diagnosis or procedure code.

**UHDDS** Uniform Hospital Discharge Data Set
**CDC** Centers for Disease Control and Prevention

## Comparative Analysis

Coded data are used to compare facility-specific, regional, national, and international health care observations.

● **Healthcare Common Procedure Coding System (HCPCS)** A coding system, of which CPT-4 is level one, used for drugs, equipment, supplies, and other auxiliary health care services rendered.

**Current Procedural Terminology (CPT)** A coding system used to bill for physician services, developed and maintained by the AMA.

**payer** The individual or organization that is primarily responsible for the reimbursement for a particular health care service. Usually refers to the insurance company or third party.

## Reimbursement

One of the most common uses of coded data today is reimbursement. HCPCS/CPT codes, for example, were developed specifically for the purpose of communicating to payers information about services rendered by the provider. Chapter 7 discusses reimbursement in detail.

### EXERCISE 6-3

#### Specialty Code Sets

1. What coding system is used to develop cancer mortality statistics?
2. DSM-5 is sponsored by what organization?
3. CDT codes are used in what patient setting?

## WORKS CITED

American Dental Association: Code on Dental Procedures and Nomenclature. http://www.ada.org/3827.aspx. Copyright 1995-2011. Accessed July 15, 2011.

American Health Information Management Association: AHIMA Standards of Ethical Coding. http://library.ahima.org/xpedio/groups/public/documents/ahima/bok2_001166.hcsp?dDocName=bok2_001166. Revised September 2008. Accessed July 20, 2011.

American Medical Association: CPT Process—How a Code Becomes a Code. http://www.ama-assn.org/ama/pub/physician-resources/solutions-managing-your-practice/coding-billing-insurance/cpt/cpt-process-faq/code-becomes-cpt.page. Copyright 1995-2012. Accessed May 11, 2012.

American Medical Association: About CPT. http://www.ama-assn.org/ama/pub/physician-resources/solutions-managing-your-practice/coding-billing-insurance/cpt/about-cpt.page?Copyright1999-2011.Accessed August 5, 2011.

American Psychiatric Association: DSM-IV-TR. http://www.psych.org/practice/dsm/dsm-iv-tr. Accessed September 12, 2012.

American Psychiatric Association: DSM-5 Development: DSM-5: The Future of Psychiatric Diagnosis. http://www.dsm5.org/. Copyright 2010. Accessed August 5, 2011.

Canadian Institute for Health Information: Standards: classification and coding: CCI coding structure. http://www.cihi.ca/CIHI-ext-portal/internet/en/document/standards+and+data+submission/standards/classification+and+coding/codingclass_ccistruct. Copyright 1996-2011. Accessed July 15, 2011.

Centers for Disease Control and Prevention, National Center for Health Statistics: Classification of Diseases, Functioning, and Disability: International Classification of Diseases, Tenth Revision, Clinical Modification (ICD-10-CM). http://www.cdc.gov/nchs/icd/icd10cm.htm. Updated March 1, 2011. Accessed July 15, 2011.

Center for Medicare and Medicaid Services: Healthcare Common Procedure Coding System (HCPCS) Level II Coding Procedures. http://www.cms.gov/Medicare/Coding/MedHCPCSGenInfo/Downloads/HCPCSLevelIICodingProcedures7-2011.pdf

Centers for Medicare and Medicaid Services. ICD-10 PCS Final Report. https://www.cms.gov/ICD10/Downloads/pcs_final_report2012.pdf. Accessed May 11, 2012.

Centers for Medicare and Medicaid Services: Transactions and code set regulations. http://www.cms.gov/TransactionCodeSetsStands/02_TransactionsandCodeSetsRegulations.asp#TopOfPage. Modified July 14, 2011. Accessed August 5, 2011.

Centers for Medicare and Medicaid Services: HCPCS Level II Coding Process & Criteria. http://www.cms.gov/MedHCPCSGenInfo/02_HCPCSCODINGPROCESS.html. Modified July 27, 2011. Accessed August 5, 2011.

Centers for Medicare and Medicaid Services: ICD-10. Overview. http://www.cms.gov/ICD10/01_Overview.asp#TopOfPage. Modified May 5, 2011. Accessed August 5, 2011.

International Health Terminology Standards Development Organisation: About IHTSDO. http://www.ihtsdo.org/about-ihtsdo/. Accessed August 10, 2012.

International Health Terminology Standards Development Organisation: SNOMED CT Browser. http://www.snomedct.nu/SNOMEDbrowser. September 12, 2012.

National Center for Biomedical Ontology: NCI Thesaurus. http://bioportal.bioontology.org/ontologies/46317/?p=terms&conceptid=International_Medical_Terminology? Accessed May 10, 2012.

U.S. Food and Drug Administration: National Drug Code Directory. http://www.accessdata.fda.gov/scripts/cder/ndc/default.cfm. Accessed August 15, 2011.

U.S. National Institutes of Health, National Cancer Institute: Surveillance Epidemiology and End Results. http://seer.cancer.gov/. Accessed July 15, 2011.

World Health Organization: Classifications: International Classification of Diseases for Oncology, 3rd Edition (ICD-O-3). http://www.who.int/classifications/icd/adaptations/oncology/en/index.html. Accessed August 1, 2011.

World Health Organization: History of the Development of the ICD. http://www.who.int/classifications/icd/en/HistoryOfICD.pdf. Accessed August 5, 2011.

## SUGGESTED READING

CMS: NCCI Policy Manual for Medicare Services, 2012. http://www.cms.hhs.gov/Medicare/Coding/NationalCorrectCodInitEd/Downloads/NCCI_Policy_Manual.zip.

# CHAPTER ACTIVITIES

## CHAPTER SUMMARY

Coding is an increasingly important function in health care. Guided by a strict code of ethics, coders in a variety of settings use different nomenclature and classification systems to facilitate communication among providers, payers, and other users of health care data. These systems include ICD-9, ICD-10-CM, ICD-10-PCS, HCPCS/CPT-4, ICD-O-3, DSM-5, and CDT. Because these systems are required for use in electronic data interchange, the coder assumes the important role of ensuring that the data derived from the systems are complete and accurate.

Other systems without direct coder involvement include SNOMED-CT and NDC. These systems are important because of their use in the electronic health record and as HIPAA transaction code sets. Different coding systems currently in use satisfy the need to capture coded data for different uses by different providers. Some systems are very specialized, whereas some systems, such as SNOMED-CT, are far more comprehensive, with a broader range of users. Each system has its own unique uses. In most provider settings today, such as physician offices and acute care hospitals, there are two important coding systems currently in use: ICD-9-CM (ICD-10-CM after October 1, 2014) and HCPCS/CPT.

## REVIEW QUESTIONS

1. Describe reasons why is it important to have knowledge of ICD-9-CM.
2. What main advantage does ICD-10-CM have over ICD-9-CM?
3. Describe how the structure of ICD-10-PCS enables the addition of new codes.
4. Describe the process of "building" ICD-10-PCS codes.
5. Discuss the key differences, including structure and use, between HCPCS/CPT and ICD-10-PCS.
6. What is reimbursed with the use of HCPCS Level I codes? Level II codes?
7. Describe why and how SNOMED-CT is used in the electronic health record.
8. Explain the terms "topography" and "morphology" as they are applied in ICD-O.

### ● CAREER TIP

Inpatient coding experience as well as experience coding in a variety of settings is essential for a position in coder training. A college degree in a related field and supervisory or management experience are competitive advantages. To expand your skill set, offer to guest lecture in a local coding program or to speak at a local professional association meeting. Take continuing education courses that teach training and professional development leadership skills. Consider a master's degree in education, focusing on adult learning.

## ● PROFESSIONAL PROFILE

### Corporate Trainer—Coding Specialist Division

My name is Charlene, and I am employed in the Corporate Training Department of a large, multicampus medical center. In addition to our six inpatient facilities, we see hundreds of patients on a daily basis in our outpatient clinics, including behavioral health, and our same-day surgery centers. We are also affiliated with a dental school.

The Coding Specialist Division of the Corporate Training Department provides the coding training for all of our facilities, clinics, and outpatient programs. As a trainer within this division, I am responsible for training all new employees on the specific code sets they need to learn for their jobs as well as training existing employees on coding updates and changes in coding regulation.

Because we offer so many services in different settings, I must know ICD-10-CM, ICD-10-PCS, CPT-4, HCPCS, DSM-5, and CDT. I need to have an in-depth knowledge of all of these code sets in order to be an effective trainer. I must keep abreast of all changes and revised coding and reporting guidelines for all the services the medical center provides and provide in-service training to all of our coders accordingly.

I also act as a resource for the Patient Financial Services Department when there are code-based reimbursement issues. When chargemasters are updated, I am part of a team that reviews all new and revised codes to ensure they are current and correctly applied. This may sound tedious, but our work is extremely important if our medical center is to receive the reimbursement that we are entitled to for services provided.

I was promoted to this position because of my years of experience coding in one of our inpatient facilities and in several outpatient clinics. I am a Registered Health Information Technician (RHIT), Certified Coding Specialist (CCS), and Certified Coding Specialist–Physician Based.

I enjoy my job very much because my needed knowledge base is so varied, even though it is all "coding." It is personally rewarding to be able to share my enthusiasm with the new coders and set them on the right track for a successful career with our medical center.

## PATIENT CARE PERSPECTIVE

**Olga (Dr. Lewis's Practice Manager)**

When we were transitioning from ICD-9-CM to ICD-10-CM, I needed to plan how to train my staff. Diamonte Hospital is owned by a company that has a corporate training department. That department offered orientation classes and some physician office–based classes in ICD-10-CM. I was able to take advantage of those classes and obtained a great deal of information. This enabled me to plan my staff training as well as review our internal documentation and ancillary order sheets. So our patients were not disadvantaged by our inability to communicate with the hospital once we went live with ICD-10-CM.

## APPLICATION

*Standards of Ethical Coding*

AHIMA's *Standards of Ethical Coding* was first published in 1999 as a statement of principles that reflected the expectations of a professional coder. In 2008 the *Standards of Ethical Coding* was revised to reflect the current health care environment and modern coding practices. These Standards are intended to be relevant to all health care settings and applicable to all coders, regardless of whether they are members of AHIMA.

By following the *Standards of Ethical Coding,* the coding professional agrees to ethical principles that may have legal and reimbursement implications. If you were the coding supervisor, what emphasis would you put on the *Standards of Ethical Coding* in your area? Would you include the *Standards of Ethical Coding* in your policy and procedure manual? Would you review the *Standards of Ethical Coding* on a regular basis? If yes how often? What disciplinary action would you take if you found that a coder violated the *Standards of Ethical Coding*? Would the severity of the disciplinary action depend on which standard was violated? Why or why not?

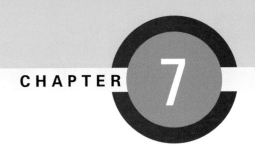

# REIMBURSEMENT

Marion Gentul

## CHAPTER OUTLINE

## VOCABULARY

# CHAPTER OBJECTIVES

*By the end of this chapter, the student should be able to:*
1. List and describe the types of health insurance.
2. List and describe the major reimbursement methodologies.
3. Describe different prospective payment systems and the settings in which they are used.
4. Identify and explain the major components of the UB-04 (CMS-1450).
5. Identify and explain the major components of the CMS-1500.
6. Explain the role of the coder in reimbursement and data quality.
7. Describe the revenue cycle and the role of coding in the revenue cycle process.

Patients and providers were, historically, the two main parties involved in a health care relationship. Patients were free to seek whatever services they were able to afford, and providers could charge whatever the market would bear. This one-on-one relationship has been split into a multiparty, complex system. The following section explores this system.

## PAYING FOR HEALTH CARE

The party (person or organization) from whom the provider is expecting payment for services rendered (reimbursement) is called the **payer**. The payer is frequently an insurance company. It may also be a government agency, such as Medicare or Medicaid. The term **reimbursement** is something of a misnomer. It is generally used today to refer to the payment provided to a physician or other health care provider in exchange for services rendered. With respect to reimbursement in health care, one of following two reimbursement scenarios typically occurs:
1. A patient pays a health care provider directly for services rendered and then that patient requests reimbursement from the insurance company (the insurer).
2. The health care provider renders services and requests reimbursement (bills) for those services directly from the insurer (the payer).

In a hospital setting, for example, a hospital provides services and supplies to a patient, thus incurring costs, under the assumption that it will be reimbursed for these costs after the patient has been discharged. The payer is billed at a later date. Insurance plans today do not typically require a patient to reimburse a hospital and then submit a **claim** to the insurance company for reimbursement. Patients without some form of third party payment relationship are called **self-pay** patients and are billed directly for services rendered.

## TYPES OF REIMBURSEMENT

Reimbursement takes many different forms. In the past, it was not uncommon for a physician to be "paid in kind." For example, a physician might have made a house call to treat a patient and then received chickens as compensation. These types of bartering arrangements were mutually acceptable to both physician and patient. Reimbursement today is generally monetary, especially for hospitalization services, but in many parts of the world and in the United States, bartering for health care services is common and acceptable.

Historically, a physician did not necessarily receive the payment that he or she charged but rather the payment that the patient thought the physician's services were worth. In the early twentieth century, this practice changed to paying what the physician charged. More recently, the amount of compensation given to the physician or health care provider is decided not by the patient or physician but by the third party payer. **Third party payers** have assumed the risk that a particular group of patients will require health care services and therefore incur the cost of paying for the services. In the following discussion, reimbursement is categorized according to the control that the health care provider exerts over the fees that are charged.

---

**payer** The individual or organization that is primarily responsible for the reimbursement for a particular health care service. Usually refers to the insurance company or third party.

**Medicare** Federally funded health care insurance plan for older adults and for certain categories of chronically ill patients.

**Medicaid** A federally mandated, state-funded program providing access to health care for the poor and the medically indigent.

**reimbursement** The amount of money that the health care facility receives from the party responsible for paying the bill.

**claim** The application to an insurance company for reimbursement.

**self-pay** A method of payment for health care services in which the patient pays the provider directly, without the involvement of a third party payer (e.g., insurance).

**insurer** The party that assumes the risk of paying some or all of the cost of providing health care services in return for the payment of a premium by or on behalf of the insured.

**third party payer** An entity that pays a provider for part or all of a patient's health care services; often the patient's insurance company.

# Insurance

**Insurance** is a contract between two parties in which one party assumes the risk of loss on behalf of the other party in return for some, usually monetary, compensation. The **insurer** receives a premium payment, often on a monthly basis, and in return it pays for some of all of the cost of health services.

## History

Insurance companies have existed for centuries. Notably, Lloyds of London insured cargoes on merchant ships, which were frequently subject to loss from piracy, inclement weather, and other catastrophes. The beginnings of insurance in health care date only to the mid-nineteenth century, when companies insured railroad and paddleboat employees in the event of catastrophic injury or death. A lump sum was paid to an employee or employee's family after such an event.

The origins of modern health care insurance, as we know it today in the United States, begin during the Great Depression in the 1930s. A decline in health care industry income prompted the development of hospital-based insurance plans. For a payment of a small sum, a hospital guaranteed a specific number of days of hospital care at no additional charge. The most successful of these plans was developed at Baylor University by Justin Ford Kimball (Sultz, Young, 2006; Blue Cross, 2011)—Baylor's plan eventually became the model for what we know today as Blue Cross Plans. Table 7-1 contains definitions of several terms that are useful during any discussion of health insurance.

In the early days of the industry, health care insurance was paid for by the recipient, sometimes through the employer, union, or other organization. In the original Baylor University scheme, teachers paid $0.50 a month, which entitled them to 21 days of hospital care should they need it (Sultz, Young, 2006). The insurance company became a third party payer in the relationship between the provider and patient.

Many patients have more than one payer. The primary payer is billed first for payment. A secondary payer is approached for any amount that the primary payer did not remit, and so on. For example, patients who are covered by Medicare may have supplemental or secondary insurance with a different payer. The physician first sends the bill to Medicare. Any amount that Medicare does not pay is then billed to the secondary payer.

Ultimately, the patient is financially responsible for payment of services that he or she has received. Depending on the type of insurance, the patient may have automatic responsibilities, such as *copays, co-insurance,* or *deductibles.* A **copay** is a fixed amount that a patient remits at the time of service. Copays typically vary according to the service rendered. For example, a copay may be $20 for a physician visit and $100 for an emergency department visit. **Co-insurance** is the percentage of the payment for which the patient is responsible. The payer may have 80% responsibility for the payment, and the patient 20%. A **deductible** is a fixed amount of patient responsibility that must be incurred before the third party payer is responsible. For example, if the patient has a $500 deductible, then the patient must spend $500 for health care services first. After $500 is expended, the third party payer will begin to reimburse for services rendered. In all cases, payment by third party payers depends on the contractual relationship between the third party and the patient. Third party payers will reimburse only for services that are covered in that contract.

If the patient is a dependent, a person other than the patient may be ultimately responsible for the bill. The person who is ultimately responsible for paying the bill is called the **guarantor**. For example, if a child goes to the physician's office for treatment, the child, as a dependent, cannot be held responsible for the invoice. Therefore the parent or legal guardian is responsible for payment and is the guarantor. Figure 2-6 lists financial data required by a health care provider.

After World War II, employers began offering their employees certain benefits, including health insurance. Benefits packages became useful in enabling employers to hire and retain employees. Employees benefited because they did not need to spend money on **premiums**, and employers benefited because health insurance benefits were a relatively low-cost way to attract quality employees. Insurance companies benefited from an

---

**insurance** A contract between two parties in which one party assumes the risk of loss on behalf of the other party in return for some, usually monetary, compensation.

**insurer** The party that assumes the risk of paying some or all of the cost of providing health care services in return for the payment of a premium by or on behalf of the insured.

**copay** A fixed amount paid by the patient at the time of service.

**co-insurance** A type of third party payer arrangement in which an individual is responsible for a percentage of the amount owed to the provider.

**deductible** A specified dollar amount for which the patient is personally responsible before the payer reimburses for any claims.

**Go To** This data is typically collected at registration, which is discussed in greater detail in Chapter 4.

**guarantor** The individual or organization that promises to pay for the rendered health care services after all other sources (such as insurance) are exhausted.

**financial data** Elements that describe the payer. For example, the name, address, and telephone number of the patient's insurance company, as well as the group and member numbers that the company has assigned to the patient.

**premium** Periodic payment to an insurance company made by the patient for coverage (an insurance policy).

## TABLE 7-1

### TERMINOLOGY COMMON TO HEALTH INSURANCE POLICIES

| TERM | DESCRIPTION |
| --- | --- |
| Benefit | The payment for specific health care services, or the health care services that are provided from an insurance policy or a managed care organization |
| Beneficiary | One who receives benefits from an insurance policy or a managed care program, or one who is eligible to receive such benefits |
| Benefit period | A period of time during which benefits are available for covered services, and which varies among payers and policies |
| Claim | The application to an insurance company for reimbursement of services rendered |
| Copayment (copay) | A fixed amount paid by the patient (or the subscriber to insurance policy) at the time of the health care service |
| Coverage | The health conditions, diagnostic procedures, and therapeutic treatments for which the insurance policy will pay |
| Deductible | A specified dollar amount for which the patient is personally responsible before the payer reimburses for any claims |
| Exclusions | Medical conditions or risks not covered by an insurance policy; preexisting conditions and experimental therapy are common exclusions to standard policies |
| Fiscal intermediary | An entity that administers the claims and reimbursements for a funding agency (i.e., an insurer or payer) |
| Insurance | A contract (policy) made with an insurer to assume the risk of paying some or all of the cost of providing health care services in return for the payment of a premium by or on behalf of the insured |
| Out-of-pocket costs | Costs not covered by an insurer, which are in turn paid by the patient directly to the provider |
| Payer | The individual or organization that is primarily responsible for the reimbursement for a particular health care service. Usually refers to the insurance company or third party |
| Premium | Periodic payments to an insurance company made by the patient for coverage under a policy |
| Preexisting condition | A medical condition identified as having occurred before a patient obtained coverage within a health insurance plan |
| Reimbursement | The amount of money that the health care facility receives from the party responsible for paying the bill |
| Rider | An adjustment to a policy that increases or decreases coverage and benefits, corresponding in an increase or decrease in the cost to the insured |
| Policy | Written contract detailing the coverage, benefits, exclusions, premiums, copays, deductibles, and other terms of the health plan |
| Subscriber | A person who purchases insurance |
| Third party payer | An entity that pays a provider for part or all of a patient's health care services; often the patient's insurance company |

increased client base. However, this thrust a fourth party into the provider/patient relationship: the employer.

Originally, the focus of insurance was on the coverage of services at the health care provider's fee. If the provider raised the fee, the insurance company raised its premiums to cover these fees. As health care costs increased, premiums also increased dramatically, becoming too expensive for many employers to pay in full. Currently, many employers pay only a part of the premiums, with employees bearing the rest of the expense.

### Assumption of Risk

Health care providers render services for which they expect to be fairly compensated. Patients need these services, but their high cost is largely unaffordable. Insurance companies are willing to assume the **risk** of having to pay for expensive services, but they cannot spend more than they earn in premiums. To avoid this, insurance companies try to balance their risk by insuring a large number of patients, many of whom will likely not need health care services at all. This assumption of risk is the foundation of the concept of insurance.

Insurance companies negotiate contracts with both the patient (usually via the employer) and the provider. Each party would like to minimize its financial loss. The provider wants to minimize the chances of receiving less payment for services than it costs to provide those services. The insurance company wants to minimize the potential loss of paying out more

● **risk** The potential exposure to loss, financial expenditure, or other undesirable events; used to determine potential reimbursement of health care services.

for health care than it receives in premiums. The patient wants to minimize the cost of health care. Each party negotiates contracts and attempts to minimize its risks by taking all potential treatment costs and circumstances into consideration.

Insurance companies serve the public by assuming the risk of financial loss. Automobile owners probably have auto insurance. They pay periodic premiums to the auto insurance company, which in turn covers all or part of the costs incurred in an accident. The auto insurance company, although assuming the risk of financial loss in the event of an accident, is gambling that its customers will not have one. In fact, it goes to great lengths to predict the likelihood of accidents in certain populations, geographical areas, and types of vehicles. If one pays $1000 per year in auto insurance premiums for 40 years and never has an accident, then the insurance company keeps the $40,000 (plus interest) accumulated over the life of the policy. If the auto insurance company insures a very large number of drivers, in theory and under normal circumstances, only a small percentage of them will ever have a costly accident. In some states, auto insurance companies are permitted to choose which drivers they wish to insure. Obviously, they would prefer to choose drivers with good driving records and no history of accidents. In other states, insurers may not pick and choose and must offer insurance to anyone who applies for it. This requirement raises the risk that the insurer will be required to pay for the costs of accidents and resultant settlements, in turn raising the cost of auto insurance for all, unless the premiums of the high-risk drivers are increased significantly to compensate.

Health insurance works in a similar way. In a system in which employers provide most private insurance plans, health insurers have fewer ways to limit their exposure to "high-risk" patients. Nevertheless, this model remains attractive to health insurers: they want to cover large numbers of individuals so that the cost of very expensive care is offset by premiums collected from many others requiring less expensive care. The health insurer wants to cover large numbers of individuals so that the risk that someone will require expensive medical care is offset by the large numbers of individuals who require less expensive care (Figure 7-1).

When the employer pays the cost (premium) of the health care insurance, it is the employer who negotiates what will be covered. Although there are some federal mandates regarding what must be covered and under what circumstances, in general it is the employer's decision—generally based on what the employer can afford to pay in premiums for the group. **Group plans**, such as those negotiated through employers, consist of pools of potential patients (in this case, employees) whose risk can be averaged by the third party payer.

**group plan** A pool of covered individuals that averages the risk for a third party payer, used to leverage lower premiums for the group as a whole.

**payer** The individual or organization that is primarily responsible for the reimbursement for a particular health care service. Usually refers to the insurance company or third party.

## HIT-bit

### RISK: THE BIG PICTURE

Risk is the danger that an activity will lead to an undesired outcome. In health care, risk applies to the patient, the physician, and the insurance company. The physician risks making an error in either the diagnosis or the treatment of the patient (obviously, this also presents a risk to the patient). There is also the risk that the physician will not be paid for the services rendered. The patient faces the risk that the cost of health care will be greater than the patient can bear, which would lead to excessive debt. For the payer, the risk is that claims for payment and administrative costs will exceed the premiums received. The payer may raise premiums to compensate; however, in so doing, the payer may lose subscribers. Overall, the financial risks and rewards in the health care industry are a delicate balancing act.

In an environment of rising health care costs, increases in payments to providers trigger increases in premiums to the insured. But the insertion of the employer into the patient/provider relationship has at least two effects: loss of control over the choice of individuals to cover and loss of total freedom to raise premiums. The insurer is pressured to accept all employees, reducing the insurer's ability to control risk. If one individual cancels a policy,

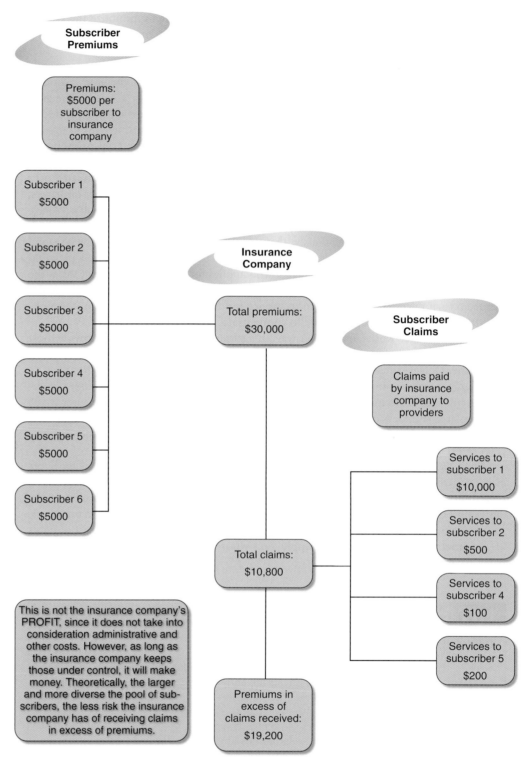

**Figure 7-1** How insurance companies reduce risk.

the financial impact is far less dramatic than if an employer cancels a *group policy*. In this way, an employer can pressure the health insurer to keep premiums low so as not to lose the employer's account.

**reimbursement** The amount of money that the health care facility receives from the party responsible for paying the bill.

## Types of Health Insurance

There are many different insurance plans, with an almost endless variety of benefits and reimbursement rules. Plans may set dollar-amount limits or usage limits on the benefits used in a certain amount of time. Nevertheless, plans fall into one of two basic categories: indemnity and managed care. Managed care plans are further divided into two major types: preferred provider organizations (PPOs) and health maintenance organizations (HMOs). The major features of these plans are discussed later in this chapter. The plans differ in the relationships among the physician, patient, and insurer and affect the way patients access care.

### Indemnity

A typical insurance arrangement requires the patient to pay the physician or other health care provider and then submit the bills to the insurance company for reimbursement. Under the terms of the insurance contract is a list of services for which the insurance company agrees to pay, called the covered services. If the patient receives a covered service, then the insurance company reimburses the patient. Some insurance companies pay 100% of the cost of certain covered services and a lower percentage of the cost of other covered services. This type of insurance, called **indemnity insurance**, was the predominant type of health insurance for many years, and patients generally paid the premiums. Indemnity insurance plans still exist, but managed care plans have become more prevalent.

An important feature of indemnity insurance is the deductible. A deductible is the amount for which the patient is personally responsible before any insurance benefits are paid. If a patient incurs medical expenses of $5000, and her policy includes a deductible of $300, she pays the first $300 out-of-pocket (from her personal funds). The insurer then pays the portion of the remaining $4700 covered by the policy. After that, the patient is responsible for any amount not covered by her policy.

Depending on the insurance company plan, a deductible could apply for every encounter, every visit, or every hospitalization, or it could be applied on an annual basis. If the insurance plan covers a whole family, the deductible could be per person or per family. One effect of the deductible is that routine health care costs often do not exceed the deductible amount. In these instances, the insurance company ultimately covers and pays for only unusual or extraordinary expenses. Conversely, indemnity contracts often specify limits for certain covered services. If the benefit limit is $3000 for physician office visits and the patient's care (after the deductible) is $4000, then the patient is responsible for the additional $1000.

Indemnity insurance plans led to an increase in the amount of money spent on health care. In a simple physician-patient relationship, the patient bears the cost of the care and therefore has some influence on the fees. Individuals may choose not to go to the physician in the first place because they feel the fee is too high and they cannot afford it, or they might be able to afford only some services. But because indemnity insurance plans, even with the deductible, reduce the out-of-pocket expense to the patient, they increase the likelihood that the services of the provider will be used regardless of the fees. Consequently, the number of people using health care services has increased. In addition, if the insurance company reimburses for services without reviewing the need for those services, then physicians have no incentive to be conservative in their diagnostic and treatment plans. The costs have risen still further with advances in diagnostic and therapeutic technologies, many of which are extremely costly in their initial phases. As these technologies become more widely used, the cost of providing health care increases.

In addition to the technology-driven expenses, health care costs have risen because a small portion of the health care community provided an excessive number of services to their patients. Two radiographs may have been taken when one would have sufficed, or computed tomography or magnetic resonance imaging was used when a simple radiograph would have been sufficient to achieve the same diagnostic goal. Often it is not entirely the provider's fault when these excesses occur. Some patients may feel entitled to the newest technologies even if they are not necessary, and so they pressure their physicians into ordering them. The physician may not want to lose the patient's business or to be subjected to a lawsuit for failure to use all available diagnostic means.

To meet the rising costs of health care, insurance companies raised health care premiums. Eventually, some employers could no longer afford to offer health insurance as a benefit. Many employers began shifting the cost of insurance to the employees. Other

**indemnity insurance** Assumption of the payment for all or part of certain, specified services. Characterized by out-of-pocket deductibles and caps on total covered payments.

**deductible** A specified dollar amount for which the patient is personally responsible before the payer reimburses for any claims.

**out-of-pocket** Payment from personal funds.

**encounter** A patient's health care experience; a unit of measure for the volume of ambulatory care services provided.

**plan of treatment** The diagnostic, therapeutic, or palliative measures that are taken to investigate or treat the patient's condition or disease.

**premiums** Periodic payments to an insurance company made by the patient for coverage (an insurance policy).

employers solved the escalating premium problem by hiring more part-time employees, who were not eligible for benefits. Still other employers hired outside contractors to perform noncritical functions.

With costs rising, health insurance companies had to find ways to control their expenses. Certain steps, such as imposing higher deductibles and strictly limiting the number and types of covered services, could help lower their costs. However, insurance becomes less attractive under these circumstances, and insurance companies want to remain in business. The insurance industry responded to these circumstances and factors, opening the door to the concept of managed care plans.

### Managed Care

The term **managed care**, in general, refers to the control that an insurance company or other payer exerts over the reimbursement process and over the patient's choices in selecting a health care provider.

In the pure physician-patient relationship, the patient uses the physician of his or her choice. The patient arrives at the office with a medical concern, and the physician determines a diagnosis and develops a treatment plan. The patient agrees (or declines) to undergo the treatment plan, the physician bills the patient, and the patient pays the physician.

Under managed care, the insurer (payer) and the health care provider have a contractual arrangement with each other. The providers participate in a particular managed care plan, which means that they are under contract with the managed care plan insurer to provide services to the insurer's patients. Managed care patients are referred to, depending on the insurer, as members, enrollees, or covered lives. The primary insured member is the subscriber, with those covered under the subscriber's policy referred to as dependents or additional insured. The insurer's patients must choose their providers from those participating in the managed care plan. The scope of services paid for is determined by the insurer's contract with the subscriber (or the subscriber's employer or group manager). Decisions about the medical necessity of specific services are made by the managed care organization. For example, a physician may write an order for a blood test to determine whether the patient has a vitamin D deficiency. The managed care organization may have determined that it will pay for vitamin D blood tests only if the patient is known or suspected to have a bone loss condition, such as osteopenia or osteoporosis.

---

**managed care** A type of insurer (payer) focused on reducing health care costs, controlling expensive care, and improving the quality of patient care provided.

**payer** The individual or organization that is primarily responsible for the reimbursement for a particular health care service. Usually refers to the insurance company or third party.

**reimbursement** The amount of money that the health care facility receives from the party responsible for paying the bill.

**diagnosis** The name of the patient's condition or illness, or the reason for the health care encounter.

---

## HIT-bit

### THE INSURANCE CONTRACT

An insurance contract is essentially the promise to pay for certain health care costs incurred by the subscriber in return for the payment of a premium to the insurer by either the subscriber or another party. When the subscriber contracts directly with the insurer, the premium is not usually negotiable. However, when the subscriber is a member of a larger group, such as that provided by an employer, both the premium and the services for which the insurer will pay may be subject to negotiation.

Insurance companies (particularly managed care organizations) also negotiate with each provider to determine the services that apply to that provider, how much the insurer is willing to pay for those services, and under what circumstances the provider may render those services. Providers apply to be included in insurers' lists of in-plan providers. Because subscribers are encouraged to choose providers from those lists, being on multiple lists is theoretically a good business decision for providers. However, if insurers reduce payments and restrict services, providers may decide to avoid these payer relationships entirely. In fact, physicians may elect not to accept insurance at all, requiring patients to file cumbersome claims for reimbursement with their insurers.

In a managed care scenario, the patient goes to the primary care physician (PCP), whom the patient has chosen from a list of participating physicians. The physician diagnoses and treats the patient according to the guidelines from the managed care plan. The patient may pay the physician a small copay. The physician bills the managed care insurer directly for the visit. The managed care insurer may refuse to pay the physician if the physician does not obtain preapproval or authorization for some treatments, such as hospitalization. If the patient sees a physician outside the plan, the patient may not be covered at all and may have to pay the physician himself or herself. In many instances, the patient cannot go to a specialist directly but must visit the PCP first. After examination and discussion with the patient, the PCP must justify the necessity for the involvement of a specialist and must refer the patient to a specialist participating in the plan.

Managed care organizations seek to reduce costs by controlling as much of the health care delivery system as possible. The underlying rationale for managed care is to reduce overall costs by eliminating unnecessary tests, procedures, visits, and hospitalizations through financial incentives if the plan is followed and financial penalties or sanctions if the plan is not followed. A major controversy in this strategy lies in the definition of what constitutes unnecessary health care and who makes this determination. Traditionally, physicians have determined the care that they provide to patients, whereas managed care has shifted that determination somewhat to the insurer. To emphasize: The managed care organization does not dictate what care will be rendered; it dictates what care it will pay for. It is the prohibitive cost of care that drives a patient to elect only that care for which third party payment is available.

It should be noted that managed care plans employ physicians who assist in making determinations. For example, many managed care insurers did not consider preventive care to be necessary and would not pay for it. It was only through years of study, investigation, and trial and error that they discovered that preventive care was one of the best ways to reduce health care costs. This fact is particularly salient with regard to obstetrical care. The costs of treating a pregnant woman through prenatal testing, education, and regular examinations, with the goal of delivering a healthy newborn, are significantly less than those of treating a newborn or new mother with complications that could have been prevented or treated earlier at less cost. The same holds true for dental care. Theoretically, if teeth are examined and cleaned routinely, expensive fillings and root canal treatments will not be needed because the dentist will help detect and treat those problems early.

Individuals who change jobs are often forced to find new health care providers if their previous physicians are not included in the new insurer's plan. The same may be true if the employer changes insurers. Patients who live at the outskirts of a plan's primary service area may be required to travel unacceptably long distances to receive covered health care services.

Physicians may feel a loss of control in the treatment process. They are sometimes frustrated by the emphasis on medical practice standards, what some call "cookbook medicine," and resistance to what they may see as individualized, alternative approaches of care. Managed care organizations focus heavily on statistical analysis of treatment outcomes and scrutinize physicians whose practices appear to vary significantly from the norm. Managed care has forced physicians to become more aware of and active in managing their own resources by employing reimbursement methods other than fee for service that shift some financial risk to the physician.

Despite controversy and criticism, managed care has become an important presence in the health care arena. Managed care takes a number of different forms, and there are many variations in the relationship among managed care organizations and physicians and other health care providers who deliver their services. At the heart of managed care is the idea that the insurer can gain better control over cost of health care by delivering the services directly. The U.S. Congress supported this concept with the Health Maintenance Organization Act of 1973, which encouraged the development of **health maintenance organizations** (**HMOs**) and mandated certain employers to offer employees an HMO option for health care delivery.

**primary care physician (PCP)** In insurance, the physician who has been designated by the insured to deliver routine care to the insured and to evaluate the need for referral to a specialist, if applicable. Colloquial use is synonymous with "family doctor."

**copay** A fixed amount paid by the patient at the time of service.

**outcome** the result of a patient's treatment.

**fee for service** The exchange of monies, goods, or services for professional services rendered at a specific rate, typically determined by the provider and associated with specific activities (such as a physical examination).

**health maintenance organization (HMO)** Managed care organization characterized by the ownership or employer control over the health care providers.

**network** A group of providers serving the members of a managed care organization; the payer will generally not cover health care services from providers outside the network.

**staff model HMO** An HMO in which the organization owns the facilities, employs the physicians, and provides essentially all health care services.

**group practice model HMO** An HMO that contracts with a group or network of physicians and facilities to provide health care services.

**independent practice association (IPA) model HMO** An HMO that contracts with individual physicians, portions of whose practices are devoted to the HMO.

**preferred provider organization (PPO)** A managed care organization that contracts with a network of health care providers to render services to its members.

**primary care physician (PCP)** In insurance, the physician who has been designated by the insured to deliver routine care to the insured and to evaluate the need for referral to a specialist, if applicable. Colloquial use is synonymous with "family doctor."

**claim** The application to an insurance company for reimbursement.

**flexible benefit account** A savings account in which health care and certain child-care costs can be set aside and paid using pretax funds.

## Health Maintenance Organizations

An HMO is a managed care organization that has ownership or employer control over the health care provider. Essentially, the HMO is the insurer (payer) and the provider. Members must use the HMO for all services, and the HMO will generally not pay for out-of-plan (also called out of **network**) services without prior approval. In some plans, approval to obtain health care services outside the plan is granted only in emergency situations.

In the **staff model HMO**, the organization owns the facilities, employs the physicians, and provides essentially all health care services. In a **group practice model HMO**, the organization contracts with a group or a network of physicians and facilities to provide health care services. Finally, in an **independent practice association (IPA) model HMO**, the HMO contracts with individual physicians, portions of whose practices are devoted to the HMO. Regardless of the HMO model, an HMO generally does not reimburse for services provided by providers who are not in the HMO's network.

## Preferred Provider Organizations

A **preferred provider organization (PPO)** is another managed care approach in which the organization contracts with a network of health care providers who agree to certain reimbursement rates. It is from this network that patients are encouraged to choose their primary care physician and any specialists. If a patient chooses a provider who is not in the network, the PPO reimburses in the same manner as an indemnity insurer: for specified services, with specific dollar amounts or percentage limits, and after any deductible is paid by the insured.

A PPO is a hybrid plan that gives patients the option of choosing physicians outside the plan without totally forfeiting benefits. In addition, PPOs may offer patients a certain degree of freedom to self-refer to specialists. For example, some plans allow patients to visit gynecologists and vision specialists directly, without referral from the PCP.

## Self-Insurance

Although not specifically a type of insurance, self-insurance (or self-funded insurance) is an alternative to purchasing an insurance policy. The term *self-insurance* should not be confused with patients who "self-pay" or those who have no insurance or coverage plan at all. Self-insurance is really a savings plan in which an individual or employer puts aside funds to cover health care costs. In this way, the individual or company assumes the financial risk associated with health care. Because the assumption of risk rests with the company or the individual, this is not so much a type of insurance as it is an alternative to shifting the risk to an insurer.

An employer may choose to self-insure for all health care benefits, or it may self-insure to provide specific benefits that its primary insurance plan does not cover. For example, an insurance plan may cover preventive care, hospital and physician services, and diagnostic tests. However, it may not cover vision or dental care. The employer may designate to each employee a certain dollar amount with which the employee may then be reimbursed for these other services. Ordinarily, if the annual dollar amount is not spent, it is lost to the employee. Because the issue of confidentiality is so important, employers may choose to contract with an insurer to process health care claims, even if the employer self-insures.

Individuals may self-insure by saving money on a regular basis through their employer. These savings are designated for health care expenses. One formal plan that enables individuals to save in this manner is a **flexible benefit account** (or medical savings account). A flexible benefit account provides the individual with a savings account, usually through payroll deduction, into which a set amount determined by the employee can be deposited routinely. These funds can then be drawn on to pay out-of-pocket health care and some child-care expenses. The advantage to a flexible benefit account is that the funds are withdrawn from the individual's salary on a pretax basis, thereby reducing the individual's income tax liability. The disadvantage is that nondisbursed funds are forfeited at the end of the year. Table 7-2 summarizes the four types of insurance that have been discussed.

**TABLE 7-2**

**SUMMARY OF HEALTH INSURANCE RELATIONSHIPS**

| INSURANCE | MAJOR FEATURES |
|---|---|
| Indemnity | Employer maintains group policy with insurer, thereby spreading the risk among many. |
| | Employer may pay all or part of the premium. |
| | Employer sets policy as to classification of eligible employees and collects employee share of premium, if any. |
| HMO (health maintenance organization) | Providers are limited to those in the plan. |
| | Patient pays small copayment. |
| | Covered services must be medically necessary. |
| | Providers tend to be employees of the HMO or to have exclusive contracts with HMO. |
| | Primary care physician acts as gatekeeper, evaluating the need for specialized care and providing referrals. |
| PPO (preferred provider organization) | Combination of HMO and indemnity features. |
| | Providers are independent contractors. |
| Self-insurance | Employer may reserve funds to cover projected medical expenses. |
| | Covered employees may contribute to fund. |
| | Insured sets aside pretax dollars to cover specific medical expenses, such as vision care. Unused funds are lost. |

## Clinical Oversight

In Chapter 1, a collaborative process of patient care involving the physicians, nurses, and other allied health professionals was described. This patient care plan is more than just a series of instructions or recommendations for an individual patient. Clinicians typically follow established patterns of care that are based on experience, successful outcomes, and research. The formal description of these patterns of care is the clinical pathway. Each discipline has a specific clinical pathway that describes the appropriate steps to take, given a specific diagnosis or a specific set of signs and symptoms and based on the answers to critical questions. For example, a patient with high blood glucose (hyperglycemia) must be tested to determine whether the patient is diabetic. If the patient is diabetic, further studies will identify whether the condition is insulin dependent or not. The physician will prescribe the appropriate medications and other regimens on the basis of that determination. Nursing staff will assess the patient's level of understanding of his or her condition and take the appropriate steps to educate the patient and possibly the family. Figure 7-2 illustrates a clinical pathway.

### Case Management

The responsibility for patient care rests with the provider, but often multiple providers, and possibly multiple facilities, are involved in a patient's care. From the payer's perspective, **case management** is necessary to coordinate the approval of and adherence to the care plan. From the provider's perspective, case managers are necessary to facilitate the continuity of care. Thus a patient may have multiple case managers working from different perspectives, all helping to ensure that the patient is cared for appropriately and efficiently.

### Utilization Review

Understanding clinical pathways and payer issues enables a facility to evaluate patient care, control the use of facility resources, and measure the performance of individual clinical staff. In a hospital, the **utilization review (UR)** department works closely with all health care disciplines involved in caring for a patient who has been admitted. UR

**patient care plan** The formal directions for treatment of the patient, which involves many different individuals, including the patient.

**outcome** The result of a patient's treatment.

**clinical pathway** A predetermined standard of treatment for a particular disease, diagnosis, or procedure designed to facilitate the patient's progress through the health care encounter.

**case management** The coordination of the patient's care and services, including reimbursement considerations.

**continuity of care** The coordination among caregivers to provide, efficiently and effectively, the broad range of health care services required by a patient during an illness or for an entire lifetime. May also refer to the coordination of care provided among caregivers/services within a health care organization.

**utilization review (UR)** The process of evaluating medical interventions against established criteria, on the basis of the patient's known or tentative diagnosis. Evaluation may take place before, during, or after the episode of care for different purposes.

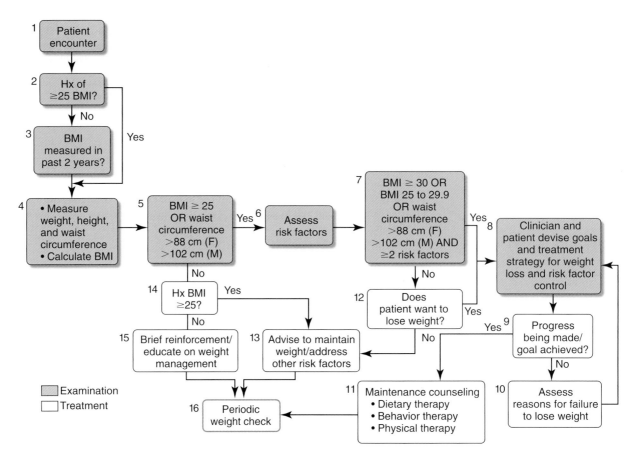

**Figure 7-2** Clinical pathway for obesity. (From National Institutes of Health, National Heart, Lung, and Blood Institute in cooperation with The National Institute of Diabetes and digestive and Kidney Diseases: "Clinical guidelines on the identification, evaluation, and treatment of overweight and obesity in adults": The evidence report. NIH Publication No. 98-4083. http://www.nhlbi.nih.gov/guidelines/obesity/ob_gdlns.pdf. Published September 1998.)

**intensity of service** In utilization review, a type of criteria, consisting primarily of monitoring and diagnostic assessments, that must be met in order to qualify a patient for inpatient admission.

**discharge planning** The multidisciplinary, coordinated effort to ensure that a patient is discharged to the appropriate level of care and with the appropriate support.

**UR** utilization review

**admission denial** Occurs when the payer or its designee (such as utilization review staff) will not reimburse the facility for treatment of the patient because the admission was deemed unnecessary.

staff members (also known as case management personnel) are responsible, with physician oversight, for performing an admission review that covers the appropriateness of the admission itself, certifying the level of care for an admission (e.g., acute, skilled nursing), monitoring the *intensity of services* provided, and ensuring that a patient's length of stay is appropriate for that level of care. UR staff members may have daily contact with a patient's insurance company during the patient's admission to verify that the correct level of care payment will be received for the anticipated length of stay. UR staff may also make provisions for aftercare once the patient is discharged; this is called **discharge planning**.

For example, suppose a patient with Type 1 diabetes mellitus is admitted because the patient performed a self-check at home and could not control his blood glucose level even while taking the prescribed amounts of daily insulin. UR staff members will be notified that the patient has been admitted, and they will perform an admission review. This admission review entails an evaluation of the patient's medical record, including physician orders and any test results. In some cases, the admission will be deemed unnecessary. The admission might be unnecessary if the patient's blood glucose levels were all normal on admission. At that point, UR staff members would not certify the admission for reimbursement; this is called an **admission denial**.

If UR staff members deem the admission necessary, they will certify the admission. UR staff may contact the patient's insurer, verify the diagnosis of uncontrolled Type 1 diabetes mellitus, and determine that the anticipated length of stay for that diagnosis is 2 to 3 days. The insurer agrees to reimburse the hospital for 3 days of acute care as certified by UR staff. During the hospitalization, UR staff members will discuss the aftercare, or discharge plan, with the attending physician. In this case, perhaps more home health care services are warranted. On the third day, the patient is expected to be discharged. If the patient is not discharged on day 3, members of the UR staff must review documentation and discuss the case further with the physician to justify additional hospitalization. If the additional days are not justified by the documentation in the health record, the additional days may not be reimbursed by the insurer; this is called a **continued stay denial**. In these instances, the patient will be notified that he or she no longer needs to be in the hospital, that the insurer will not reimburse the hospital for any additional costs, and that the patient is responsible for all further costs. When a continued stay denial occurs, the physician is also notified. The physician will either concur with the continued stay denial and discharge the patient or provide documentation justifying the additional care.

## EXERCISE 7-1

### Insurance

1. Each type of reimbursement has unique characteristics and a different approach to risk. Compare and contrast the four types of reimbursement, identifying the financial risk to the parties involved.
2. Health care insurance involves the assumption of the risk of financial loss by a party other than the patient. Describe how insurance companies can afford to assume such risk.
3. The text discussed three different types of health insurance. List them, and describe how they are different.

## Entitlements

Although the United States does not have universal health care (i.e., government-subsidized health care for all citizens), the various levels of government do serve as the largest payer for health care services. Because eligibility for certain government-sponsored programs is automatic, being based on age, condition, or employment, they are called **entitlement programs** rather than insurance.

### Federal Coverage for Specific Populations

The U.S. government has historically allocated funds for the benefits of specific populations. In the case of health care, target populations of chronically ill or indigent patients have received low-cost or free health care. Until the 1960s, funding was not entirely predictable and health care providers were often required to provide a certain amount of charity care. In addition, large groups of individuals with limited incomes were not eligible for federal assistance. The federal government took the plunge in the mid-1960s with the enactment of legislation that made it the largest single payer in the health care industry: *Title XVIII* and *Title XIX of the Social Security Act*, which established the Medicare and Medicaid programs.

In addition to Medicare and Medicaid, the federal government administers **TRICARE** (formerly called CHAMPUS), which provides health benefits for military personnel, their families, and military retirees. The federal government provides health services to veterans through the Veterans Health Administration (VHA). The Civilian Health and Medical Program of the Veterans Administration (CHAMPVA) was created in 1973 to provide health services for spouses and children of certain deceased or disabled veterans. TRICARE, VHA, and CHAMPVA are service benefits, not insurance, and are included here to illustrate the extent of the federal government's financial involvement in health care. (See the TRICARE and CHAMPVA Web sites for additional information.) Table 7-3 provides a summary of this involvement.

---

**attending physician** The physician who is primarily responsible for coordinating the care of the patient in the hospital; it is usually the physician who ordered the patient's admission to the hospital.

**home health care** Health care services rendered in the patient's home.

**health record** Also called *medical record*. It contains all of the data collected for an individual patient.

**continued stay denial** Similar to admission denial; however, it is the additional payment for the length of stay that is not approved rather than the entire admission.

**entitlement programs** In health care, government-sponsored programs that pay for certain services on the basis of an individual's age, condition, employment status, or other circumstances.

**Medicare** Federally funded health care insurance plan for older adults and for certain categories of chronically ill patients.

**Medicaid** A federally mandated, state-funded program providing access to health care for the poor and the medically indigent.

**TRICARE** A U.S. program of health benefits for military personnel, their families, and military retirees, formerly called *CHAMPUS*.
TRICARE on the Web: www.tricare.mil
CHAMPVA on the Web: http://www.va.gov/hac/forbeneficiaries/champva/champva.asp

| TABLE 7-3 | | |
|---|---|---|
| **SUMMARY OF FEDERAL INVOLVEMENT IN HEALTH CARE** | | |
| **ACRONYM** | **DESCRIPTION** | **COVERED LIVES** |
| Medicare | Title XVIII of the Social Security Act (1965) | Older adult, disabled, renal dialysis, and transplant patients<br>Part A: inpatient services<br>Part B: outpatient services and physician claims<br>Part C: managed care option<br>Part D: prescription drug benefit |
| Medicaid | Title XIX of the Social Security Act (1965) | Low-income patients |
| TRICARE | Medical services for members of the armed services, their spouses, and their families | Administered by the Department of Defense and applying to members of the Army, Air Force, Navy, Marine Corps, Coast Guard, Public Health Service, and National Oceanic and Atmospheric Administration |
| VHA | Veterans Health Administration | Health services for veterans |
| CHAMPVA | Civilian Health and Medical Program of the Department of Veterans Affairs (CHAMPVA) | Programs administered by the U.S. Department of Veterans Affairs (Health Administration Center) for veterans and their families |
| IHS | Indian Health Service | Provides, or assists in providing and organizing, health care services to American Indians and Alaskan Natives |

**Title XVIII of the Social Security Act** Amendment to the Social Security Act that established Medicare.

**inpatient** An individual who is admitted to a hospital with the intention of staying overnight.

**ambulatory surgery** Surgery performed on an outpatient basis; the patient returns home after the surgery is performed. Also called *same-day surgery*.

**claim** The application to an insurance company for reimbursement of services rendered.

**Medicare administrative contractor (MAC)** Regional, private contractor who processes reimbursement claims for CMS.

The Indian Health Services (IHS) provides care for American Indians and Alaska Natives. The IHS provides a comprehensive health service delivery system for approximately 1.9 million American Indians and Alaska Natives who belong to 564 federally recognized tribes in 35 states (Indian Health Services, 2012).

### Medicare

**Title XVIII of the Social Security Act** established the Medicare program in 1965. Originally enacted to provide funding for health care for older adults, Medicare has grown to include individuals with certain disabilities or with end-stage renal disease requiring dialysis or kidney transplantation. Medicare represents more than 50% of the income of some health care providers. Medicare is an extremely important driving force in the insurance industry because many insurance companies follow Medicare's lead in adopting reimbursement strategies. For example, if Medicare decides that a particular surgical procedure will be reimbursed only if is it performed in the inpatient setting (as opposed to ambulatory surgery), other insurance companies may choose to enforce the same rule.

The Medicare program, although funded by the federal government and administered by the Centers for Medicare and Medicaid Services (CMS), does not process its own claims reimbursements. Reimbursements are processed by **Medicare administrative contractors (MACs)** located in different regions throughout the country.

---

**HIT-bit**

### ANCILLARY AND PHYSICIAN BILLING

Not all diagnostic testing and other services are billable by the health care facility. For example, a facility may not have a magnetic resonance imaging (MRI) machine. If this is the case, the patient is transported to the MRI provider, who bills either the payer or the original facility separately for both the diagnostic procedure and its interpretation, depending on the reimbursement method and payer. Additionally, unless the physician is an employee of the hospital, physicians bill separately for their services.

Medicare coverage applies in four categories: Parts A, B, C, and D. Part A covers inpatient hospital services and some other services, such as hospice. Part B covers physician claims and outpatient services. Part C is a voluntary managed care option. Part D, implemented in 2006, is a prescription drug program.

Because there are limits to Medicare coverage, many beneficiaries choose to purchase additional insurance; such plans, called **wraparound policies** (supplemental policies), are aimed at absorbing costs not reimbursed by Medicare. Many end-of-life hospital stays generate costs in the hundreds of thousands of dollars. Therefore wraparound policies can help preserve estates and save surviving spouses from financial ruin. Medicare may also be the secondary payer for enrollees who are still employed and covered primarily by the employer's insurance plan.

Medicare beneficiaries also may enroll in a Medicare HMO program, called Medicare+Choice. Different HMOs have contracted with the federal government under the Medicare+Choice program to provide health services to these beneficiaries.

## Medicaid

In 1965, Congress enacted **Title XIX of the Social Security Act**, which created a formal system of providing funding for health care for low-income populations. Also administered by CMS, Medicaid, which is sometimes also called "Medical Assistance," is a shared federal and state program designed to shift resources from higher-income to lower-income individuals. Funds are allocated according to the average income of the residents of the state. Unlike Medicare, which reimburses through **fiscal intermediaries**, Medicaid reimbursement is handled directly by each individual state. The reimbursement guidelines vary from state to state. Some states have contracted with insurers to offer HMO plans to Medicaid beneficiaries.

Eligibility for Medicaid is determined by the individual states on the basis of the state's income criteria. The federal government mandates that the following services be included in each state's program: hospital and physician services, diagnostic services, home health, nursing home, preventive care, family planning, pregnancy care, and child care (see the CMS Web site for more information: http://www.cms.hhs.gov).

## Tax Equity and Fiscal Responsibility Act of 1982

With the federal government's entry into the reimbursement arena, more citizens had access to health care services than ever before. The use of health care services rose accordingly, in turn driving health care costs upward at an alarming rate. Improved access for older adults meant better care and therefore longer life expectancy, which further increased costs. Thus cost containment became a critical issue. In the early 1970s, Professional Standards Review Organizations (PSROs) were established. PSROs conducted local peer reviews of Medicare and Medicaid cases for the purpose of ensuring that only medically necessary services were being rendered and appropriately reimbursed. Under the Peer Review Improvement Act of 1982, PSROs were replaced by Peer Review Organizations (PROs) through a federal law called the **Tax Equity and Fiscal Responsibility Act of 1982 (TEFRA)**. TEFRA included a broad array of provisions, many of which had nothing to do with health care. For example, TEFRA raised taxes by eliminating previous tax cuts. In 2002, PROs were replaced by (or, more accurately, renamed) Quality Improvement Organizations (QIOs). Many HIM professionals are employed in QIOs because certain specialized skills, such as data analysis and coding expertise, are necessary to support various federal initiatives delegated to QIOs. TEFRA's impact on health care included a modification of Medicare reimbursement for inpatient care to include a **case mix** adjustment based on diagnosis related groups (DRGs). In 1983, Medicare adopted the *Prospective Payment System (PPS)*, which uses the DRG classification system as the basis of its reimbursement methodology. **Prospective payment systems (PPS)** are discussed at length later in the chapter, but in the broadest terms, they operate on the assumption that patients with the same diagnoses will require roughly the same level of care, therefore consuming roughly the same resources and incurring roughly the same costs. Of course, the focus of treatment, patient length of stay, and the individuals involved in the care plan differ from setting to setting. Because

**hospice** Palliative health care services rendered to the terminally ill, their families, and their friends.

**outpatient** A patient whose health care services are intended to be delivered within 1 calendar day or, in some cases, a 24-hour period.

**wraparound policy** Insurance policies that supplement Medicare coverage. Also called *secondary insurance*.

**HMO** health maintenance organization

**Title XIX of the Social Security Act** Amendment to the Social Security Act that established Medicaid.

**Medicaid** A federally mandated, state-funded program providing access to health care for the poor and the medically indigent.

**fiscal intermediaries** Organizations that administer the claims and reimbursements for the funding agency. Medicare uses fiscal intermediaries to process its claims and reimbursements.

**CMS** Centers for Medicare and Medicaid Services

**Go To** More information about QIOs can be found in Chapter 11 and on the CMS Web site, with links to local QIOs.

**Tax Equity and Fiscal Responsibility Act of 1982 (TEFRA)** A federal law with wide-reaching provisions, one of which was the establishment of Medicare PPS.

**case mix** Statistical distribution of patients according to their utilization of resources. Also refers to the grouping of patients by clinical department or other meaningful distribution, such as health insurance type.

**prospective payment system (PPS)** A system used by payers, primarily CMS, for reimbursing acute care facilities on the basis of statistical analysis of health care data.

**QOI** Quality Improvement Organizations

**DRGs** diagnosis related groups

prospective reimbursement systems are based on just these types of factors, different systems were developed for each health care setting.

Paying for health care is an ever-changing subject. HIM professionals must be aware of new developments that pertain to their practice and keep abreast of general reimbursement issues.

## ■ EXERCISE 7-2

### Government Influence on Reimbursement

1. What is the difference between Medicare and Medicaid?
2. What is the difference between the VHA and TRICARE?
3. Who benefits from the Indian Health Services?
4. Explain the impact of TEFRA on health care.

## REIMBURSEMENT METHODOLOGIES

**coding** The assignment of alphanumerical values to a word, phrase, or other nonnumerical expression. In health care, coding is the assignment of alphanumerical values to diagnosis and procedure descriptions.

This section provides a general discussion of how reimbursement is accomplished in the health care industry, who is involved in the reimbursement process, what methodologies are used to calculate reimbursement, and how HIM professionals are involved in the process. One of the most visible roles that HIM professionals play in health care today involves the reimbursement process (e.g., as coding professionals or clinical data managers).

## FEE FOR SERVICE

**fee for service** The exchange of monies, goods, or services for professional services rendered at a specific rate, typically determined by the provider and associated with specific activities (such as a physical examination).

**charges** Fees or costs for services rendered.

As previously mentioned, a physician or other health care provider does not necessarily need to receive money as compensation. Perhaps chickens, bread, or other food is acceptable under certain circumstances. In other circumstances, services might be bartered (e.g., "You treat my pneumonia, and I will take care of your plumbing."). This is known as an *exchange of services*, or *reciprocal services*. The parties involved decide the value of each service (e.g., how many hours of plumbing would be equal in value to how many hours of physician treatment). However, monetary compensation is the generally accepted reimbursement method in the United States.

**Fee for service** is the term assigned to the payment for services rendered by a physician, health care provider, or facility. It is sometimes referred to as "pay as you go" because this is how many patients without any insurance pay for treatments. The patient is essentially "buying" services or supplies. For example, a patient goes to, or "visits," the physician's office because of a runny nose. The physician examines the patient and determines that the patient is allergic to a house pet. This service, which comprises an office visit and examination, is billed at $100. This $100 is the "fee." Suppose this same patient also needs an allergy shot, and this shot has a fee of $20. In this case, the total fee for the visit is $120. As this example shows, fees correspond to the services rendered, "fee for service." Health care provider fees are also called **charges**. Note that costs and charges are different. Cost is what the health care provider expended in the process of rendering services. Costs include time, supplies, and expenses such as rent and utilities. Charges are the fees that are billed for the services. The term "cost" is often used to refer to the overall expenditures for health care, but the narrow definition is used for this discussion.

**usual and customary fees** Referring to health care provider fees, the rates established by an insurance company on the basis of the regional charges for the particular services.

**payer** The individual or organization that is primarily responsible for the reimbursement for a particular health care service. Usually refers to the insurance company or third party.

Comparing the fees charged by physicians in a particular state or geographical area, one finds that the fees for services are similar. Ignoring the very high and very low fees, one would be able to determine the **usual and customary fees (UCFs)** charged by physicians in that area. To determine usual and customary fees, it is necessary to compare not only the services but also the specialties of the physicians providing the services. The term *usual and customary fees* commonly appears in the language of insurance contracts because this is the fee that third party payers are willing to reimburse for services. For example, a physician may decide to charge $100 for an office visit, but the insurer will reimburse only $80, if $80 is the usual and customary fee for that specialty in that area.

## DISCOUNTED FEE FOR SERVICE

Within this category of reimbursement are other negotiated fees. In a typical **discounted fee for service** arrangement, the third party payer (in this case, the insurer) negotiates a payment that is less than the provider's normal rate. For example, the provider may charge $100 for a service. The insurer assumes that the volume of patients added to the provider's business would warrant a 10% discount from the normal rate. Therefore the payment for the service would be $90.

Some insurers reimburse at flat rates, known as per diem (daily) rates, for service. A per diem rate is basically a flat fee, negotiated in advance, that an insurer will pay for each day of hospitalization. For inpatient health care providers or facilities, per diem rates may represent a significant discount from the actual accumulated fees for each service performed, but again, the provider or facility benefits by gaining that payer's business. Per diem rates are most commonly negotiated with providers who serve a limited patient population, such as providers of rehabilitation services.

**discounted fee for service** The exchange of cash for professional services rendered, at a rate less than the normal fee for the service.

## PROSPECTIVE PAYMENT

**Prospective payment** is a method of determining the payment to a health care provider on the basis of predetermined factors, not on individual costs for services. Numerous insurers and government agencies use prospective payment systems for reimbursement, most notably the Medicare Prospective Payment System (PPS), which is discussed in detail later in this chapter. PPSs are based on the statistical analysis of large quantities of historical health care data for the purpose of evaluating the resources used to treat specific diagnoses and effect certain treatments. On the basis of this evaluation, it has been determined that certain diagnoses and procedures consume sufficiently similar resources, such that reimbursement to the facility for all patients with such diagnoses and undergoing such procedures should be the same. For this purpose, resources are measured in both costs and days. Essentially, the provider receives a payment that represents the historical average cost of treating patients with that particular combination of diagnoses and procedures.

For example, suppose a review of 10,000 uncomplicated appendectomies reveals that the patients were hospitalized for an average of 2 days. The statistical average charge for these hospitalizations, based on the 10,000 uncomplicated appendectomy cases, is $5000. An insurer who uses a prospective payment system to reimburse a facility will pay that facility $5000, regardless of how long a given patient who received an uncomplicated appendectomy was actually hospitalized or what the actual charges were. If the charges for that hospitalization were actually $4500, the facility would still receive $5000. If the charges for that hospitalization were actually $5500, the facility would still receive $5000. The use of the term "prospective" in this type of reimbursement system means that both the facility and the insurer know, in advance, how much each type of case will be reimbursed.

From the payer's perspective, prospective payment can be an extremely effective budgeting tool. Utilization trends can be followed, types of cases can be analyzed in groups, and reimbursement costs can be better controlled through rate setting for each type of case. From the perspective of the provider or facility, there is greater motivation to keep costs under tight control. If there are inefficiencies within the facilities or among physicians, facilities may lose income. However, critics of PPSs, including some physicians, maintain that prospective payment focuses only on the financial aspects of treating a patient and does not take into consideration individual, case-by-case clinical management.

**prospective payment** Any of several reimbursement methods that pay an amount predetermined by the payer on the basis of the diagnosis, procedures, and other factors (depending on setting) rather than actual, current resources expended by the provider.

**diagnosis** The name of the patient's condition or illness, or the reason for the health care encounter.

**procedure** A process that describes how to comply with a policy. Also, a medical or surgical treatment. Also refers to the processing steps in an administrative function.

## CAPITATION

Another type of payment is capitation. **Capitation** requires payment to a health care provider regardless of whether the patient is seen or how frequently the patient is seen during

**capitation** A uniform reimbursement to a health care provider based on the number of patients contractually in the physician's care, regardless of diagnoses or services rendered.

**primary care physician (PCP)**
The physician who has been designated by the insured to deliver routine care to the insured and to evaluate the need for referral to a specialist, if applicable.

a given period. For example, a physician might receive $10 a month for each patient under an insurance plan whose patients choose him or her as their primary care physician. If 100 patients choose this physician as their primary care physician, the physician receives $1000 a month for those patients—even if no one comes in for a visit. If all 100 patients are seen in one month, the physician still receives $1000. Generally, however, the more patients who choose this physician under a capitation plan, the greater the odds that that physician will receive adequate overall payment for his or her services, especially if that group of patients is relatively healthy and does not make many office visits. The insurer will still benefit if it is less expensive to pay a known monthly capitation fee rather than reimburse an unpredictable amount of money to the physician each month (Figure 7-3).

## COMPARISON OF REIMBURSEMENT METHODS

Table 7-4 summarizes the four methods of reimbursement previously discussed: fee for service, discounted fee for service, prospective payment, and capitation. To distinguish among these methods, remember the previous example of the patient's visit to the doctor's office for an allergy shot. Say the charge for that visit, under fee-for-service reimbursement, is $100. Under discounted fee-for-service reimbursement, a contract may be negotiated for payment based on a discount of 10% of the fee for service; therefore the charge for the same visit would still be $100, but the reimbursement would be $90. The $10 difference is a contractual allowance, enabling the provider to keep track of the discount for accounting purposes. Under a PPS, the insurance company may reimburse the physician $85 on the

---

**TABLE 7-4**

**COMPARISON OF REIMBURSEMENT METHODS**

| METHOD* | DESCRIPTION |
|---|---|
| Fee for service | Payment for services rendered |
| Discounted fee for service | Payment for services rendered but at a rate lower than the usual fee for a service |
| Prospective payment | Payment of a flat rate on the basis of diagnoses, procedures, or a combination of the two |
| Capitation | Payment of a regular, flat rate to the provider regardless of whether services are rendered |

*There are numerous variations on these methods, and exceptions to a normal method of payment are made under certain circumstances. For example, under prospective payment, additional compensation can sometimes be obtained if it is medically necessary for the patient to be hospitalized far in excess of the average length of stay for the diagnosis or procedure.

---

There are 20 patients in the physician's panel
No one received treatment in June

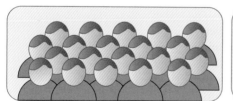

The payer pays $10 for each patient this month.

Physician receives $200 with no expenses

In July, 2 of the 20 patients receive treatment

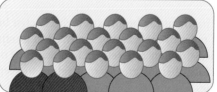

The payer pays $10 for each patient in July, regardless of whether they came in for a visit.

If each visit costs $12, the physician receives $176 in July

$10 × 20 patients   =   $200
$12 × 2 patients seen = −$ 24
                        $176 net profit

All 20 patients come in for treatment

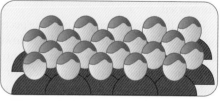

The rate does not change in August. The payer pays a total of $200 for the panel.

Because the physician's expenses outweigh his payment for August, the physician loses $40 this month

$10 × 20 patients        =   $200
− $12 × 20 patients seen = − $240
                           $40 net loss

**Figure 7-3** Capitation scenarios with a pool of 20 patients.

basis of a statistical analysis of costs associated with office visits for allergy shots. Under capitation reimbursement, the insurance company would not pay the physician anything for a particular visit, paying instead $10 each month for that patient. The total reimbursement for that patient under capitation amounts to $120 annually: a financial advantage to the provider if the patient visits once or not at all, but a disadvantage if the patient visits more than once.

These methods vary widely, and exceptions to a normal method of payment are made under certain circumstances. For example, under PPS, additional reimbursement can sometimes be obtained if it is medically necessary for the patient to be hospitalized far in excess of the average length of stay for the medical service.

## EXERCISE 7-3
### Reimbursement

1. The payer had an agreement with the physician to pay the usual and customary fee less 10%. This is an example of _____.

2. What incentive do physicians have to operate under each of the four methods of reimbursement discussed?

*Use the following scenario to answer Questions 3 and 4:*
   The 82-year-old patient came to the physician's office for a routine physical examination. He gave the receptionist two cards proving his primary, government-funded insurance plan, which pays for most of the bill, and an additional private plan that covers the remaining charges.

3. The patient's primary insurance is most likely _____.
4. The patient's secondary insurance is called _____.
5. The physician charged the patient $75 for the office visit. The patient paid the physician $5, and the patient's insurance company paid the physician $70. This method of reimbursement is called _____.
6. The physician charged the patient $75 for the office visit. The patient paid the physician $5, and the patient's insurance company paid the physician $70. The patient's portion of the payment is called _____.

*Match the definition on the left with the health insurance terminology on the right.*

_____ 1. Amount of cost that the beneficiary must incur before the insurance will assume liability for the remaining cost

_____ 2. Contractor that manages the health care claims

_____ 3. One who is eligible to receive or is receiving benefits from an insurance policy or a managed care program

_____ 4. Party who is financially responsible for reimbursement of health care costs

_____ 5. Payer's payment for specific health care services or, in managed care, the health care services that will be provided or for which the provider will be paid

_____ 6. Payment by a third party to a provider of health care

_____ 7. Request for payment by the insured or the provider for services covered

A. Beneficiary
B. Benefit
C. Claim
D. Deductible
E. Fiscal intermediary
F. Payer
G. Reimbursement

## PROSPECTIVE PAYMENT SYSTEMS

Prospective Payment Systems (PPSs), as they apply to inpatient acute care, are based on diagnosis related groups (DRGs). Medicare inpatients under PPS are grouped, and hospitals reimbursed, through the use of the MS-DRG grouper. The MS-DRG grouper is a DRG grouper that incorporates a patient's medical severity (MS) into its assignments and reimbursement calculation. The MS-DRG grouper is one of several DRG **groupers**. For example, the AP-DRG grouper is a grouper used by some payers other than Medicare. "AP" stands for All Payer. In general, DRGs classify, or group, patients by common type according to diagnosis, treatments, and resource intensity. The statistical foundation of DRGs is based on the assumption that the same diagnosis requires the same type of care

○ **Prospective Payment System (PPS)**
   A system used by payers, primarily CMS, for reimbursing acute care facilities on the basis of the statistical analysis of health care data.

**diagnosis related groups (DRGs)**
   A collection of health care descriptions organized into statistically similar categories.

**grouper** The software used to derive the DRG from the ICD-10-CM diagnoses and procedures.

**resource intensity (RI)** A weight of the resources used for the care of an inpatient in an acute care setting that result in a successful discharge.

**DRG** diagnosis related group
**PPS** prospective payment system

**case mix** Statistical distribution of patients according to their utilization of resources. Also refers to the grouping of patients by clinical department or other meaningful distribution, such as health insurance type.
**Medicare** Federally funded health care insurance plan for older adults and for certain categories of chronically ill patients.

for all patients. The term **resource intensity (RI)** generally refers to demands and costs associated with treating specific types of patients: how much it costs to treat a particular disease or condition, depending on what types of resources that type of patient consumes and in some instances factoring in the age and gender of the patient. For example, if a patient is being treated in the hospital for congestive heart failure and nothing else, then that patient will probably consume the same amount of resources, have the same procedures performed, require the same number of consultations, and have the same intensity of nursing care as any other patient coming into the hospital with the same diagnosis, barring complications. Statistically, on the basis of review of hundreds of thousands of records, this assumption proves to be true, allowing for the classification of the patient's stay into a DRG assignment.

Classifying types of patients into DRGs and predicting their expected resource consumption provide the basis for assigning monetary amounts for each MS-DRG in Medicare PPS. For example, even though a normal newborn and a patient scheduled for a cholecystectomy (gallbladder removal) may both stay in the hospital for 3 days, the normal newborn will not consume as much in the way of resources as a patient who required use of the operating room and postoperative care. Both patients, having different diagnoses and treatments, would be assigned to two different MS-DRGs, with the amount reimbursed for the newborn's hospitalization less than the amount reimbursed for the patient who had gallbladder surgery.

## History of Diagnosis Related Groups and Impact on Health Information Management and the Coding Function

Currently, the DRG system is known as a "patient classification scheme, which provides a means of relating the type of patients a hospital treats (i.e., its case mix) to the costs incurred by the hospital" (Diagnosis Related Groups Definitions Manual, 1989). It also serves as a basis for hospital reimbursement by Medicare and certain other payers. However, DRG classifications were originally developed by Yale University in the 1960s as a tool to ensure quality of care and appropriate utilization. DRG classifications were separate from reimbursement until the late 1970s, when the New Jersey Department of Health mandated use of the system for reimbursement. In New Jersey, DRG-based methodology reimbursement applied to all patients and all payer classifications; DRG reimbursement classifications were adopted with the goal of containing overall inpatient health care costs, which were rapidly increasing. Because the DRG classification system in New Jersey applied to all inpatients and payers, even self-pay patients, it has been referred to as an "all payer" prospective payment system. (This is a historical reference, as the New Jersey systems have since changed.)

---

### HIT-bit

#### CASE MIX GROUPS

It should be noted that there are many grouper systems in use in the United States and, in fact, the world. In 1983, the Canadian Institute for Health Information developed case mix groups.

The prospective payment system does not apply to Canadian hospitals. Instead, hospitals in Canada operate under a global budget. Each hospital receives a sum of money according to its size and the types of services it provides. A large hospital that performs organ transplants, for example, would receive a higher monetary global budget than a small community hospital would.

---

Later in this chapter, you will read in greater detail how patients are classified in groups according to the DRG classification system, with coding being the main critical element. Without assigned codes for each patient, there cannot be a DRG assignment. Without a DRG assigned, a hospital cannot receive reimbursement. When the coding function became linked to reimbursement, coders and HIM personnel (e.g., medical records staff) made enormous gains in importance and stature. There was a saying at the time that medical records professionals came "out of the basement and into the board room." For the first time ever, a national health care publication featured a medical records director on its cover, when it published a feature article about DRGs. With the advent of the DRG system, HIM professionals basked in the national health care spotlight and embraced their new leadership roles and responsibilities.

Again, the coding function had comparatively fewer pressures before the implementation of prospective payment systems and DRGs. Coders were focused on assigning codes for statistical purposes, such as analysis of resource utilization in the facility. The accuracy of codes, although important, was not so closely scrutinized, and coders were under less pressure to perform their tasks in a timely manner. Most hospital administrators would try to complete the previous month's cases no later than 2 weeks into the following month. Coding was considered just another function in a medical records department, perhaps on par with the analysis function. Coders were trained primarily by their employers, and some were credentialed as either registered record administrators (RRAs) or accredited record technicians (ARTs), which were the only two credentials offered at the time. People earning either credential did not specialize in coding but rather took one or two courses in coding. Today, coding has become a highly specialized and desirable profession in itself, with several credentials offered solely for coding by different organizations.

With the evolution of coding and the coding profession, tremendous changes occurred in hospital computer systems. In the late 1970s, most medical records departments did not have computers or even access to their hospital computers. In some instances, DRG grouping was actually done by using a large paper manual that outlined the DRG grouper program. In most cases, however, coders dialed into a system off-site, entered codes and other data elements for each patient, and received a DRG assignment over the telephone connection. This was not even an Internet connection but rather a telephone modem connection to an off-site computer, originally the one at Yale University, where DRGs were developed. One advantage (possibly the only one) in grouping cases this way was that the coder truly understood the software program and could therefore provide feedback and suggestions. Because today all grouping is computerized, coders may not be as familiar with all of the nuances and elements of grouping. On the other hand, computerized grouping is certainly far more accurate than grouping with a paper manual. In any event, coders not only began to take greater responsibility for timely and accurate coding because of the DRG system but also learned more about information technology and health information. Eventually, computerization and the data collection activities required to support coding, DRG assignment, and reimbursement moved facilities closer to what will eventually become an electronic health record (EHR).

Overall, the impact of DRGs and the prospective payment system on health care was enormous. In addition to New Jersey, a number of states soon adopted prospective payment systems, or "all payer" systems, requiring all payers, including Medicare, to use DRGs as a reimbursement methodology for hospital inpatients. Because the prospective payment system was a completely new reimbursement model, its adoption had a dramatic financial impact on facilities during the initial years. Patients were also affected because lengths of stay were gradually decreased. Before the adoption of prospective payment systems, there were no financial incentives to reduce a patient's length of stay. For example, it was once common for a new mother and baby to stay in the hospital for a week; today it would be unusual for a healthy mother and baby to stay more than 2 or 3 days.

## Diagnosis Related Group Assignment

DRGs, including MS-DRGs, were initially developed with some basic characteristics in mind (Figure 7-4). Put in simple terms, modern DRG grouping software gathers certain demographic and clinical data from the patient abstract and uses those data to assign a three-digit code. It uses the patient's gender, diagnosis code(s), procedure codes(s), any hospital-acquired conditions, and discharge status to determine the appropriate group. Prior to the implementation of ICD-10-CM and PCS, MS-DRGs were derived from

**analysis** The review of a record to evaluate its completeness, accuracy, or compliance with predetermined standards or other criteria.

**DRG** diagnosis related group

**electronic health record (EHR)** A secure real-time, point-of-care, patient centric information resource for clinicians allowing access to patient information when and where needed and incorporating evidence-based decision support.

**prospective payment system (PPS)** A system used by payers, primarily CMS, for reimbursing acute care facilities on the basis of statistical analysis of health care data.

**inpatient** An individual who is admitted to a hospital with the intention of staying overnight.

**demographic data** Data elements that distinguish one patient from another, such as name, address, and birth date.

**clinical data** All of the medical data that have been recorded about the patient's stay or visit, including diagnoses and procedures.

**abstract** A summary of the patient record.

**ICD-10-CM** code set mandated by HIPAA for reporting diagnoses and reasons for healthcare encounters in all settings.

**ICD-10-PCS** classification system used in the U.S. for reporting procedures used in inpatient settings.

| Characteristics | Explanation |
|---|---|
| "The patient characteristics used in the definition of the DRGs should be limited to information routinely collected on hospital abstract systems." | This information consists of the patient's principal diagnosis code, secondary diagnosis code or diagnoses codes, procedure code or codes, the patient's age, sex, and discharge status. In some DRG groupers, a newborn's birth weight must also be included. |
| "There should be a manageable number of DRGs which encompass all patients seen on an inpatient basis." | The point of this is so that meaningful comparative analyses of DRGs can be performed and patterns detected in case mix and costs. |
| "Each DRG should contain patients with a similar pattern of resource intensity." | Clinical coherence means that patients in a particular DRG share a common organ system or condition and/or procedures, and that typically a specific medical or surgical specialty would provide services to that patient. For example, one would expect a psychiatrist to treat all patients in DRGs created for mental diseases and disorders. |
| "Each DRG should contain patients who are similar from a clinical perspective (i.e., each class should be clinically coherent)." | This is so that a hospital can establish a relationship between their case mix and resource consumption. |

**Figure 7-4** Characteristics of DRGs. (From All patient refined diagnosis related groups [APR-DRGs], methodology overview, version 20.0. Wallingford, CT, 2003, 3M Health Information Systems.)

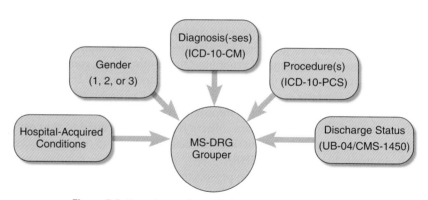

**Figure 7-5** Data inputs for an MS-DRG grouping program.

**Uniform Hospital Discharge Data Set (UHDDS)** The mandated data set for hospital inpatients.
**Uniform Bill (UB-04)** The standardized form used by hospitals for inpatient and outpatient billing to CMS and other third party payers.

**CMS** Centers for Medicare and Medicaid Services

ICD-9-CM diagnosis (Volumes I and II) and procedure (Volume III) codes. Effective October 1, 2014, the MS-DRGs are based on ICD-10-CM and ICD-CM-PCS codes. The patient's gender is entered with a valid range of 1 to 3, in which 1 is male, 2 is female, and 3 is unknown. Discharge status is coded with use of Uniform Hospital Discharge Data Set (UHDDS) standards, as defined for the UB-04 by the The National Uniform Billing Committee (NUBC). Figure 7-5 illustrates the data elements of MS-DRG grouping.

DRG assignment can proceed once all of the necessary information is abstracted into the hospital's information system. Grouper software is used to assign each DRG. 3M Health Information Systems is the Grouper Contractor for CMS. Medicare patients under the Inpatient Prospective Payment System (IPPS) are grouped into MS-DRGs. Patients that self-pay or have other insurance may be grouped into a different DRG, such as the AP-DRG. Except for Medicare IPPS patients, the use of other DRG groupers may vary from state to state. Table 7-5 compares various DRG grouping systems.

## TABLE 7-5

### COMPARISON OF DIAGNOSIS RELATED GROUP GROUPERS FOR A SPECIFIC DIAGNOSIS, HEART FAILURE AND SHOCK, IN A 60-YEAR-OLD WOMAN

**First Grouper**

| | |
|---|---|
| Principal Diagnosis | Combined systolic and diastolic heart failure, acute on chronic |
| Secondary Diagnoses | Pneumonia, not otherwise specified |
| | Obstructive chronic bronchitis with acute exacerbation |

| | | |
|---|---|---|
| MS-DRG | 291 | HEART FAILURE & SHOCK W MCC |
| AP-DRG | 544 | CHF & CARDIAC ARRHYTHMIA W MAJOR CC |
| APR-DRG | 194 | HEART FAILURE |
| | | 2 Moderate Severity of Illness |
| | | 1 Minor Risk of Mortality |

**Second Grouper**

| | |
|---|---|
| Principal Diagnosis | Combined systolic and diastolic heart failure, acute on chronic |
| Secondary Diagnosis | Obstructive chronic bronchitis with acute exacerbation |

| | | |
|---|---|---|
| MS-DRG | 292 | HEART FAILURE & SHOCK W CC |
| AP-DRG | 127 | HEART FAILURE AND SHOCK |
| APR-DRG | 194 | HEART FAILURE |
| | | 2 Moderate Severity of Illness |
| | | 1 Minor Risk of Mortality |

**Third Grouper**

| | |
|---|---|
| Principal Diagnosis | Combined systolic and diastolic heart failure, acute on chronic |
| Secondary Diagnosis | No secondary diagnosis |

| | | |
|---|---|---|
| MS-DRG | 293 | HEART FAILURE & SHOCK W/O CC/MCC |
| AP-DRG | 127 | HEART FAILURE AND SHOCK |
| APR-DRG | 194 | HEART FAILURE |
| | | 1 Minor Severity of Illness |
| | | 1 Minor Risk of Mortality |

CC, comorbidity or complication; CHF, congestive heart failure; DRG, diagnosis related group; MCC, major comorbidity or complication; w/o, without.

## Grouping

The MS-DRG grouper software follows a process that resembles a flowchart, much like any flowchart created to track a process or procedure. This particular flowchart is referred to as a *decision tree diagram*. DRG grouper programs vary depending on the DRG system in use, but some generalizations may be made about the basic formats.

The process begins with examination of the **principal diagnosis** code. The principal diagnosis is defined in the UHDDS as the reason, after study, that the patient was admitted to the hospital. Codes must be currently valid and accepted as a principal diagnosis code by the **Medicare Code Editor (MCE)**. The MCE is essentially a list of codes that would not make sense if used as a principal diagnosis in an acute care facility. For example, many "Z codes" are on this list, such as ICD-10-CM code Z85.3, "history of breast cancer." The codes must also, when applicable, align with the sex of the patient. For example, a patient who is abstracted as male cannot then be assigned pregnancy codes.

If you examine an ICD-10-CM code book, you will see that the codes are divided into chapters or sections, primarily according to body system. In similar fashion, once the principal diagnosis code is accepted, the grouping process begins by assigning patients into basic sections, also primarily by body system, called **major diagnostic categories (MDCs)**. Whereas hundreds of DRGs exist, there are 25 MDCs in the Medicare MS-DRG grouper that resemble the chapters in ICD-10-CM, although not necessarily in the same order.

The MDCs are listed in Table 7-6. The complete list as well as the appendices can be seen on the CMS Web site: http://www.cms.gov/icd10manual/fullcode_cms/p0001.html.

**principal diagnosis** According to the UHDDS, the condition that, after study, is determined to be chiefly responsible for occasioning the admission of the patient to the hospital for care.

**Medicare Code Editor (MCE)** A part of grouping software that checks for valid codes in claims data.

**acute care facility** A health care facility in which patients have an average length of stay less than 30 days and that has an emergency department, operating suite, and clinical departments to handle a broad range of diagnoses and treatments.

**UHDDS** Uniform Hospital Discharge Data Set

**major diagnostic categories (MDCs)** Segments of the DRG assignment flowchart (grouper).

**DRG** diagnosis related group

## TABLE 7-6

### MAJOR DIAGNOSTIC CATEGORIES FOR MS-DRGs

| MDC NUMBER | DESCRIPTION |
| --- | --- |
| 1 | Diseases & Disorders of the Nervous System |
| 2 | Diseases & Disorders of the Eye |
| 3 | Diseases & Disorders of the Ear Nose Mouth & Throat |
| 4 | Diseases & Disorders of the Respiratory System |
| 5 | Diseases & Disorders of the Circulatory System |
| 6 | Diseases & Disorders of the Digestive System |
| 7 | Diseases & Disorders of the Hepatobiliary System & Pancreas |
| 8 | Diseases & Disorders of the Musculoskeletal System & Conn Tissue |
| 9 | Diseases & Disorders of the Skin Subcutaneous Tissue & Breast |
| 10 | Endocrine Nutritional & Metabolic Diseases & Disorders |
| 11 | Diseases & Disorders of the Kidney & Urinary Tract |
| 12 | Diseases & Disorders of the Male Reproductive System |
| 13 | Diseases & Disorders of the Female Reproductive System |
| 14 | Pregnancy Childbirth & the Puerperium |
| 15 | Newborns & Other Neonates with Condtn Orig in Perinatal Period |
| 16 | Diseases & Disorders of Blood Blood Forming Organs Immunolog Disord |
| 17 | Myeloproliferative Diseases & Disorders Poorly Differentiated Neoplasm |
| 18 | Infectious & Parasitic Diseases Systemic or Unspecified Sites |
| 19 | Mental Diseases & Disorders |
| 20 | Alcohol/Drug Use & Alcohol/Drug Induced Organic Mental Disorders |
| 21 | Injuries Poisonings & Toxic Effects of Drugs |
| 22 | Burns |
| 23 | Factors Influencing Hlth Stat & Other Contacts with Hlth Servcs |
| 24 | Multiple Significant Trauma |
| 25 | Human Immunodeficiency Virus Infections |

From Centers for Medicare and Medicaid Services: MDC Description File. https://www.cms.gov/AcuteInpatientPPS/FFD/itemdetail.asp?filterType=none&filterByDID=-99&sortByDID=2&sortOrder=ascending&itemID=CMS1247844&intNumPerPage=10. Published 2008. Accessed September 10, 2011.

Once the patient is assigned to an MDC, the grouper examines any procedure codes. Not all procedure codes are used for MS-DRG assignment. For example, codes for ultrasound examinations are diagnostic radiology and are essentially ignored during the grouping process. Procedure codes that are recognized and used for grouping are categorized as either OR (operating room) or Non-OR. An OR procedure code indicates that the patient has undergone a procedure requiring the use of an operating room: for example, a gastric bypass or open fracture reduction. Non-OR procedures include procedures or treatments such as paracentesis or nonexcisional débridements. Figure 7-6 shows an example of an MDC decision tree.

Most MDCs have two main sections, one for medical patients and one for surgical patients. The two sections are referred to as medical partitioning and surgical partitioning. Once a case is assigned to an MDC, the case is sorted or assigned to one of these main sections. Note that in Figure 7-6, the first question is whether the patient had an operation (OR procedure). If the answer is yes, then the correct MS-DRG is found in the surgical partitioning. If the answer is no, then the decision tree sends the user to the medical partitioning.

For cases sorted into the medical partition, the grouper looks for, depending on the MDC, the patient's age. The MCE detects instances in which a patient's age does not correspond with the principal or secondary coded diagnoses. For example, an 80-year-old woman with pregnancy codes would not pass the edit and would not be grouped until a correction was made in abstracting.

Next, depending on the MDC, the grouper will search the secondary diagnosis codes for a comorbidity or complication (CC) and major comorbidity or complication (MCC). The list of CCs and MCCs can be seen on the CMS Web site listed previously, in Appendix G, Diagnoses Defined as Complications or Comorbidities, and Appendix H, Diagnoses

**MDC** major diagnostic category
**CMS** Centers for Medicare and Medicaid Services

**MCE** Medicare Code Editor

**abstracting** The recap of selected fields from a health record to create an informative summary. Also refers to the activity of identifying such fields and entering them into a computer system.

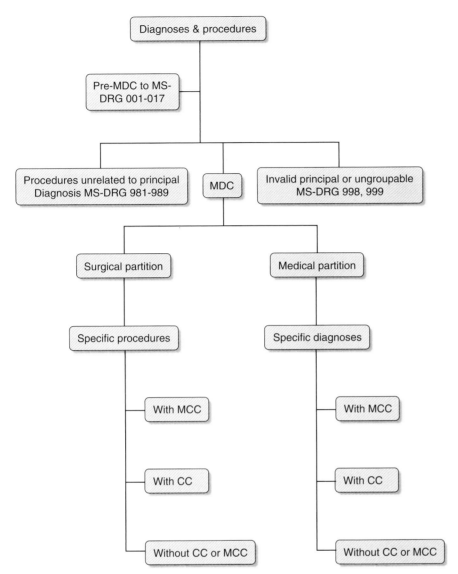

**Figure 7-6** Overview of MS-DRG assignment logic. Adapted from Centers for Medicare and Medicaid Services: Acute Inpatient Prospective Payment System Fiscal Year 2013 Final Rule, Table 5. http://www.cms.gov/Medicare/Medicare-Fee-for-Service-Payment/AcuteInpatientPPS/FY-2013-IPPS-Final-Rule-Home-Page-Items/FY2013-Final-Rule-Tables.html. Published 2012.

Defined as Major Complications or Comorbidities. Major comorbidity or complication (MCC) codes are complications or comorbidities of greater severity than CC codes. MCC codes, when applied in the MS-DRG calculation, "adjust" the DRG assignment and reimbursement to account for this greater severity.

A **comorbidity** is a condition that was present upon admission, whereas a **complication** is a condition that arose during the hospitalization. If a secondary diagnosis code, when matched with a certain principal diagnosis code, is statistically proved to extend a patient's length of stay by at least 1 day in 75% of cases, that secondary diagnosis is considered a CC in combination with that principal diagnosis. For example, suppose a patient has a principal diagnosis of pneumonia (J18.9) and also has hyponatremia (E87.1). It has been statistically demonstrated that 75% of patients with pneumonia and a secondary diagnosis of hyponatremia must remain in the hospital at least 1 day longer than patients with pneumonia alone. Therefore E87.1 is considered an applicable CC code when J18.9 is the principal diagnosis code.

The list of CC and MCC codes are reviewed and revised each year by CMS and published in the *Federal Register* and on the CMS Web site previously listed, usually at the same time as any DRG revisions.

**CC** comorbidity or complication
**MCC** major comorbidity or complication

**comorbidity** A condition that affects the patient's care and/or length of stay and exists at the same time as the principal diagnosis.
**complication** A condition that arises during hospitalization, or as a result of the health care encounter.
**principal diagnosis** According to the UHDDS, the condition that, after study, is determined to be chiefly responsible for occasioning the admission of the patient to the hospital for care.
*Federal Register* The publication of the proceedings of the United States Congress.

Not all CC codes appearing in the CC or MCC list apply in all instances. Certain CC codes are not considered CCs with certain principal diagnoses codes because the secondary diagnosis code is a condition that has been determined to not significantly affect length of stay or treatment. A list of all CC codes and MCC codes can be seen in Appendix C (of the *Federal Register* publication), Complications or Comorbidities Exclusion List. Each CC or MCC code listed is followed by a code or codes that, when assigned as principal diagnoses, exclude that CC or MCC from affecting MS-DRG assignment. For example, I09.81, rheumatic heart failure, is a CC. If I09.81 is assigned as a secondary diagnosis code with a principal diagnosis of I50.1 Left Ventricular failure, it will not "count" as a CC because I09.81 is on the CC exclusion list for code I50.1.

CC and MCC codes are important to MS-DRG assignment because the presence of a CC or MCC code can determine the final MS-DRG assigned. The final stage in the MDC tree diagram is frequently a choice between an MS-DRG with a CC and an MS-DRG without a CC, or a MS-DRG with an MCC or without an MCC. For example, MS-DRG 290 is "Acute and subacute endocarditis w/o (without) CC/MCC," MS-DRG 289 is "Acute and subacute endocarditis w (with) CC," and MS-DRG 288 is "Acute and subacute endocarditis with MCC." The MS-DRG with the CC is reimbursed at a higher rate than the MS-DRG without the CC. The MS-DRG with the MCC is reimbursed at a higher rate than the MS-DRG with the CC. Multiple CC or MCC codes do not have any impact because only one CC or MCC code is needed for the case to be assigned to the MS-DRG with the higher rate of reimbursement.

Cases assigned to the surgical partitioning section of an MDC essentially follow the same format for MS-DRG assignment as those in the medical partitioning section but must account for instances in which more than one procedure performed (from the OR or Non-OR List) on the same patient during the same admission. Only one MS-DRG is assigned for each admission, even if multiple procedures are performed. In these cases, the grouper reviews all of the procedure codes assigned and identifies the single procedure that required the most resource intensity. Each surgical partition is sequenced according to a surgical hierarchy. When multiple procedures have been performed, the procedure code that is highest in the surgical hierarchy is selected by the grouper for MS-DRG assignment. On the MDC tree diagram, the surgical hierarchy lists procedures in descending order, with the procedure requiring the greatest resource intensity at the top. For example, assume that a patient in MDC 8 ("Diseases and disorders of the musculoskeletal system and connective tissue") undergoes a total hip replacement. This case would group to MS-DRG 470, "Major joint replacement or reattachment of lower extremity w/o MCC." In another case, a patient undergoes a shoulder arthroscopy. That case would group to MS-DRG 512, "Shoulder, forearm or shoulder procedure excluding major joint procedure w/o/ CC/MCC." Now, suppose that a patient who was admitted for and underwent total hip replacement later complained of severe shoulder pain and was returned to the OR during the same admission for a shoulder arthroscopy. The MS-DRG for this admission would be MS-DRG 470, because a total hip replacement is higher on the surgical hierarchy than a shoulder arthroscopy. The arthroscopy has no influence on MS-DRG assignment in this case because it is superseded by the total hip replacement in resource intensity. When abstracting a case, even if the arthroscopy was listed first as **principal procedure**, the grouper would still select the total hip replacement for MS-DRG assignment. This is a major difference from cases in the medical partition, in which the principal diagnosis selected by the coder is used for MS-DRG assignment.

Exceptions to the program format described in the preceding paragraphs include organ transplantation cases and patients who have had a tracheostomy and a certain diagnosis. These cases are not assigned to an MDC first but rather directly assigned to each respective MS-DRG. Examples of these MS-DRGs include MS-DRG 002, "Heart transplant or implant of heart assist system," and DRG 013, "Tracheostomy for face, mouth, and neck diagnosis." As of fiscal year (FY) 2011, there were 11 DRGs grouped into these "Pre-MDCs."

There are other exceptions in which a case is grouped directly to a MS-DRG without first being assigned to an MDC. Unusual, unpredictable, or unique circumstances occasionally occur during hospitalization, making such cases exceptions to the usual rules of MS-DRG assignment. These exceptions are categorized into the following MS-DRGs:

**CC** comorbidity or complication
**MCC** major comorbidity or complication

**MDC** major diagnostic category

**resource intensity** A weight of the resources used for the care of an inpatient in an acute care setting that result in a successful discharge.
**abstracting** The recap of selected fields from a health record to create an informative summary. Also refers to the activity of identifying such fields and entering them into a computer system.
**principal procedure** According to the UHDDS, the procedure that was performed for definitive treatment, rather than one performed for diagnostic or exploratory purposes or necessary to take care of a complication. If two procedures appear to meet this definition, then the one most related to the principal diagnosis should be selected as the principal procedure.
**grouper** The software used to derive the DRG from the ICD-10-CM diagnoses and procedures.

**major diagnostic categories (MDCs)** Segments of the DRG assignment flowchart (grouper).

*DRG 981, "Extensive OR procedure unrelated to principal diagnosis w MCC," DRG 982, "Extensive OR procedure unrelated to principal diagnosis w CC," and DRG 983, "Extensive OR procedure unrelated to principal diagnosis w/o CC/MCC":* An example would be a patient admitted for a myocardial infarction. During her hospitalization, a breast lump is noticed, the patient is found to have breast cancer, and a mastectomy is performed. The myocardial infarction as principal diagnosis is not associated with or related to the mastectomy, so the case is grouped to DRG 983.

*DRG 998, "Principal diagnosis invalid as discharge diagnosis":* A code, such as Z93.8, "Colostomy status," was submitted as principal diagnosis for an inpatient admission.

*DRG 984, "Prostatic OR procedure unrelated to principal diagnosis w MCC," DRG 985, "Prostatic OR procedure unrelated to principal diagnosis w CC," and DRG 986, "Prostatic OR procedure unrelated to principal diagnosis w/o CC/MCC":* An example would be a patient who was admitted for exacerbation of chronic obstructive pulmonary disease and underwent a transurethral prostatectomy. This case would group to DRG 986.

*DRG 987, "Non-extensive OR procedure unrelated to principal diagnosis w MCC," DRG 988, "Non-extensive OR procedure unrelated to principal diagnosis w CC," and DRG 989, "Non-extensive OR procedure unrelated to principal diagnosis w/o CC/MCC":* These DRGs are similar to DRGs 981 to 983, except that the procedure is, as it states, non-extensive. An example would be if the previously mentioned patient with a myocardial infarction had a breast biopsy instead of a mastectomy. The myocardial infarction as principal diagnosis is not associated with or related to the breast biopsy, and the breast biopsy is a non-extensive procedure, unlike the mastectomy, so the case is grouped to DRG 989.

A complete list of DRGs and related information is published yearly, in late summer, as a Final Rule in the *Federal Register* on the CMS Web site in conjunction with ICD-10-CM/PCS updates, effective each October 1.

Understanding how DRGs are assigned helps coders to properly sequence their code assignments and focus on the correct principal diagnosis. Box 7-1 summarizes the steps in DRG assignment.

### Diagnosis Related Group (MS-DRG) Reimbursement Calculation

Medicare reimbursements for MS-DRGs are based on two components: the national numerical value or **relative weight (RW)** of each MS-DRG and each hospital's **Prospective Payment System (PPS) blended rate.** The blended rate consists of the hospital-specific rate, which is based on historical financial data provided annually to CMS by the hospital, and additional factors such as regional labor costs and graduate medical education. The blended rate is expressed in a dollar amount specific to each hospital. All hospitals are reimbursed on the basis of the same national RW for each MS-DRG multiplied by the

**relative weight (RW)** A number assigned yearly by CMS that is applied to each DRG and used to calculate reimbursement. This number represents the comparative difference in the use of resources by patients in each DRG.

**Prospective Payment System (PPS) blended rate** A weighted component of MS-DRG assignment that consists of the hospital-specific rate and additional factors such as regional labor costs and graduate medical education.

---

**BOX 7-1   ASSIGNMENT OF THE DRG**

Most cases in various grouper programs follow the following format:

- Search for clinical procedures: transplants, ventilators, and tracheotomies, and group immediately to the appropriate DRG, if detected.
- The principal diagnosis code assigns a case to MDC.
- The grouper reviews all diagnoses and procedure codes and then assigns the case to either the medical or surgical portion of the MDC.
- The grouper, using the Medicare code edits, makes sure that the principal diagnosis code is appropriate for an inpatient admission.
- The grouper, using the Medicare code edits, makes sure that the patient's age and sex are appropriate for the diagnoses and procedures assigned.
- The grouper may further process the case according to the patient's age.
- The grouper reviews all secondary diagnoses codes for the presence of a comorbidity or complication.
- If the case is surgical the grouper reviews all procedure code assigned and bases the DRG selection on the procedure code highest in the surgical hierarchy.

DRG, diagnosis related group; MDC, major diagnostic category.

**outlier payment** An unusually high payment within a given case mix group.

**RW** relative weight

**principal diagnosis** According to the UHDDS, the condition which, after study, is determined to be chiefly responsible for occasioning the admission of the patient to the hospital for care.

**case mix index (CMI)** The arithmetic average (mean) of the relative DRG weights of all health care cases in a given period.

**provider number** The number assigned to a participating facility by Medicare for identification purposes.

individual hospital's blended rate. For example, suppose MS-DRG 999 (fictional) has a national RW of 3.0000. Hospital A has a blended rate of $5000, and hospital B has a blended rate of $4500. Hospital A will receive $15,000 for each case in MS-DRG 999 (3.0000 × $5000). Hospital B will receive $13,500 for each case in MS-DRG 999 (3.0000 × $4500).

There are variations to this basic calculation for cases incurring extraordinarily high costs. These cases may qualify for **outlier payment**. "To qualify for outlier payments, a case must have costs above a fixed-loss cost threshold amount (a dollar amount by which the costs of the case must exceed payments in order to qualify for outliers)" (Centers for Medicare and Medicaid Services, 2005). Several calculations to determine outlier payments depend on the hospital's specific operating and capital cost factors.

The fact that each MS-DRG has its own RW used to calculate reimbursement makes the importance of correctly assigning codes for each case to group into the correct DRG apparent. For example, suppose that you are a coder at Hospital A. Your fictional MS-DRG 924 has an RW of 3.0000. MS-DRG 924 happens to be a pair MS-DRG (i.e., there is another similar MS-DRG, MS-DRG 925, that resembles MS-DRG 924 except MS-DRG 925 denotes that a CC code is present). Suppose MS-DRG 925 has an RW of 4.0000. If you do not correctly code and do not include the CC code for MS-DRG assignment, the case would group to MS-DRG 924. If the CC code were included, the case would group to MS-DRG 925. In this example, the absence or presence of the CC code would have the following effect on reimbursement with Hospital A's blended rate of $5000:

MS-DRG 925 "With CC" RW: 4.0000 × $5000 = $20,000 reimbursement
MS-DRG 924 "Without CC" RW: 3.0000 × $5000 = $15,000 reimbursement

Consider how the MS-DRG grouper assigns cases to a MS-DRG and the great importance of assigning the correct principal diagnosis. If the incorrect principal diagnosis is assigned, it is highly likely that the MS-DRG will also be incorrect. The resultant incorrect MS-DRG assignment may be reimbursed at either a higher or lower rate than the correct MS-DRG assignment would have been. In either case, the hospital will not receive the appropriate reimbursement. When such errors in MS-DRG assignment are found, the hospital must rebill or reconcile the reimbursement amount with Medicare and other affected providers. In addition, the hospital's statistics will be negatively affected if cases are not correctly assigned. One important statistic is the hospital's *case mix index (CMI)*.

### Case Mix Index

A hospital's **case mix index** (**CMI**) is a number derived by adding the RWs of all of the actual MS-DRG cases and then dividing by the total number of cases discharged in a given period.

A hospital uses the CMI to monitor its performance: the higher the number, the greater the reimbursement received. Fluctuations in CMI indicate incorrect coding, changes in patient populations, changes in physician practices and personnel, or other conditions.

For example, Hospital A discharged 54 patients in January. Each of the 54 MS-DRG RWs is added together, with a combined total of 43.9675. To calculate its CMI for January, Hospital A divides 43.9675 by 54; the CMI for January is 0.81421. Hospital A then decides to do a 6-month comparison and calculates its CMI for June. In June, 47 patients were discharged with a combined RW of 41.5482. The CMI for June is calculated by dividing 41.5484 by 47; the CMI for June is 0.88400. Hospital A must decide whether the difference in the CMI from January to June is significant enough to warrant further investigation. In this example, the CMI was higher in June than January, so the hospital received more reimbursement on average per patient in June.

The CMI for all hospitals is published yearly by CMS on its Web site in the Public Use Files. Each hospital has its own unique **provider number** that can be referenced on a chart. The chart notes the total number of Medicare cases discharged in the previous fiscal year (FY) and the CMI for that FY. The federal FY begins October 1 and ends September 30. The chart is useful in that hospitals can use it as a reference to compare their CMIs with those of other hospitals that have a similar number of cases. The provider number must be known in order to identify a specific hospital. For example, an employee at Hospital A checks the chart and goes to the hospital's provider number, 000099. The chart shows that Hospital A had 808 Medicare cases discharged in the previous FY and that Hospital A had a CMI of 1.023784 for that period. Next, the Hospital A employee checks the chart for hospitals that had a similar number of discharges and sees that provider number 000054 had 812 cases and a CMI of 2.371271, significantly higher than that of Hospital A. The employee reviews the chart again and in each instance notes that the CMI for similar providers is higher than the CMI for Hospital A. Hospital A administrators may elect to perform an internal investigation, such as a coding audit.

**CMI** case mix index

### The Coder's Role in Diagnosis Related Group (MS-DRG) Assignment

The coder must be able to properly apply current coding rules and coding conventions to each case. Although this section focuses on the Medicare PPS system, all cases, regardless of payer, should be coded with equal care, even if payment is not affected, if a hospital's statistics are to be accurate and useful. As previously emphasized, complete and accurate coding is necessary to generate data and statistics beyond MS-DRGs and other DRG grouper assignments.

It is unethical and fraudulent to deliberately code a case incorrectly so that it may be placed into a MS-DRG with a higher reimbursement rate. This practice is sometimes referred to as "upcoding," maximizing, or "DRG creep." Some coding software includes prompts that alert the coder that a case would group to a higher-paying MS-DRG if a CC or MCC were added or if a different principal diagnosis were assigned. The coder may wish to review the medical record to search for a CC or MCC or confirm that there is no CC or MCC. Under no circumstances should the coder simply add a CC or MCC without confirming that the CC or MCC is documented in the medical record. Likewise, the principal diagnosis code should not be changed unless an error was made in the original assignment. The coding software prompts are intended to assist the coder in ensuring proper coding and sequencing; this process is sometimes referred to as optimizing. The prompts should never be interpreted as directives to code or sequence a certain way simply to obtain higher reimbursement when no supporting documentation exists.

**maximization** The process of determining the highest possible DRG payment.
**optimization** The process of determining the most accurate DRG payment.

**CC** comorbidity or complication
**MCC** major comorbidity or complication

In all cases, without exception, coding and sequencing must be supported by documentation in the medical record. To code otherwise is considered fraudulent by the federal government under the Civil False Claims Act and may subject the hospital to considerable monetary penalties if a pattern of fraud and abuse is demonstrated.

Under the auspices of the U.S. Department of Health and Human Service's Office of the Inspector General (OIG), the federal government released Compliance Program Guidance for Hospitals, which addresses coding issues. Coders should be familiar with this publication as well as their own hospital's compliance program. The OIG publishes a Work Plan every year that includes coding projects focused on particular MS-DRGs and patterns of MS-DRG assignment.

**Go To** Refer to Chapter 6, Figure 6-1.

Usually, medical records are coded and MS-DRGs are assigned after the patient is discharged. The hospital cannot submit a claim for reimbursement until after the patient is discharged. To minimize the time between discharge and claims submission, some facilities perform coding concurrently—that is, while the patient is still in the hospital. The coder may review the medical record when the patient is admitted and every day or every other day thereafter until discharge. Temporary codes are assigned as well as a temporary MS-DRG. This concurrently assigned MS-DRG is often referred to as a **working MS-DRG**. The coder has the opportunity to question the physician about documentation and potentially facilitate coding and MS-DRG assignment accuracy; these efforts may shorten the time between discharge and claims submission. Coding concurrently does present some disadvantages, however. More coding staff may be needed, and some necessary information, such as pathology reports, may not yet be available. In effect, concurrent coding may be a duplication of effort since the post-discharge coding must still take place.

**discharged** The status of a patient after leaving the care of the facility.
**claim** The application to an insurance company for reimbursement of services rendered.
**working DRG** The concurrent DRG. The DRG that reflects the patient's current diagnosis and procedures while still an inpatient.

One way to obtain both the advantages of concurrent coding and the resolution of physician queries prior to discharge is through a Clinical Documentation Improvement (CDI) program. In a CDI program, improving the quality of the physician documentation is the primary goal. Developing a working MS-DRG is important; however, the entire chart is not coded. A CDI program can be an effective and efficient way to ensure that the documentation accurately reflects the patient's severity of illness as well as the medical decision making involved in directing the care of the patient. This effort can support both case

**CDI** clinical documentation improvement

**severity of illness (SI)** In utilization review, a type of criteria, based on the patient's condition, that is used to screen patients for the appropriate care setting.

management, ensuring the documentation of the medical necessity of the inpatient stay, and postdischarge coding, obtaining the highest degree of specificity in the documentation. CDI specialists are usually nurses who have been trained to code or experienced coders with extensive clinical knowledge.

## Ambulatory Payment Classification

As is true for inpatient services, the costs for outpatient, or ambulatory, services has risen. In addition, many patient care services have shifted from inpatient to outpatient settings, thus increasing the amount of reimbursement from outpatient/ambulatory services. In ambulatory health care, a number of different reimbursement methodologies apply; fee for service and discounted fee for service are most commonly used. A number of insurers are participating in capitation as well.

In the 1990s, the federal government was spending billions of dollars on outpatient services using a cost-based system. In an attempt to cut or at least control the costs of these services and as part of the Balanced Budget Act of 1997, Congress mandated that CMS (at that time the HCFA) develop a PPS for Medicare outpatient services, referred to as the **Outpatient Prospective Payment System (OPPS)**. Just as DRGs are used for reimbursement for Medicare inpatient services under PPS, the OPPS uses **ambulatory payment classifications (APCs)** to reimburse for Medicare outpatient services. Originally, this system was called ambulatory payment groups (APGs), but the HCFA changed the name when it modified APGs in 1998. The OPPS and APCs were implemented for services provided on or after August 1, 2000. The Final Rule for implementation and subsequent updates can be found on the CMS Web site and in the *Federal Register* (Medicare, 2000). APCs are updated annually to include additions, deletions, and modifications. Updates occur each calendar year (CY).

The APC system uses HCPCS/CPT procedure, service, or item codes to group patients. ICD-10-CM codes are used not for grouping but to indicate the medical necessity of the procedure, service, or item provided. For example, if a claim were submitted for reimbursement of an electrocardiogram, there should be a logical corresponding cardiac ICD-10-CM code that indicates the reason that the electrocardiogram was performed. ICD-10-PCS (procedure) codes are not used in OPPS and the APC system, although they are sometimes assigned.

Under the APC classification system, patients are grouped on the basis of clinical similarities and similar costs or resource consumption. There are approximately 2000 APCs, a figure subject to change depending on the yearly modifications. APCs are categorized as follows:

- Significant procedures, therapies, or services
- Medical visits
- Ancillary tests and procedures
- Partial hospitalization
- Drugs and biologicals
- Devices

Consideration of these categories makes it easier to envision how one outpatient visit can result in the assignment of multiple APCs. That more than one APC can be assigned per visit is a major difference between APCs and MS-DRGs, in which only one MS-DRG is assigned per inpatient hospitalization. For example, suppose a man is found unconscious on the sidewalk and brought to the hospital's emergency department by the police. The emergency department physician performs a workup, discovers that the patient is in a diabetic coma, and gives him insulin to bring his glucose level under control. In addition, the emergency physician notes that the patient injured his arm after falling on the sidewalk and orders a radiograph to rule out a fracture. In such a scenario, there will be an APC for the emergency visit, an APC for the administration of the drug insulin, and an APC for the radiograph. Each APC has its own payment. The facility is reimbursed in an amount equal to all three APCs added together or, in some instances, receives a reduced or discounted payment for one of the services. For example, if a patient requires the use of a minor surgery suite for multiple procedures, the patient probably uses fewer resources

---

**outpatient** A patient whose health care services are intended to be delivered within 1 calendar day or, in some cases, a 24-hour period.

**capitation** A uniform reimbursement to a health care provider based on the number of patients contractually in the physician's care, regardless of diagnoses or services rendered.

**CMS** Centers for Medicare and Medicaid Services

**HCFA** Health Care Financing Administration

**Outpatient Prospective Payment System (OPPS)** A Medicare prospective payment system (PPS) used to determine the amount of reimbursement for outpatient services.

**ambulatory payment classifications (APCs)** A prospective payment system for ambulatory care based on medically necessary services.

**Healthcare Common Procedure Coding System (HCPCS)** A coding system, of which CPT-4 is level one, used for drugs, equipment, supplies, and other auxiliary health care services rendered.

**Current Procedural Terminology (CPT)** A nomenclature and coding system developed and maintained by the American Medical Association to facilitate billing for physicians and other services.

**claim** The application to an insurance company for reimbursement.

**APC** ambulatory payment classification

overall than if the procedures were performed separately at different times. Therefore a reduced payment is warranted. By the same logic, if a procedure is terminated or discontinued, the payment is reduced or discounted, depending on whether anesthesia was started.

Final payment for APCs is based on a complex set of edits and payment rules that include, for example, HCPCS/CPT codes, code modifiers, and revenue codes. The coder is usually responsible only for assigning the HCPCS/CPT codes and modifiers, and the other billing elements are the responsibility of other departments where charges have been incurred.

A code **modifier** is a two-digit number added to a HCPCS/CPT code that provides additional information regarding the procedure or service performed. A modifier may be used, for example, to indicate a right, left, or bilateral body part; a specific appendage; extent of anesthesia; limited or reduced services; and other situations or circumstances. A **revenue code** is a three-digit code that denotes the department in which a procedure, service, or supply item was provided. Revenue codes are in the **Chargemaster**, which is discussed later in this chapter. Some modifiers are classified as "pricer modifiers"; others are considered "informational" or "statistical" modifiers.

On the basis of the HCPCS/CPT code or codes, each APC is assigned a payment status indicator (SI) that determines reimbursement under OPPS. For example, SI T indicates "significant procedure, multiple-procedure reduction applies." SI V indicates "clinic or emergency department visit," and SI X indicates "ancillary service." The entire list of APCs and each SI can be found on the CMS Web site along with the RW for each APC, each payment rate, national unadjusted copayment, and minimum unadjusted copayment. CPT/HCPCS codes and APCs are updated each CY; therefore it is important to note any changes because reimbursements may be affected.

## Payment Denials and Claims Rejections

Coding professionals in various settings, from ambulatory hospital settings to physician offices, are frequently involved in responding to payment denials or claims rejections. As noted in this brief overview of APCs, the system undergoes changes yearly and is complicated on several levels, from coding to billing. When claims are submitted through the Medicare Administrative Contractors (MACs), the claims are subjected to a number of edits that include the outpatient code editor (OCE) and National Correct Coding Initiative (NCCI) edits. The OCE and NCCI edits flag coding errors in the claims. Until the errors are corrected, the claim is rejected and reimbursement is denied for that claim.

Avoidance of payment denials or claims rejections is of paramount concern because income is adversely affected. One way to avoid these rejections is to understand the reasons for the rejections. Each MAC uses a **local coverage determination (LCD)** definition to determine if a service is covered for payment. These LCDs are derived from the CMS (Medicare) **national coverage determination (NCD)**. The NCD is a general discussion of the service and what it is useful in determining. The LCD lists the specific diagnosis codes that justify the medical necessity of the service. The LCD is available to providers, usually on the MAC's Web site. The LCD is extremely useful in that the policy defines covered services and details concerning exactly what diagnosis codes are needed for a service, procedure, or item to be deemed medically necessary. Coders familiar with the LCD, as well as the OCE and NCCI edits, can be proactive in avoiding payment denials and claims rejections.

For example, general medical examination is not sufficient justification for Medicare to pay for a blood test for vitamin D deficiency. Osteoporosis and osteopenia, on the other hand, will justify the vitamin D test. A provider who is performing the laboratory test upon a physician's order must query the physician to determine the reason for the test. If the diagnosis does not meet the LCD requirement for performing the test, then the provider should obtain a signed Advance Beneficiary Notice (ABN) from the patient. Completion of an ABN obligates the patient to pay for the test if Medicare does not. It is important to note that there is no prohibition on performing the test itself. If the physician feels the test is necessary and the patient is willing to pay for it, then the provider can certainly perform it.

---

**modifier** A two-digit addition to a CPT or HCPCS code that provides additional information about the service or procedure performed.

**revenue code** A Chargemaster code required for Medicare billing.

**Chargemaster** The database that contains the detailed description of charges related to all potential services rendered to a patient.

**RW** relative weight

**Medicare Administrative Contractor (MAC)** Regional, private contractor who processes reimbursement claims for CMS.

**local coverage determination (LCD)** A list of diagnostic codes used by Medicare contractors to determine medical necessity.

**national coverage determination (NCD)** A process using evidence-based medicine to determine whether Medicare will cover an item or service on the basis of medical necessity.

**OCE** outpatient code editor
**NCCI** National Correct Coding Initiative

**OPPS** Outpatient Prospective Payment System

**LCD** local coverage determination

**MAC** Medicare Administrative Contractor

**CMS** Centers for Medicare and Medicaid Services

**CC** comorbidity or complication

**per diem** Each day, daily. Usually refers to all-inclusive payments for inpatient services.

**patient assessment instrument (PAI)** A tool used to identify patients with greater needs and for the treatment of whom the long-term care or skilled nursing facility will receive higher reimbursement.

**comorbidity** A condition that affects the patient's care and/or length of stay and exists at the same time as the principal diagnosis.

**etiology** The cause or source of the patient's condition or disease.

**Uniform Bill (UB-04)** The standardized form used by hospitals for inpatient and outpatient billing to CMS and other third party payers.

**principal diagnosis** According to the UHDDS, the condition that, after study, is determined to be chiefly responsible for occasioning the admission of the patient to the hospital for care.

OCE and NCCI details can be found on the CMS Web site in the Medicare section under OPPS. LCDs are issued by the regional MACs and are described in detail on the MACs' Web sites.

## Additional Prospective Payment Systems

### Inpatient Psychiatric Facility Prospective Payment System

CMS recognized that providing services for psychiatric patients is unique and not readily comparable to providing services for medical or surgical patients. The psychiatric setting is often more difficult to manage in terms of resources and length of stay. The Inpatient Psychiatric Facility Prospective Payment System (IPF PPS) was designed to address these issues beginning January 1, 2005. The major change concerning reimbursement is that under IPF PPS, payment is made on a per diem rate based on a federal rate. The federal rate is based on various factors and adjustments. There are two levels of adjustments: patient level and facility level. The patient level includes length of stay and patient age, and the facility level includes the geographical location of the facility and whether the facility is a teaching hospital.

IPF PPS will be based on ICD-10-CM coding, and, as was the case under MS-DRGs, all of the coding rules will apply. A difference that coders will notice is that CC codes play a larger role than in the psychiatric MS-DRGs in the PPS MS-DRG system. The addition of these CC codes under IPF PPS will cause a case to fall into additional adjustment categories. It is important for psychiatrists to fully document all secondary diagnoses, including all medical diagnoses, in addition to psychiatric diagnoses.

### Inpatient Rehabilitation Facility Prospective Payment System

The Balanced Budget Act of 1997 also required CMS to establish a PPS for Inpatient Rehabilitation Facilities (IRF PPS). The Final Rule for IRF PPS was published in the *Federal Register* on August 1, 2000, and became effective January 1, 2002. IRF PPS replaced a cost-based payment system. IRF PPS reimburses on a per-discharge basis addresses both the costs of inpatient rehabilitation services as well as the unique needs of each patient that a facility admits. A comprehensive **patient assessment instrument (PAI)**, called the Inpatient Rehabilitation Facility Patient Assessment Instrument (IRF-PAI), is used to assess each patient with the intent that patients with greater needs will be identified and that the facility will receive higher payment for these individuals. IRF-PAI includes sections on, for example, bowel continence, impairments, infections, and pressure ulcers. Two sections of IRF-PAI require the use of ICD-10-CM codes. Patients are grouped into case mix groups (CMGs). Each CMG has four possible weights; the final weight is determined by the patient's comorbidities.

Unique to IRF PPS is that two types of coding practice are applied: one type for IRF-PAI and one type for billing. IRF PPS requires coding of the etiology diagnoses, essentially the same diagnoses that would have been coded in the acute setting even though the patient is no longer receiving acute care. For reporting purposes on the Uniform Bill (UB-04), standard coding rules and conventions are applied. For example, suppose a patient admitted to the hospital was diagnosed with type 1 diabetes mellitus with severe peripheral angiopathy and gangrene and had to have his leg amputated. The ICD-10-CM diagnosis code assigned for the inpatient stay is E10.52, Type 1 diabetes mellitus with diabetic peripheral angiopathy with gangrene. After the amputation, the patient was transferred to an inpatient rehabilitation facility to learn how to use an artificial leg. The same code, E10.52, would be used for IRF-PAI, but a rehabilitation code, code Z47.81, Encounter for orthopedic aftercare following surgical amputation, would be reported as the principal diagnosis on the UB-04.

### Long-Term Care Hospital Prospective Payment System

The Long-term Care Prospective Payment System (LTCH-PPS) became effective for cost reporting periods beginning on or after October 1, 2002. Medicare regulations define long-term care hospitals as hospitals that have an average inpatient length of stay greater than 25 days. Patients in long-term care hospitals have multiple acute and chronic complex conditions and may need, for example, comprehensive rehabilitation services, respiratory therapy, cancer treatment, and pain management. LTCH-PPS is based on DRGs, but these DRGs are modified to reflect patient acuity and the greater costs involved in treating the complex conditions of these patients, which require longer lengths of stay. This modification is accomplished through the identification of a **Resource Utilization Group (RUG)** category. A Minimum Data Set (MDS), which includes the MS-DRG, is completed for the patient at various intervals during the stay. MDS 3.0 is included in Appendix C of this text book. The data are entered into a grouper that determines the RUG.

## Home Health Prospective Payment System

The Home Health Prospective Payment System (HH PPS) applies to reimbursement for services rendered by home health care providers. Payments are in units, each unit being a 60-day episode, and are distributed to the provider in two split payments. The case mix system used is called Home Health Resources Groups (HHRGs), and the level of the HHRGs determines the payment. A comprehensive patient assessment tool, OASIS (Outcomes and Assessment Information Set), is used with ICD-10-CM codes to group these patients into HHRGs.

## Skilled Nursing Facility Prospective Payment System and Resource Utilization Groups

RUGs are the basis for payment for skilled nursing facility (SNF) services for Medicare patients. RUGs are currently in their fourth version and referred to as RUG-IV. Unlike DRGs and APCs, RUGs are not a retrospective reimbursement system for an entire stay or visit. Reimbursement based on RUGs is a daily, or per diem, rate based on the admission assessment of the patient. A review of data sets may help in a discussion of this concept.

As discussed in Chapters 2, 4, and 5, specific data sets are abstracted and reported retrospectively for both ambulatory and hospital care: the UACDS and the UHDDS, respectively. In long-term care, the Minimum Data Set (MDS) is collected as part of the **Resident Assessment Instrument (RAI)**. The MDS, currently in version 3.0, contains far more data than the UHDDS or the UACDS. It includes the patient's cognitive and medical condition as well as his or her ability to perform self-care and other activities of daily living. Assessment therefore is performed at the beginning of the patient's stay, not at the end. Reimbursement is then based on the patient's care needs, consisting of 1 of 44 groups within seven broad categories: rehabilitation, extensive services, special care, clinically complex, impaired cognition, behavioral problems, and reduced physical function. Although there are other RUG systems in existence, Medicare reimbursement is determined using the RUG-IV system.

In most SNF settings, much of the information collected has been under the domain of the nursing department. Nursing staff members usually collect and record the MDS data, largely composed of diagnostic statements and including the ICD-10-CM codes associated with the patient's medical condition. This is not to imply that health information professionals are incapable of performing this task.

PPSs continue to evolve and expand into various patient settings, primarily as a result of legislation and instruction from Congress. Although these PPSs are initiated and developed for reimbursing services for Medicare patients, other payers and insurers often use or modify these systems for their patients as well. To code accurately and in compliance with regulations, all coding professionals should be aware of what PPSs apply, and to whom, in the setting in which they are employed. Table 7-7 contains a summary of the previously discussed PPSs.

## Resource-Based Relative Value System

The **resource-based relative value system (RBRVS)** is the basis of reimbursement to physicians for services rendered to Medicare patients. Because the reimbursement is for physician services, the location where services were provided can be the physician's office, a hospital, or a nursing home—essentially anywhere that a patient can be treated. Physicians submit claims for reimbursement using HCPCS/CPT codes. Each HCPCS/CPT code has

---

- **DRG** diagnosis related group

- **Resource Utilization Groups (RUGs)** These constitute a prospective payment system for long-term care. Current Medicare application is a per diem rate based on the RUG III grouper.
- **Minimum Data Set (MDS)** The detailed data collected about patients receiving long-term care. It is collected several times, and it forms the basis for the Resource Utilization Group.

- **home health care** Health care services rendered in the patient's home; or an agency that provides such services.
- **Outcome and Assessment Information Set (OASIS)** Data set most associated with home health care. This data set monitors patient care by identifying markers over the course of patient care.

- **Skilled nursing facility (SNF)** A long-term care facility providing a range of nursing and other health care services to patients who require continuous care, typically those with a chronic illness.

- **Resident Assessment Instrument (RAI)** A data set collected by skilled nursing facilities (SNFs) that includes elements of MDS 3.0, along with information on patient statuses and conditions in the facility.

- **UHDDS** Uniform Hospital Discharge Data Set
- **UACDS** Uniform Ambulatory Care Data Set

- **SNF** skilled nursing facility

- **PPS** prospective payment system

- **resource-based relative value system (RBRVS)** The system used to determine reimbursements to physicians for the treatment of Medicare patients.
- **Healthcare Common Procedure Coding System (HCPCS)** A coding system, of which CPT-4 is level one, used for drugs, equipment, supplies, and other auxiliary health care services rendered.
- **Current Procedural Terminology (CPT)** A nomenclature and coding system developed and maintained by the American Medical Association to facilitate billing for physicians and other services.

## TABLE 7-7

### SUMMARY OF PROSPECTIVE PAYMENTS SYSTEMS (PPSs)

| SYSTEM | SETTING | CODE SYSTEM | BASIS OF REIMBURSEMENT |
|---|---|---|---|
| MS-DRG (medical severity–diagnosis related group) | Short-stay facility, inpatient acute care, Medicare patient | ICD-10-CM diagnosis and ICD-10-PCS procedure codes | Diagnoses and procedures<br>Single MS-DRG assignment<br>Retrospective |
| APC (ambulatory payment classification) | Ambulatory care, outpatient services, emergency departments | CPT-4<br>HCPCS<br>ICD-10-CM diagnosis codes | Procedures<br>Diagnoses used for validation<br>May have multiple APCs<br>Retrospective |
| Inpatient Psychiatric Facility (IPF) PPS | Inpatient psychiatric | ICD-10-CM | Per diem and federal rate |
| Inpatient Rehabilitation Facility (IRF) PPS | Inpatient rehabilitation facilities | ICD-10-CM | Per discharge<br>Inpatient Rehabilitation Facility Patient Assessment Instrument (IRF-PAI)<br>Case mix groups |
| Long-term Care Hospital (LTCH) PPS | Hospitals with average length of stay >25 days | ICD-10-CM | DRGs<br>Patient acuity |
| Home Health care (HH) PPS | Home health care providers | ICD-10-CM | Home Health Resources Groups (HHRGs)<br>Payment units<br>Oasis |
| Resource Utilization Group, version 4 (RUG-IV) | Medicare Skilled nursing facility services | ICD-10-CM | Per diem rate<br>Not retrospective<br>Minimum data set data |

**fee schedule** The list of charges that a physician expects to be paid for services rendered. Also, a list of the amounts a payer will remit for certain services.

three relative value units (RVUs). Each RVU corresponds to the complexity of the service provided, the consumption of resources incurred by the service provided, and the relation of the service provided in comparison with other services provided. Physicians receive reimbursement on the basis of a national Medicare physician **fee schedule** that is adjusted according to the physician's geographical location. Physicians located in different areas of the United States receive varying reimbursement amounts for identical services because Medicare recognizes that operating costs vary by location.

## ▪ EXERCISE 7-4

### ▪ Prospective Payment System

1. If patients are grouped into the same MS-DRG, it is because they have what three criteria in common?
2. What is meant by the term "resource intensity"?
3. Describe how a case is assigned to a major diagnostic category (MDC).
4. After assignment of the MDC, what occurs next in the grouping process?
5. What patient attributes are important to grouper assignment?
6. What is a CC code, and why is it significant?
7. What is the difference between a comorbidity and a complication?
8. What is a MCC code, and why is it significant?
9. What does the Medicare Code Editor do?
10. Describe two types of coding errors that may affect MS-DRG assignment.
11. What coding classification or nomenclature system is used to indicate medical necessity?
12. What is a modifier, and for what is it used?

# BILLING

To be reimbursed for services rendered to a patient, a facility must alert the payer that payment is due. This is accomplished by filing a claim with the patient's health insurance carrier, which is also called **billing**. In an acute care facility, the billing function is performed in a department that is often called patient accounting or patient financial services.

Coding and billing are key components of the *revenue cycle management* process. **Revenue cycle management (RCM)** is composed of all the activities that connect the services being rendered to a patient with the provider's reimbursement for those services.

## PATIENT FINANCIAL SERVICES

The **patient financial services** department is responsible for ensuring that accurate claims are sent for each patient's account, that they are sent in the correct format to the correct payers, and that the facility receives the correct reimbursement. A patient's bill includes a compilation of charges for items used and services rendered. Each patient is assigned an account number for items received and services rendered during a particular visit or stay. The account number, unlike the patient's medical record number, changes for each encounter. In this way, charges can be accurately assigned, or "posted," to each specific encounter so that the bill reflects the charges for each individual account. For example, a patient may visit a hospital three times in one month: once as an inpatient, then as a clinic patient, and later as an emergency department patient. The hospital does not combine all three visits into one monthly bill. Instead, a different account number is assigned for each encounter, and a separate bill is sent for each account that reflects the charges incurred for each individual visit. A bill that is produced and sent is called a "dropped," or final, bill. A bill that has been dropped is pending payment. Once the dropped bill has been paid, the account is closed to any further activity.

To use an acute care inpatient as an example, three key steps must happen in order to produce and drop a bill: (1) The patient's charges must be entered into, or posted to, the account; (2) the patient must have been discharged so that the account reflects the charges accumulated for the patient's entire length of stay; and (3) the medical record must be coded. Whether or not payers use MS-DRGs or another DRG grouper as a method of reimbursement, they still want to see the ICD-10-CM and ICD-10-PCS codes related to the clinical stay, and these codes must appear on the UB-04, a billing form discussed later in this chapter. It is through the coding of the diagnoses and procedures that the payer often gets the first impression of what actually should have happened in terms of services rendered.

Beginning at discharge and until a final bill is dropped, hospitals monitor the accounts that have not been billed. This list of undropped bills is called by a variety of names, including the *unbilled list* or the *DNFB* ("discharged, no final bill" or "discharged, not final billed"). Regardless of the name used, this list of delayed payments can add up to millions of dollars. Because the delays are partially due to the fact that coding has not occurred on some of the accounts, the HIM department proactively and aggressively monitors the DNFB on a regular basis. Management of the coding function and the DNFB is often complex, with many factors contributing to uncoded medical records that then result in unbilled accounts. Because the patient accounting and HIM departments both have the same goal of reducing or eliminating unnecessary unbilled accounts, the departments ideally assist each other in reducing the factors contributing to payment delays.

## CHARGEMASTER (CHARGE DESCRIPTION MASTER)

Whether a facility is reimbursed using PPS or another system, a variety of procedures must be in place to ensure the accurate accumulation of charges and the accurate

**billing** The process of submitting health insurance claims or rendering invoices.

**acute care facility** A health care facility in which patients have an average length of stay less than 30 days and that has an emergency department, operating suite, and clinical departments to handle a broad range of diagnoses and treatments.

**revenue cycle management (RCM)** All the activities that connect the services being rendered to a patient with the provider's reimbursement for those services.

**patient financial services** The department in a health care facility that is responsible for submitting bills or claims for reimbursement. Also called *patient accounts* or *patient accounting*.

**encounter** A patient's health care experience; a unit of measure for the volume of ambulatory care services provided.

**charges** Fees or costs for services rendered.

**grouper** The software used to derive the DRG from the ICD-10-CM diagnoses and procedures.

**Uniform Bill (UB-04)** The standardized form used by hospitals for inpatient and outpatient billing to CMS and other third party payers.

**DNFB** "discharged, no final bill"

**PPS** prospective payment system

### TABLE 7-8

#### SAMPLE FIELDS IN A CHARGE DESCRIPTION MASTER

| FIELD | DESCRIPTION |
|---|---|
| General ledger code | Internal code used by the facility's accounting department to track revenue and expenses |
| CPT/HCPCS code | Billing code for transmission to the insurer |
| Cost basis | The cost of the item to the facility |
| Charge | The amount that the facility charges for the item or service |
| Description | Definition or description of the item or service |
| Date | Date of the most recent update of the aforementioned fields for the item or service |

**coding** The assignment of alphanumerical values to a word, phrase, or other nonnumerical expression. In health care, coding is the assignment of alphanumerical values to diagnosis and procedure descriptions.

**clinical data** All of the medical data that have been recorded about the patient's stay or visit, including diagnoses and procedures.

**fee schedule** The list of charges that a physician expects to be paid for services rendered. Also, a list of the amounts a payer will remit for certain services.

**Chargemaster** The database that contains the detailed description of charges related to all potential services rendered to a patient.

**charge capture** The systematic collection of specific charges for services rendered to a patient.

**encounter form** A data collection device that facilitates the accurate capture of ambulatory care diagnoses and services.

**superbill** An ambulatory care encounter form on which potential diagnoses and procedures are preprinted for easy check-off at the point of care.

coding of the clinical data. Charges are the facility's individual fees, or the dollar amount for items or services provided to a patient and owed to the facility. Each item or service is assigned a charge, which is usually reviewed and adjusted or changed annually. Charges may be set on the basis of fee schedules or contractual arrangements with certain payers or may be determined internally through the use of the facility's cost-accounting system. The actual charges are not always equal to the amount that the payer reimburses a facility; the payment received depends on contractual agreements and may be discounted accordingly, as discussed earlier in this chapter. A facility compares its charges with actual reimbursements to determine the impact of contractual arrangements and whether they allow the facility to operate profitably (i.e., earn more money than it spends).

The report of the data fields that contain a facility's charges or costs for services and items is called a Chargemaster. Other terms that are sometimes used include Charge Data Master and Charge Description Master (CDM). Table 7-8 illustrates key data fields that usually appear in a Chargemaster. The Chargemaster must be updated regularly so that fees and costs are accurate. Because HCPCS/CPT codes are included in the Chargemaster, these codes must also be updated when changes or revisions occur. All the services that a facility provides, from adhesive bandages to intravenous drips and room and board, must appear on the Chargemaster, or they cannot be billed. Coding professionals often initiate or assist in making the updates to the CDM and informing departments about changes.

## CHARGE CAPTURE

As previously discussed, charges must be posted to a patient's account in order for proper billing to occur. This process is called **charge capture**.

In an inpatient hospital setting, charges are usually posted to the patient's account electronically, using order-entry software, each time a service or item is provided. If the hospital does not use order-entry software or does not use the software for all types of charges, these charges still must be captured on a paper form called a charge ticket. All charge tickets must be forwarded to the accounting or billing department at the end of each business day and manually posted to the correct account. As one can imagine, manual charge capture is extremely laborious and vulnerable to human error.

Depending on factors such as length of stay, each account may have hundreds of posted charges. Most facilities allow time between discharge and submission of the bill so that all charges can be posted. This period, called the bill-hold period, usually ranges from 1 to 5 days after discharge, perhaps longer for outpatient or ambulatory services. In smaller facilities, posting delays may occur because of reduced staff on weekends. Charges posted after the final bill drops are considered late charges. Because late charges must be submitted separately and some insurers do not pay late charges at all or only after a certain time, it is essential that charges be posted no later than the end of the bill-hold period.

In an ambulatory setting, charges are often captured, by service, on an **encounter form**, or **superbill**. An encounter form may be in electronic format or a single sheet of paper, sometimes double-sided, that contains a list of the most common patient complaints, diagnoses, procedures, and services provided by the facility. The paper form must be

**Figure 7-7** Ambulatory care encounter form/superbill. (From Abdelhak M, Grostick A, Hanken MA, Jacobs H: Health information: management of a strategic resource, ed 2, Philadelphia, 2001, Saunders, p 244. CPT copyright 2012 American Medical Association. All rights reserved. CPT is a registered trademark of the American Medical Association.)

transferred into an electronic billing format in order to submit the claim electronically. Some insurers provide their own encounter forms. A comprehensive encounter form includes ICD-10-CM diagnoses codes and HCPCS procedure codes. Encounter forms facilitate communication between the physician or other health care provider and the administrative personnel who are responsible for coding and billing. Because it is not the encounter form but the health record that supports the reimbursement claim, care must be taken to ensure that the health record indicates all services provided. Figure 7-7 is an example of an encounter form (superbill).

In a physician's office, the process of obtaining reimbursement may rest with the administrative personnel (e.g., the medical secretary, medical assistant, or practice manager). The role of these employees is to determine which services were provided for which patient and

**Healthcare Common Procedure Coding System (HCPCS)** A CMS coding system, of which CPT is level one, used for physician services, drugs, equipment, supplies, and other auxiliary health care services rendered.

**claim** The application to an insurance company for reimbursement.

which insurer or insurers should receive a bill and to ensure that all services provided are billed correctly.

In some situations, such as in a solo practitioner's office, the physician may file the claims directly to the insurer for payment. Because the insurance industry is so complex and there are many different types of payers, all with their own rules, many physicians rely on billing services to perform the administrative tasks of charge capture and billing. Performing all of these tasks is critical to accurate and timely reimbursement.

## THE UNIFORM BILL

**NUBC** National Uniform Billing Committee
**AHA** American Hospital Association
**UB** Uniform Bill

**Uniform Bill (UB-04)** The standardized form used by hospitals for inpatient and outpatient billing to CMS and other third party payers.

**UHDDS** Uniform Hospital Discharge Data Set

**Federal Register** The publication of the proceedings of the United States Congress.

The National Uniform Billing Committee (NUBC) is responsible for developing and implementing a single billing form and standard data set to be used nationwide by providers/hospitals and payers/insurers for handling inpatient health care claims. The NUBC comprises representatives from all the major provider and payer organizations, including the American Hospital Association (AHA) and Medicare, the public health sector, and electronic standards development organizations.

The first standard Uniform Bill appeared in 1982 and was referred to as the UB-82. Representatives from across the country were surveyed to seek improvements on the UB-82, and the UB-92 was the result of their efforts. At this time claims are submitted electronically using the UB-04, also known as the Form CMS-1450. Although the UB was originally used for claims reimbursement only, the NUBC has recognized that it contains a wealth of data that can be used for additional purposes. The data captured on the UB are now also used by health researchers to gauge the delivery of health care services to patients and to set future policy.

Figure 7-8 shows a UB-04 form. Notice that the Uniform Bill itself is composed of the UHDDS demographic and financial data elements as well as many additional data fields that are useful for communication between the provider and the payer. Coding professionals should be aware that fields on the UB-04 form include the admitting diagnosis code, distinct fields for the patient's reason for visit, and expanded diagnosis and procedure fields to accommodate ICD-10-CM and ICD-10-PCS codes (American Hospital Association, 2010). The UB-04 is the paper representation of the electronic 837I billing file.

UHDDS definitions allow standardized reporting of specific data elements collected by all acute care short-term hospitals. These data elements and their definitions can be found in the July 31, 1985, *Federal Register* (Health Information Policy Council, 1985). Figure 7-9 illustrates the data elements of the UHDDS and their relationship to the fields of the UB-04. The following section summarizes the UHDDS.

### Summary of UHDDS Data Elements

## Person/Enrollment Data:

1. *Personal/unique identifier:*
   The patient's full name and medical record number or other unique identifier. Although some advocate for the use of the Social Security Number in this field, there are strong arguments against it
2. *Date of birth:*
   The year, month, and day of the patient's birth
3. *Gender:*
   Male, female, or unknown/not stated
4. *Race and ethnicity:*
   Race: American Indian/Eskimo/Aleut; Asian or Pacific Islander; Black; White; Other; Unknown/not stated
   Ethnicity: Hispanic Origin; Other; Unknown/not stated
5. *Residence:*
   Full address and ZIP code of the patient's usual residence

1

2

3a PAT. CNTL #

b. MED. REC. #

4 TYPE OF BILL

5 FED. TAX NO.

6 STATEMENT COVERS PERIOD  FROM  THROUGH

7

8 PATIENT NAME  a

9 PATIENT ADDRESS  a

b

b

c  d  e

10 BIRTH DATE  11 SEX  12 DATE  ADMISSION 13 HR  14 TYPE  15 SRC  16 DHR  17 STAT  18  19  20  21  CONDITION CODES 22  23  24  25  26  27  28  29 ACDT STATE  30

31 OCCURRENCE CODE  DATE  32 OCCURRENCE CODE  DATE  33 OCCURRENCE CODE  DATE  34 OCCURRENCE CODE  DATE  35 CODE  OCCURRENCE SPAN FROM  THROUGH  36 CODE  OCCURRENCE SPAN FROM  THROUGH  37

38

39 CODE  VALUE CODES AMOUNT  40 CODE  VALUE CODES AMOUNT  41 CODE  VALUE CODES AMOUNT

a

b

c

d

42 REV. CD.  43 DESCRIPTION  44 HCPCS / RATE / HIPPS CODE  45 SERV. DATE  46 SERV. UNITS  47 TOTAL CHARGES  48 NON-COVERED CHARGES  49

| 1 | | | | | | | 1 |
| 2 | | | | | | | 2 |
| 3 | | | | | | | 3 |
| 4 | | | | | | | 4 |
| 5 | | | | | | | 5 |
| 6 | | | | | | | 6 |
| 7 | | | | | | | 7 |
| 8 | | | | | | | 8 |
| 9 | | | | | | | 9 |
| 10 | | | | | | | 10 |
| 11 | | | | | | | 11 |
| 12 | | | | | | | 12 |
| 13 | | | | | | | 13 |
| 14 | | | | | | | 14 |
| 15 | | | | | | | 15 |
| 16 | | | | | | | 16 |
| 17 | | | | | | | 17 |
| 18 | | | | | | | 18 |
| 19 | | | | | | | 19 |
| 20 | | | | | | | 20 |
| 21 | | | | | | | 21 |
| 22 | | | | | | | 22 |
| 23 | | | | | | | 23 |

PAGE ____ OF ____  CREATION DATE  TOTALS ➡

50 PAYER NAME  51 HEALTH PLAN ID  52 RES. INFO  53 ASG. BEN.  54 PRIOR PAYMENTS  55 EST. AMOUNT DUE  56 NPI

57 OTHER PRV ID

A  B  C

58 INSURED'S NAME  59 P. REL  60 INSURED'S UNIQUE ID  61 GROUP NAME  62 INSURANCE GROUP NO.

A  B  C

63 TREATMENT AUTHORIZATION CODES  64 DOCUMENT CONTROL NUMBER  65 EMPLOYER NAME

A  B  C

66 DX  68

69 ADMIT DX  70 PATIENT REASON DX  71 PPS CODE  72 ECI  73

74 PRINCIPAL PROCEDURE CODE  DATE  a. OTHER PROCEDURE CODE  DATE  b. OTHER PROCEDURE CODE  DATE  75  76 ATTENDING  NPI  QUAL

LAST  FIRST

c. OTHER PROCEDURE CODE  DATE  d. OTHER PROCEDURE CODE  DATE  e. OTHER PROCEDURE CODE  DATE  77 OPERATING  NPI  QUAL

LAST  FIRST

80 REMARKS  81CC a  78 OTHER  NPI  QUAL

b  LAST  FIRST

c  79 OTHER  NPI  QUAL

d  LAST  FIRST

UB-04 CMS-1450  APPROVED OMB NO.  THE CERTIFICATIONS ON THE REVERSE APPLY TO THIS BILL AND ARE MADE A PART HEREOF.

NUBC™ National Uniform Billing Committee  LIC9213257

Figure 7-8 UB-04.

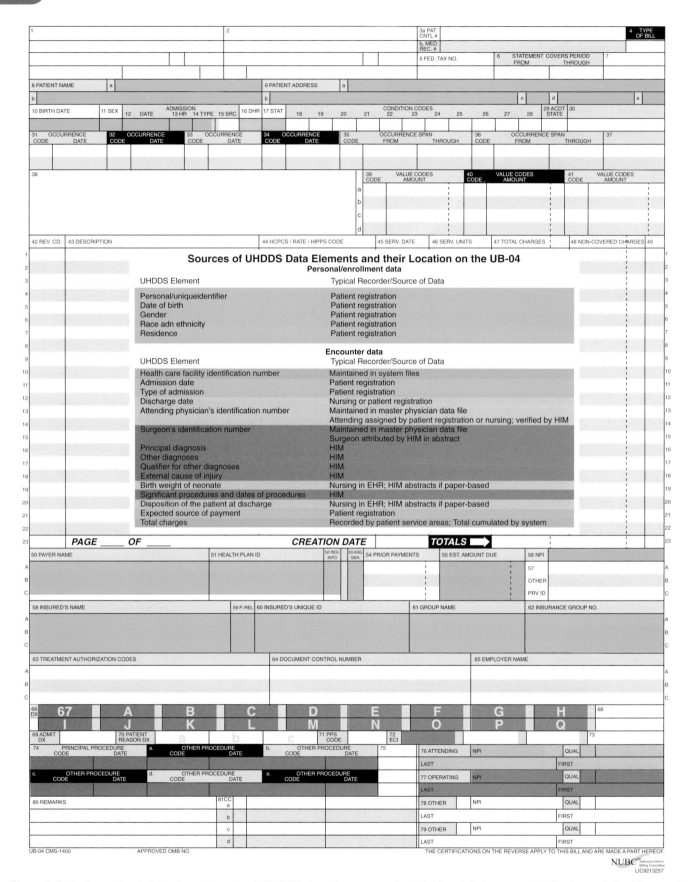

**Figure 7-9** Uniform Hospital Discharge Data Set (UHDDS) data elements on the UB-04 and their sources. EHR, electronic health record; HIM, health information management (department).

## Encounter Data:

6. *Health care facility identification number:*
   Identification number of the facility that treated the patient
7. *Admission date:*
   The year, month, and day of admission for the current episode of care
8. *Type of admission:*
   Was the admission expected or unexpected?
9. *Discharge date:*
   The year, month, and day of discharge for the current episode of care
10. *Attending physician's identification number:*
    The unique national identification number assigned to the clinician of record at discharge who is responsible for the discharge summary
11. *Surgeon's identification number:*
    The unique national identification number assigned to the clinician who performed the principal procedure
12. *Principal diagnosis:*
    The condition established after study to be chiefly responsible for occasioning the admission of the patient to the hospital (ICD-10-CM code)
13. *Other diagnoses:*
    All conditions that coexist at the time of admission, or develop subsequently, that affect the treatment received, the length of stay, or both (also an ICD-10-CM code)
14. *Qualifier for other diagnoses:*
    For each other diagnosis, was the onset prior to admission? (Yes or No)
15. *External cause-of-injury code:*
    The cause of an injury, poisoning, or adverse effect that has been recorded as the principal or other diagnosis (also an ICD-10-CM code)
16. *Birth weight of neonate:*
    If the patient is a newborn, the actual birth weight in grams is reported
17. *Principal procedure and date of procedure:*
    The procedure that was performed for definitive treatment, rather than one performed for diagnostic or exploratory purposes, or was necessary to take care of a complication. If more than one procedure qualifies, the one most closely related to the principal diagnosis should be selected (ICD-10-PCS code)
18. *Other procedure(s) and the date(s) of the procedure(s):*
    All other procedures that qualify (see 17)
19. *Disposition of the patient at discharge (see examples):*
    Discharged alive:
    • Discharged to home or self care (routine discharge)
    • Discharged/transferred to another short-term general hospital for inpatient care
    • Discharged/transferred to skilled nursing facility (SNF)
    • Discharged/transferred to an intermediate care facility (ICF)
    • Discharged/transferred to another type of institution for inpatient care or referred for outpatient services to another institution
    • Home under care of organized home health service organization
    • Home under care of a Home IV (home intravenous therapy) provider
    • Left against medical advice or discontinued care
    Expired
    Status not stated
20. *Expected source of payment:*
    • Primary source of payment. The primary source is expected to be responsible for the largest percentage of the patient's current bill
    • Secondary sources of payment
21. *Categories of source of payment are as follows:*
    • Self-pay
    • Workers' compensation
    • Medicare

- Medicaid
- Maternal and child health
- Other government payments
- Blue Cross
- Insurance companies
- No charge (free, charity, special research, or teaching)
- Other
- Unknown/not stated

22. *Total charges:*
    All charges for procedures and services rendered to the patient during a hospitalization or encounter

## CMS-1500

The CMS-1500 form is the paper data collection form used for transmittal of billing information for ambulatory/outpatient claims and physician's office claims. The CMS-1500 form has fewer fields that the UB-04 but it contains much of the same information. Figure 7-10 shows a CMS-1500 form. The CMS-1500 is the paper representation of the 837P electronic billing file.

## CLAIMS REJECTIONS

**payer** The individual or organization that is primarily responsible for the reimbursement for a particular health care service. Usually refers to the insurance company or third party.

**local coverage determination (LCD)** A list of diagnostic codes used by Medicare contractors to determine medical necessity.

**Medicare** Federally funded health care insurance plan for older adults and for certain categories of chronically ill patients.

**ED** emergency department

Optimally, the facility or provider has recorded all of the required billing data accurately, and the claim drops to the payer without human intervention. However, the potential for human error requires that all claims be reviewed prior to being submitted to the payer. The provider, or provider's billing service, will examine the claims for errors such as missing fields, LCD errors, and invalid data. Claims that are rejected must be corrected prior to resubmission.

An example of a claim rejection is the failure to combine an outpatient account with an inpatient visit that occurs within 3 days prior to the inpatient visit. Consider a patient who is treated for congestive heart failure in the emergency department and is admitted to that hospital 2 days later—also for congestive heart failure. Because the admission is within 3 days, Medicare will not pay separately for the emergency department visit. All diagnostic testing and all related therapeutic services must be combined into the inpatient visit. It is the responsibility of the hospital to support the rationale for not combining therapeutic visits. An example of therapeutic services that might not be combined is an ED visit for a broken leg, which would likely not be combined with a subsequent unrelated inpatient visit for pneumonia (CMS Three Day Payment Window, 2012).

## CLAIMS DENIALS

**claim** The application to an insurance company for reimbursement of services rendered.

**ABN** advance beneficiary notice

Once the claim is submitted, there is an additional layer of review by the payer. The payer may refuse to pay the claim for a variety of reasons; examples are services not covered by the patient's insurance plan, service overlaps another provider's bill, codes submitted on the bill do not match the preauthorized services, lack of medical necessity for the services provided, and untimely filing.

Some errors, such as untimely filing and lack of medical necessity, cannot be corrected. Such claims will be adjusted to a zero balance and the provider will receive no payment for the services. If the provider has obtained an ABN or waiver from the patient in advance of the services, the patient may be billed for the services directly. In some cases, the provider may file an appeal with the payer to challenge the payer's denial. There may also be the opportunity for the patient to appeal.

## 1500

# HEALTH INSURANCE CLAIM FORM

APPROVED BY NATIONAL UNIFORM CLAIM COMMITTEE 08/05

PICA

1. MEDICARE   MEDICAID   TRICARE CHAMPUS   CHAMPVA   GROUP HEALTH PLAN   FECA BLK LUNG   OTHER
   (Medicare #)   (Medicaid #)   (Sponsor's SSN)   (Member ID#)   (SSN or ID)   (SSN)   (ID)

1a. INSURED'S I.D. NUMBER          (For Program in Item 1)

2. PATIENT'S NAME (Last Name, First Name, Middle Initial)

3. PATIENT'S BIRTH DATE        SEX
MM   DD   YY      M     F

4. INSURED'S NAME (Last Name, First Name, Middle Initial)

5. PATIENT'S ADDRESS (No., Street)

6. PATIENT RELATIONSHIP TO INSURED
Self   Spouse   Child   Other

7. INSURED'S ADDRESS (No., Street)

CITY                    STATE

8. PATIENT STATUS
Single   Married   Other

CITY                    STATE

ZIP CODE     TELEPHONE (Include Area Code)
(      )

Employed   Full-Time Student   Part-Time Student

ZIP CODE     TELEPHONE (Include Area Code)
(      )

9. OTHER INSURED'S NAME (Last Name, First Name, Middle Initial)

10. IS PATIENT'S CONDITION RELATED TO:

11. INSURED'S POLICY GROUP OR FECA NUMBER

a. OTHER INSURED'S POLICY OR GROUP NUMBER

a. EMPLOYMENT? (Current or Previous)
YES   NO

a. INSURED'S DATE OF BIRTH        SEX
MM   DD   YY      M     F

b. OTHER INSURED'S DATE OF BIRTH    SEX
MM   DD   YY     M     F

b. AUTO ACCIDENT?     PLACE (State)
YES   NO

b. EMPLOYER'S NAME OR SCHOOL NAME

c. EMPLOYER'S NAME OR SCHOOL NAME

c. OTHER ACCIDENT?
YES   NO

c. INSURANCE PLAN NAME OR PROGRAM NAME

d. INSURANCE PLAN NAME OR PROGRAM NAME

10d. RESERVED FOR LOCAL USE

d. IS THERE ANOTHER HEALTH BENEFIT PLAN?
YES   NO   *If yes*, return to and complete item 9 a-d.

**READ BACK OF FORM BEFORE COMPLETING & SIGNING THIS FORM.**
12. PATIENT'S OR AUTHORIZED PERSON'S SIGNATURE I authorize the release of any medical or other information necessary to process this claim. I also request payment of government benefits either to myself or to the party who accepts assignment below.

SIGNED _____   DATE _____

13. INSURED'S OR AUTHORIZED PERSON'S SIGNATURE I authorize payment of medical benefits to the undersigned physician or supplier for services described below.

SIGNED _____

14. DATE OF CURRENT:   ILLNESS (First symptom) OR
MM   DD   YY   INJURY (Accident) OR PREGNANCY(LMP)

15. IF PATIENT HAS HAD SAME OR SIMILAR ILLNESS. GIVE FIRST DATE   MM   DD   YY

16. DATES PATIENT UNABLE TO WORK IN CURRENT OCCUPATION
MM   DD   YY   TO   MM   DD   YY
FROM

17. NAME OF REFERRING PROVIDER OR OTHER SOURCE

17a.
17b.   NPI

18. HOSPITALIZATION DATES RELATED TO CURRENT SERVICES
MM   DD   YY   TO   MM   DD   YY
FROM

19. RESERVED FOR LOCAL USE

20. OUTSIDE LAB?     $ CHARGES
YES   NO

21. DIAGNOSIS OR NATURE OF ILLNESS OR INJURY (Relate Items 1, 2, 3 or 4 to Item 24E by Line)

1. |___.___|      3. |___.___|

2. |___.___|      4. |___.___|

22. MEDICAID RESUBMISSION CODE     ORIGINAL REF. NO.

23. PRIOR AUTHORIZATION NUMBER

| 24. A.   DATE(S) OF SERVICE | | | B. PLACE OF SERVICE | C. EMG | D. PROCEDURES, SERVICES, OR SUPPLIES (Explain Unusual Circumstances) | | E. DIAGNOSIS POINTER | F. $ CHARGES | G. DAYS OR UNITS | H. EPSDT Family Plan | I. ID. QUAL. | J. RENDERING PROVIDER ID. # |
|---|---|---|---|---|---|---|---|---|---|---|---|---|
| From MM DD YY | To MM DD YY | | | | CPT/HCPCS | MODIFIER | | | | | | |
| 1 | | | | | | | | | | | NPI | |
| 2 | | | | | | | | | | | NPI | |
| 3 | | | | | | | | | | | NPI | |
| 4 | | | | | | | | | | | NPI | |
| 5 | | | | | | | | | | | NPI | |
| 6 | | | | | | | | | | | NPI | |

25. FEDERAL TAX I.D. NUMBER   SSN EIN

26. PATIENT'S ACCOUNT NO.

27. ACCEPT ASSIGNMENT? (For govt. claims, see back)
YES   NO

28. TOTAL CHARGE   $

29. AMOUNT PAID   $

30. BALANCE DUE   $

31. SIGNATURE OF PHYSICIAN OR SUPPLIER INCLUDING DEGREES OR CREDENTIALS (I certify that the statements on the reverse apply to this bill and are made a part thereof.)

SIGNED _____   DATE _____

32. SERVICE FACILITY LOCATION INFORMATION

a.      b.

33. BILLING PROVIDER INFO & PH # (      )

a.      b.

NUCC Instruction Manual available at: www.nucc.org

APPROVED OMB-0938-0999 FORM CMS-1500 (08/05)

CARRIER — PATIENT AND INSURED INFORMATION — PHYSICIAN OR SUPPLIER INFORMATION

**Figure 7-10** CMS-1500 health insurance claim form.

**HIM** health information management

**ambulatory surgery** Surgery performed on an outpatient basis; the patient returns home after the surgery is performed. Also called *same-day surgery*.

**revenue cycle** The groups of processes that identify, record, and report the financial transactions that result from the facility's clinical relationship with a patient.

## ERROR CORRECTION

There is a great deal of pressure on both HIM professionals and billing professionals to submit claims that will be paid. Great care must be taken to ensure that only accurate, verifiable, and valid data are submitted on claims. If a claim is denied for codes submitted that do not match the preauthorized services, the case could be sent to a coding supervisor for review. Perhaps the case was coded incorrectly. If the coder made an error, the case can be recoded, re-abstracted, and rebilled. However, in some cases the codes provided to the payer at preregistration are NOT the codes for the services that were ultimately provided. For example, an ambulatory surgery case may have been preauthorized for a dilation & curettage without indicating that intrasurgical decision making could result in a hysterectomy. If the hysterectomy is performed and that is what the coder entered, then the case cannot be recoded, because there was no coding error.

## COLLECTION

Coding and billing processes may take place without error and yet the provider has one major step left in the revenue cycle process: follow-up and collections. Medicare and most major commercial payers remit payment on a relatively predictable schedule. However, some payers delay reimbursement as long as possible. When patients are responsible for all or part of the payment, further delays may ensue. Providers must be diligent in following up and seeking payment for services so that cash is received as timely as possible.

## EXERCISE 7-5
### Billing

1. What are some possible reasons that a bill has not been dropped?
2. What management tool is used to track unbilled accounts?
3. How would someone use the tool described in Question 2?
4. The charges or costs for a vaccination are listed in a facility's

   _____.

5. For the vaccination charge to appear on a patient's bill, how does the charge get to the patient's account?
6. In an ambulatory setting, an encounter form is often used for charge capture. Name three items that would be on an encounter form.

## IMPACT OF CODING ON REIMBURSEMENT

In any discussion of the various reimbursement methodologies, the importance of accurate ICD-10-CM, ICD-10-PCS and HCPCS/CPT-4 coding cannot be overstated. Because the codes determine the payment and facilitate the claim, the accuracy and timeliness of the coding function are critical.

### Coding Quality

**postdischarge processing** The procedures designed to prepare a health record for retention.
**charge capture** The systematic collection of specific charges for services rendered to a patient.
**assembly** The reorganization of a paper record into a standard order.
**analysis** The review of a record to evaluate its completeness, accuracy, or compliance with predetermined standards or other criteria.

The timeliness and completeness of the postdischarge processing of a record are important. In addition to charge capture, all pertinent medical record data must have been collected for correct assignment of codes, and the processing cycle must facilitate efficient, timely coding. For example, if a paper-based medical record must be assembled and analyzed before it is given to a coder, and if the assembly and analysis sections are 5 or 6 days behind the current discharge date, then medical records may not be coded until 7 days after the discharge date. Even factoring in the bill-hold period, a week is a long time for a facility to go without dropping a bill for a patient's stay. Facilities sometimes choose to code the record before it is assembled or analyzed so that the bill may be dropped more quickly.

Although this sequence expedites payment, it can also lead to coding errors if the medical record is incomplete because missing elements are not clearly identified or if important reports are misplaced in the wrong sections of the record.

The issues surrounding a paper-based medical record will generally be eliminated with the electronic health record (EHR). The EHR will permit access to patient information immediately upon its entry. Information cannot be "lost" once it is entered into the EHR. Coders may access the EHR at any point after patient admission and after discharge. In addition, computer-assisted coding (CAC) programs embedded in the EHR may facilitate the coding process in terms of speed and accuracy.

Coding must be reliable and valid, both individually and collectively within a facility or group. A coder or group of coders is said to demonstrate **reliability** when codes are consistently assigned for similar or identical cases. **Validity** of coding refers to the degree of accuracy of the codes assigned.

## Regulatory Issues

Effective each October, an updated version of the "ICD-10-CM Official Guidelines for Coding and Reporting" is issued by CMS and the **National Center for Health Statistics (NCHS)** and approved by the Cooperating Parties for the ICD-10-CM. The Cooperating Parties for ICD-10-CM are the American Hospital Association (AHA), the American Health Information Management Association (AHIMA), CMS, and NCHS. The "Official Guidelines for Coding and Reporting" can be found in its entirety at http://www.cdc.gov/nchs/data/icd10/icdguide.pdf. Adherence to these guidelines is required under HIPAA (see Chapter 12). The following statement is made in the Guidelines regarding coding, provider documentation, and incomplete medical records: "The importance of consistent, complete documentation in the medical record cannot be overemphasized. Without such documentation the application of coding guidelines is a difficult, if not impossible, task."

Accurate coding is necessary for **optimization** of reimbursement, particularly in a PPS, and is best achieved through coding from a complete medical record. Optimization occurs when the coding results in the MS-DRG that most accurately represents the facility's utilization of resources, on the basis of the diagnoses and procedures, and is completely substantiated by documentation. **Maximization,** on the other hand, is simply assigning and sequencing codes to obtain the highest-paying MS-DRG. Optimization is highly desirable; maximization is illegal and unethical. Patterns of maximization could be considered abuse. Patterns of maximization that intentionally result in excessive payments to the provider are considered fraud. Under the U.S. government's National Correct Coding Initiative (NCCI), as well as fraud and abuse audits, patterns of maximization, if proved, can result in the criminal prosecution of facility administrators as well as individual complicit employees.

## Coding Compliance

A comprehensive coding compliance plan is an important part of a facility's corporate compliance plan. The coding compliance plan should include regular internal audits and audits performed by objective external reviewers who have no vested interest in the facility's profit margin. Coding audits performed by payers are not necessarily useful in determining coding accuracy because their overall goal is to find only those coding errors that adversely affect the payer. In any type of audit, however, results should be shared and discussed with the coding staff.

There are two fundamentally different approaches to coding audits: general reviews of all records of all payer types to identify potential problems and targeted reviews of known or potential problem areas. In general reviews, records are selected by a statistical method or by any method that captures a representative sample of records. All coders, all record types, and all payers should be included in a general review. The audit results can be used to determine coding error rates by coder or more generally.

**electronic health record (EHR)** A secure real-time, point-of-care, patient centric information resource for clinicians allowing access to patient information when and where needed and incorporating evidence-based decision support.

**CAC** computer-assisted coding

**reliability** A characteristic of quality exhibited when codes are consistently assigned by one or more coders for similar or identical cases.
**validity** The data quality characteristic of a recorded observation falling within a predetermined size or range of values.

**National Center for Health Statistics (NCHS)** A member of the Cooperating Parties. Sponsored by the Centers for Disease Control, a health care agency that reports on current public health care concerns.
**Cooperating Parties** The four organizations responsible for maintaining the ICD-10-CM: CMS, NCHS, AHA, and AHIMA.

**optimization** The process of determining the most accurate DRG payment.
**Prospective Payment System (PPS)** A system used by payers, primarily CMS, for reimbursing acute care facilities on the basis of statistical analysis of health care data.
**maximization** The process of determining the highest possible DRG payment.

**coding compliance plan** The development, implementation, and enforcement of policies and procedures to ensure that coding standards are met.

**Go To** See Chapter 12 for more information on compliance.

**DRG** diagnosis related group
**OIG** Office of the Inspector General

**Quality Improvement Organization (QIO)** An organization that contracts with payers, specifically Medicare and Medicaid, to review care and reimbursement issues.
**Recovery Audit Contractors (RACs)** Entities contracting with CMS that audit providers, using DRG assignment and other data to identify overpayments and underpayments.

**CMS** Centers for Medicare and Medicaid Services

Targeted reviews may be aimed at specific coders, codes, DRGs, MS-DRGs, or other factors or elements of coding. For example, the OIG develops a list of so-called targeted MS-DRGs, which are MS-DRGs that have a history of aberrant coding (i.e., inaccurate coding leading to Medicare overpayments). **Quality Improvement Organizations (QIOs)** monitor and assess facility data and may perform reviews of cases assigned to these targeted MS-DRGs. **Recovery Audit Contractors (RACs)** are another group that reviews cases on behalf of CMS. RACs request records on the basis of targeted cases, including the DRG assignment as well as medical necessity. RACs review all providers, including physicians, durable medical equipment providers, and hospitals. Regardless of audit findings, coding error rates are not applicable to targeted reviews because such audits are not based on a random selection.

Throughout this chapter, the importance of the coding function and reimbursement has been emphasized. The essence of being a professional coder entails training and development, continuous education, knowledge and application of current rules, regulations, and guidelines, and ethical conduct, in spite of daily challenges and pressures. Performing the coding function well makes the professional coder a valuable member of the health care team.

## EXERCISE 7-6

### Impact of Coding

1. Why is the timing of postdischarge processing important to a coder?
2. What is a coding compliance plan?
3. Explain the difference between optimization and maximization.
4. Compare and contrast two different approaches to high-quality coding audits.

## WORKS CITED

American Hospital Association, National Uniform Billing Committee: The History of the NUBC. http://www.nubc.org/history.html. Published 2010. Accessed October 22, 2012.

Blue Cross. About the Blue Cross Association: The Prototype. http://www.bcbs.com/about-the-association/ Accessed November 19, 2012.

Centers for Medicare and Medicaid Services: Acute Inpatient Prospective Payment System— Outlier Payments. http://cms.gov. Published 2005. Accessed July 12, 2006.

Centers for Medicare and Medicaid Services: Three Day Payment Window. https://www.cms.gov/Medicare/Medicare-Fee-for-ServicePayment/AcuteInpatientPPS/Three_Day_Payment_Window.html. Accessed August 28, 2012.

Diagnosis related groups definitions manual, 6th revision, Number 89-009 Rev.00, New Haven, CT, 1989, Health Systems International.

Health Information Policy Council: 1984 Revision of the Uniform Hospital Discharge Data Set. Federal Register 50:31038–31040, 1985.

Indian Health Services: Indian Health Service Introduction: The Prototype. http://ihs.gov/index.cfm?module=ihsIntro. Published 2012. Accessed October 22, 2012.

Medicare: Hospital outpatient services; prospective payment system. Federal Register 65(68):18433–18820, 2000.

Sultz H, Young K: Health care USA: understanding its organization and delivery, ed 5, Sudbury, MA, 2006, Jones & Bartlett.

## SUGGESTED READING

AHIMA Coding Practice team: Internet resources for accurate coding and reimbursement practices. (AHIMA Practice Brief), J AHIMA 75:48A–48G, 2004.

American Hospital Association: Coding clinic for ICD-9-CM. Chicago, published quarterly, American Hospital Association.

Averill, RF, Grant TM, Steinbeck BA: Preparing for the outpatient prospective payment system, J AHIMA 71:35–43, 2000.

Bowman S: Coordination of SNOMED-CT and ICD-10: Getting the most out of electronic health record systems, Perspect Health Inf Manag 65(68), 2005.

Brown F: ICD-9-CM coding handbook, with answers, Chicago, 2006, American Hospital Association.

Cade T: A comparison of current prospective payment system methodologies in the United States. In 2004 IFHRO Congress & AHIMA Convention Proceedings. Washington, D.C., October 2004.

CPT assistant, Chicago: American Medical Association, 2006. Accessed August 22, 2012.

Schraffenberger LA, Keuhn L, editors: Effective management of coding services, ed 3, Chicago, 2007, American Health Information Management Association.

Scichilone R: Getting ready for APCs, J AHIMA 70:84–92, 1999.

## CHAPTER ACTIVITIES

## CHAPTER SUMMARY

One of the key uses for coded data is reimbursement. Medicare prospective payment systems arose out of cost-control measures and are based on code systems originally designed for other purposes. Inpatient hospitals are reimbursed using Medical Severity–Diagnosis Related Groups (MS-DRGs). Medicare outpatient services are reimbursed under Ambulatory Patient Classifications (APCs). Additional Prospective Payment Systems include Inpatient Psychiatric Facility Prospective Payment System (IPF PPS), Inpatient Rehabilitation Facility Prospective Payment System (IRF PPS), Long-Term Care Hospital Prospective Payment System (LTCH-PPS), Home Health Prospective Payment System (HH PPS), Skilled Nursing Facility Prospective Payment System (SNF PPS), and Resource Utilization Groups (RUGs).

Billing in a hospital is generally the responsibility of the patient accounts department. Charges are posted to the patient's account on the basis of data maintained in the facility's Chargemaster, or Charge Description Master. Hospital-based services are submitted for payment using a Uniform Bill, currently UB-04. Outpatient services are billed using the CMS-1500 form. Because of the importance of the coded data in correct billing and collections, health information professionals must maintain a strong working relationship with the patient accounts professionals.

Coders are an integral part of maintaining the quality of a facility's coded clinical data, ensuring compliance with regulatory mandates, and facilitating optimal reimbursement.

## REVIEW QUESTIONS

1. What are the financial risks in health care delivery for providers, third party payers, and patients?
2. List, compare, and contrast four reimbursement methodologies.
3. Compare and contrast indemnity health insurance plans with managed care plans.
4. Describe government involvement in health insurance.
5. Discuss the impact of the prospective payment system on the coding function.
6. List three prospective payment systems, and describe how reimbursement is obtained in each.
7. Discuss the significance of a hospital's case mix index and reasons that it should be monitored.
8. What are the major differences between MS-DRGs and ambulatory patient classifications (APCs)?
9. Discuss the relationship between the HIM department and the patient accounts department with regard to unbilled accounts in an acute care hospital.
10. Provide an example of how incorrect inpatient coding would financially affect a hospital.
11. Distinguish between the UB-04 and the CMS-1500.
12. Describe how charges are captured in an inpatient setting, and compare this process with charge capture in an ambulatory setting.
13. Describe and discuss an example of an unethical coding practice.
14. What is the difference between optimization and maximization?
15. Name two types of coding audits. When would you use each?

● **CAREER TIP**
The level of skill needed to manage a physician group practice depends on the size and scope of the practice. A bachelor's degree in a health care–related field, such as HIM, is a good start. Experience in a physician office setting is helpful, particularly demonstrating progressive increase in responsibility. For very large practices, a master's degree may be required.

● **PROFESSIONAL PROFILE**

### Practice Manager

My name is Sherri, and I am the Practice Manager for a group partnership of six physicians who specialize in internal medicine, Ridgewood Medical Associates. I use my expertise in physician billing and contract negotiations to ensure that Ridgewood Medical Associates receives the appropriate payments and reimbursement from our patients and insurers after services are rendered.

I began my career in health care by taking a coding certificate course at my local community college. Our course work included coding all types of patient records and outpatient encounters, and I realized that I preferred outpatient coding. After I completed the course, I sat for the American Health Information Management Association (AHIMA) Certified Coding Specialist—Physician-based (CCS-P) exam, passed it, and earned my credential as a CCS-P. I was fortunate to find a position working for a physician billing company.

As a physician biller, I applied my knowledge of HCPCS/CPT-4 and ICD-9-CM coding, adding the correct codes to billing claims so that physicians could be reimbursed for services rendered. After a few years as a physician biller, I was ready for new challenges to further my career. I applied for the position of practice manager for Ridgewood Medical Associates and was hired.

To perform my job well, I must manage and oversee the many daily tasks and functions of a busy medical practice. First, I must make sure that every new and existing patient is registered in our patient billing system with the correct information according to insurance type. Because we accept all types of patient insurance and also accept self-pay patients, we need to know who must pay a deductible, who must pay a copay, and who will pay out-of-pocket fees. We store this information and patient demographic details electronically, and we anticipate adding clinical information as we move toward adopting an electronic health record (EHR). Our goal is to become a paperless office within 5 years. I keep abreast of the latest information concerning the EHR through my professional association, AHIMA. I am also a member of the Medical Group Management Association (see http://www.mgms.com).

Patients who are in managed care plans may require from one of our physicians a referral to see a specialist. It is my job to see that the referral process does not inconvenience either our patients or our physicians. To accomplish this goal, I need to know which managed care plans require a referral and for which specialties. I access referral forms from each managed care plan's Web site and download them from my computer. These referral forms are made accessible to our physicians at all times; they can either retrieve the forms online or use one of the hard copies that are readily available in patient treatment areas. If our physician orders a referral to a different specialist outside our group practice, I assist our patient by making appointment and ensuring that our referral form and any necessary medical records are forwarded to the specialist in time for the appointment.

I supervise our billing staff and perform periodic audits of the codes submitted to insurers on claims submissions. We must submit accurate claims, including codes, to insurers to be properly reimbursed and also to avoid claims rejections. We submit most of our claims electronically. As a CCS-P, I stay abreast of any code changes or changes in claims submission requirements. I must also periodically remind our physicians to provide our billing staff with documentation that is complete and legible.

I also supervise our accounting staff. I receive detailed monthly reports that include an analysis of each insurer's payments to us. If I see that our expenses to treat a certain insurer's patients are not covered under the reimbursement we receive, I will negotiate with that insurer for a higher reimbursement to be applied for the next contract period. I must be able to review each insurer's contract and understand contract language so that I go into negotiations well prepared.

As a practice manager, I am involved in every nonclinical aspect of Ridgewood Medical Associates. I look forward to going to work each day because of the variety of functions that I oversee, and I also feel that I am helping our patients. The physicians value my work because I minimize the time that they must spend filling out paperwork and worrying about reimbursement. When I perform my job well, I enable our physicians to devote their time and clinical expertise to our patients.

## PATIENT CARE PERSPECTIVE

**Maria**

Recently, I received an explanation of benefits from our insurance company that denied payment for my radiology test because the insurance company had not given authorization for the test that the hospital had coded. I didn't know what that meant, so I called Sherri in the doctor's office to help me make sense of it. She was able to coordinate a conversation with the hospital pre-registration department and the insurance company, and they solved the problem together.

## APPLICATIONS

### TIMELY BILLING AND QUALITY CODING

HIM departments are frequently under intense pressure to code medical records as soon as possible after patient discharge so that the hospital may be reimbursed. Pressure may come from patient accounts department staff members, who may not completely understand the myriad reasons that all medical records cannot be accurately coded or even coded at all immediately after discharge. If you were the coding supervisor at a hospital, how would you describe the reasons for delays in coding with patient accounts department staff members? How would you discuss the DNFB (discharged, no final bill) and coding requirements under HIPAA with patient accounts staff members in a collaborative, rather than adversarial, way? Can you identify ways in which patient accounts staff members might help HIM employees decrease delays?

### PATIENT REGISTRATION

You are the manager of patient registration at a community hospital. When registering patients, your staff is required to obtain insurance information. The largest employer in your town has recently changed its employee benefit plan from an indemnity plan to a managed care plan. As manager of patient registration, you must educate your staff as to the differences in registering patients in a managed care plan versus an indemnity plan. For example, what will be your process for obtaining copays? How will your staff handle cash or checks? How will you ensure that cash or check copays are correctly credited to each patient's account? What will you instruct your staff to do if a patient with managed care insurance comes to the hospital for admission but the physician is not a participant in the patient's managed care plan?

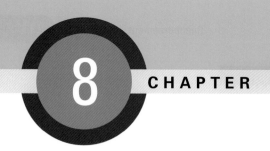

# 8 CHAPTER

# HEALTH INFORMATION MANAGEMENT ISSUES IN OTHER CARE SETTINGS

Angela Kennedy

## CHAPTER OUTLINE

**AMBULATORY CARE**
PHYSICIANS' OFFICES
  Settings
  Services
  Care Providers
  Data Collection Issues
  Data Sets
  Licensure and Accreditation
EMERGENCY DEPARTMENT
  Settings
  Services
  Care Providers
  Data Collection Issues
  Data Sets
  Licensure and Accreditation
RADIOLOGY AND LABORATORY
  SERVICES
  Settings
  Services
  Care Providers
  Data Collection Issues
  Licensure and Accreditation
AMBULATORY SURGERY
  Length of Stay

Settings
Services
Care Providers
Data Collection Issues
Data Sets
Licensure and Accreditation
**OTHER INPATIENT HEALTH CARE
SETTINGS**
LONG-TERM CARE
  Length of Stay
  Settings
  Services
  Care Providers
  Data Collection Issues
  Data Sets
  Licensure and Accreditation
BEHAVIORAL HEALTH FACILITIES
  Length of Stay
  Settings
  Behavioral Health Services
  Drug and Alcohol
    Rehabilitation
  Care Providers
  Data Collection Issues

Data Sets
Licensure and Accreditation
REHABILITATION FACILITIES
  Length of Stay
  Settings
  Services
  Care Providers
  Data Collection Issues
  Data Sets
  Licensure and Accreditation
HOSPICE
  Length of Stay
  Services
  Care Providers
  Data Collection Issues
  Licensure and Accreditation
**OTHER SPECIALTY CARE**
HOME HEALTH CARE
  Settings
  Services
  Care Providers
  Data Collection Issues
  Data Sets
  Licensure and Accreditation

## VOCABULARY

Accreditation Association
  for Ambulatory
  Health Care
  (AAAHC)
ambulatory care
ambulatory care facility
ambulatory surgery
ambulatory surgery center
  (ASC)
baseline
cancer treatment center
clinic
cognitive remediation
Commission on
  Accreditation of

Rehabilitation Facilities
  (CARF)
Community Health
  Accreditation Program
  (CHAP)
Data Elements for
  Emergency Department
  Systems (DEEDS)
dialysis
dialysis centers
electronic data interchange
  (EDI)
encounter
group practice
home health care

hospice
laboratory
long-term care facility
mobile diagnostic
multispecialty group
National Center for Injury
  Prevention and Control
  (NCIPC)
National Committee for
  Quality Assurance
  (NCQA)
Outcome and Assessment
  Information Set (OASIS)
pain management
  treatment center

palliative care
physiatrist
physician's office
picture archiving and
  communication system
  (PACS)
primary care physician
  (PCP)
primary caregiver
radiology
Resident Assessment
  Instrument
  (RAI)
Resident Assessment
  Protocol (RAP)

respite care
retail care
skilled nursing facilities
  (SNFs)

Substance Abuse and
  Mental Health Services
  Administration
  (SAMHSA)

triage
Uniform Ambulatory
  Care Data Set
  (UACDS)

Urgent Care Association of
  America (UCAOA)
urgent care center
visit

## CHAPTER OBJECTIVES

*By the end of this chapter, the student should be able to:*

1. List and describe four ambulatory care facilities.
2. List and describe three types of long-term care settings.
3. Describe the behavioral health care setting including the type of care provided.
4. Describe the rehabilitation health care setting including the type of care provided

5. Describe home health care and hospice care, including the difference in the type of care provided by each.
6. Compare and contrast the data collected in acute care facilities with data collected in non-acute care facilities.
7. List and describe the data sets unique to non-acute care facilities.

So far, this text has addressed what occurs in an acute care facility, including how data are collected and by whom. Previous chapters mentioned the special data requirements of certain diagnoses and other health care facilities. In this chapter these other health care facilities—ambulatory care, long-term care (LTC), behavioral health, rehabilitation, home health, and hospice—are described in more detail. The most important thing to remember is that the skills and the knowledge presented thus far in this text are applicable to any health care delivery system. Demographic, financial, socioeconomic, and clinical data are collected in all settings. The volume and types of physician data, nursing data, and data from therapy, social services, and psychology vary significantly, depending on the diagnosis and the setting. In addition to discipline-specific data requirements, health care facilities must also comply with the licensure regulations of the state in which they operate. The regulations may include very specific documentation requirements based on the type of care provided. Further, all facilities seeking full Medicare reimbursement must comply with the Medicare Conditions of Participation. The Centers for Medicare and Medicaid Services (CMS) Web site should be consulted for detailed information about those requirements. Health information management (HIM) professionals who are employed in special health care settings should become familiar with the unique data requirements of those settings. The Joint Commission (TJC) offers accreditation to all providers discussed in this chapter, either independently or in conjunction with the host facility.

> **acute care facility** A health care facility in which patients have an average length of stay less than 30 days and that has an emergency department, operating suite, and clinical departments to handle a broad range of diagnoses and treatments.
>
> **licensure** The mandatory government approval required for performing specified activities. In health care, the state approval required for providing health care services.
>
> **Centers for Medicare and Medicaid Services (CMS)** The division of the U.S. government's Department of Health and Human Services that administers Medicare and Medicaid.

**Go To** Review demographic, financial, socioeconomic, and clinical data Chapter 2.

### HIT-bit

**OUTPATIENT**

When ambulatory services are offered by an otherwise inpatient facility, the patients receiving them are also called outpatients.

## AMBULATORY CARE

Ambulatory, or outpatient, care is provided in a brief period, typically in 1 day or in less than 24 hours. This timing distinguishes it from inpatient care, in which the patient is admitted and is expected to stay overnight. As discussed in Chapter 1, a physician's office is only one type of ambulatory care setting. Although other types of ambulatory care settings provide different services from a physician's office, the basic clinical flow of events is similar. Ambulatory care services are the most frequently utilized patient care service in the health care industry. Changes in reimbursement methodologies and innovations in technology and medicine during the 1980s and 1990s can explain the shift from care provided in acute, inpatient to ambulatory settings.

> **outpatient** A patient whose health care services are intended to be delivered within 1 calendar day or, in some cases, a 24-hour period.
>
> **reimbursement** The amount of money that the health care facility receives from the party responsible for paying the bill.

**ambulatory care** Care provided on an outpatient basis, in which the patient is not admitted: arriving at a facility, receiving treatment, and leaving within 1 day.

**encounter** A patient's health care experience; a unit of measure for the volume of ambulatory care services provided.

**visit** In ambulatory care, a unit of measuring the number of patients who have been served.

The term **ambulatory care** refers to a wide range of preventive and therapeutic services provided at a variety of facilities. Patients receive those services in a relatively short time. Facilities render services on the same day that the patient arrives for treatment or, in some cases, within 24 hours. Therefore the terms *admission* and *discharge* have little or no relevance in ambulatory care. In the ambulatory care environment, the interaction between patient and provider is referred to as an **encounter** or a **visit**.

## HIT-bit

### QUANTITY OF SERVICES

To determine the quantity of services rendered, we count the number of visits or encounters. *Visits* and *encounters* may mean the same thing. For example, think of a patient who goes to a physician's office to see the doctor and undergoes a chest radiograph at the same time in the same facility. The patient interacted with the facility in two ways: an examination by the doctor and a chest radiograph. Think of it another way: The patient *visited* the facility and *encountered* the doctor and the radiology technician. Thus the visit represents the number of times that the patient interacted with the facility as a whole. The encounter represents the number of different areas of the facility that were used or services provided. As the different ambulatory care settings are explored in this chapter, think about the ways to count the quantity of services rendered.

**ambulatory care facility** An outpatient facility, such as an emergency department or physician's office, in which treatment is intended to occur within 1 calendar day.

**retention** The procedures governing the storage of records, including duration, location, security, and access.

**analysis** The review of a record to evaluate its completeness, accuracy, or compliance with predetermined standards or other criteria.

Beyond the time frame stated previously, the services rendered in **ambulatory care facilities** vary widely. Each type of facility has its own specific data collection, retention, and analysis needs. However, the general flows of patient care are similar. The patient initiates the interaction, gives demographic and financial data to the facility, meets with the provider, who documents the clinical care, and the patient then implements any follow-up instructions, such as diagnostic testing or a visit to a specialist.

## PHYSICIANS' OFFICES

### Settings

**physician's office** A setting for providing ambulatory care in which the primary provider is the physician.

**Go To** Chapter 1 introduces many different types of physicians.

A **physician's office** is one type of ambulatory care facility. Some physicians have offices attached to their homes; others have space in office buildings or in a medical mall (a building that contains only health care practitioners in a variety of specialties). Still others are associated with different types of facilities and, as employees, maintain offices in those facilities. Some physicians do not see patients at all. For example, a pathologist examines tissue samples in a laboratory. Some radiologists examine only radiographs and other types of imaging results. In general, these physicians give results of those examinations to another physician to discuss with the patient. For the purposes of this section, only physicians who see patients in their offices are discussed.

**continuity of care** The broad range of health care services required by a patient during an illness or for an entire lifetime. May also refer to the continuity of care provided by a health care organization. Also called *continnuum of care.*

**group practice** Multiple physicians who share facilities and resources and may also cooperate in rendering patient care.

### Group Practice

Sometimes physicians share office space and personnel with other physicians to reduce the cost of maintaining an office, to share financial risk, to increase flexible time, and to improve continuity of care. This type of physician's office is called a **group practice**. For example, several physicians working together may need only one receptionist. Sharing office space and personnel also provides increased opportunities for professional collaboration among physicians and can improve the continuity of care for the patients served by the practice. Administrative responsibilities of the practice may be shared by all physicians in the practice. Physicians in a group practice share the burden of being "on call" or available 24 hours a day and are afforded emergency, vacation, and holiday coverage by their colleagues. Physicians in a group practice can distribute the cost of capital investments, innovations, and technology across the practice and reduce the individual financial burdens. Physicians may share a physician's assistant or nurse practitioner. Staffing of this nature may be cost prohibitive in a solo practice.

Group practices may have only one type of physician, such as a group of family practitioners. Frequently, these physicians not only share office space and personnel but also see one another's patients. To help one another with their patient loads, the physicians must also collaborate in developing and maintaining relationships with insurance companies.

Another combination of physicians may consist of several different specialties; this arrangement is called a **multispecialty group**. A family practice physician may be in a group with a pediatrician and a gynecologist, for example. One of the advantages of a multispecialty group practice is the convenience of centralized care that it provides for the patient.

Another administrative advantage of a group practice is the ability to centralize record keeping. Whether the patient records are maintained in paper or electronic form, centralization offers substantial cost savings and efficiency.

## HIT-bit

### OPEN-ACCESS PHYSICIAN OFFICES

Some physicians rely solely on appointments for scheduling office time. Other physicians employ open-access techniques. In open access, some appointments are made, but time is allowed for patients who call for a same-day appointment. Scheduling appointments requires knowledge of time budgeting, and implementation of open-access methods requires a firm understanding of the demand for time in relation to the number of patients per doctor.

## Clinic

A **clinic** is a facility-based ambulatory care service that provides general or specialized care such as those provided in a physician's office. Clinics may be funded or established by charitable organizations, the government, or different types of health care facilities. For example, a community health center is a type of clinic that provides primary or secondary care in a specific geographical area. Many of these centers are located in areas accessible to populations that have challenges with accessing health care. Many acute care facilities have developed clinics that resemble physicians' office services. A hospital may have primary care and specialty clinics that serve particular patient populations, such as an infectious disease clinic or an orthopedic clinic. Clinics may also closely resemble multispecialty group practices. Large teaching facilities may be affiliated with many clinics. The clinic may be part of the physicians' general practice, the physicians may be employees of the parent facility, or they may donate their time, often called *in-kind service*.

## Urgent Care Center

An **urgent care center** provides unscheduled care outside the emergency department (ED) on a walk-in basis. An urgent care center treats injuries and illnesses that are in need of immediate attention but are not life threatening. Urgent care centers are usually stand-alone facilities equipped with on-site diagnostics and point-of-care medication dispensing. Use of urgent care centers is encouraged by payers and managed care organizations. The centers may be stand-alone or affiliated with a clinic, group practice, or hospital.

In 2009, the **Urgent Care Association of America (UCAOA)** established criteria for urgent care centers. The American Medical Association grants the specialty in urgent care medicine (UCM) to physicians who choose to specialize in the discipline. Practitioners are licensed in the state in which they operate. Urgent care accreditation is offered by TJC. The Comprehensive Accreditation Manual for Ambulatory Care (CAMAC) and National Patient Safety Goals to Reduce Medical Errors guide the accreditation process.

---

**Physician's Office Coding Notes**
Diagnosis Code is ICD-10-CM.
Procedure Code is HCPCS/CPT.*
Example:
- **E11.9** Type 2 diabetes mellitus without complications
- **99203** Office visit, established patient
- Bill format: CMS-1500

*CPT copyright 2012 American Medical Association. All rights reserved. CPT is a registered trademark of the American Medical Association.

**multispecialty group** In ambulatory care, a group practice consisting of physicians with different specialties.

**clinic** A facility-based ambulatory care department that provides general or specialized services, such as those provided in a physician's office.

**urgent care center** A facility that treats patients whose illness or injury requires immediate attention but that is not life threatening.

**payer** The individual or organization that is primarily responsible for the reimbursement for a particular health care service. Usually refers to the insurance company or third party.

**managed care** A type of insurer (payer) focused on reducing health care costs, controlling expensive care, and improving the quality of patient care provided.

**Urgent Care Association of America (UCAOA)** A professional organization representing those working in urgent care settings, serving as an advocate for the role of urgent care facilities in health care delivery.

**accreditation** Voluntary compliance with a set of standards developed by an independent agent, who periodically performs audits to ensure compliance.

**National Patient Safety Goals** Guidance created by TJC to recommend patient saftey measures in accredited facilities.

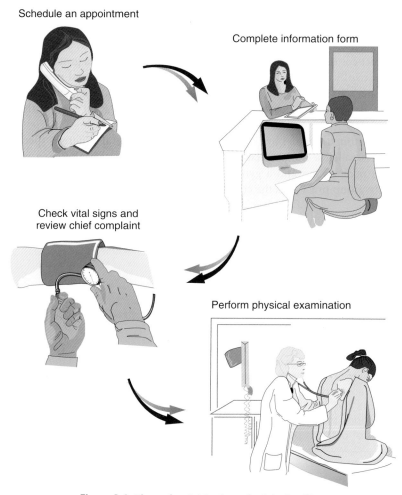

Schedule an appointment

Complete information form

Check vital signs and review chief complaint

Perform physical examination

Figure 8-1 Flow of activities in a physician's office.

## Services

The following sections describe a hypothetical visit to a physician's office to trace the clinical flow of a patient's data through the office and list the data that are collected. This visit is a general guide to the events to illustrate the flow of health information in the ambulatory care settings as previously mentioned. Figure 8-1 shows the flow of activities in a typical physician's office.

A patient can generally choose the physician he or she will visit as long as the physician chosen is accepting new patients. However, a patient who expects his or her insurance plan to pay all or part of the cost of the visit must take into consideration whether the physician is included in the insurance plan. If payment is an issue, the first step in selecting a physician is to determine whether that physician participates in the patient's insurance plan. The patient may also ask friends and family members for recommendations. If the patient needs to see a specialist, such as a cardiologist, some insurance plans require that the **primary care physician** (**PCP**) refer the patient to a specific physician. Some specialists, such as thoracic surgeons, see only those patients who have been referred by other physicians. Thus the visit is initiated either by the patient or by referral and may be influenced by the patient's insurance plan. Some insurance plans allow patients to self-refer for certain services, such as obstetrics and gynecology.

## Care Providers

After choosing a physician, the patient calls the office for an appointment. Very likely, the patient will speak to someone who works with the physician. The individual who answers

**visit** In ambulatory care, a unit of measuring the number of patients who have been served.

**primary care physician (PCP)** In insurance, the physician who has been designated by the insured to deliver routine care to the insured and to evaluate the need for referral to a specialist, if applicable. Colloquial use is synonymous with "family doctor."

the telephone and handles the appointments may be any one of a number of different allied health professionals, such as a receptionist, a medical secretary, or a medical assistant. A *receptionist* usually handles the telephones, does some filing, and schedules appointments. A *medical secretary* has a more detailed knowledge of office procedures, scheduling, filing, and billing. A *medical assistant* has all of that similar knowledge and some basic clinical knowledge, such as measuring and recording blood pressure and temperature, changing dressings, and assisting the physician in examining and treating the patient. Medical secretaries and medical assistants have generally received formal training, particularly if they are certified in their fields.

Other personnel who support the physician include physician's assistants, nurses, and advanced practice registered nurses. A physician's assistant (PA) is a highly trained clinical professional who collect a variety of data, including the medical history, and assist the physician in diagnosing and treating patients. PAs undergo at least 2 years of training, including rotations through multiple specialties. An Advanced Practice Registered Nurse (APRN) has completed either a Master of Nursing or a Doctor of Nursing degree and additional training in their speciality. APRNs include certified registered nurse anesthetists, certified nurse-midwives, clinical nurse specialists, and certified nurse practitioners. APRNs may deliver primary care and often work in areas where there are not enough physicians. PAs and APRNs require state licensure to practice and the extent to which they may practice is determined by state regulations. Individual facilities further specify practice within the facility. Figure 8-2 shows some employees common in a physician's office.

## Data Collection Issues

Suppose that a physician's office has a number of different staff members and employs a receptionist to handle telephone calls and appointments. When the patient calls for an appointment, the receptionist asks for the patient's name and telephone number and inquires whether he or she is a current patient. The patient's status will be verified, often while he or she is still on the phone. It is very important to know whether the patient is a current patient, because a new patient requires more data collection, which takes more of the staff's time, and a longer appointment with the physician. Also, if the physician is not taking new patients, the patient must be directed to another physician. The receptionist also asks why the patient wants to see the physician, information that aids in scheduling. A regular patient coming in for a flu shot takes far less of the physician's time than does a new patient who complains of stomach pains. Identification of a new versus an established

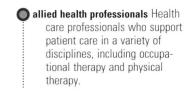

**allied health professionals** Health care professionals who support patient care in a variety of disciplines, including occupational therapy and physical therapy.

**PA** physician's assistant
**APRN** Advanced Practice Registered Nurse

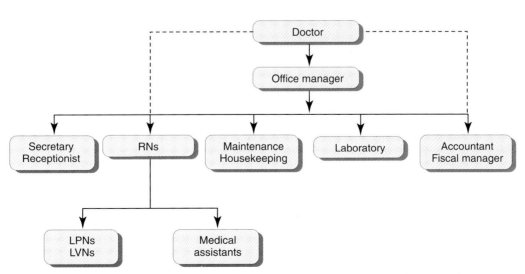

**Figure 8-2** Sample of employees in a physician's office. LPN, Licensed Practical Nurse; LVN, Licensed Vocational Nurse; RN, Registered Nurse. (From Simmers L: *Diversified health occupations,* ed 4, Albany, 1998, Delmar Publishers, Inc.)

**billing** The process of submitting health insurance claims or rendering invoices.

**medical record number (MR#)** A unique number assigned to each patient in a health care system; this code will be used for the rest of the patient's encounters with that specific health system.

**point-of-care documentation** Clinical data recorded at the time the treatment is delivered to the patient.

**Go To** Chapter 12 discusses this authorization and other types of consents and releases.

**baseline** A beginning value; the value at which an activity is originally measured, such as the first blood pressure reading at an initial physician's office visit.

**history and physical (H&P)** Health record documentation comprising the patient's history and physical examination; a formal, dictated copy must be included in the patient's health care record within 24 hours of admission for inpatient facilities.

**copay** A fixed amount paid by the patient at the time of service.

patient is also important for billing of physician services. The receptionist will ask the patient whether he or she is insured and who the payer is. If the physician does not accept the patient's insurance, it is preferred that the patient know this before the visit so that the method of payment can be determined or an alternate physician may be chosen. The office staff will verify the patient's insurance before the visit—protecting the patient from incurring unnecessary bills.

When the patient gets to the office, the receptionist asks the patient to fill out some forms. On these forms, the patient provides personal data: name and address, past medical history, emergency contact, and how the patient intends to pay for the services. The receptionist or a medical secretary may then enter some or all of this data into the electronic registration system. Some electronic record systems allow the patient to complete the forms online, eliminating the paper and data entry step. Patients will sign forms that authorize the physician to treat them, to release information to their insurance companies, and to acknowledge their receipt of the physician's statement of privacy policies.

In a paper-based environment, a folder is created for each new patient, labeled by name and medical record number, and used to hold the personal data form as well as any other documentation, such as a copy of the insurance card, the clinical notes, and copies of reports and test results. At each subsequent visit, the folder would be retrieved and visit data added. Historically, the folder has been the only record; however, capturing the administrative and clinical data in a point-of-care information system instead of on paper is becoming increasingly common. Computerization offers options for alerts and reminders for patient health care maintenance and provides easy access for staff and clinicians for patient care and billing purposes.

Once the administrative record-keeping processes are completed, a medical assistant or nurse measures and records the patient's temperature, blood pressure, height, and weight—all data that develop a profile of information about the patient and the visit. If this is the patient's first visit, this profile is called the **baseline**. It is the information against which all future visits will be compared.

Eventually, the physician meets the patient and performs and documents the appropriate level of history and physical. Perhaps the physician recommends tests to determine the extent of disease or to help determine the diagnosis. If the diagnosis is clear, the physician prescribes therapeutic treatment at this visit, which could be medications (prescription), therapy services, diagnostic procedures (radiology, laboratory) or referral to another physician. Before the patient leaves the physician's office, he or she either remits payment for the visit or signs a release for the insurance company. For managed care patients, a copay may be required, which is paid at the time of the visit.

Table 8-1 contrasts care events in acute care and ambulatory care settings.

**TABLE 8-1**

**CONTRAST BETWEEN KEY AMBULATORY AND ACUTE CARE EVENTS**

| | AMBULATORY CARE (PHYSICIAN'S OFFICE) | ACUTE CARE (HOSPITAL) |
|---|---|---|
| How to choose | Referral, advertisement, or investigation | Choices limited to facilities in which physician has privileges |
| | Choices sometimes limited by insurance plan | Choices sometimes limited by insurance plan |
| Initiate contact | Call for an appointment; walk in, if permitted | Emergency department or attending physician orders admission |
| Collection of demographic and financial data | Receptionist, medical secretary | Patient registration, patient access, or admissions department personnel |
| Initial assessment | Vital signs and chief complaint recorded by physician, nurse, or medical assistant | Nursing assessment |
| | | Physician responsible for history and physical examination |
| Plan of care | Prescriptions, instructions, diagnostic tests, and therapeutic procedures performed on an ambulatory basis | Medication administration, instructions, and diagnostic tests performed on an inpatient basis |

## TABLE 8-2

### SUMMARY OF MINIMUM DATA SETS

| DATA SET | SETTING |
|---|---|
| Uniform Hospital Discharge Data Set (UHDDS) | Acute care |
| Uniform Ambulatory Care Data Set (UACDS) | Ambulatory care |
| Minimum Data Set (MDS) | Long-term care |
| Outcome and Assessment Information Set (OASIS) | Home health care |
| Data Elements for Emergency Department Systems (DEEDS) | Emergency departments |

---

**BOX 8-1**  **SECTIONS I, II, AND III OF THE UNIFORM AMBULATORY CARE DATA SET (UACDS)**

SECTION I: PATIENT DATA ITEMS
1. Personal Identification (including name and facility reference number)
2. Residence
3. Date of birth
4. Sex
5. Race and ethnicity
6. Living arrangements and marital status (optional)

SECTION II: PROVIDER DATA ITEMS
7. Provider identification
8. Location or address
9. Profession

SECTION III: ENCOUNTER DATA ITEMS
10. Date, place or site, and address of encounter
11. Patient's reason for encounter (optional—problem, diagnosis, or assessment)
12. Services
13. Disposition
14. Patient's expected source of payment
15. Total charges

---

## Data Sets

Minimum data sets are the key data elements about the patient and the health care he or she received. Table 8-2 contains a summary of the data sets discussed in this chapter for use in various health care settings. In ambulatory care, the minimum data set is called the **Uniform Ambulatory Care Data Set (UACDS)**. The UACDS was developed in 1989 by committees working under the auspices of the U.S. Department of Health and Human Services. Reporting of this data is mandatory for facilities who accept Medicare and Medicaid payments. The data set was approved by the National Committee on Vital and Healthcare Statistics (NCVHS) in 1989 and is utilized to improve data comparison of ambulatory and outpatient facilities. The data set provides uniform definitions to aid in analyzing patterns of care. Box 8-1 lists the 15 elements of the UACDS; Figure 8-3 shows the UACDS data elements in relation to the CMS-1500 form.

## Licensure and Accreditation

Practitioners are licensed in the state in which they operate. Ambulatory care accreditation is offered by TJC and the **Accreditation Association for Ambulatory Health Care (AAAHC)**.

**Uniform Ambulatory Care Data Set (UACDS)** The mandated data set for ambulatory care patients.

**Medicare** Federally funded health care insurance plan for older adults and for certain categories of chronically ill patients.

**Medicaid** A federally mandated, state-funded program providing access to health care for the poor and the medically indigent.

**accreditation** Voluntary compliance with a set of standards developed by an independent agent, who periodically performs audits to ensure compliance.

**Accreditation Association for Ambulatory Health Care (AAAHC)** An organization that accredits ambulatory care facilities.

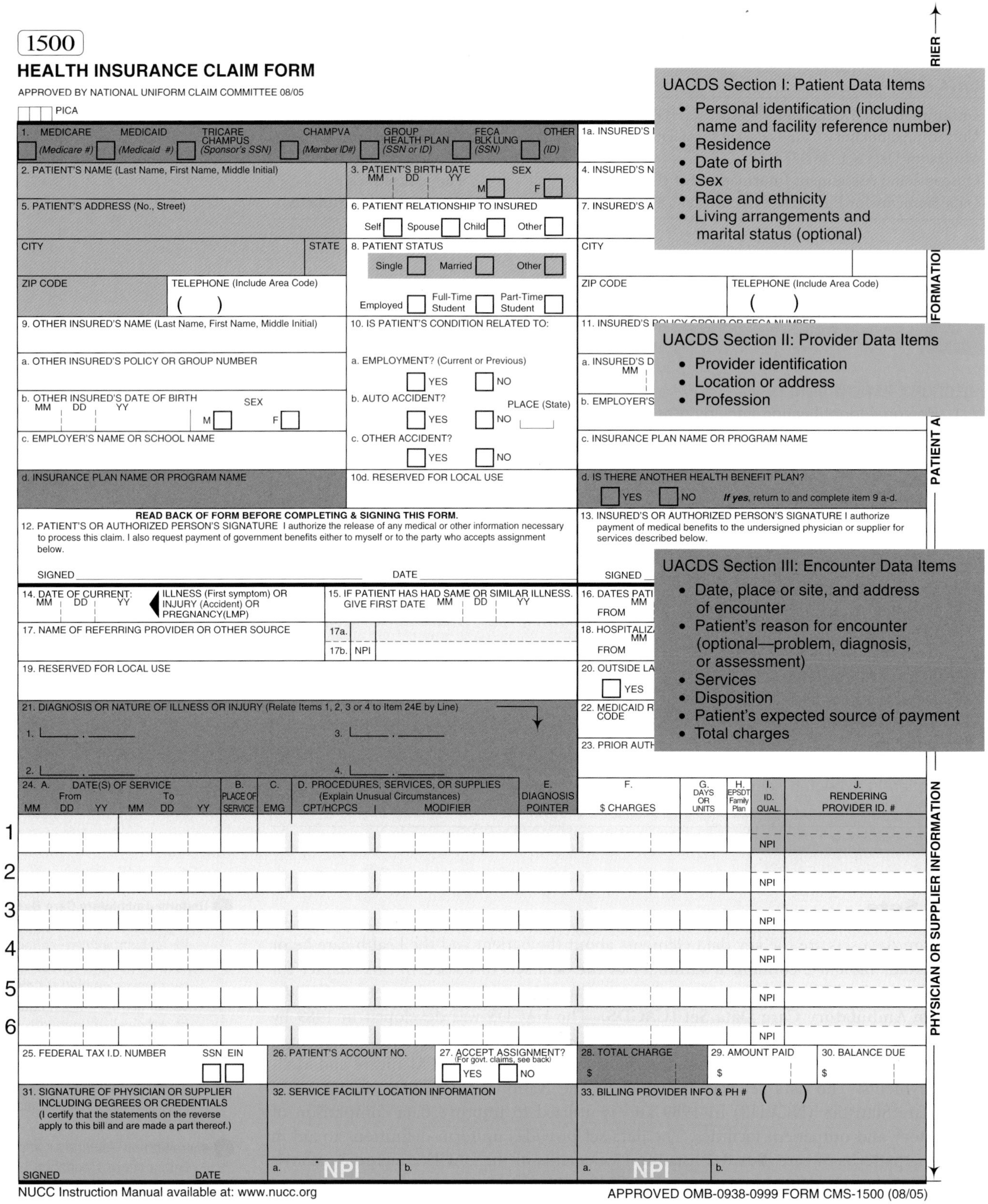
1500

HEALTH INSURANCE CLAIM FORM

APPROVED BY NATIONAL UNIFORM CLAIM COMMITTEE 08/05

PICA

1. MEDICARE (Medicare #) MEDICAID (Medicaid #) TRICARE CHAMPUS (Sponsor's SSN) CHAMPVA (Member ID#) GROUP HEALTH PLAN (SSN or ID) FECA BLK LUNG (SSN) OTHER (ID)

1a. INSURED'S I

2. PATIENT'S NAME (Last Name, First Name, Middle Initial)

3. PATIENT'S BIRTH DATE MM DD YY SEX M F

4. INSURED'S N

5. PATIENT'S ADDRESS (No., Street)

6. PATIENT RELATIONSHIP TO INSURED Self Spouse Child Other

7. INSURED'S A

CITY STATE

8. PATIENT STATUS Single Married Other

CITY

ZIP CODE TELEPHONE (Include Area Code) ( )

Employed Full-Time Student Part-Time Student

ZIP CODE TELEPHONE (Include Area Code) ( )

9. OTHER INSURED'S NAME (Last Name, First Name, Middle Initial)

10. IS PATIENT'S CONDITION RELATED TO:

11. INSURED'S POLICY GROUP OR FECA NUMBER

a. OTHER INSURED'S POLICY OR GROUP NUMBER

a. EMPLOYMENT? (Current or Previous) YES NO

a. INSURED'S D MM

b. OTHER INSURED'S DATE OF BIRTH MM DD YY SEX M F

b. AUTO ACCIDENT? YES NO PLACE (State)

b. EMPLOYER'S

c. EMPLOYER'S NAME OR SCHOOL NAME

c. OTHER ACCIDENT? YES NO

c. INSURANCE PLAN NAME OR PROGRAM NAME

d. INSURANCE PLAN NAME OR PROGRAM NAME

10d. RESERVED FOR LOCAL USE

d. IS THERE ANOTHER HEALTH BENEFIT PLAN? YES NO *If yes,* return to and complete item 9 a-d.

READ BACK OF FORM BEFORE COMPLETING & SIGNING THIS FORM.

12. PATIENT'S OR AUTHORIZED PERSON'S SIGNATURE I authorize the release of any medical or other information necessary to process this claim. I also request payment of government benefits either to myself or to the party who accepts assignment below.

SIGNED DATE

13. INSURED'S OR AUTHORIZED PERSON'S SIGNATURE I authorize payment of medical benefits to the undersigned physician or supplier for services described below.

SIGNED

14. DATE OF CURRENT: MM DD YY ILLNESS (First symptom) OR INJURY (Accident) OR PREGNANCY(LMP)

15. IF PATIENT HAS HAD SAME OR SIMILAR ILLNESS. GIVE FIRST DATE MM DD YY

16. DATES PATI MM FROM

17. NAME OF REFERRING PROVIDER OR OTHER SOURCE

17a.

17b. NPI

18. HOSPITALIZ MM FROM

19. RESERVED FOR LOCAL USE

20. OUTSIDE LA YES

21. DIAGNOSIS OR NATURE OF ILLNESS OR INJURY (Relate Items 1, 2, 3 or 4 to Item 24E by Line)

1. 3.

2. 4.

22. MEDICAID R CODE

23. PRIOR AUTH

24. A. DATE(S) OF SERVICE From To MM DD YY MM DD YY | B. PLACE OF SERVICE | C. EMG | D. PROCEDURES, SERVICES, OR SUPPLIES (Explain Unusual Circumstances) CPT/HCPCS MODIFIER | E. DIAGNOSIS POINTER | F. $ CHARGES | G. DAYS OR UNITS | H. EPSDT Family Plan | I. ID. QUAL. | J. RENDERING PROVIDER ID. #

1 NPI

2 NPI

3 NPI

4 NPI

5 NPI

6 NPI

25. FEDERAL TAX I.D. NUMBER SSN EIN

26. PATIENT'S ACCOUNT NO.

27. ACCEPT ASSIGNMENT? (For govt. claims, see back) YES NO

28. TOTAL CHARGE $

29. AMOUNT PAID $

30. BALANCE DUE $

31. SIGNATURE OF PHYSICIAN OR SUPPLIER INCLUDING DEGREES OR CREDENTIALS (I certify that the statements on the reverse apply to this bill and are made a part thereof.)

SIGNED DATE

32. SERVICE FACILITY LOCATION INFORMATION

a. NPI b.

33. BILLING PROVIDER INFO & PH # ( )

a. NPI b.

NUCC Instruction Manual available at: www.nucc.org

APPROVED OMB-0938-0999 FORM CMS-1500 (08/05)

CARRIER — PATIENT AND INSURED INFORMATION — PHYSICIAN OR SUPPLIER INFORMATION



**Figure 8-3** Uniform Ambulatory Care Data Set (UACDS) data elements included in the form fields of the CMS-1500 claim form.

# EMERGENCY DEPARTMENT

## Settings

Emergency departments (EDs) are unique to hospitals, specifically acute care facilities. They are designed to handle patients in life-threatening situations or crises. Acutely ill patients who are admitted to the hospital from the ED will become inpatients.

---

**HIT-bit**

### AMBULATORY CARE

*Ambulatory* literally means the "process of walking." Therefore an ambulatory care patient is theoretically walking in and out. However, the name is a little misleading. Ambulatory care patients are not always ambulatory. *Ambulatory* also refers to a patient who is able to walk. However, patients in wheelchairs can visit a physician at the office. Some patients are driven to the physician's office in special vans that resemble ambulances. Clearly, in neither case do the patients actually walk into the office, but they are nonetheless ambulatory care patients.

---

In rural and community health settings, the ED is often utilized to host clinics and visiting physicians who provide specialty services. Access to diagnostic equipment and personnel make it an attractive location to host services not otherwise provided to the community. These encounters are scheduled during non-peak, routine daytime hours. These visits often lead to inpatient admissions.

The Emergency Medical Treatment and Active Labor Act (EMTALA) of 1986 was enacted in response to the practice of hospitals refusing to treat indigent patients and transferring such patients to charity care hospitals. EMTALA requires hospitals with EDs to conduct a medical screening examination on any individual who presents for such a purpose. The hospital is obligated by law to stabilize the patient, which may result in the treatment of the patient's condition. Because EMTALA prohibits the hospital from refusing to treat an emergency patient who cannot pay for the services provided, hospitals comply with EMTALA by deferring the request for insurance information until after the medical screening examination. It should be noted that EMTALA does not prohibit billing of the patient subsequent to the visit.

## Services

Emergency department services vary dramatically. Broken legs and heart attacks are typical cases. A *trauma patient* is defined as a patient with a serious illness who has a high risk of dying or suffering morbidity from multiple and severe injuries. Trauma patients often are treated first in the ED and are stabilized there before being admitted to the hospital as inpatients. Because the services vary so much, the facility must determine the order in which to treat the patients. The policy of "first come, first served" does not make much sense when the first patient has strained a ligament and the second patient is experiencing a myocardial infarction. Therefore patients are screened as part of the registration process to determine the priority with which they will be treated. This prioritization process is called **triage** and is generally performed by a registered or advanced practice nurse. In some emergency departments, a separate section of the department is set aside for noncritical services. Noncritical services in this scenario may include minor wound repair, for example.

## Care Providers

The ED is staffed with physicians, nurses, and medical secretaries/unit clerks. The physicians in this department are highly qualified to handle the various types of illnesses and

---

**acute care facility** A health care facility in which patients have an average length of stay less than 30 days and that has an emergency department, operating suite, and clinical departments to handle a broad range of diagnoses and treatments.

**inpatient** An individual who is admitted to a hospital with the intention of staying overnight.

**encounter** A patient's health care experience; a unit of measure for the volume of ambulatory care services provided.

**admission** The act of accepting a patient into care in a health care facility, including any nonambulatory care facility. Admission requires a physician's order.

**EMTALA** Emergency Medical Treatment and Active Labor Act

**ED** emergency department

**Emergency Department Coding Notes**
Diagnosis Code is ICD-10-CM.
Procedure Code is HCPCS/CPT.*
Example:
- **R11.2** Nausea and vomiting
- **99283** Emergency Department Visit
- Bill format: UB-04

*CPT copyright 2012 American Medical Association. All rights reserved. CPT is a registered trademark of the American Medical Association.

**morbidity** A disease or illness.

**triage** In emergency services, the system of prioritizing patients by severity of illness.

**physician's orders** The physician's directions regarding the patient's care.

**allied health professional** Health care professionals who support patient care in a variety of disciplines, including occupational therapy and physical therapy.

**National Center for Injury Prevention and Control (NCIPC)** A component of the CDC that focuses on reducing injuries and the diseases associated with, death from, and sequelae of injuries.

**Data Elements for Emergency Department Systems (DEEDS)** Minimum data set for emergency services.

**electronic data interchange (EDI)** A standard in which data can be transmitted, communicated, and understood by the sending and receiving computer systems, allowing the exchange of information.

**UACDS** Uniform Ambulatory Care Data Set

injuries of the patients who seek treatment in the ED. In one room a physician may treat a child with a bead stuck in the ear and in the very next room may diagnose and treat a patient who was involved in a major traffic accident and is unconscious and bleeding internally. The nurses also have a high level of skills in order to provide nursing care for these patients. The unit secretary in this department is very helpful in facilitating the flow of patient care, making sure that the physician's orders are followed in timely fashion, requesting patient records from the HIM department, and following up with other departments for diagnostic tests that need to be performed or obtaining test results that are needed for diagnosis and subsequent treatment. Because the ED is located within a hospital, other allied health professionals are available for radiology, laboratory, respiratory, and other services required by the patients.

## Data Collection Issues

Because the pace in the ED is fast, data collection must be fast. In a paper-based environment, menu-based forms have long been the standard for data collection. This menu-driven data collection has facilitated the implementation of computer data collection in the ED environment. Data collection unique to the ED includes the method and time of arrival.

## Data Sets

The **National Center for Injury Prevention and Control (NCIPC)** has developed a uniform data set for EDs. The **Data Elements for Emergency Department Systems (DEEDS)** apply to hospital-based EDs (Figure 8-4). DEEDS supports the uniform collection of data in hospital-based emergency departments to improve continuity among emergency room records. DEEDS incorporates national standards for **electronic data interchange (EDI)**, allowing diverse computer systems to exchange information. The Essential Medical Data Set (EMDS) complements DEEDS and provides medical history data on each patient to improve the overall effectiveness of care provided in the ED. In comparison with UACDS, the elements of DEEDS are more concise and specific to the services and treatment provided in the ED.

## Licensure and Accreditation

An ED accounts for most unscheduled admissions to the hospital. The ED is licensed and accredited under the umbrella of its host facility. An ED is licensed according to the type of services available and the capacity to provide trauma services, which is a special level of licensing. Some EDs are actual *trauma centers*, which are specially equipped to treat patients who have suffered traumatic injuries, such as in a car accident or a violent assault. Designation of an ED as a trauma center is by state licensure. Additionally, the presence of specific trauma resources may be verified by the American College of Surgeons as either a level I, level II, or level III; with level I trauma centers providing the highest level of care.

## EXERCISE 8-1

### Ambulatory Care Facilities

1. Describe the experiences of a patient in a physician's office.
2. What professionals is the patient likely to encounter in a physician's office?
3. What role do those professionals play in caring for the patient?
4. What role does urgent care play in health care delivery?
5. List and describe the elements of the UACDS.
6. What is the data set used in hospital-based emergency departments?

**Section 1: Patient Identification**

Internal ID
Name
Alias
Date of Birth
Sex
Race
Ethnicity
Address
Telephone Number

Account Number
Social Security Number
Occupation
Industry
Emergency Contact Name
Emergency Contact Address
Emergency Contact Telephone Number
Emergency Contact Relationship

**Section 2: Facility and Practitioner Identification**

ED Facility ID
Primary Practitioner Name
Primary Practitioner ID
Primary Practitioner Type
Primary Practitioner Address
Primary Practitioner Telephone Number
Primary Practitioner Organization

ED Practitioner ID
ED Practitioner Type
ED Practitioner Current Role
ED Consultant Practitioner ID
ED Consultant Practitioner Type
Date/Time ED Consult Request Initiated
Date/Time ED Consult Starts

**Section 3: ED Payment**

Insurance Coverage or Other Expected
    Source of Payment
Insurance Company
Insurance Company Address
Insurance Plan Type
Insurance Policy ID
ED Payment Authorization
    Requirement
Status of ED Payment
    Authorization Attempt

Date/Time of ED Payment
    Authorization Attempt
ED Payment Authorization Decision
Entity Contacted to Authorize ED Payment
ED Payment Authorization Code
Person Contacted to Authorize ED Payment
Telephone Number of Entity of Person
    Contacted to Authorize ED Payment
Total ED Facility Charges
Total ED Professional Fees

**Section 4: ED Arrival and First Assessment**

Date/Time First Documented in ED
Mode of Transport to ED
EMS Unit that Transported ED Patient
EMS Agency that Transported ED Patient
Source of Referral to ED
Chief Complaint
Initial Encounter for Current Instance of
    Chief Complaint
First ED Acuity Assessment
Date/Time of First ED Acuity Assessment
First ED Acuity Assessment Practitioner ID
First ED Acuity Assessment Practitioner type
First ED Responsiveness Assessment
First ED Glasgow Eye Opening Component
    Assessment
First ED Glasgow Verbal Component Assessment
First ED Glasgow Motor Component Assessment

Date/Time of First ED Glasgow Coma
    Scale Assessment
First ED Systolic Blood Pressure
Date/Time of First ED Systolic Blood Pressure
First ED Diastolic Blood Pressure
First ED Heart Rate
First ED Heart Rate Method
Date/Time of First ED Heart Rate
First ED Respiratory Rate
Date/Time of First ED Respiratory Rate
First ED Temperature Reading
First ED Temperature Reading Route
Date/Time of First ED Temperature Reading
Measured Weight in ED
Pregnancy Status Reported in ED
Date of Last Tetanus Immunization
Medication Allergy Reported in ED

**Figure 8-4** Data elements for emergency department systems (DEEDs). ED, emergency department; ID, identification. (From Centers for Disease Control and Prevention: Data Elements for Emergency Department Systems, Release 1.0 [DEEDS], 1997. http://www.cdc.gov/ncipc/pub-res/pdf/deeds.pdf.)

## RADIOLOGY AND LABORATORY SERVICES

**Radiology** and **laboratory** facilities serve both the inpatient and outpatient settings with services authorized through their license and trained personnel. Diagnostic radiology (CT, radiograph, MRI, PET scan, ultrasonograph) and laboratory services are routinely offered on an ambulatory basis depending on the resources of the facility. Patients are not admitted; they are tested. There may be serial visits for patients who are in need of therapeutic radiology or laboratory studies, which may result in an admission,

**radiology** Literally, the study of radiographs. In a health care facility, the department responsible for maintaining radiographic and other types of diagnostic and therapeutic equipment as well as analyzing diagnostic films.

**laboratory** The physical location of the specialists who analyze body fluids.

**Section 5: H&P Exam Data**

Date/Time of First Ed Practitioner Evaluation
Date/Time of Illness or Injury Onset
Injury Incident Description
Coded Cause of Injury
Injury Incident Location type
Injury Activity
Injury Intent
Safety Equipment Use
Current Therapeutic Medication
Current Therapeutic Medication Dose

Current Therapeutic Medication Dose Units
Current Therapeutic Medication Schedule
Current Therapeutic Medication Route
ED Clinical Finding Type
ED Clinical Finding
Date/Time ED Clinical Finding Obtained
ED Clinical Finding Practitioner ID
ED Clinical Finding Practitioner Type
ED Clinical Finding Data Source

**Section 6: ED Procedure and Result Data**

ED Procedure Indication
ED Procedure
Date/Time ED Procedure Ordered
Date/Time ED Procedure Starts
Date/Time ED Procedure Ends
ED Procedure Practitioner ID

ED Procedure Practitioner Type
Date/Time ED Diagnostic
   Procedure Result Reported
ED Diagnostic Procedure Result Type
ED Diagnostic Procedure Result

**Section 7: ED Medication Data**

Date/Time ED Medication Ordered
ED Medication Ordering
   Practitioner ID
ED Medication Ordering
   Practitioner Type
ED Medication
ED Medication Dose
ED Medication Dose Units

ED Medication Schedule
ED Medication Route
Date/Time ED Medication Starts
Date/Time ED Medication Stops
ED Medication Administering
   Practitioner ID
ED Medication Administering
   Practitioner Type

**Section 8: Disposition and Diagnosis Data**

Date/Time of Recorded ED
Disposition
ED Disposition
Inpatient Practitioner ID
Inpatient Practitioner Type
Facility Receiving ED Patient
Date/Time Patient Departs ED
ED Follow-Up Care Assistance
Referral at ED Disposition
ED Referral Practitioner Name
ED Referral Practitioner ID
ED Referral Practitioner Type
ED Referral Organization
ED Discharge Medication Order Type
ED Discharge Medication Ordering
   Practitioner ID
ED Discharge Medication Ordering
   Practitioner Type
ED Discharge Medication
ED Discharge Medication Dose
ED Discharge Medication Dose Units

ED Discharge Medication Schedule
Ed Discharge Medication Route
Amount of ED Discharge Medication to
   Be Dispensed
Number of ED Discharge Medication Refills
ED Disposition Diagnosis Description
ED Disposition Diagnosis Code
ED Disposition Diagnosis Practitioner ID
ED Disposition Diagnosis Practitioner Type
ED Service Level
ED Service Level Practitioner ID
ED Service Level Practitioner Type
Patient Problem Assessed in ED
   Outcome Observation
ED Outcome Observation
Date/Time of ED Outcome Observation
ED Outcome Observation Practitioner ID
ED Outcome Observation Practitioner Type
ED Patient Satisfaction Report Type
ED Patient Satisfaction Report

**Figure 8-4, cont'd**

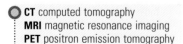

**CT** computed tomography
**MRI** magnetic resonance imaging
**PET** positron emission tomography

and the length of stay depends on the tests/procedure being performed. All radiology and laboratory tests require a physician order and diagnosis to support the purpose of the test.

## Settings

Radiology and laboratory services are maintained in acute care and inpatient rehabilitation facilities. These services are often available to the general public and can be obtained through a physician's order. Some of these hospitals do not maintain the services by using their own employees but rather lease the space to organizations that agree to provide the services to the hospitals. Radiology and laboratory services may also be offered in free-standing facilities.

Mobile laboratories are common and began with mobile blood and plasma services. **Mobile diagnostic** services provide convenient access to patient testing and diagnostics, offering convenience and cost efficiency by eliminating unnecessary travel and stress for the patient. These services are widely utilized by older adults and home bound patients because of their convenience. Mobile diagnostics services can provide specialty tests that, due to facility requirements, cannot be performed within a hospital or clinic setting. They can provide radiography, electrocardiography, mammography, ultrasound scanning, Holter heart monitoring, and bone density tests, and some units offer basic blood pressure and cholesterol screenings. Occupational health testing units offer flu shots and private drug screenings. These services are often located near clinics and nursing homes, in rural communities, in heavily populated areas, and near large businesses. Mobile eye and dental units are common in areas where access to care is limited and where demand for convenience is high. These services are covered by federal and private providers. TJC provides accreditation for mobile diagnostic services. Ambulance service is the most common type of mobile diagnostic service.

## Services

Diagnostic radiology services include radiography, CT, MRIs, and PET scanning. Three-dimensional ultrasound scans may be used to visualize a fetus in utero. Therapeutic radiology (also known as radiation therapy) is most closely associated with the treatment of certain types of cancers. Services are provided on the order of a physician.

Laboratory services include examinations of blood, urine, specimens, and other bodily secretions for the diagnosis, treatment, and prevention of disease. Hematology, serology, cytology, bacteriology, biochemistry, and blood and organ banking are functions of the clinical laboratory.

An interesting recent phenomenon, though, is the increased frequency in the marketing of radiology and laboratory services to the general public as a prophylactic diagnostic measure. For example, a PET scan may be advertised as providing the patient with peace of mind. Laboratory tests for vitamin D deficiency may be advocated as a general screening measure. Marketing of health care services of this nature encourages patients to advocate for their personal health and well-being; however, the physician is the arbiter of whether such tests are beneficial in each case and payers do not necessarily cover such services in the absence of a specific diagnosis or suspected condition.

## Care Providers

Radiologic technologists or radiographers produce images of anatomical structures. Radiographers are typically trained in hospital-based training programs, community colleges, or 4-year baccalaureate degree programs. Their training is accomplished on state-of-the-art equipment that allows them to obtain clear and accurate images. Physicians who work in a radiology department are called radiologists. They interpret the images and dictate the reports associated with the interpretation. Front-end voice recognition software is often used by radiology departments to communicate radiological findings. The voice recognition software allows radiologists to review radiology images and speak their findings into the software to create reports, eliminating the need for someone to transcribe the reports.

Laboratories are staffed with a variety of personnel, including pathologists, microbiologists, histotechnologists, cytotechnologists, medical laboratory technicians, and phlebotomists. These lab professionals work with microscopes, computers, and instruments to process body fluids, tissues, and cells that help physicians detect, diagnose, treat, and prevent disease. The phlebotomists draw blood using a procedure called venipuncture.

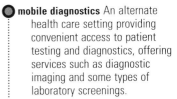

**Radiology and Laboratory Coding Notes**
Diagnosis Code is ICD-10-CM.
Procedure Code is HCPCS/CPT.*
Example:
- **M81.0** Osteoporosis
- **82652** Vitamin D deficiency
- Bill format: UB-04

*CPT copyright 2012 American Medical Association. All rights reserved. CPT is a registered trademark of the American Medical Association.

**mobile diagnostics** An alternate health care setting providing convenient access to patient testing and diagnostics, offering services such as diagnostic imaging and some types of laboratory screenings.

**TJC** The Joint Commission

**Go To** Review Chapter 3 for more information about PACS and how it works.

**release of information (ROI)** The term used to describe the HIM department function that provides disclosure of patient health information.

**picture archiving and communication system (PACS)** A system that allows many different kinds of diagnostic images (e.g., radiographs, magnetic resonance images, ultrasound scans, computed tomography scans) produced by many different kinds of machines to be archived and accessed from any computer terminal in the network.

**electronic health record (EHR)** A secure real-time, point-of-care, patient-centric information resource for clinicians allowing access to patient information when and where needed and incorporating evidence-based decision support.

**Conditions of Participation** The terms under which a facility is eligible to receive reimbursement from Medicare.

**AAAHC** Accreditation Association for Ambulatory Health Care
**NIAHO** National Integrated Accreditation for Healthcare Organizations
**CMS** Centers for Medicare and Medicaid Services

**reimbursement** The amount of money that the health care facility receives from the party responsible for paying the bill.

**ASC** ambulatory surgery center

**ambulatory surgery** Surgery performed on an outpatient basis; the patient returns home after the surgery is performed. Also called *same-day surgery*.

## Data Collection Issues

Radiology and laboratory services generate various forms of documentation and reports. The original material (radiographic film, digital image, or fluid sample) is retained in the testing department or facility. The report of the analysis of the material is maintained in the testing department. A copy of the report is sent to the requesting physician and to the facility that ordered the procedure. The report will become a part of the patient's health record in the facility that ordered the test.

Radiology services typically handle their own release of information (ROI). Currently, radiological images are captured in digital format. These digital images captured and shared using a system called the **picture archiving and communication system (PACS)**, can be given to patients and their physicians on computer disk along with the program to view the image, integrated into an electronic health record (EHR), or shared over a network. This arrangement facilitates communication with the physician and provides the patient with a valuable tool for developing and maintaining a personal health record, so the patient may retain a copy of the results for future health care encounters.

## Licensure and Accreditation

Facilities are licensed by the departments of health and human services of the states in which they operate and must adhere to the guidelines outlined in the Conditions of Participation. Accreditation is available for these facilities through TJC, AAAHC, and NIAHO. Clinical laboratories are regulated by the CMS under the Clinical Laboratories Improvement Amendments (CLIAs). For current information about this program, refer to the CMS Web site: http://www.cms.hhs.gov/clia.

### EXERCISE 8-2

**Ambulatory Care: Radiology and Laboratory**

1. What services are provided by radiology and laboratory facilities?
2. Describe the unique data collection issues in radiology and laboratory facilities.
3. What services are provided by mobile diagnostics?
4. What is the purpose and function of PACS?

## AMBULATORY SURGERY

As health care costs rise, providers are under increasing pressure to offer surgical services on an ambulatory basis. Because of lower overhead costs, ambulatory surgery centers are able to perform surgical procedures at lower costs than hospitals. Also contributing to the rise in ambulatory surgical services is improved technology that allows for less postsurgical recovery time. The CMS maintains a list of surgical procedures that Medicare will reimburse only if they occur in an inpatient setting. All other procedures are designated as appropriate to ambulatory surgery. Although an ambulatory surgery center may operate as a functional unit of a facility, such as a hospital, it is considered a separate entity. The surgery center must maintain individual governance, professional supervision, administrative services, clinical functions, record keeping, and financial and accounting systems. The distinction between an ambulatory surgery center (ASC) and an ambulatory surgery department of a hospital is important. ASCs are individually licensed and accredited.

## Length of Stay

**Ambulatory surgery** patients technically have a length of stay of 1 day. In other words, they are treated and released on the same day. Patients who require additional care beyond the day of surgery may be held overnight under the same day surgery status, transferred to observation status, or admitted to inpatient status. A hysterectomy, for example, is a common ambulatory surgery procedure; however, if the patient's vital signs are unstable for a significant amount of time post-surgery, the surgeon will write an order to hold the patient overnight for observation or to admit the patient for inpatient care. In a standalone ASC, the patient would be transferred to an acute care facility and then admitted as an inpatient.

## Settings

Ambulatory surgery may take place in an acute care facility or a freestanding **ambulatory surgery center (ASC)**. Sometimes the ASC specializes in a specific type of surgery (i.e., eye operations, orthopedic surgery). Some large health care companies, like Surgical Care Affiliates—formerly a division of HealthSouth—own and operate hundreds of ASCs, both freestanding and located within hospitals. Alternatively, a group of surgeons may form a partnership with one another or may combine with a health care management services company to create an ASC. ASCs look to engage in contractual agreements with hospitals and health systems by providing nonemergency procedures. The ASC can offer the hospital skilled physicians and state-of-the-art technology, allowing the hospital to stay competitive, as well as to satisfy care requirements imposed by CMS and managed care organizations. In return, the ASC has the support of the hospital, which may include the use of its facilities, staff, and services, if an ASC patient requires admission.

## Services

ASCs provide surgical procedures that do not require inpatient hospitalization. Ambulatory surgery is just that: surgery. The types of procedures performed in this environment are limited only by the postsurgical care required. Cataract removal, colonoscopy, removal of skin lesions, cholecystectomy, appendectomy, and carpal tunnel release are examples of procedures that are typically performed on an ambulatory basis.

## Care Providers

Care providers in this setting are generally limited to:
- Physicians
- Nurses
- General medical office personnel
- Surgical technicians
- Anesthesiologists

## Data Collection Issues

The volume of data collected for an ambulatory surgery case is relatively low compared with that for inpatient surgical procedures. Preadmission testing may include laboratory work and radiological services as well as an anesthesia consultation. The history and physical must be completed. The surgical report may be brief and may contain substantial menu-based data (Figure 8-5). The data are always focused on the reason for the surgical encounter. Anesthesia would include preoperative, intraoperative, and postoperative evaluations and postanesthesia recovery.

## Data Sets

In ambulatory surgery, the Uniform Ambulatory Care Data Set (UACDS) applies (see Box 8-1).

## Licensure and Accreditation

An ASC is considered a separate entity under Medicare and must maintain separate licensure and accreditation even if it is acting as a functional unit within

---

**ambulatory surgery center (ASC)** A surgical facility that performs procedures that do not require an inpatient stay.

**managed care** A type of insurer (payer) focused on reducing health care costs, controlling expensive care, and improving the quality of patient care provided.

**ASC** ambulatory surgery center
**CMS** Centers for Medicare and Medicaid Services

**Ambulatory Surgery Coding Notes**
Diagnosis Code is ICD-10-CM.
Procedure Code is HCPCS/CPT.*
MDS RUG code is reported.
Example:
- **K35.80** Appendicitis
- **44970** Laparoscopic appendectomy
- Bill format: UB-04

*CPT copyright 2012 American Medical Association. All rights reserved. CPT is a registered trademark of the American Medical Association.

**Uniform Ambulatory Care Data Set (UACDS)** The mandated data set for ambulatory care patients.

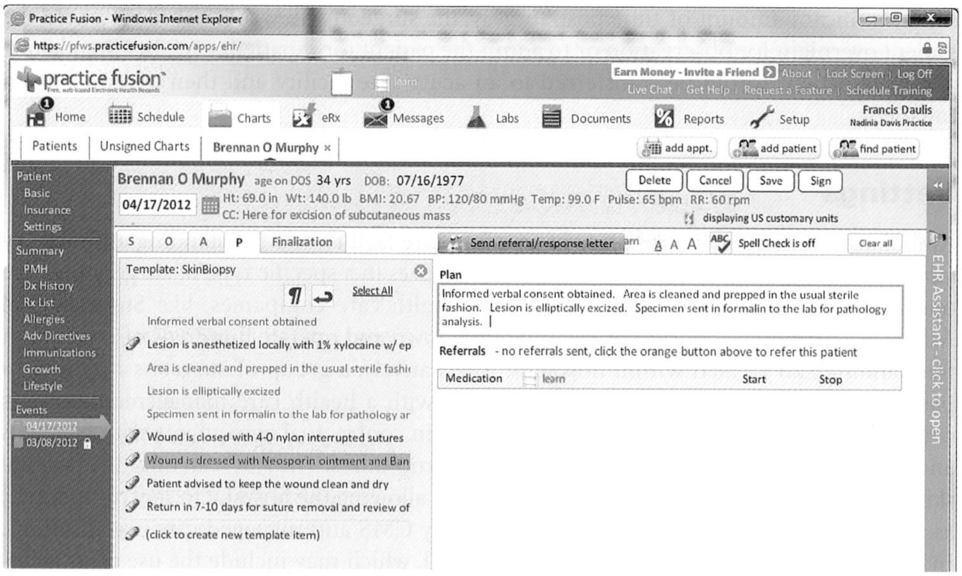

**Figure 8-5** Using menu-driven choices from a template on the left, the surgeon can quickly populate the operative reports with data common to this ambulatory surgery center procedure, the removal of a skin lesion. ED, emergency department; H&P, history and physical examination; ID, identification. (Courtesy Practice Fusion, Inc., San Francisco, CA.)

---

**TJC** The Joint Commission
**AAAHC** Accreditation Association for Ambulatory Health Care
**NIAHO** National Integrated Accreditation for Healthcare Organizations

---

▌▌▌

**Long-Term Care Coding Notes**
Diagnosis Code is ICD-10-CM.
Limited procedures, usually therapies and charge items.
MDS RUG Code is reported.
Global billing—most services covered by PPS payment.
Example:

- **Z51.89** Encounter for other specified aftercare
- **M62.82** Rhabdomyolysis
- **I10** Hypertension
- **F32.9** Major depressive disorder, single episode, unspecified
- **97001** PT Eval
- **97110** PT Therapy
- **97116** PT Gait training
- **RUB01** RUG code
- Bill format: UB-04

---

**long-term care (LTC) facility** A hospital that provides services to patients over an extended period; an average length of stay is in excess of 30 days. Facilities are characterized by the extent to which nursing care is provided.

**activities of daily living (ADLs)** Refers to self-care, such as bathing, as well as cooking, shopping, and other routines requiring thought, planning, and physical motion.

---

another facility, such as a hospital. Outpatient surgical services provided by a hospital are different from an ASC. ASCs are licensed by the departments of health and human services of the states in which they operate. Accreditation is offered by TJC, the AAAHC, Healthcare Facilities Accreditation Program (HFAP), and the NIAHO.

▪ **EXERCISE 8-3**

▪ **Ambulatory Care: Ambulatory Surgery**

1. Define and give examples of ambulatory surgery.
2. Describe the unique data collection issues in ambulatory surgery.
3. Who accredits ambulatory surgery facilities?
4. What happens in the ambulatory surgery setting when the patient requires "emergency" acute care services?

## OTHER INPATIENT HEALTH CARE SETTINGS

### LONG-TERM CARE

In addition to length of stay, there are other fundamental differences between **long-term care (LTC) facilities** and acute care facilities. Although both care for inpatients, they differ significantly in focus and delivery of quality health care. Long-term care is non-acute care consisting of rehabilitative and supportive services. Patients receiving long-term care are considered residents of the facility; they are not only being treated there—they actually live there. Thus there is a greater emphasis on comfort, activities of daily living (ADLs), and recreational activities, such as games and crafts. Group activities are common ways to facilitate residents' interaction and socialization.

### Length of Stay

Many state licensure documents define a LTC as one in which the average length of stay exceeds 30 days. In practice, the length of stay varies significantly, depending on the needs of the patient. It is not unusual for patients to require long-term care for months or years.

## Settings

A wide variety of facilities are considered long-term care. Some of these facilities, such as assisted living facilities, are not as strictly regulated as others. Table 8-3 contains a brief description of LTC facilities.

### Skilled Nursing Facility

**Skilled nursing facilities (SNFs)** are health care facilities that offer both short- and long-term care options for those with temporary or permanent health problems too complex or serious for home care or an assisted living setting. SNFs are designed for very sick patients. Services that a skilled nursing facility offers may vary, but they normally provide the following: medical treatment prescribed by a doctor, physical therapy, speech therapy, occupational therapy, assistance with personal care activities such as eating, walking, bathing, and using the restroom, case management, and social services.

### Nursing Home

A nursing home is a facility for patients who need constant care and/or help with daily living activities, but at a lesser level of care than a skilled nursing facility. Services are offered to older adults and to individuals who may have physical disabilities. Nursing homes may also offer rehabilitative services after an accident or illness, such as physical therapy and occupational therapy.

**skilled nursing facility (SNF)** A long-term care facility providing a range of nursing and other health care services to patients who require continuous care, typically those with a chronic illness.

**case management** The coordination of the patient's care and services, including reimbursement considerations.

| TABLE 8-3 | |
|---|---|
| **EXAMPLES OF LONG-TERM CARE FACILITIES** | |
| **FACILITY** | **TYPE OF CARE** |
| Independent living | Residents are housed in apartment settings. Health care is provided on site; however, residents are independent in their activities of daily living (ADLs) and do not require medical supervision on a 24-hour basis. Some meals may be provided in a cafeteria or restaurant atmosphere. |
| Assisted living | Residents are housed in apartment-like setting, often with limited food preparation equipment, or in dormitory rooms—usually with private bath. Health care is provided on site. Residents have varying degrees of independence in their ADLs and need for medical supervision. Some or all meals may be provided in a communal or restaurant atmosphere. Ancillary services may include computer labs, chapel, spa services, entertainment and activity rooms, and laundry facilities. |
| Subacute care | This is usually a transitional level of care between acute care and either home care or other long-term care. Subacute care may be offered in acute care facilities or in long-term care facilities. Patients require substantial treatment but no longer need the 24-hour supervision of an acute care facility. |
| Transitional | Generally offered in an acute care facility, patients require up to 8 hours of nursing care per day. Average length of stay is within acute care definition. |
| General | Patients require up to 5 hours of care per day and typically stay from 10 to 40 days in a long-term care facility. |
| Chronic | Patients require up to 5 hours of care per day and typically stay from 60 to 90 days in a long-term care facility. |
| Long-term transitional | Patients require up to 9 hours of care per day and typically stay more than 25 days in an acute care facility. |
| Intermediate care | Patients do not require 24-hour supervision. Cognitive or motor impairment contraindicates independent living. |
| Skilled nursing | Residents require substantial assistance with ADLs. Frequent therapies from a variety of professionals are needed to maintain status. |
| Long-term acute care | Patients require an acute level of care over an extended period. The average length of stay is more than 25 days. Services may be provided in an acute care, long-term care, or rehabilitation hospital. Medicare considers this long-term care. |

These are general categories of care provided to help the reader understand the environment of long-term care. Facility, licensure, and regional differences in terminology exist. Many facilities offer multiple levels of care and are not distinguishable as a specific type of facility. For example, some organizations offer lifetime care that transitions from independent to assisted to intermediate to skilled care as the patient's condition deteriorates.

**LTAC** long-term acute care

### Long-Term Acute Care

Long-term acute care (LTAC) facilities focus on treating patients who need special, intense care for a longer time than is customary in an acute care hospital; their stay is usually no less than 25 days. Patients in an LTAC facility could consist of older adults, patients from a nursing home, and those who have serious medical problems, such as patients who need long-term ventilator assistance.

### Community-Based Services

Community-based services are programs or care offered to people of all ages who are either disabled or need home assistance. Services normally include nursing, transportation, personal support, and other rehabilitation services. Individuals who qualify for these services usually receive it for free or at a low cost.

**activities of daily living (ADLs)** Refers to self-care, such as bathing, as well as cooking, shopping, and other routines requiring thought, planning, and physical motion.

### Board and Care Homes

Board and care homes are basically group living arrangements. The arrangements usually consist of four to six residents whose care is provided by live-in staff. The residents do not need nursing home care but need help with ADLs. Care rendered at many such facilities are custodial in nature as opposed to medical.

### Assisted Living

**assisted living** A type of long-term care in which the resident is significantly independent in activities of daily living and does not need high levels of skilled nursing.

Assisted living is also considered a group living arrangement. It offers help with ADLs and monitors the residents to ensure their health, safety, and well-being. Residents live in apartments that typically have limited kitchen facilities. There are community dining rooms and residents generally have meal plan options. Most assisted living facilities have worship, entertainment, and personal care services available on site.

### Continuing Care Retirement Communities

Continuing care retirement communities offer help with the process of coping with aging and/or change in general. There are different levels of care, depending on the individual's needs. Considering one's health, they may be able to live independently or in a more assisted facility.

## Services

LTC facilities typically offer rehabilitation services, such as occupational therapy and physical therapy, in addition to nursing care, housing, and activities associated with daily living.

## Care Providers

Patients entering an LTC facility are evaluated by a physician to ensure that the facility is appropriate for the patient's optimal care. The physician is responsible for ensuring that the patient meets the goals established by the patient's care plan. Once the patient is admitted, the physician plays a small role in the patient's daily life. Unless there is a change in the patient's medical condition or the patient's care plan, the physician routinely sees the patient only once every month.

**skilled nursing facility (SNF)** A long-term care facility providing a range of nursing and other health care services to patients who require continuos care, typically those with a chronic illness.

The level of nursing care required by the patient is the key to determining what type of facility the patient needs. In a skilled nursing facility, the patient typically needs 24-hour supervision with skilled nursing personnel at both the Registered Nurse and Licensed Vocational Nurse (LVN) levels. In an assisted living facility, a resident may need only a nurse on call.

### Registered Dietitian

Nutrition is an important part of managing an older adult patient's health care. It is important to make sure the patient receives the appropriate nutrition via diet or supplements to support his or her health care. A registered dietitian (RD) manages food services and evaluates patients' nutritional needs. They plan menus and special diets, and educate patients and families. RDs are primarily employed in health care facilities. A bachelor's degree in dietetics from an accredited program and 1200 hours of clinical practice are minimum requirements to apply for the national registration examination, which is offered by the Commission on Dietetic Registration. The American Dietetic Association, which has been the primary professional association for registered dietitians, is now called the Academy of Nutrition and Dietetics.

As with other professions described in this chapter, there is another level of dietitian practice, a dietetic technician, registered (DTR). There are several pathways to the DTR, all of which require training in an approved program and clinical practice (American Dietetic Association, 2011).

## Data Collection Issues

LTC facilities generate voluminous amounts of data on their patients. Much of the data consist of nursing notes and medication sheets. Therapies also add to the volume. In a paper-based environment, the records must be periodically thinned of older documentation. Older documentation is analyzed, completed, and coded before being transferred to storage, leaving relevant and current documentation at the nursing unit. Retention standards for medical records are specific by each state and should be followed when one is thinning, storing, or destroying patient information.

## Data Sets

Long-term care facilities seeking reimbursement from Medicare must complete the Minimum Data Set (MDS) for each of their patients, currently version 3.0. This lengthy data set is initiated upon admission and contains detailed clinical data about the patient. It must be submitted to the facility's state repository within 14 days of admission, updated quarterly for specific sections, and resubmitted at least annually. The MDS is one component of a series of data collected when the health care professional assess the type of care the patient will need in the long-term care setting. Combined with the **Resident Assessment Instrument (RAI)**, the RAI-MDS is a comprehensive assessment that measures physical, psychological, and psychosocial functioning of the resident. Mandated by the Nursing Home Reform Act (1987), this data collection identifies "residents' strengths, weaknesses, preferences, and needs in key areas of functioning. It is designed to help nursing homes thoroughly evaluate residents and provides each resident with a standardized, comprehensive, and reproducible assessment." (U.S. Department of Health and Human Services, 2001). The goal of this volume of documentation is to ensure a high quality of care in LTC settings. Information gathered by this data set can trigger a more detailed assessment using **Resident Assessment Protocols (RAPs)**, which will help establish the patient plan of care in the long-term care setting on a continuing basis, in which the patient's condition is regularly reevaluated. The RAI-MDS is of interest because it illustrates the volume and type of data that are collected in long-term care, which is mirrored in other non-acute care settings as well.

## Licensure and Accreditation

LTC facilities are licensed in the states in which they operate. Each state has different licensure and accreditation laws for SNFs, LTACs, and nursing homes, depending on numerous factors. Licensing will define the types of LTC that can be provided, such as skilled, subacute, or rehabilitation services. Each of these specialties and LTC environments requires specially trained personnel and must adhere to specific guidelines. **The Commission on Accreditation of Rehabilitation Facilities (CARF)** accredits LTC facilities offering rehabilitation services; however, not all states require accreditation from that specific organization. For example, an SNF in Illinois must be accredited by TJC, the CARF, or the Continuing Care Accreditation Commission (CCAC); and must be provided to Medicare and Medicaid patients. ABC Nursing Home in Mississippi, however, is accredited by TJC and is licensed by the Mississippi State Department of Health Division of Licensure and Certification and the CMS.

**LTC** long-term care

**Go To** Chapter 9 details health record retention processes.

**Minimum Data Set (MDS)** The detailed data collected about patients receiving long-term care. It is collected several times, and it forms the basis for the Resource Utilization Group.

**Resident Assessment Instrument (RAI)** A data set collected by skilled nursing facilities (SNFs) that includes elements of MDS 3.0 along with information on patient statuses and conditions in the facility.

**Resident Assessment Protocols (RAP)** A detailed, individualized evaluation and plan for patients in long-term care.

**Go To** Review the MDS 3.0 in Appendix C of this text.

**LTAC** long-term acute care

**skilled nursing facility (SNF)** A long-term care facility providing a range of nursing and other health care services to patients who require continous care, typically those with a chronic illness

**Commission on Accreditation of Rehabilitation Facilities (CARF)** An organization that accredits behavioral health and rehabilitation facilities.

**CMS** Centers for Medicare and Medicaid Services

## EXERCISE 8-4

### Long-Term Care Facilities

1. When does a patient require long-term care?
2. What services are provided by long-term care workers?
3. List three types of long-term care.
4. Describe the unique data collection issues in a long-term care environment.
5. What minimum data set is associated with long-term care?
6. Who accredits long-term care facilities?

## BEHAVIORAL HEALTH FACILITIES

**behavioral health facility** An inpatient or outpatient health care facility that focuses on the treatment of psychiatric conditions.

Behavioral health facilities and behavioral health services housed in other types of facilities focus on the diagnosis and treatment of psychological and substance abuse disorders such as drug and alcohol addiction, eating disorders, schizophrenia, bipolar disorders, and chronic cognitive impairment. These services may be residential or nonresidential, ambulatory or inpatient.

### Length of Stay

**Behavioral Health Coding Note**
**Inpatient**
Diagnosis Code is ICD-10-CM.
Procedure Code is ICD-10-PCS.
Example:
- **F10.20** Alcoholism without remission
- **HZ2ZZZZ...** Detoxification
- **HZ33ZZZ...** Individual counseling
- Bill format: UB-04

**Outpatient**
Diagnosis Code is ICD-10-CM.
Procedure Code is HCPCS/CPT.*
Example:
- **F33.2** Major depressive disorder, recurrent severe without psychotic features
- **90870** Electroconvulsive therapy
- Bill format: usually UB-04 for facility-based; CMS-1500 for practitioner

*CPT copyright 2012 American Medical Association. All rights reserved. CPT is a registered trademark of the American Medical Association.

The length of stay for behavioral health services offered on an inpatient basis depends on the diagnosis and the individual patient's response to the therapeutic plan. Behavioral health services are also offered on an outpatient basis in a day hospital or day treatment program.

### Settings

Behavioral health services are offered in all health care settings. In the acute care setting, services may be provided by consultation; there are also likely to be psychiatrists on staff. In the rehabilitation setting, behavioral health services are vital for *cognitive remediation* (discussed in more detail later in this chapter). Behavioral health services are also offered in psychiatric hospitals, freestanding outpatient clinics, and physician office settings.

### Behavioral Health Services

Behavioral health services address a wide range of issues and disorders. Services include counseling, psychotherapy, occupational therapy, psychological testing, therapy, pharmaceutical interventions, and respite for children and adults.

### Drug and Alcohol Rehabilitation

Although treatment is referred to as rehabilitation, drug and alcohol abuse or dependence is considered a psychological condition. There are two phases of treatment: detoxification and rehabilitation. *Detoxification* refers to the treatment of a patient who is going through withdrawal of substances from his or her body. This withdrawal may take 3 or 4 days. *Rehabilitation* is the treatment of the patient by psychiatrists, psychologists, drug and alcohol counselors, and social workers that teaches the patient ways to resist drugs and alcohol in the future. Although treatment varies, initial rehabilitation may take weeks or months, with continuing treatment throughout the patient's life. A drug and alcohol rehabilitation facility may be freestanding or may be connected with another facility, such as a psychiatric hospital or an acute care facility.

### Care Providers

Although some patients in behavioral health facilities may have additional medical conditions that require treatment, the primary thrust of care is delivered by psychiatrists (physicians), psychologists (non-physician specialists), and social services personnel. Additionally, in an inpatient facility, there may also be a physician known as a family care physician, primary care physician, or internist who is responsible for treating any medical conditions that may occur during the patient's course of treatment.

### Social Workers

Social workers are among the behavioral health specialists who work with individuals with special needs. For example, a patient who leaves the hospital after surgery may need to rest. This is a problem if the patient lives alone and has no caregiver at home. A social worker helps the patient identify and obtain the needed assistance. Social workers also provide education and assistance to individuals with chronic illnesses, including human immunodeficiency virus (HIV), and substance abuse problems. The National Association of Social Workers promotes high professional standards and public awareness and administers the credentialing process (National Association of Social Workers, 2011). Some states offer licensure of trained social workers with master's degrees under a variety of different designations. The LMSW (Licensed Master Social Worker) and the LCSW (Licensed Clinical Social Worker), for example, are designations offered by the state of New York (New York State Education Department, 2011).

## Data Collection Issues

Much of the data collection in behavioral health is free text. Psychology notes tend to be voluminous and detailed and do not lend themselves to menu-driven data collection. Of particular concern are psychology notes and documentation of restraints. Because of changing regulations and the process for billing services, many point-of-care systems are helping to define the content of a clinical note, enabling better management and production of data reports for patient populations.

Psychology notes may include results of testing instruments and extensive interview notes. Many of these notes are retained in the psychology department and do not become part of the patient's legal health record. Confidentiality must be maintained for psychological testing documents as required by the developer/publisher. A summary of the results may be retained in the record. Only specially trained psychology staff may access testing instruments and their scoring and interpretation guidelines. Standards for records retention are established for each state by its department of health and human services. Accreditation agencies also provide standards for records retention. The facility must have a policy specifically dealing with the storage of, retention of, and access to psychological records. The facility should adopt the standard that is the most stringent if following both state and accreditation guidelines. Separate guidelines may apply to testing instruments and patient records.

Unfortunately, at times, a client may require restraints because he or she would otherwise become harmful to self or others and cannot be controlled with less restrictive options. The use of restraints requires a physician's order. Restraints include not only physical restraints but also confinement in protective enclosures or chemical restraint through the administration of strong psychotropic drugs. Documentation—of a complete assessment, less restrictive methods attempted, interventions attempted, consent from the patient for restraints, the restraint order specific for type of restraint (i.e., four-point, wrist, ankle, vest, seclusion, type of medication), the application of restraints, the monitoring of a restrained patient, and the timely release from restraints—is required. Guidelines vary from state to state on the use of restraints. Restraints may be applied for 12 to 24 hours. Strict guidelines on patient monitoring apply. Some facilities require that patients be checked every 5 minutes. Accreditation and licensure standards offer clear guidelines for the application, use, and monitoring of restraints.

## Data Sets

There is no specific data set unique to behavioral health, so the data collected reflect the setting in which the services are provided. The National Institute of Mental Health offers

**primary care physician (PCP)**
In insurance, the physician who has been designated by the insured to deliver routine care to the insured and to evaluate the need for referral to a specialist, if applicable. Colloquial use is synonymous with "family doctor."

**point-of-care documentation**
Clinical data recorded at the time the treatment is delivered to the patient.

**Go To** Explore preemption in Chapter 12.

**physician's orders** The physician's directions regarding the patient's care. Also refers to the data collection device on which these elements are captured.

**Diagnostic and Statistical Manual of Mental Disorders, Fifth Edition (DSM-5)** Diagnostic and Statistical Manual of Mental Disorders, 5th edition, used for coding behavior and mental health care encounters in a structured format.

**National Committee for Quality Assurance (NCQA)** A nonprofit entity focusing on quality in health care delivery that accredits managed care organizations.

**Substance Abuse and Mental Health Services Administration (SAMHSA)** An agency under the U.S. Department of Health and Human Services (DHHS) facilitating research and care for the treatment of patients with substance abuse and mental health problems.

**CARF** Commission on Accreditation of Rehabilitation Facilities

**Go To** See Chapter 12.

a limited data set for reporting and surveillance. The CMS inpatient psychiatric facility prospective payment system (IPF PPS) provides a Case Mix Assessment Tool (CMAT). The CMAT includes detailed information about the patient. In the absence of a data set, behavioral health utilizes the DSM-5 (*Diagnostic and Statistical Manual*, 5th edition), which provides data elements based on a five-axis format as follows:

- *Axis I:* Specific major mental, clinical, learning, or substance abuse disorders
- *Axis II:* Personality disorders and intellectual disabilities
- *Axis III:* Acute medical conditions and physical disorders
- *Axis IV:* Psychosocial and environmental factors contributing to the above disorders
- *Axis V:* Functional assessment

DSM-5 is published by the American Psychiatric Association (APA) and provides diagnostic criteria for psychiatric diagnosis to enhance clinical practice. DSM-5 also serves as a common language for communicating with third parties such as governmental agencies and insurance companies. At the time of writing, DSM-5 is scheduled for release in May 2013.

## Licensure and Accreditation

Behavioral health facilities are licensed by the states in which they operate. In addition to TJC, accreditation is available from the Commission on Accreditation of Rehabilitation Facilities (CARF) and the **National Committee for Quality Assurance (NCQA)**. The **Substance Abuse and Mental Health Services Administration (SAMHSA)** is a governmental agency that provides key resources on behavioral health issues.

An additional layer of regulation in behavioral health is the release of patient information. Release of information is strictly protected by law, over and above the rules that apply to protected health information in general, and release requires special authorization.

### EXERCISE 8-5
#### Behavioral Health Facilities

1. Describe conditions that would require behavioral health treatment.
2. What services are provided by behavioral health workers?
3. Describe the unique data collection issues in a behavioral health environment.
4. What minimum data set is associated with behavioral health?
5. Who accredits behavioral health facilities?

## REHABILITATION FACILITIES

Rehabilitation facilities offer care to patients who need specific therapies as a result of illness or injury. Patients recovering from respiratory failure, cerebrovascular accident, joint replacement surgery, traumatic head injury, or spinal cord injury are examples of typical rehabilitation patients. Therapies include respiratory therapy, physical therapy, occupational therapy, speech therapy, and *cognitive remediation*. **Cognitive remediation** is used to improve memory, judgment, reasoning, or perception impairments that make it difficult for a person to achieve functional goals. Cognitive remediation includes practice and adaptive strategies to help patients improve memory, attention, and problem-solving skills.

**cognitive remediation** A type of therapy for judgment, reasoning, perception, or memory impairments.

## Length of Stay

The length of stay in a rehab facility will be determined by the patient's diagnosis and care plan. For example, a patient who needs rehabilitation following a total hip replacement may stay only a few days to a week in the facility in order to improve mobility, function, and range of motion. However, a patient who survived a gunshot wound to the head may need extensive rehabilitation to relearn major motor function and life skills. Rehabilitation is offered on an inpatient or outpatient basis, depending on the needs of the patient. Rehabilitation services are offered in acute care facilities and long-term care facilities.

## Settings

To qualify for reimbursement of costs at this level of service, patients must participate in a specific number of hours of therapy. For Medicare patients, 3 hours of therapy daily is required.

Outpatient services may be housed in an inpatient facility, a stand-alone outpatient facility, or a related facility. For example, a growing number of outpatient rehabilitation services are associated with exercise facilities.

## Services

Respiratory care, occupational therapy, physical therapy, speech therapy, and cognitive remediation are common services utilized by rehabilitation patients. Ventilation and dialysis services are provided at some facilities. Social services are an additional service offered to such patients. They play an important role in helping patients find the additional services that they may need; that is, DME following discharge to the home, home health visits, and assistance with meals. In inpatient facilities, recreation therapy may play a role in helping patients increase their ability to accomplish their ADLs. Social interaction and physical exercise are important aspects of recreational therapy for patient independence and restoration.

A unique aspect of rehabilitation, in comparison with acute care, is the ability of the care providers to focus on preparing the patient to return to the workplace. Industrial rehabilitation, a holistic program of multiple therapies and evaluation techniques, plays an important role in this process. Further, the patient may need to be redirected in his or her employment goals as a result of the sequelae of the illness or injury.

## Care Providers

As with patients receiving behavioral health services, rehabilitation patients may have medical conditions that require treatment while they are in therapy. There is an internist on staff at inpatient facilities to treat these conditions. However, the thrust of treatment is the therapy.

Rehabilitation physical therapy occurs under the direction of a **physiatrist**, a physician who specializes in physical medicine and rehabilitation. Respiratory therapists (RTs), physical therapists (PTs), occupational therapists (OTs), speech/language pathologists (SLPs), social workers, and psychologists participate to varying degrees in the rehabilitation of individual patients.

### Occupational Therapist

Occupational therapists (OTs) are clinical professionals who focus on returning the patient to his or her maximal functions in activities of daily living (ADLs). The American Occupational Therapy Association (2011a) refers to ADLs as "skills for the job of living," which include but are not limited to self-care, driving, and shopping. OTs are primarily employed in rehabilitation facilities but may work in virtually any health care environment. They serve a wide variety of clients, including those suffering from traumatic injuries, the after-effects of stroke, and the loss of limbs. OTs may specialize in the treatment of specific conditions or specific age groups. The increasing life span and greater activity of today's older adults are important factors in the demand for OTs.

Occupational therapists are required to hold a master's degree in occupational therapy. Certification (registration) can be obtained from the American Occupational Therapy Association. The Association defines professional practice domains for education, practice, and licensure. Licensure is required in most states as a prerequisite for practicing occupational therapy.

Occupational therapy professionals also include occupational therapy assistants (OTA) and aides. OTAs have completed training in accredited programs and have passed a national certification examination. Occupational therapy aides receive on-the-job training and are not eligible for certification or licensing (American Occupational Therapy Association, 2011b).

---

**Rehabilitation Facility Coding Notes**

**Inpatient**

Diagnosis Code is ICD-10-CM. Procedure Code is ICD-10-PCS.

Example:

- **Z51.89** Encounter for other specified aftercare
- **I69.351** Hemiplegia due to cerebrovascular accident, affecting right dominant side
- **F021DYZ** Neuromotor development assessment of neurological system upper back/upper extremity
- **F022DYZ** Neuromotor development assessment of neurological system upper back/upper extremity
- Bill format: UB-04

**Outpatient**

Diagnosis Code is ICD-10-CM. Procedure Code is HCPCS/CPT.*

Example:

- **I69.951** Hemiplegia due to cerebrovascular accident, affecting right dominant side
- **97535** Self-care/home management training
- Bill format: UB-04 for facility and CMS-1500 for practitioner

*CPT copyright 2012 American Medical Association. All rights reserved. CPT is a registered trademark of the American Medical Association.

**Medicare** Federally funded health care insurance plan for older adults and for certain categories of chronically ill patients.

**dialysis** The extracorporeal elimination of waste products from bodily fluids (e.g., blood).

**DME** durable medical equipment

**ADLs** activities of daily living

**physiatrist** A physician who specializes in physical medicine and rehabilitation.

**activities of daily living (ADLs)** Refers to self-care, such as bathing, as well as cooking, shopping, and other routines requiring thought, planning, and physical motion.

### Physical Therapist

Physical therapists (PTs) focus on strength, gait, and range-of-motion training to return patients to maximum functioning, reduce pain, and manage illness. They are employed primarily in rehabilitation facilities but may work in virtually any health care environment. A master's or doctoral degree from an accredited program is required to become a PT. In order to practice, PTs must take a national licensing examination. Practice requirements vary from state to state (American Physical Therapy Association, 2011).

The practices of occupational therapy and physical therapy overlap somewhat, and patients may receive treatment from both in the same period. For example, a patient who has had a hip replacement may undergo physical therapy in order to learn to walk with the new joint, to increase range of motion, and maintain stability. At the same time, the patient might receive occupational therapy to practice getting in and out of a car, making a bed, or bending and stretching to clean house or cook.

## Data Collection Issues

In a paper-based inpatient environment, the patient's record may travel with the patient from one therapy to the next; this may be accomplished by transporting the charts on a cart or with the patient's transporter. Many rehabilitation patients are moved from unit to unit by wheelchair, and the chart can be placed on the back of the chair.

With a large number of patients and little time between appointments, therapists may have insufficient time to adequately document treatments. Delays in charting may increase errors in documentation. A moving medical chart arrangement also exposes the facility to the risk of incorrect handling of the patient's chart. Incomplete documentation may result in decreased reimbursement or denial of reimbursement.

Some facilities retain the medical portion of the paper record (physician's orders, progress notes, medication administration records) at the nursing unit for physician and nursing documentation, and only the therapy notes travel with the patient. This strategy hampers communication among the care team, however.

An EHR solves the logistical problem of physically moving the chart because it can be accessed electronically via computer terminals in the health care facility. Therapists log all notes directly into the computer. The electronic format allows for convenient and timely access to information and reduces the bulk associated with a paper record. However, the time allotted for entry of notes must be sufficient to accommodate the documentation requirements.

## Data Sets

Facilities seeking reimbursement from Medicare must complete the Inpatient Rehabilitation Facility–Patient Assessment Instrument (IRF-PAI) data set. This data set is composed of detailed clinical data about the patient similar to those required by long-term care.

## Licensure and Accreditation

Rehabilitation facilities are licensed by the states in which they operate. Accreditation is available from TJC and CARF. Some facilities choose to seek accreditation from both organizations.

---

**reimbursement** The amount of money that the health care facility receives from the party responsible for paying the bill.

**physician's orders** The physician's directions regarding the patient's care. Also refers to the data collection device on which these elements are captured.

**progress notes** The physician's record of each interaction with the patient.

**medication administration** Clinical data including the name of the medication, dosage, date and time of administration, method of administration, and the nurse who administered it.

**electronic health record (EHR)** A secure real-time, point-of-care, patient centric information resource for clinicians allowing access to patient information when and where needed and incorporating evidence-based decision support.

**Medicare** Federally funded health care insurance plan for older adults and for certain categories of chronically ill patients.

**CARF** Commission on Accreditation of Rehabilitation Facilities

---

## ▪ EXERCISE 8-6

### Rehabilitation Facilities

1. When is a patient eligible for rehabilitation?
2. What services are provided by rehabilitation workers?
3. Describe the unique data collection issues in a rehabilitation environment.
4. What minimum data set is associated with home health care?
5. Who accredits rehabilitation facilities?

## HOSPICE

**hospice** Palliative health care services rendered to the terminally ill, their families, and their friends.

**palliative care** Health care services that are intended to soothe, comfort, or reduce symptoms but are not intended to cure.

As discussed in Chapter 1, **hospice** care is focused on the terminally ill patient and his or her friends and family members. The focus of hospice is to provide **palliative care**, aid and comfort rather than curative treatment. According to the National Hospice and Palliative Care Organization (NHPCO), as of 2010 there were more than 5000 hospice providers serving about 1.56 million patients in the United States. Of the 2,450,000 persons who died in the United States in 2009, more than 1 million received hospice care (National Hospice and Palliative Care Association, 2010). A physician must order and help coordinate hospice care.

### Length of Stay

The duration of hospice care varies depending on the life expectancy of each patient and the friends' and family's need for support after the patient's death. The patients themselves are in the end stage of illness and have a life expectancy of less than 6 months. (Although care could be rendered to patients with a longer expected life, reimbursement entities typically look to the 6-month rule, as certified by the physician.) Friends and family members may receive bereavement services during the illness and for up to a year after the patient's death. The NHPCO states that in 2009, the average length of service for a hospice patient was 69.0 days, with a more representative median of 21.1 days (National Hospice and Palliative Care Association, 2010).

Hospice services may be provided at the patient's residence or in an inpatient/long-term care setting. Hospice inpatient facilities may resemble group homes because they are specifically designed to give comfort rather than to render acute treatment.

### Services

Hospice staff members are on call 24 hours a day. Available services include medical, nursing, counseling, legal, pharmaceutical, and bereavement services.

### Care Providers

Volunteers play a major role in assisting patients and family members in a hospice setting. Volunteers run errands for the family or the patient, spend time with the patient for the patient's enjoyment, provide the caregiver with respite, may help the patient write letters or with hobbies, and provide bereavement services. Physicians, nurses, and therapists are involved to the extent needed to make the patient comfortable. Medicare benefits cover the following therapies (National Hospice and Palliative Care Association, 2006):

- Physician services for the medical direction of the patient's care
- Regular home visits by registered nurses and licensed practical nurses
- Home health aides and homemakers for services such as dressing and bathing
- Social work and counseling
- Medical equipment such as hospital beds
- Medical supplies such as bandages and catheters
- Drugs for symptom control and pain relief
- Volunteer support to assist patients and loved ones
- Physical therapy, speech therapy, occupational therapy, and dietary counseling

### Data Collection Issues

The initial palliative plan of care is required within 48 hours of admission. Continuous nursing care, when provided, must be documented to facilitate reimbursement. A report of patient progress is also required for reimbursement.

**NHPCO** National Hospice and Palliative Care Organization

**Hospice Coding Notes**
Diagnosis Code is ICD-10-CM.
Procedure Code is HCPCS/CPT.*
Example:
- **C43.8** Malignant melanoma of overlapping sites of skin
- **C79.81** Secondary malignant neoplasm of breast
- **C79.51** Secondary malignant neoplasm of bone
- **96374** Injection, intravenous push
- **J2271** Injection, morphine
- Bill format: UB-04 for facility and CMS-1500 for practitioner

*CPT copyright 2012 American Medical Association. All rights reserved. CPT is a registered trademark of the American Medical Association.

## Licensure and Accreditation

**NHPCO** National Hospice and Palliative Care Organization

Licensure requirements vary by state, and not all states license hospice providers. The NHPCO offers accreditation.

### EXERCISE 8-7

**Hospice**

1. Who receives hospice care?
2. Describe palliative care.
3. When is a patient eligible for hospice care?
4. What role do volunteers play in hospice care?
5. Who accredits hospice organizations?

# OTHER SPECIALTY CARE

Other types of facilities are defined by medical specialty or by the types of patients that they treat. Some specific examples are adult day care, respite care, and dialysis centers and home health care. Adult day care is usually rendered on an outpatient basis in a rehabilitation or LTC facility. It provides care for adults who need supervision during the day when their primary caregivers are not available—for example, because of full-time jobs. Adult day care provides activities, social interaction, some therapies, and some medical treatment. Medical treatment usually consists of ensuring that the patient takes the proper medication at the appropriate time.

**respite care** Services rendered to an individual who is not independent in activities of daily living, for the purpose of temporarily relieving the primary caregiver.

**primary caregiver** The individual who is principally responsible for the daily care of a patient at home; usually a friend or family member.

**Respite care** is any care that is provided to give relief to the **primary caregiver**. Caring for the chronically ill can be stressful and exhausting. Respite care gives the primary caregiver temporary relief from caring for the patient. The primary caregiver may need a break to simply take care of personal business or may require physical and emotional support. Respite services are planned short-term breaks. The temporary caregiver learns the patient's routine and identifies medication regimens and cares for the patient while the primary caregiver is absent.

**dialysis center** An ambulatory care facility that specializes in blood-cleansing procedures to treat, for example, chronic kidney (renal) failure.

**dialysis** The extracorporeal elimination of waste products from bodily fluids (e.g., blood).

**Dialysis centers** provide renal **dialysis** services to patients with chronic renal failure. When a patient who receives ongoing dialysis is admitted for an acute condition, the dialysis may be performed on an inpatient basis. Patients who are critically ill may require inpatient bedside dialysis. In both instances, mobile dialysis services can be provided in the patient's room. Some health care facilities are equipped with a dialysis unit. In such a facility, stable patients are transferred to the dialysis unit for care and then returned to their rooms for continued treatment.

**retail care** Preventive health services and treatment for minor illnesses offered in large retail stores, supermarkets, and pharmacies.

**urgent care center** A facility that treats patients whose illness or injury requires immediate attention but that is not life threatening.

**Retail care** centers, also known as convenient care clinics (CCCs), are clinics located in large retail stores, pharmacies, and supermarkets. CCCs offer preventive health services and treat minor illnesses such as cold, flu, allergies, sore throat, ear infections, urinary tract infections, head lice, and ringworm. Nurse practitioners and physician assistants provide diagnosis, treatment, and coordination of care. Typically, retail clinics provide care for a fraction of the cost of a visit to the physician's office or to an urgent care center.

Medical malls offer convenient access to a variety of medical specialties and services for the health care consumer in one location. Medical malls are located in underserved and growing communities. These facilities are often found near hospitals. Multi specialty, diagnostic, therapeutic, pharmacy, wellness, fitness, and personal services make it a "one-stop" center for medical care.

**pain management treatment center** A specialty setting that provides care and intervention procedures to alleviate acute and chronic pain.

**Pain management treatment centers** provide highly specialized care and interventional procedures aimed to alleviate acute and chronic pain. They provide care to patients when pain fails to respond to traditional medicine and surgery. These freestanding facilities offer medical, surgical, psychological, diagnostic, and therapeutic services to patients.

Cancer treatment centers provide innovative, multidisciplinary outpatient and inpatient services aimed at cancer treatment and management. These state-of-the-art facilities provide oncology, surgical, radiation, hematology, and reconstructive services. Conventional and comprehensive therapies are provided for treatment, to boost immunity, to reduce pain, and to improve the quality of life. Cancer treatment centers offer pastoral care and counselors to assist patients and families. Onsite accommodations, pharmacies, and activities for patients and families are available at most centers. Cancer treatment centers are accredited by TJC.

**cancer treatment centers** A facility that specializes in cancer treatment and management.

**TJC** The Joint Commission

## EXERCISE 8-8

### Other Specialty Care

1. Explain respite care.
2. Describe retail care and medical malls.
3. Explain the care provided by a pain management center and a cancer treatment center.

## HOME HEALTH CARE

An increasingly important segment of health care is focused on delivery of services in the home. **Home health care** is significantly less expensive than inpatient care.

Typically, home health care patients receive services at their residences. Patients may reside at home or in a health care facility, such an assisted living or other LTC facility. The duration of home health care is usually measured in visits by specific therapies (such as two visits per week by physical therapist for 14 weeks) or by specific dates (such as 4 weeks of assistance from a live-in home health aide). A physician will write an order for home health care services and specify the special types of services to be provided.

**home health care** Health care services rendered in the patient's home; or, an agency that provides such services.

### Settings

Home health care is generally rendered by an agency that provides multiple services. For Medicare reimbursement, the home health care facility should offer nursing plus at least one additional rehabilitation therapy, the patient must be confined to the place of residence, and the patient must be under the care of a physician who determines what services are needed. Home health care agencies also assume the responsibility for arranging durable medical equipment (DME) that has been ordered by the physician. The DME companies work with the home health agency to provide specialized services such as oxygen, walkers, wheelchairs, and home hemodialysis equipment.

**DME** durable medical equipment

### Services

Most services available on an outpatient/ambulatory care basis can be offered as home health care. Rehabilitation services, nursing care, and even physician visits can be accomplished in the home health care facility. Table 8-4 lists the types of services provided in the home health care setting.

### Care Providers

In addition to nursing and therapies, home health providers also render assistance to the patient for a variety of ADLs. Care providers include housekeepers and companions.

**ADLs** activities of daily living

### Data Collection Issues

In the home health care environment, data collection and documentation should be completed at the time of service. This principle poses a problem because care providers are

| TABLE 8-4 | |
| --- | --- |
| **HOME HEALTH CARE SERVICES** | |
| **CAREGIVER** | **ROLE IN HOME HEALTH** |
| Home care providers | These caregivers deliver a wide variety of health care and supportive services, ranging from professional nursing and home care aide (HCA) care to physical, occupational, respiratory, and speech therapies. They also may provide social work and nutritional care as well as laboratory, dental, optical, pharmacy, podiatry, radiograph, and medical equipment and supply services. Services for the treatment of medical conditions are usually prescribed by an individual's physician. Supportive services, however, do not require a physician's orders. An individual may receive a single type of care or a combination of services, depending on the complexity of his or her needs. |
| Physician | Physicians visit patients in their homes to diagnose and treat illnesses just as they do in hospitals and private offices. They also work with home care providers to determine which services are needed by patients, which specialists are most suitable to render these services, and how often these services must be provided. With this information, physicians prescribe and oversee patient plans of care. Under Medicare, physicians and home health agency personnel review these plans of care as often as required by the severity of patient medical conditions or at least once every 62 days. |
| Interdisciplinary teams | Interdisciplinary teams review the care plans for hospice patients and their families at least once a month or as frequently as patient conditions or family circumstances require. |
| Nurses | Registered nurses (RNs) and licensed practical nurses (LPNs) provide skilled services that cannot be performed safely and effectively by nonprofessional personnel. Some of these services include injections and intravenous therapy, wound care, education on disease treatment and prevention, and patient assessments. RNs may also provide case management services. RNs have received 2 or more years of specialized education and are licensed to practice by the state. LPNs have 1 year of specialized training and are licensed to work under the supervision of RN. The intricacy of a patient's medical condition and required course of treatment determine whether care should be provided by an RN or can be provided by an LPN. |
| Physical therapists (PTs) | PTs work to restore the mobility and strength of patients who are limited or disabled by physical injuries through the use of exercise, massage, and other methods. PTs often alleviate pain and restore injured muscles with specialized equipment. They also teach patients and caregivers special techniques for walking and transfer. |
| Social workers | Social workers evaluate the social and emotional factors affecting individuals with illnesses or disabilities and provide counseling. They also help patients and their family members identify available community resources. Social workers often serve as case managers when patients' conditions are so complex that professionals are needed to assess medical and supportive needs and coordinate a variety of services. |
| Speech/language pathologists (SLPs) | SLPs work to develop and restore the speech of individuals with communication disorders; usually these disorders are the result of traumas such as surgery or stroke. Speech therapists also help retrain patients in breathing, swallowing, and muscle control. |
| Occupational therapists (OTs) | OTs help individuals who have physical, developmental, social, or emotional problems that prevent them from performing the general activities of daily living. OTs instruct patients on using specialized rehabilitation techniques and equipment to improve their function in tasks such as eating, bathing, dressing, and basic household routines. |
| Dietitians | Dietitians provide counseling services to individuals who need professional dietary assessment and guidance to properly manage an illness or disability. |
| HCAs/home health aides | These caregivers assist patients with activities of daily living such as getting in and out of bed, walking, bathing, toileting, and dressing. Some aides have received special training and are qualified to provide more complex services under the supervision of a nursing professional. |
| Homemakers and chore workers | These caregivers perform light household duties, such as laundry, meal preparation, general housekeeping, and shopping. Their services are directed at maintaining patient households rather than providing hands-on assistance with personal care. |
| Companions | These caregivers provide companionship and comfort to individuals who, for medical and/or safety reasons, cannot be left at home alone. Some companions may help clients with household tasks, but most are limited to providing "sitter" services. |
| Volunteers | Volunteers meet a variety of patient needs. The scope of a volunteer's services depends on his or her level of training and experience. Volunteer activities include, but are not limited to, providing companionship, emotional support, and counseling and helping with personal care, paperwork, and transportation. |

From National Association for Home and Hospice Care. 2012: http://www.nahc.org/famcar_types.html.

with the patient and not at the agency that is responsible for the record. Multiple care providers for the same patient have competing needs to review the patient record. In a paper environment, agencies should have policies that require all documentation for a patient's record to be returned to the agency within a short time frame, such as 24 hours after service is rendered. However, a patient may need multiple visits from other caregivers in that time frame. For that reason, a copy of the documentation of service provided is often left at the patient's residence for reference by other caregivers.

It is this logistical problem that drives the development of electronic record keeping in home health care. Increasingly, agencies are requiring real-time data entry at the time of service to facilitate communication and coordination of services among care providers and to expedite payment.

All orders for home health care must be given by a physician. The physician must review the plan of care every 62 days or whenever there is a significant change in patient status.

## Data Sets

The **Outcome and Assessment Information Set (OASIS)** applies in home health care. A copy of this data set can be obtained from the Center for Health Services Research, in Denver, Colorado.

## Licensure and Accreditation

Home health care agencies must be licensed in the state in which they operate. The **Community Health Accreditation Program (CHAP)** and TJC both offer accreditation opportunities for home health agencies.

**patient care plan** The formal directions for treatment of the patient.

### Home Health Care Coding Notes
Diagnosis Code is ICD-10-CM. Diagnosis is a component of the patient assessment, which is the foundation for the Health Insurance Prospective Payment System (HIPPS) codes.
• Bill format: UB-04

**Outcome and Assessment Information Set (OASIS)** Data set most associated with home health care. This data set monitors patient care by identifying markers over the course of patient care.

**Community Health Accreditation Program (CHAP)** An organization that accredits home health care agencies.

## EXERCISE 8-9
### Home Health Care

1. What services are provided by home health care workers?
2. Describe the unique data collection issues in a home health care environment.
3. What minimum data set is associated with home health care?
4. Who accredits home health care agencies?

## WORKS CITED

American Dietetic Association: The Basics. http://www.eatright.org/students/education/. Published 2011. Accessed August 6, 2011.

American Occupational Therapy Association: About Occupational Therapy. http://www.aota.org/About/AboutOT.aspx. Published 2011. Accessed August 6, 2011.

American Physical Therapy Association: About PT/PTA Careers. http://www.apta.org/Careers/. Published 2011. Accessed August 6, 2011.

National Association of Social Workers: About NASW. https://www.socialworkers.org/nasw/default.asp. Published 2006. Accessed June 6, 2006.

National Hospice and Palliative Care Association: How Does Hospice Work? http://www.caringinfo.org/i4a/pages/index.cfm?pageid=3467. Published 2006. Accessed July 7, 2006.

National Hospice and Palliative Care Association: NHPCO Facts and Figures. http://www.nhpco.org/files/public/Statistics_Research/Hospice_Facts_Figures_Oct-2010.pdf. Published 2010. Accessed December 30, 2011.

New York State Education Department, Office of the Professions: LMSW License Requirements. http://www.op.nysed.gov/prof/sw/. Published 2011. Accessed August 6, 2011.

U.S. Department of Health and Human Services, Office of Inspector General: Nursing Home Resident Assessment Quality of Care. http://oig.hhs.gov/oei/reports/oei-02-99-00040.pdf. Published 2001. Accessed April 10, 2012.

## SUGGESTED READING

Abraham PR: Documentation and reimbursement for home care and hospice programs, Chicago, 2001, American Health Information Management Association.

American Health Information Management Association: Ambulatory care documentation, ed 2, Chicago, 2001, AHIMA.

American Health Information Management Association: Documentation and reimbursement for behavioral healthcare services, Chicago, 2005, AHIMA.

Clark JS: Documentation for acute care, revised edition, Chicago, 2004, American Health Information Management Association.

James E: Documentation and reimbursement for long-term care, Chicago, 2004, American Health Information Management Association.

Manger BJ: Documentation requirements in non-acute care facilities & organizations, Pearl River, NY, 2001, Parthenon Publishing Group, Inc.

Peden AH: Comparative health information management, ed 3, Clifton Park, NY, 2011, Delmar Cengae Learning.

# CHAPTER ACTIVITIES

## CHAPTER SUMMARY

Health care is delivered in a multitude of inpatient and outpatient settings. Ambulatory care is rendered in physicians' offices as well as EDs, surgery centers, urgent care centers, radiology and laboratory facilities, rehabilitation facilities, and home care facilities. Specialty therapeutic services are offered both in hospitals and on an outpatient basis, including physical, occupational, and psychological therapies.

In general, health care facilities are licensed in the states in which they operate. Accreditation is offered by the TJC, HFAP, ACS, AAAHC, CHAP, and CARF.

Important data sets include UACDS, DEEDS, OASIS, and MDS.

All facilities seeking Medicare reimbursement are regulated by CMS. The CMS Web site should be consulted for detailed information on those regulations. HIM professionals who are employed in special health care settings must become familiar with the unique data requirements of those settings.

## REVIEW QUESTIONS

1. Describe four different types of ambulatory care.
2. Compare rehabilitation facilities with the various types of LTC facilities, including the specific data collection issues.
3. Identify and describe five allied health professions and their principal occupational settings.
4. What is the difference between occupational therapy and physical therapy? If you have trouble explaining the difference, try finding Web sites for their national professional associations. What do those sites have to offer the public in terms of information about the profession?
5. Describe the difference between the behavioral health care setting and the rehabilitation health care setting, including the type of care provided.
6. Describe home health care and hospice care, including the differences in the type of care provided by each.
7. What services are available on a home health basis?
8. Compare and contrast the data collected in acute care facilities with data collected in non-acute care facilities.
9. List and describe the data sets unique to non-acute care facilities.

## ● PROFESSIONAL PROFILE

### Medical Records Manager

 My name is Francis, and I work in a 120-bed subacute/long-term care center. Subacute care centers are rehab and nursing inpatient care facilities that treat patients who no longer need or qualify for acute care but who still are unable to return to their homes or previous care settings because of the severity of their illness or injury. We also accept long-term care patients who are on ventilators permanently as well as those who are considered weanable from ventilators.

My job duties include, but are not limited to, discharge processing, correspondence, utilization review, auditing and thinning of medical records, and general management of the medical records department.

The major differences between working in a subacute care center and working in an acute care center include the absence of large volumes of coding and transcription. We use the MDS (Minimum Data Set) for billing purposes. Generally speaking, there is an interdisciplinary team that meets once a week to assess the patient and complete an MDS on the basis of that assessment, which is then electronically submitted to Medicare, Medicaid, or other third party payers. Also, although our turnover rate is one to two charts per day, our charts are significantly larger than those in a typical acute care hospital. I also have to manage a whole file area for thinned records only (mainly for our long-term care patients).

I enjoy my position because I really feel that I'm a part of the team here and I'm helping the patients as well as the staff.

## PATIENT CARE PERSPECTIVE

### Maria

My mother, Isabel, needed to be in a nursing home for a little while after her stroke last year. I wanted to get a copy of her medical records so that I could work with a private patient advocate to find rehabilitation and home care afterwards that met our needs. Because my mother signed herself in to the nursing home and didn't list me as a contact, I had some difficulty getting the records. I contacted Francis, the medical records manager, who helped obtain consent from my mother to release the records. I really appreciated his compassion in understanding our issues and respecting my mother's dignity and right to privacy.

## APPLICATION ●

### New Challenges

Fred has been working in acute care facilities for the past 5 years in progressively responsible positions. After he graduated from his HIT program and passed the RHIT exam, he was offered a position as the HIM manager in his organization's new long-term care center, which was recently purchased. Fred has heard through the grapevine that the center's records have not been strictly maintained and that the new manager will be expected to organize the records and to ensure that the facility's documentation policies are in compliance with all regulatory and accrediting bodies.

If Fred decides to accept this position, what can he do to ensure that he is prepared for the challenges of his new position?

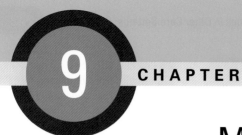

**9** CHAPTER

# MANAGING HEALTH RECORDS

Melissa LaCour

## CHAPTER OUTLINE

MASTER PATIENT INDEX
 Development
 Maintenance
 Retention
IDENTIFICATION OF PHYSICAL
 FILES
 Alphabetical Filing
 Unit Numbering
 Serial Numbering
 Serial-Unit Numbering
 Family Unit Numbering
 Patient Accounting
LEGACY SYSTEMS

Filing Methods
Paper Record Storage Methods
Offsite Storage
CHART LOCATOR SYSTEMS
 Manual Systems
 Computerized Systems
INFORMATION SYSTEMS
 Hardware and Software
 Storage
 Scanned Imaging and Electronic
  Storage
 Cloud Computing

SECURITY OF HEALTH
 INFORMATION
 Disaster Planning
 Theft and Tampering
 Destruction of Health Information
 Restoration of Information Lost
  Inadvertently
RECORD RETENTION
 Retention Policy
 Facility Closure

## VOCABULARY

chart locator system
cloud computing
computer output to laser
 disk (COLD)
enterprise master patient
 index (EMPI)
family unit numbering
 system

file folder
index
master patient index (MPI)
medical record number
 (MR#)
microfiche
microfilm
middle-digit filing system

optical disk
outguide
patient account number
record retention schedule
redundant arrays of
 independent disks
 (RAIDs)
retention

scanner
serial numbering system
serial-unit numbering
 system
storage area network (SAN)
straight numerical filing
terminal-digit filing system
unit numbering system

## CHAPTER OBJECTIVES

*By the end of this chapter, the student should be able to:*
1. Explain the purpose of the master patient index.
2. Maintain the accuracy of a master patient index.
3. Determine whether a patient has a previous health record at the facility.
4. Compare and contrast numbering systems for identification of patient records.
5. Compare and contrast filing systems for patient records.
6. File health records appropriately according to the file system used by the facility.
7. Maintain accuracy of filing methods.

8. Identify the alternative storage system best suited for a particular health care facility.
9. Explain a chart locator system.
10. Determine the appropriate file space for a given set of circumstances.
11. Compare various computer storage architectures.
12. Identify ways to ensure the physical security of health information.
13. Determine the retention schedule for specific health care records.

Earlier chapters discussed the recording of patient data for communication. The accuracy, validity, and completeness of health data are all necessary in order for the data to be useful. Yet storage, too, is an important aspect of managing health records. HIM departments must have the appropriate shelf space and furniture to accommodate paper records as well as the computer hardware and software to facilitate workflow, efficient access, and secure storage for vast amounts of electronic files. Previous patient data may communicate to a physician important information necessary for treatment. A patient's health care may depend on the physician's review of the patient's previous health records. Therefore it is important to make sure the patient's health data are recorded, organized, and analyzed in the health record and stored in a way that allows the information to be retrieved when the patient returns to the facility for follow-up care.

What happens if the physician cannot locate the patient's health record from the last visit? What if comparison of the notes from the previous visit with the present information reflects a significant weight loss for the patient, or a current test result must be compared with a previous result? This information may be important in the care and treatment of the patient. For example, it could change the patient's dosage of a particular medication or indicate a new diagnosis.

**data accuracy** The quality that data are correct.

**data validity** The quality that data reflect the known or acceptable range of values for the specific data.

**completeness** The data quality of existence. If a required data element is missing, the record is not complete.

**health data** Elements related to a patient's diagnosis and procedures as well as factors that may affect the patient's condition.

**treatment** A procedure, medication, or other measure designed to cure or alleviate the symptoms of disease.

**analysis** The review of a record to evaluate its completeness, accuracy, or compliance with predetermined standards or other criteria.

**HIM** health information management

**diagnosis** The name of the patient's condition or illness.

**Go To** Chapter 12 details the release of information (ROI) process.

**continuity of care** The broad range of health care services required by a patient during an illness or for an entire lifetime. May also refer to the continuity of care provided by a health care organization. Also called *continuum of care*.

**reimbursement** The amount of money that the health care facility receives from the party responsible for paying the bill.

**accreditation** Voluntary compliance with a set of standards developed by an independent agent, who periodically performs audits to ensure compliance.

**litigation** The term used to indicate that a matter must be settled by the court and the process of engaging in legal proceedings.

**hybrid record** A record in which both electronic and paper media are used.

---

## HIT-bit

### RETRIEVAL OF HEALTH INFORMATION

Other reasons that a health record may be retrieved include the following:
- Physician specialists may review a patient's record before providing care.
- Insurance companies request copies of reports before paying the claim (reimbursement).
- Facilities review their own records to assess quality of care.
- Accrediting bodies review records to evaluate compliance with standards.
- Lawyers present health records during lawsuits to represent their clients.
- Researchers may use health records to investigate disease trends.

---

HIM professionals systematically collect and organize a patient's health information to create a timely, accurate, and complete record. Health information is vital not only to the patient but also to the health care provider and the community. HIM departments routinely provide health information on request to authorized users. The patient's health record, whether paper or electronic, must be retained for the continuity of patient care, and for reimbursement, accreditation, potential litigation, research, and education purposes. This information must be stored in a secure, organized environment and accessible to those who need it. This chapter explores the issues of health record storage for electronic and paper records, including computer hardware and storage capacity, file identification, filing systems, filing furniture, scanning, and security of the file environment. It also discusses alternative storage methods, including offsite storage and microfilm.

The organized storage of the health record begins with appropriate identification of each patient's record. Whether the facility maintains paper health records or works in a hybrid or electronic environment, the master patient index (MPI) is the primary tool for identifying a file for each patient the facility has seen.

**master patient index (MPI)**
A system containing a list of patients who have received care at the health care facility and their encounter information, often used to correlate the patient with the file identification.

**health record** Also called *record* or *medical record*. It contains all of the data collected for an individual patient.

**medical record number (MR#)** A unique number assigned to each patient in a health care system; this code will be used for the rest of the patient's encounters with that specific health system.

## MASTER PATIENT INDEX

The **master patient index** (**MPI**) is used to maintain the information and location of each patient admitted to the facility. Originally, before computers, an MPI was a manual system maintained on index cards organized in a file cabinet in alphabetical and numerical order; today it is a computerized system.

The data contained in the MPI are the data collected during the patient registration process. At registration, an identification number and a **medical record number** (**MR#**) are assigned. This unique number is used to individually identify each patient within that health care facility. The process of recording the registration data into the MPI and generating the MR # initiates the patient's health record.

### HIT-bit

#### LOCATION LOCATION LOCATION

To envision an MPI, consider how a book is located in the library. To locate the book, first access the catalog to determine whether the book is available in the library. If it is available, the catalog number is necessary to find the book on the library shelf. The library catalog index correlates the book with its catalog number, which is necessary to locate the book on the shelf in the library, where the books are organized by catalog number.

Each health care facility has an MPI. The MPI is a list of all patients who have received health care services at the facility. When looking for the health record of a particular patient, staff in the patient registration department must first find out whether the patient has previously received services at the health care facility and then determine the patient's medical record number. They use the MPI to obtain this information. The MPI correlates the patient with the facility's medical record number to identify the patient's health record. Box 9-1 lists the recommended and optional contents of an MPI. The information contained in the MPI is a combination of the demographic, financial, and clinical data.

Each patient is entered only once in the MPI. All visits for a particular patient are listed in the MPI under the patient's name. HIM professionals are very careful to prevent duplication of patients within the MPI, because it may cause confusion and delay in retrieval of patient files.

---

**BOX 9-1    CONTENTS OF A MASTER PATIENT INDEX**

**RECOMMENDED DATA ELEMENTS**
- Patient's name
- Alias/previous name(s)
- Address
- Date of birth
- Social security number
- Gender
- Race
- Ethnicity
- Medical record number and any duplicates
- Hospital identification number
- Patient account number
- Payer
- Admission date(s)
- Discharge date(s)
- Type of service for the encounter
- Patient disposition

**OPTIONAL DATA ELEMENTS**
- Marital status
- Physician
- Telephone number
- Mother's maiden name
- Place of birth
- Advance directive and surrogate decision making
- Organ donor status
- Emergency contact
- Allergies/reactions
- Problem list

*Note:* In the capturing of dates, it is important to record the year as four numbers, i.e., MMDDYYYY or YYYYMMDD.
Modified from AHIMA Practice Brief No. 433. http://library.ahima.org/xpedio/groups/public/documents/ahima/bok1_048390.hcsp?dDocName=bok1_048390

Last Name, First Name, Middle Initial    Date of Birth    Medical Record #

_____    __/__/__    _____

Address    Phone #    Married    Death

_____    (   )  -    _____    _____

City, State _____ Zip Code _____

Gender _____    Social Security # _____-_____-_____

Race _____    Financial Class _____

| Admit Date | Discharge Date | Service | Physician | Patient Account # |
|---|---|---|---|---|
|  |  |  |  |  |
|  |  |  |  |  |
|  |  |  |  |  |
|  |  |  |  |  |

Figure 9-1  MPI card in a manual system.

## Development

### Manual Master Patient Index

In previously used manual MPI systems, as patients were registered in the facility, the HIM department was notified of the admission. The notification might have been a copy of the face sheet, a computer printout of the admission, or the admit log. The HIM department created an index card in the MPI for each patient who was registered in the health care facility. If the patient had been treated at the facility on a previous occasion, the patient's MPI card was retrieved from the card file, reviewed to make sure the patient's information was correct, and the new admission information added (date of admission, type of service, account number for that visit, attending physician, discharge date). The MPI had to be updated each time the patient was admitted to the health care facility so that all health care services were listed on the card. Figure 9-1 illustrates a manual MPI card.

### Computerized Master Patient Index

Today, the MPI is computerized even if the HIM department maintains paper health records. A modern, computerized MPI is more robust than a manual system. It captures more patient information and can be accessed from areas outside the HIM department, such as the emergency department and patient registration. A computerized MPI system uses software to capture and store patient identification and admission information. The computerized MPI software is typically one feature of a larger electronic health record (EHR) system or is interfaced with other information systems in the health care facility.

Information entered into a computerized MPI creates a history for each patient. At registration, the admitting clerk searches the MPI history files to determine whether the patient has been treated at the facility on a previous occasion. If the patient is new, a new history is created by entering the information listed in Box 9-1. If the patient has been treated at the facility on a previous occasion, the admitting clerk identifies the patient's history and reviews it to ensure the accuracy of all of the information. Any changes to the patient's address, phone number, or health insurance should be documented in the MPI.

Figure 9-2 shows a computerized MPI screen, the results of a search for patient Mary Davidson. Notice that there are two results. The example shown is an MPI for a multihospital system in which all of the facilities share an MPI. This system is commonly called an **enterprise master patient index (EMPI)**. This particular MPI indicates that that Mary Davidson has been a patient in two different health care facilities within the multihospital

**face sheet** The first page in a paper record. Usually contains at least the demographic data and contains space for the physician to record and authenticate the discharge diagnoses and procedures. In many facilities, the admission record is also used as the face sheet.

**attending physician** The physician who is primarily responsible for coordinating the care of the patient in the hospital; it is usually the physician who ordered the patient's admission to the hospital.

**MPI** master patient index

**electronic health record (EHR)** A secure real-time, point-of-care, patient centric information resource for clinicians allowing access to patient information when and where needed and incorporating evidence-based decision support.

**interface** Computer configuration allowing information to pass from one system to another.

**enterprise master patient index (EMPI)** A master patient index shared across a multihospital system, such as an HIE.

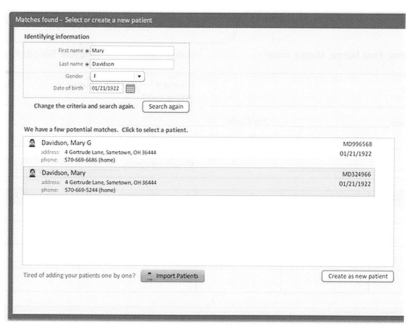

**Figure 9-2** Computerized MPI results. (Courtesy Practice Fusion, Inc., San Francisco, CA.)

system. The EMPI improves access to records and allows for easy retrieval of the patient's health information when authorized. Though each facility within the multi-hospital system maintains its own patient health records, the facilities share an EMPI in order to manage patient encounters. The computerized MPI can also help resolve the use of an alias (AKA, or also known as) and "merges" for a particular patient. The AKA feature links any other names for this patient (e.g., maiden name). The merge feature can identify whether any duplicate numbers have been assigned to a patient; this knowledge can be helpful if a chart was incorrectly filed under a duplicate patient number.

---

### HIT-bit

#### ENTERPRISE MASTER PATIENT INDEX

An EMPI is one that lists all patients for a health care system that consists of two or more hospitals or health care facilities. This type of MPI allows employees at each facility to determine whether a patient has been treated at one of the health care facilities in the system. The arrangement enables health records to be retrieved for patient care and related for continuity of care or longitudinal use. Another important use of this EMPI involves billing, discussed in Chapter 7. The accuracy of the EMPI is very important and must be monitored and maintained to ensure that patients receive proper care and compliance with billing guidelines.

---

There are advantages and disadvantages to a computerized MPI. The computerized MPI provides the opportunity to store more patient identification information for each admission—for example, patient financial class, marital status, social security number, and AKA functions, which link the patient to another name resulting from divorce or marriage or to a pseudonym. More information is stored in a smaller space combined with greater search capabilities to access possible matches for a name using phonetics, date of birth, Social Security number, or age. Information systems also allow the MPI to be linked to other departments. The disadvantage of a computerized MPI is that it is not available during computer down time or power outages. Therefore, a printout of key fields for emergency lookup or locally installed backup are "manual" solutions that provide access to the data when the system is not available.

## Maintenance

Regardless of format or type, it is necessary to maintain an accurate MPI. The most common errors include duplication of patient entries and misspelling of patient names. When they are identified, an HIM professional must carefully follow procedures to correct each error and to properly identify the patient in the MPI and with the correlating record. If a patient has more than one entry in the MPI, the HIM professional must be sure to correct all associated records to reflect the accurate number and patient. If the patient's name is incorrect, this information must also be corrected wherever it appears to ensure accurate retrieval of patient information. Failure to maintain an accurate MPI can impact patient care because information may be unavailable or incomplete and not accessible when needed at the point of care. Inaccuracies can also impact reimbursement and compliance if the MPI is used to correlate patient visits with appropriate billing or claims processing.

> **reimbursement** The amount of money that the health care facility receives from the party responsible for paying the bill.
>
> **compliance** Meeting standards. Also the development, implementation, and enforcement of policies and procedures that ensure that standards are met.
>
> **claim** The application to an insurance company for reimbursement of services rendered.

### HIT-bit

#### MEDICAL RECORD NUMBER

Medical record numbers (MR#) are assigned by the facility in which the patient is registered to receive health care. Patients do not have the same MR# for their files when receiving care at another facility. However, if a patient receives care in a large multifacility health care system, one that is owned and operated by the same organization, the patient may be assigned a system-wide MR# that is used in all the facilities.

### HIT-bit

#### NEW VERSUS OLD RECORDS

How does a facility distinguish a new patient from a patient who already has a record (has received care) at the facility?
- **New:** new to the facility as a patient; not registered or treated at the facility on a prior occasion
- **Old:** returning patient; has been treated previously in the facility and has a MR# and is listed in the MPI; new visit added to patient's existing MPI

## Retention

The MPI must be retained by the health care facility permanently. This index is extremely important in the everyday operations of the health care facility and the HIM department. In a numerical filing system (discussed later in this chapter), the medical record number (MR#) is necessary to retrieve the patient's health record. The MPI is the easiest way to access the patient's medical record number.

When a facility implements a computerized MPI, it must decide what to do with the manual system. Because the information in an MPI is never destroyed, the facility must devise a way to convert the information from the manual file into the computerized system. One method to retain the data on the manual MPI cards is to enter the MPI information in the new computerized system, allowing computer access to all MPI information. When this process is performed the facility must ensure the accuracy of the converted MPI data if it plans to dispose of the original MPI system. In other situations the MPI cards are scanned and maintained in an imaging system. This is an efficient way to maintain the original MPI system for future research if MPI data are questioned. HIM professionals should monitor the accuracy of the manual MPI conversion. If the information on even one patient or encounter is omitted or entered incorrectly, the MPI is not accurate. The

> 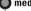 **medical record number (MR#)** A unique number assigned to each patient in a health care system; this code will be used for the rest of the patient's encounters with that specific health system.

**Go To** Microfilming as a storage solution is addressed later in this chapter.

omission or error may cause great difficulty for anyone accessing patient records. Maintenance of the original MPI information secures the validity of the data in the computerized MPI and provides a reference if a discrepancy arises in a patient's file that originated before the conversion. The ability to reference the original MPI cards allows the correction of any discrepancies caused by an error or omission. In this type of conversion, the facility should consider storing the manual MPI in the original format or microfilming the original MPI cards for future reference. The minor inconvenience caused by storing the manual system can prevent serious problems with record discrepancies in the future.

---

### HIT-bit

#### THE MASTER PATIENT INDEX

It is obvious that the manual master patient index (MPI) system is very antiquated. Today, it is rare for a facility to have a manual MPI system. This system does not allow capture of all the recommended data elements because it is limited by the size of the index card. The manual system does not typically have all of the items listed in Box 9-1. Likewise, because the index cards are filed alphabetically, it is possible for cards to be misfiled and problems to occur as they do in alphabetical filing.

---

### EXERCISE 9-1
#### Master Patient Index

1. The _____ contains patient and encounter information, which is often used to correlate the patient with the file identification.
2. The MPI is especially useful in a facility that uses a numerical system to identify patient records because the MPI _____ the patient to the MR# for the patient file.
   a. maps
   b. correlates
   c. copies
   d. registers
3. List the uses of the MPI.
4. Explain the function of an EMPI.
5. The _____ is a tool in the health care facility used to store unique identifiable information on each patient who has been registered in that facility.
6. The emergency room calls the health information management department for the old chart on Mr. Tom Jones. What is the first step in locating Mr. Jones's old record from a previous admission?

---

**EHR** electronic health record

**file folder** The physical container used to store the health record in a paper-based system.
**character** A single letter, number, or symbol.
**The Joint Commission (TJC)** An organization that accredits and sets standards for acute care facilities, ambulatory care networks, long-term care facilities, and rehabilitation facilities, as well as certain specialty facilities, such as hospice and home care. Facilities maintaining TJC accreditation receive *deemed status* from the CMS.

### IDENTIFICATION OF PHYSICAL FILES

Prior to the EHR, paper health record documents were stored in physical **file folders**. For easy identification and filing, the file folder containing the patient's health information was labeled with alphanumerical characters. In a small health care facility or a physician's office, the file folder might be identified alphabetically with the patient's name. In a large health care facility, the MR# was used to identify the patient's health record file. MR#s vary in length: Some are only six digits, others are eight or nine digits, and some may even be longer. Currently, the number of digits or type of number used by a facility is not mandated. However, accreditation agencies such as The Joint Commission (TJC) require facilities to use a system that ensures timely access to patient information when requested for patient care or other authorized use. Additionally, the facility chooses the system that best suits its purpose for identification and storage of patient files. Five types of health record identification are discussed here: alphabetical filing, unit numbering, serial numbering, serial-unit numbering, and family unit numbering. While you are learning these identification methods, keep in mind that a numbering system is not the same as a filing method.

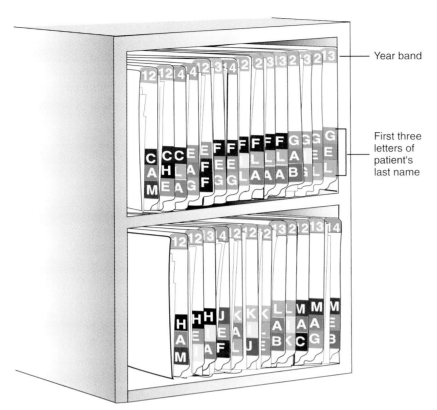

Figure 9-3 File folders in a cabinet in alphabetical order.

## Alphabetical Filing

In a small physician's office, clinic, home health care facility, or nursing home, the patient health record file folders are often labeled using the patients' names. Thus, the "numbering" and "alphabetical" filing systems are the same. The health record file for the patient John Adams is identified thus: Adams, John. File folders are arranged on the shelf in alphabetical order, beginning with the patient's last name (Figure 9-3). For those records stored on a shelf, the patient's name is color coded on the side tab, often using the first three letters of the patient's last name. The records are still filed alphabetically, but the labeling is different. In the alphabetical system in which records are filed in a cabinet, the folder is labeled with the patient's name, preferably on the top tab (Figure 9-4, *A* and *B*).

Alphabetical filing works well in health care environments where the number of patient visits or records is relatively low. The file folders are easy to label, and pulling a patient's

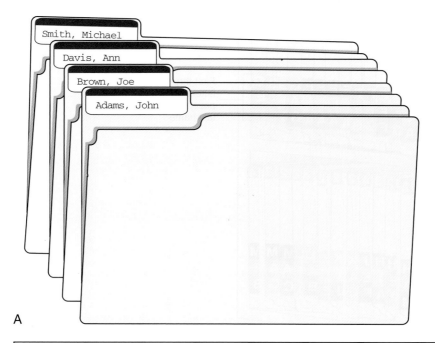

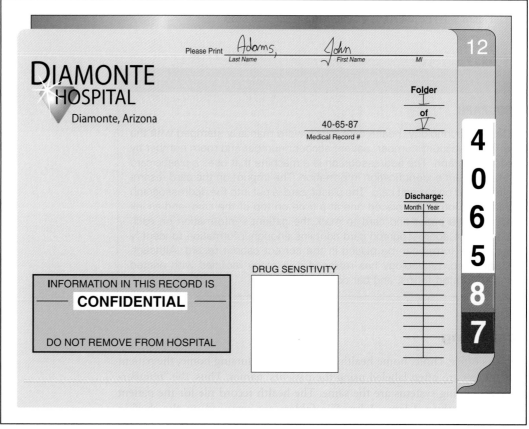

**Figure 9-4** File folder labeling showing top (**A**) and side (**B**) tabs.

file can be accomplished if the patient's name is known. Health care professionals in facilities using this system must take special care to protect the privacy of patient records because the patient health information is easily identified. Alphabetical filing does not require an additional system, such as the MPI, to correlate patient names and numbers to identify a particular file folder.

**MPI** master patient index

---

## HIT-bit

### FILE FOLDERS

Some health care environments may retain patient health records in manila folders, binders, envelopes, or expandable pocket files.

---

Problems can arise when two patients have the same name. Common names require careful attention to be certain that the correct patient record is found. Think about the names Michael, Joe, and Ann. How many other ways may these names be identified? Mike, Michael, Jo, Joe, Joseph, José, Josef, Ann, Anne, Annie, and Annette are common versions of Michael, Joe, and Ann, respectively. When duplicate names occur in an alphabetical filing system, procedures must be specified to further organize the records by the patient's middle name, by titles (Jr., Sr., III), or by the patient's date of birth (DOB). Common rules for alphabetical filing are as follows:

- Personal names are filed last name first; for example, the name John Adams is filed by Adams first, followed by John: Adams, John. The first name is followed by the middle initial (e.g., E) or name if necessary: Adams, John E.
- All punctuation and possessives are ignored. Disregard commas, hyphens, and apostrophes. In the last name, prefixes, foreign articles, and particles are combined with the name following it, omitting spaces (e.g., De Witt is filed as dewitt).
- Abbreviations, nicknames, and shortened names are filed as written (e.g., Wm, Bud, Rob).
- Suffixes are considered after the middle name or initial. Titles are considered after suffixes. Royal or religious titles follow the given name and surname; the title is indexed last.
- When identical names occur, consider the DOB for filing order and proceed chronologically.

Patients' files must be clearly labeled. It is important to print clearly when labeling the patient's file folder. This is not an occasion for fancy script or calligraphy. Illegible or fancy handwriting may cause a file folder to be misfiled. Table 9-1 lists the advantages and disadvantages of alphabetical filing.

Space is a common problem in the alphabetical filing system. The shelves or cabinets holding the files of patients' names beginning with common letters become full very quickly, so HIM departments must allow adequate file space for these letters of the

---

## TABLE 9-1

### ADVANTAGES AND DISADVANTAGES OF ALPHABETICAL FILING

| | |
|---|---|
| Advantages | Easy to learn |
| | Does not require additional cross-reference |
| | Works well in smaller facilities |
| Disadvantages | Illegible handwriting may cause problems with filing |
| | Space within the popular letters of the alphabet to locate a patient chart can fill quickly |
| | Can be inefficient for a large facility with a large patient population |
| | Many alternative spellings of names exist, which can cause problems with retrieval |

alphabet. Filing in a section that is full of records is difficult and requires shifting of the records for further filing. Alphabetical filing systems can become inefficient in a facility that serves a large population with a high volume of patient records.

Another consideration with this system is the spelling of patient names. In an alphabetical file system, a folder labeled incorrectly because of misspelling will not be filed correctly. When the HIM employee attempts to locate the patient's folder, efforts will involve searching for a misspelled, misfiled record. When unsure of the spelling of the patient's name, the person taking the information from the patient should ask for identification to clarify the spelling.

## Unit Numbering

In a **unit numbering system**, a patient receives the same medical record number for each admission to the facility. Therefore the numerical identification of each individual patient is always patient specific. For example, if a person is born in a facility that uses unit numbering, at birth (which is considered an admission) the patient is assigned a number (e.g., MR# 001234). Any subsequent admissions of this patient to the facility would use the same MR#. In a unit numbering identification system, the patient's medical record number remains the same, within the facility, throughout the lifetime of the patient. Medical record numbers are not shared and are not reused after a patient dies.

Consider the following scenario: Molly Brabant is born at Diamonte Hospital on January 1, 2001. At birth, Molly is assigned MR# 001234. Her birth record is filed in a folder identified with MR# 001234. At age 7, Molly returns to the same facility to have a tonsillectomy. Molly's new records are stored in the same folder identified as MR# 001234. Any subsequent admissions (e.g., for a hip replacement later in life) are filed under the same number (Figure 9-5).

**unit numbering system** A numerical patient record identification system in which the patient record is filed under the same number for all visits.

**medical record number (MR#)** A unique number assigned to each patient in a health care system; this code will be used for the rest of the patient's encounters with that specific health system.

**admission** The act of accepting a patient into care in a health care facility, including any nonambulatory care facility. Admission requires a physician's order.

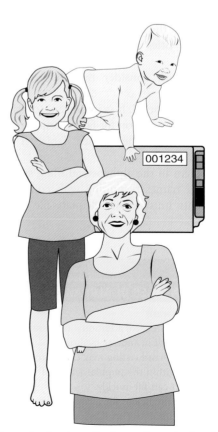

**Figure 9-5** Example of unit medical record numbering for one patient.

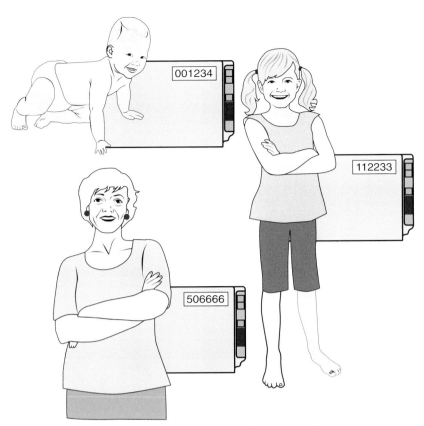

**Figure 9-6** Example of serial medical record numbering for one patient.

## Serial Numbering

In a **serial numbering system**, a new medical record number is assigned each time a patient has an encounter at the facility. In this type of system, the patient's file folders containing the health record for each encounter are not filed in the same folder. Therefore the records are not typically located together on the file shelf.

In the previous scenario but with a serial numbering system, Molly Brabant is assigned MR# 001234 at birth. However, when she returns at age 7 for a tonsillectomy, a new number, MR# 112233, is assigned (Figure 9-6). In this system, Molly's records are not stored in the same folder, and they are not located near one another on the file shelf. Molly now has two separate folders containing her health record, and she receives a third MR# and a new folder when she visits the facility for a hip replacement in later years. The number assigned during each one of Molly's encounters is recorded in the MPI under her name.

## Serial-Unit Numbering

A **serial-unit numbering system** is a combination of the previous two numbering systems. In this system, the patient receives a new medical record number each time he or she comes

**serial numbering system**
A numerical patient record identification system in which the patient is given a new number for each visit and each file folder contains separate visit information.

**MPI** master patient index

**serial-unit numbering system**
A numerical patient record identification system in which the patient is given a new number for each visit; however, with each new admission, the previous record is retrieved and filed in the folder with the most recent visit.

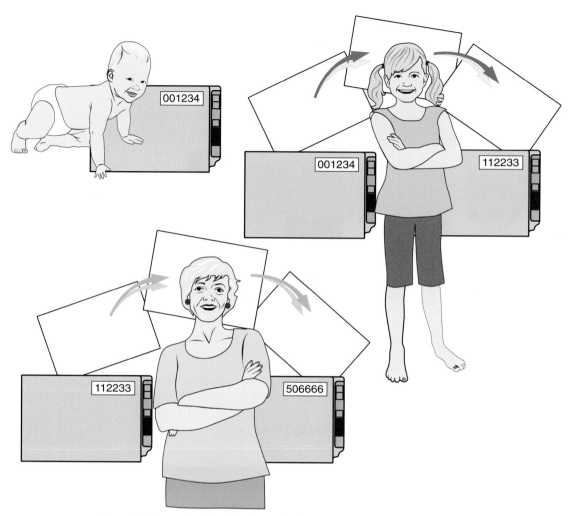

Figure 9-7 Example of serial-unit medical record numbering for one patient.

into a facility. The difference is that each time the patient receives health care, the old records are brought forward and filed with the most recent visit, under a new medical record number. This system requires a cross-reference system from the old MR# to the new number so that records can be located. For cross-referencing, the MPI must be updated so each encounter reflects the corresponding medical record number, and a file guide is placed in the old file location alerting HIM employees to look for the current MR# to locate the patient's health record.

In the previous scenario using a serial-unit numbering system, Molly is assigned MR# 001234 at birth, and on return 7 years later for a tonsillectomy, she is assigned a new number, MR# 112233. When Molly returns for the tonsillectomy, the birth record (MR# 001234) is retrieved from its place in the files and combined with the file folder MR# 112233. A cross-reference should be set up by insertion of an *outguide* (see Figure 9-16) in place of the old MR# 001234 to indicate that the record is now filed at MR# 112233 (Figure 9-7). Molly's records are transferred and cross-referenced a third time when Molly has a hip replacement later in life.

## Family Unit Numbering

In rare cases in health care settings where it is common for an entire family to visit a physician or clinic, and often to have the same insurance carrier, an entire family's records may be identified using one medical record number. Each family members file is then identified by the one medical record number to the entire family (father/husband, mother/wife, and

## TABLE 9-2

### FAMILY UNIT NUMBERING

| FAMILY MEMBER | FAMILY NUMBER | MODIFIER | PATIENT NUMBER |
|---|---|---|---|
| John Smith | 123456 | 01 | 123456-01 |
| Mary Smith | 123456 | 02 | 123456-02 |
| Molly Smith | 123456 | 03 | 123456-03 |
| Tommy Smith | 123456 | 04 | 123456-04 |

## TABLE 9-3

### ADVANTAGES AND DISADVANTAGES OF NUMBERING SYSTEMS

| SYSTEM | ADVANTAGE | DISADVANTAGE(S) |
|---|---|---|
| Unit | All patient records can be located under one number. | Filing of all encounters in one folder can cause problems with incomplete records. |
| Serial | Each admission is filed in a single folder. | Retrieving all the records for one patient involves going to multiple places in the files. |
| Serial-unit | Each admission has a unique number, but they are all filed with the most recent. | This method is time consuming. |
| Family unit | Records are files together for clinical and financial processing of claims. | Confidentiality can be compromised; divorce, remarriage, and other factors can create complications. |

children). This system is called a **family unit numbering system**. A modifier is placed at the end of the family unit number unique to each member of the family. The modifier is a number attached to the MR# using a hyphen. Each member of the family can be identified by a modifier associated with his or her position in the family: head of household, 01; spouse, 02; first born, 03; second born, 04; and so on. With this system, all of the family members' records may be contained in one file folder.

In our example, Molly's family unit number is MR# 123456. At birth, Molly, being the first-born child, is assigned MR# 123456-03. Molly's mother has MR# 123456-02. The last two numbers after the hyphen indicate to which family member the record belongs. Table 9-2 provides an example of family unit numbering.

This system is also beneficial in a small clinic or physician's office setting where clinical and financial records are combined for claims processing. There are potential problems with this numbering system, however. Families change, couples divorce, and grown children marry and adopt other names. When members of the family divorce, die, marry, or remarry, the medical records for those patients must be renumbered. This process can be quite tedious. Even in a family unit numbering system, the facility is responsible for maintaining the confidentiality of each patient's health information. Safeguards must be taken to ensure that husbands and wives are allowed access to each other's information only with appropriate authorization (see Chapter 12). Likewise, procedures should exist to safeguard the confidentiality of a child's information after he or she reaches the legal age of majority.

Each facility should examine the positive and negative aspects of each numbering identification system to choose the system that allows the most efficient delivery of health care for its patients. The system should have a positive impact on both employee and facility productivity. Table 9-3 summarizes the advantages and disadvantages of each numbering system.

## Patient Accounting

In some health care facilities the patient account number is used to identify the patient health record. The **patient account number** is unique because it is specific to the

**family unit numbering system** A numerical identification system to identify an entire family's health record using one number and modifiers.

**MR#** medical record number

**claim** The application to an insurance company for reimbursement of services rendered.

**Go To** Chapter 12 addresses the legal and regulatory environment surrounding record release.

**patient account number** A numerical identifier assigned to a specific encounter or health care service received by a patient; a new number will be assigned to each encounter, but the patient will retain the same medical record number.

**encounter** A patient's health care experience; a unit of measure for the volume of ambulatory care services provided.

**index** A system to identify or name a file or other item so that it can be located.

**EHR** electronic health record

encounter or health care service the patient receives. Patient account numbers are not typically duplicated and therefore can easily be used as an additional method of identifying a patient health record. For instance, in some facilities the number generated for the health care service may easily indicate whether a patient was treated in the emergency room, ambulatory surgery center, or outpatient clinic. In a scanned imaging system this information can be used as one of the **index** values helping HIM professionals search for a patient record or document. In the EHR the patient account number is a data field that can be used to search for patient records.

---

## HIT-bit

### PATIENT ACCOUNTING

Regardless of the identification method used by a health information management department, each health care encounter typically receives a unique patient account number. For instance, in the numbering systems discussed prior to this HIT-bit box, we mention patients having more than one encounter or visit to the same health care facility. The medical record numbering system may be used to identify the patient's health care record, but in the business office, the patient account number is the unique identifying number for organizing patient billing accounts, payments, and other information related to the financial aspects of the health care services received by the patient.

---

## LEGACY SYSTEMS

A *legacy system* is a method or computerized system formerly used by the health care facility (or any organization). As changes occur in health care, this term is used by HIM professionals to refer to the "old" way or system used. For many organizations, the manual/paper filing methods discussed in this chapter are legacy systems. It is important to recognize the value of these systems and to understand them so that the information they contain can be retrieved and used as needed for patient care.

### Filing Methods

*Filing* is the process of organizing the health record folders on a shelf, in a file cabinet, or in a computer system. There are some common methods for organizing paper-based health records in a file area: alphabetical, middle-digit, straight numerical, and terminal-digit. Alphabetical filing was described previously in the discussion on identification of files. In an electronic system, patient health information is indexed; this issue is discussed at the end of this section.

---

## HIT-bit

### PAPER RECORDS

While health care facilities are transitioning to some form of an electronic health record (EHR), it remains important for health information management (HIM) professionals to understand the issues associated with storage of the paper health record. Storage of paper health records will be an important function in the management of health information in facilities that maintain dual systems, have hybrid systems, or at least maintain filing of the older paper health records until they are transitioned to electronic format. Because an entire chapter of this text is devoted to the EHR, much (but not all) of the discussion in this chapter focuses on the management of the paper health records.

## Straight Numerical Filing

**Straight numerical filing** involves placing the folders on the shelf in numerical order (e.g., MR# 001234, MR# 001235, MR# 001522). This filing system is easy for HIM staff to understand. Straight numerical filing is best used in a system in which there is minimal activity in the records once they are filed in the permanent file area.

Straight numerical methods usually work well in long-term care facilities. In this filing method, the activity is concentrated at the end of the file shelf. The filing shelves are filled as records are added. Increased filing in the older records (lower numbers) will cause growth in shelves that may already be full, engendering a need to shift records. Shifting records involves the systematic physical relocation of files so that they are more evenly distributed on the shelves. In large file rooms, this is a time-consuming task.

## Terminal-Digit Filing

A **terminal-digit filing system** is a system in which the patient's MR# is divided into sets of digits for filing purposes. Each set of digits is used to file the health record numerically within sections of the files, beginning with the last set. Terminal-digit filing and other variations of digit filing are very common in health care facilities. The easiest example of terminal-digit filing uses a six-digit medical record number. The six-digit number is separated into three sets of two numbers before filing. For example, for MR# 012345, the sets would look like this: 01-23-45. The sets of digits have names: The first two numbers are called the *tertiary* digits, the second two numbers are called the *secondary* digits, and the last two numbers are called the *primary* digits (Table 9-4). To file in terminal-digit (TD) order, one must locate the section of files that correspond with the sets, beginning with the primary digits, then within the primary section locate the secondary digits, and finally file the record in numerical order by the tertiary digits. Filing in TD order is easy once one understands how to separate the digits in the MR# and then which digit set to use first (Figure 9-8).

In this example, one begins to file by using the last two numbers of the medical record number, the primary digits, as follows:

*Step 1:* Separate the MR# into the necessary sections. This example uses a six-digit number separated into three sections with two numbers each: MR# 012345 converts to 01-23-45. To file this health record (#01-23-45), begin with the primary digits 45, the last two digits of MR# 01-23-45. In the file area, locate the primary section 45. All files in primary section 45 will end with the number 45.

*Step 2:* In primary section 45, next search for the middle digits, 23. Remain in section 45, where the bottom two numbers are all the same, and be sure not to venture into another primary section on the shelf. Find middle digits 22 to 24 because 23 is going to be filed between middle digits 22-45 and 24-45.

*Step 3:* Once the appropriate middle-digit section is located, file the record in this TD section numerically by the first two digits.

TD filing can be modified in several different ways. Some facilities use a larger nine-digit medical record number. There are several ways to separate a nine-digit medical record number for filing. One method is to have three sections with three numbers each; for example, MR# 111222333 converts to 111-222-333 for filing.

**straight numerical filing** Filing folders in numerical order.

**long-term care (LTC) facility** A hospital that provides services to patients over an extended period; an average length of stay is in excess of 30 days. Facilities are characterized by the extent to which nursing care is provided.

**terminal-digit filing system** A system in which the patient's medical record number is separated into sets for filing, and the first set of numbers is called *tertiary*, the second set of numbers is called *secondary*, and the third set of numbers is called *primary*.

**medical record number (MR#)** A unique number assigned to each patient in a health care system; this code will be used for the rest of the patient's encounters with that specific health system.

**TD** terminal digit

| TABLE 9-4 | | |
|---|---|---|
| **TERMINAL-DIGIT SORTING OF MEDICAL RECORD NUMBER 01-23-45** | | |
| **MEDICAL RECORD NUMBER** | **NUMBER IN SECTION** | **FILING** |
| 0 | Tertiary | Finally, file in numerical order by |
| 1 | | this number. |
| 2 | Secondary | Then find number 23 in section 45. |
| 3 | | |
| 4 | Primary | First, find section 45 in the files. |
| 5 | | |

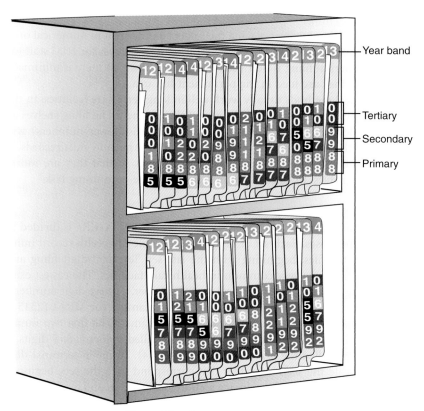

**Figure 9-8** Filing by terminal digit.

**TABLE 9-5**

**MIDDLE-DIGIT SORTING OF MEDICAL RECORD NUMBER 01-23-45**

| MEDICAL RECORD NUMBER | NUMBER IN SECTION | FILING |
|---|---|---|
| 0 | Secondary | Then find number 01 in section 23. |
| 1 | | |
| 2 | Primary | First, find section 23 in the files. |
| 3 | | |
| 4 | Tertiary | Finally, file in numerical order by this |
| 5 | | number. |

In a six-digit filing scenario, there are 100 primary sections of record, 00 through 99. In a nine-digit filing system, there are 1000 primary sections, 000 through 999. Primary sections reaching 1000 require a tremendous file area.

### Middle-Digit Filing

TD filing can be modified into another filing method, **middle-digit filing**. As in TD filing, the six-digit number is separated into three sets of two numbers before filing; MR# 012345 sets would look like this: 01-23-45. The sets of digits, however, have been renamed; the first two numbers are the secondary digits, the second two numbers are the primary digits, and the last two numbers are the tertiary digits (Table 9-5).

The following shows the process of filing MR# 012345 in a middle-digit filing system:

*Step 1:* Separate the MR# into three sections with two numbers each. MR# 012345 converts to 01-23-45. In middle-digit filing, begin with the middle set of digits and use that set as the primary digits; in our example, it is number 23. Locate the primary section (middle digits) 23 in the file area. All files in primary section 23 will have middle sets with the number 23.

*Step 2:* Remain in section 23. Be sure not to move into another primary section on the shelf. Find the secondary set of digits, 01.

**middle-digit filing system** A modification of the terminal-digit filing system in which the patient's medical record number is separated into sets for filing and the first set of numbers is called *secondary*, the second set of numbers is called *primary*, and the third set is called *tertiary*.

**TABLE 9-6**

**ADVANTAGES AND DISADVANTAGES OF FILING METHODS**

| FILING METHOD | ADVANTAGE(S) | DISADVANTAGE(S) |
|---|---|---|
| Alphabetical | Easy to learn; does not require additional cross-reference to identify a file number | Illegible handwriting can cause problems; space requirements for popular letters also problematic |
| Straight numerical | Easy to learn | File activity is concentrated |
| Terminal-digit | Equalizes filing activity throughout the filing sections | Challenging for some file clerks to learn |
| | It can be a security feature because those who are unfamiliar with terminal digit filing will be unable to identify a patient's record | Misfiles are often difficult to locate |
| Middle-digit | Equalizes filing activity throughout the filing sections | Even more challenging for some file clerks to learn; misfiles are often difficult to locate |

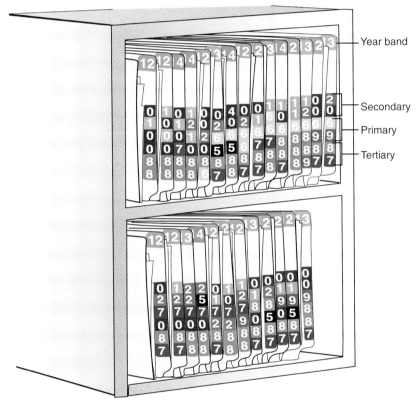

Figure 9-9 Filing by middle digit.

*Step 3:* Remain in section 01-23, and then file the record numerically by the tertiary digits 45.

Figure 9-9 shows an example of middle-digit filing.

Each facility should examine both the positive and the negative aspects of each filing method. An organized filing system allows efficient retrieval of patient health records. Quick retrieval of health records can improve the quality of patient care. A good system should have a positive impact on both employee and facility productivity. Table 9-6 lists the advantages and disadvantages of each filing method.

## Paper Record Storage Methods

The paper record requires furniture for organization and security of the files. The following discussion explains the various equipment used when an HIM department must maintain paper health record files.

**TABLE 9-7**

**ADVANTAGES AND DISADVANTAGES OF FILING EQUIPMENT**

| FILING EQUIPMENT | ADVANTAGE(S) | DISADVANTAGE(S) |
|---|---|---|
| File cabinet | Protects information from exposure to the environment | Allows access to only one drawer of information at a time |
| | Conceals information from public view | Requires additional space to open for access to information |
| | Typically provides ability to lock/secure information | |
| Open shelves | Allow easy access to records | Open to environment |
| | | Require space for aisle access to each shelf |
| Compressible shelves | Increase file space in small area | Limit access to information |
| Revolving file system | Accommodates file personnel, reducing time spent looking for file on shelf | Limits access to files |

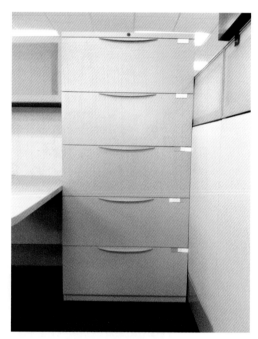

**Figure 9-10**  A filing cabinet.

### Filing Furniture

Furniture found in file areas of health care facilities includes file cabinets, open shelving, revolving systems, and movable shelves. Table 9-7 compares the advantages and disadvantages of each type of filing furniture and describes the most appropriate setting for each.

#### File Cabinets

A file cabinet (Figure 9-10) can be a vertical drawer system for filing records. This type of furniture is secure in many ways because it is easily locked, keeps records out of plain sight, and is typically a good way to secure records from fire or water damage. The disadvantages associated with this type of filing furniture are as follows:

- File cabinets are bulky and require more space than shelving systems.
- They are not efficient if the department has a large number of records that need to be accessed frequently.
- Only one drawer of records in each file cabinet can be accessed at a time.

When file cabinets face one another in rows, enough room must always be left for facing drawers to open. Approximately 5 feet between rows is necessary unless aisle space is not required.

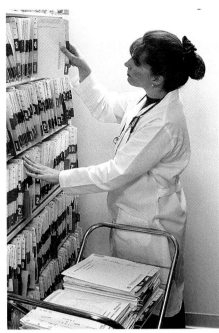

**Figure 9-11** Open shelves.

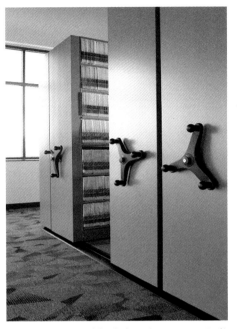

**Figure 9-12** Compressible shelves. (Courtesy Mayline Group, Sheboygan, WI.)

### Open Shelves

This type of filing furniture is simply a shelf that is always open to the file area (Figure 9-11). Open shelves allow the filing of many health records on shelves with open access to all records at all times. Open shelves require less space than filing cabinets; they may be 16 inches deep and require an aisle space of only 4 feet. Therefore two shelves can face each other and allow good access with only a 4-foot aisle. The disadvantages are that the records are always visible to visitors in the file area and they are exposed to potential fire or water damage.

### Compressible Shelves

Compressible or movable shelves allow storage of files on shelves that can be compressed so that more shelves will fit in a smaller file space (Figure 9-12). This type of shelving can move back and forth or side to side. This file furniture works well in a file room where space is limited and there are numerous patient files. The problem encountered with this filing furniture is that it provides access only to those sections of the files that are open. If a file area is very busy, compressible units may hinder filing productivity. This furniture also allows some visibility of records to visitors in the file area and potential exposure of the records to fire or water damage.

### Revolving File System

A revolving file system looks like a carousel. This system can revolve laterally or horizontally. In a horizontal revolving system, if the power supply is out, only one shelf can be accessed (Figure 9-13). A revolving file shelf works similarly to a Ferris wheel. A record cannot be retrieved until the relevant file shelf rolls around to the opening. The system may use a computer to correlate the medical record numbers to a file. When a record is needed, the file identification (MR#) is entered into the system. The revolving system presents the shelf on which the record is located so that it may be pulled from the shelf. This system provides a secure environment for storing records; however, access is limited to only one shelf at a time.

## File Rooms

Although there are many types of file furniture for storage of health records, it is important to consider the Occupational Safety and Health Administration (OSHA) space

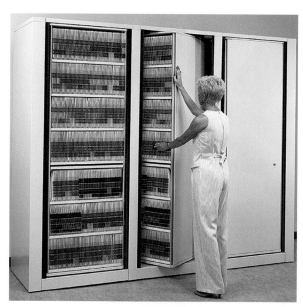

Figure 9-13 Revolving file system. (Courtesy Mayline Group, Sheboygan, WI.)

**OSHA** Occupational Safety and
Health Administration

requirements for filing areas. The OSHA requirements specify the appropriate space to provide a safe environment for employees working in the file area. OSHA mandates an aisle at least 3 feet wide between filing units or shelves, and the exit aisle must be at least 5 feet wide. Other requirements specify the amount of space required between the top shelf and the ceiling of the file room. For instance, there should be 18 inches between the top shelf and the ceiling to allow sprinkler systems to function properly if they are used as a security feature.

When designing a file area, one starts by measuring the file space. Before considering cost for filing furniture and other supplies, one must ensure that the area has adequate space to comply with OSHA guidelines to store the files. Will the files be stored in a separate room, or will they use part of the space in the department? When ordering new file furniture, care must be taken to ensure that the new furniture will accommodate all the existing files and includes room for growth. When ordering shelves or file cabinets, one must calculate the filing space within each shelf unit. Counting the number of shelves per unit, along with their width, determines the correct number of shelves to purchase. If each shelving unit has 7 shelves at a width of 36 inches, there will be 252 inches (7 shelves × 36 inches = 252 inches, or 21 feet) of file space on each shelving unit (Figure 9-14, *A*).

Calculation of file space is equally important when one is planning to enlarge or reorganize an existing file area. It may be inaccurate to assume that each record will occupy 1 inch. It is best to measure a sample of files to estimate the number of files that will fit on a shelf. Rather than counting an entire shelf, one should count the files in several 1-foot sections. For each sample section, one should note how many records were counted and average the total number (Figure 9-14, *B*).

The file space needed for the entire room can be calculated if one knows the average number of records occupying 1 foot of file space. If one uses the average in Figure 9-14, *B* (16 records per 1 foot of file space), the next information necessary to determine is the number of years of records that are stored in this location. For this example one assumes that the file area contains 3 years of files. Knowing the facility's average number of discharges (12,000) allows an approximate calculation of 36,000 files in the file area. Knowing that 1 foot equals 16 records, one divides 36,000 by 16 to determine that 2250 feet of file space is needed to accommodate 3 years of records at this facility.

Before ordering furniture, one must determine how many shelves are necessary to store 2250 feet of files, which can be done as follows: Measure the current file space to determine whether the facility can use the current furniture. If a seven-shelf unit contains 36 inches of file space on each shelf, one shelf unit (seven shelves) can hold 252 inches, or 21 feet of

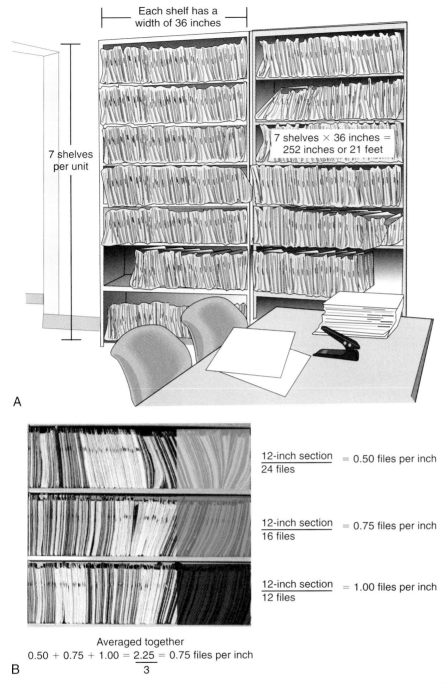

Each shelf has a width of 36 inches

7 shelves per unit

7 shelves × 36 inches = 252 inches or 21 feet

A

$$\frac{\text{12-inch section}}{\text{24 files}} = 0.50 \text{ files per inch}$$

$$\frac{\text{12-inch section}}{\text{16 files}} = 0.75 \text{ files per inch}$$

$$\frac{\text{12-inch section}}{\text{12 files}} = 1.00 \text{ files per inch}$$

Averaged together

$$0.50 + 0.75 + 1.00 = \frac{2.25}{3} = 0.75 \text{ files per inch}$$

B

**Figure 9-14  A,** Calculating total shelf space of a shelving unit. **B,** Finding the average number of files on each shelf.

records. For 2250 feet of files, 108 shelving units are needed to accommodate these files (2250 ÷ 21 feet [for one seven-shelf unit] = 107.14, or 108 shelving units). This calculation is adequate for current files but does not allow room for expansion in the future. The facility should plan for an increase in the number of patient files. Planning for an increase by overestimating the necessary space may prevent overcrowding of records in the future. To determine an appropriate amount of growing space, one should recall how much the files have grown over the past several years. This enables the projection of space needed for the future storage of records. Sometimes, a facility has a strategic plan for growth, and the financial planners in the facility can provide the HIM department with information on expected growth of discharges for the coming years.

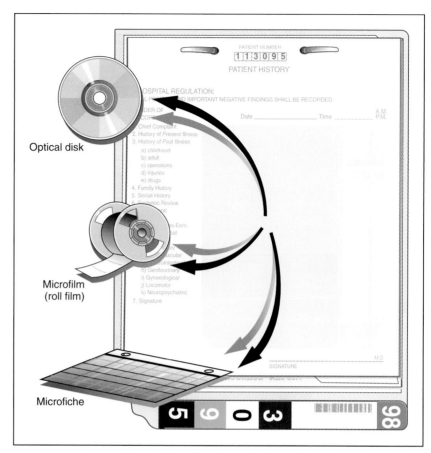

**Figure 9-15** Microfilm and microfiche.

---

**HIT-bit** ············································································

### ACTIVE VERSUS INACTIVE RECORDS

*Active records* are regularly accessed for patient care.

*Inactive records* are records that are rarely accessed for patient care or other activity.

---

**progress note** The physician's record of each interaction with the patient.

**operative report** The surgeon's formal report of surgical procedure(s) performed. Often dictated and transcribed into a formal report.

**microfilm** An alternative storage method for paper records on plastic film.

When one is planning file space in a new facility, it is best to work with estimations. An easy method for estimating is to contact the HIM professional at a local facility that provides similar health care services. The HIM professional should be able to provide information regarding the facility's chart size, which can be used to calculate an estimate. If another facility does not exist in the area, one can create a mock chart—a fake record containing an example of each document that could exist in the patient's health record. One should keep in mind that more than one page may be required for a specific document, such as progress notes or operative reports. Remember, the length of stay has an impact on the size of a record. After a mock chart is created it should be measured. How thick is the record? This measurement should be multiplied by the number of patient records estimated, with enough space allowed in the file area for a specific period.

### Microfilm

**Microfilm** is the reproduction of a complete original paper record as miniature pictures stored on plastic film, either on reels or on sheets (Figure 9-15).

At first glance, microfilm looks like a negative from pictures taken with a camera. Further study reveals that the image is a small picture of the original document that was scanned through the machine. After processing, the images were assembled on roll film or sliced into small strips of film and put into a jacket. The film that is sliced and put into jackets is also known as **microfiche**. Like other physical file formats, microfilmed records are carefully labeled with the patient's identifying name or medical record number. Each roll or sheet of film is labeled to determine which patient records are stored on that roll or sheet. In the file cabinet, microfiche records are filed in the same way that files were stored in their original format, using an alphabetical, straight numerical, or terminal-digit filing system. When microfilm is stored on roll film, the rolls may be numbered, and additional methods are necessary to correlate the records with the roll film. Also, when roll film is used, a facility may choose to have two copies of each roll available at the facility, and possibly even one master copy stored offsite as backup in case one of the rolls is spliced or splits as it is processed through the microfilm reader machine.

*Microfilm Equipment*

When microfilm is used to store records, some equipment is necessary to maintain access to the files. A printer is needed to reproduce a paper copy of the patient's record for release to another facility or authorized individual. The microfilm or microfiche health record must be maintained in appropriate storage equipment. Microfilm should be stored in a file cabinet or drawer capable of being locked or kept enclosed in a locked room. The cabinets should also protect the records from the environment and from temperature and water damage.

It is important to remember the following:

- Microfilming can be performed at an onsite or offsite location.
- If an offsite contractor is chosen, the company is responsible for maintaining the confidentiality of the information while it is being processed.
- The contracted company must also allow facility workers the necessary access to the information in a timely manner should it be required.
- The quality of the microfilm must be checked before any of the original records are destroyed.

## Offsite Storage

With offsite storage, the (paper) health record files are kept at a separate location outside the facility that may be owned and operated by a third party. The offsite storage location operates much like the file room in the health care facility. Patient health records can be requested when needed for patient care, release of information, record review, billing, or any other appropriate reason, whereupon they are brought to the facility. The records no longer take up space at the facility. The records are no longer under the direct control of the facility's HIM *custodian* but are relocated to another secure environment. Within this new environment, the facility's HIM custodian must ensure that appropriate measures are taken to secure and organize the patient records.

**microfiche** An alternative storage method for paper records on plastic sheets.

**straight-numerical filing** Filing folders in numerical order.

**terminal-digit filing system** A system in which the patient's medical record number is separated into sets for filing, and the first set of numbers is called *tertiary*, the second set of numbers is called *secondary*, and the third set of numbers is called *primary*.

**release of information (ROI)** The term used to describe the HIM department function that provides disclosure of patient health information.

**custodian** The person entrusted with the responsibility for the confidentiality, privacy, and security of medical records.

---

**HIT-bit**

**CENTRALIZED VERSUS DECENTRALIZED FILES**

In a health care facility, centralized and decentralized file areas reflect the number of separate locations within or outside the facility that store health records.

A *centralized file area* describes a single file room where all health records for the facility are stored.

A *decentralized file area* describes one or more locations outside the HIM department or outside the facility that are used to store the facility's health records.

There are many things a facility must consider before choosing to store records off site. The offsite storage facility signs a contract with the health care facility to maintain its health care records. All of the facility's concerns should be addressed in the contract. The contract must be reviewed thoroughly and clarified if anything is unclear. The following is a list of issues that should be considered before one chooses an offsite storage facility:

- Be sure that the site has appropriate security for the storage of health information.
- Personally go to the site, and examine the security system.
- What are the operating hours?
- How is a record requested in an emergency, for patient care, or for other review? Via telephone or a facsimile (fax) request, or can the record be requested online via a secure site?
- How often will the requested records be delivered to the health care facility?
- How will records be transported from the offsite facility to the health care facility and back again? In secure vehicles, taxi, fax only, courier?
- Is there a charge for immediate delivery of a record in case of emergency?
- How will the company charge for storage—by linear foot of storage space or by record storage type?
- How will the company store the records: in boxes or open shelving? Do they have a computerized chart locator system?
- Is the storage facility climate controlled?
- What are the training procedures for the storage facility's employees?
- What are the storage facility's safety and confidentiality procedures?
- Does the facility have online access to track a request or to view the history of a particular file as it moves back and forth between the offsite storage and the health care facility?
- What is the storage facility's policy for inadvertent disclosures? Does it have a disaster recovery plan?

## EXERCISE 9-2

### Filing

1. The numerical file identification system used to identify an entire family's health record using one number and modifiers is called _____.
2. The physical container used to store the paper-based health record is a _____.
3. A(n) _____ is used to identify or name a file or record so that it can be located in the computer-based health record.
4. _____ and _____ are alternative storage methods for paper records using plastic film.
5. A numerical patient record identification system that gives the patient a new number for each encounter is called _____ numbering.
6. A numerical patient record identification system in which the patient is given a new number for each visit and with each new admission the previous record is retrieved and filed in the folder with the most recent visit is called _____ numbering.
7. The filing method of organizing folders in numerical order is _____ _____ filing.
8. A filing method in which the patient's medical record number is separated into sets for filing and the first set of numbers are tertiary, the second set is secondary, and the last set is primary is called _____ filing.
9. In a _____ system, the patient record is filed under the same number for all visits.
10. Identify which of the following is not an alphabetical filing rule:
    a. Suffixes are considered after the middle name or initial.
    b. All punctuation and possessives are ignored.
    c. Abbreviations and shortened names are ignored.
    d. Personal names are filed last name, followed by first name, then middle initial.

11. Color coding of the numerical identification on the end tab of a file folder:
    a. prevents messy files.
    b. aids the identification of misfiles.
    c. is mandatory under TJC standards.
    d. warrants approval form the safety committee.
12. If a shelf unit is 36 inches wide and has 8 shelves, how many linear inches of filing space are available?
    a. 36
    b. 288
    c. 240
    d. 272
13. On a shelving unit that is 30 inches wide with 8 shelves, how many linear inches of file space are available?
    a. 240
    b. 288
    c. 24
    d. 300
14. If the average thickness of a record is 1½ inches, how many records can be stored on a shelving unit that is 30 inches wide with 8 shelves?
    a. 240
    b. 288
    c. 160
    d. 80
15. The new supervisor of Diamonte Hospital decides that new filing furniture is needed to store 12,000 annual outpatient charts. After measuring, it is determined that four charts equal 1 inch of linear file space. How many 36-inch–wide, 8-shelf units must be purchased to store these records?
    a. 288
    b. 10
    c. 11
    d. 42
16. Shelley is the new health information management file room supervisor at Diamonte Hospital. Upon entering the file room, she notices that the files are cramped and there is no room on the shelves to file any new charts. Shelley determines that it is critical to order additional shelving to increase the file shelf space so it can store all of Diamonte's records. The facility has approximately 15,000 discharges each year. They keep 2 years of paper records on site. The average thickness of a record is 1 inch. They currently have 30 shelving units, each of which has 8 shelves and is 36 inches wide. How many records can be currently stored in this filing furniture?
    a. 288
    b. 2880
    c. 8640
    d. 15,000
17. Shelley is the new health information management file room supervisor at Diamonte Hospital. Upon entering the file room she notices that the files are cramped and there is no room on the shelves to file any new charts. Shelley determines that it is critical to order additional shelving to increase the file shelf space to store all of Diamonte's records. The facility has approximately 15,000 discharges each year. They keep 2 years of paper records on site. The average thickness of a record is 1 inch. They currently have 30 shelving units that each have eight shelves and are 36 inches wide. How many additional filing units should Shelley order?
    a. 22
    b. 23
    c. 52
    d. 53
18. Compare the following file numbering or identification systems, listing the pros and cons of each: alphabetical, unit MR#, serial MR#, serial-unit MR#, family medical record number.
19. Explain how to locate a record using terminal-digit filing.

20. The file room in a recently acquired clinic that has filed records alphabetically must be converted to terminal-digit filing. List the steps involved in the conversion.
21. Given the file space area of 25 feet × 40 feet with a ceiling height of 10 feet (use grid paper, with each block equaling 1 foot), determine which filing furniture is best to store 40,000 records, averaging 1 inch in thickness. Keep in mind OSHA requirements for aisle and exit space.
22. File the following names in alphabetical order:

| | |
|---|---|
| P. B. Josh | Lauren McIntyre |
| Drew B. LaPeu | Amanda Modelle |
| Hannah Curelle | Beth Katerina Von Amberg |
| Cecelia Lower | Aubrey Bartolo, III |
| Ginger Dugas | Sister Gabrielle Brown |
| Wm. Bill Matata | Brett Thomasse, Jr. |

*Using knowledge of how numbers/identifiers are assigned to patient files in each of the numbering systems shown in the following table, read the scenario and then answer questions 26 and 27.*

| NUMBERING SYSTEM | NEXT MR# ASSIGNED |
|---|---|
| Unit | 123456 |
| Serial | 234567 |
| Serial-unit | 345678 |
| Family unit | 456789 |

*Green Oak Hospital uses a serial numbering system to identify patient health records. Jane Creason is admitted to Green Oak facility for repair of a broken ankle. On a previous admission to Green Oak for a tonsillectomy, Jane was assigned MR# 012345.*

23. What number will be assigned to Jane for the broken ankle admission?
24. If Green Oak used a unit numbering system, what medical record number would be assigned for the broken ankle admission?
25. List important things to consider before choosing an alternative storage method.

**chart locator system** A system for locating records within a facility.

**utilization review (UR)** The process of evaluating medical interventions against established criteria, on the basis of the patient's known or tentative diagnosis. Evaluation may take place before, during, or after the episode of care for different purposes.

**litigation** The term used to indicate that a matter must be settled by the court and the process of engaging in legal proceedings.

## CHART LOCATOR SYSTEMS

Health information is useful only if it is available for review. A **chart locator system** keeps track of the locations of all records in the health care facility. Many people in the health care facility have authorized need of and access to patient records. As a result, records are not always on the shelf in the permanent file location. Records may be signed out to a health care unit when a patient is readmitted. Records may be requested for research or for patient follow-up care. The utilization review (UR) department may need to review records to ensure that the care provided to the patient was appropriate. Copies of records may be requested for litigation, which requires removing the health record file from the file system in order to copy it for authorized users. Because all of these uses are necessary to the function of the facility, it is important that the HIM department be able to locate and retrieve patient records.

**CHART LOCATOR SYSTEM**

As a rule of thumb, in a large HIM department, every record should be listed in the chart locator system as the record progresses through each function in the department. When a record moves from one section, it must be "signed out" of that section and "signed in" to the new section. This method allows personnel to determine the location of a patient file without spending time searching through the various sections of the HIM department.

A chart locator system allows the HIM department to keep track of the facility's patient health records. Records that are removed from the department or from the normal processing flow in the department are "signed out" to the location to which they are being sent. Once the records are returned, they must be "signed in" to the department. This procedure allows anyone in the HIM department to easily determine when a record is available for review and when it is out of the department. A chart locator system also allows faster retrieval of a record from another location in an urgent situation—for example, for a patient care emergency. It has been said that the HIM department is only as good as the information it can provide. If the HIM department can easily access and retrieve information, then the department is functioning productively.

**AUDIT TRAIL**

Chart locator systems apply primarily to the paper health record. In a computerized or computer-based environment, records are tracked by means of an audit trail. The computer system keeps a log (known as the audit trail) of every transaction by recording the name of the employee performing the task, what information is sent and to which location, the name of the recipient, the date, the time, and other pertinent facts. This audit trail is an important tool in the computer environment for tracking the use of patient health records and information.

**Go To** Review Figure 3-7 for an example of an EHR audit trail.

## Manual Systems

Manual systems for chart location of the paper health record file use an *outguide* and a log or index card box to signify that a patient's health record file folder has been removed and sent to a new location. An **outguide** is a physical file card or jacket in place of a health record signifying that the record is away from its expected location (Figure 9-16).

The log or index card box is used as a quick alphabetical reference of all records that are signed out of the HIM department. When a patient's health record is needed in another location, the HIM file clerk completes an outguide slip, as shown in Figure 9-16, to put in place of the file when it is removed. The outguide informs anyone who looks for the patient's file that it has been moved to a new location. Outguides prevent HIM employees from spending unnecessary time searching for a file.

How does the manual system operate? When the HIM department receives a request for a health record, the clerk retrieves the patient's medical record number by looking up the patient's name in the MPI. The clerk locates the health record in the department. This may be the clerk's thought process: Is the record old enough to be in the permanent files? Is it just a week old, in which case it is probably in the incomplete record area? Is it for a recent discharge and possibly in the coding area? Once the record is located and pulled, the clerk will sign the record out to the new location, meaning that the clerk notes where the record is going. In a manual chart locator system, duplicate outguide forms are completed with the following information: medical record number, discharge date(s), the location to which the record is being sent, and the date the record was sent. The duplicate copy of the outguide is filed alphabetically in a box (or card file) for

**outguide** A physical file guide used to identify another location of a file in the paper-based health record system.

**MPI** master patient index

**medical record number (MR#)** A unique number assigned to each patient in a health care system; this code will be used for the rest of the patient's encounters with that specific health system.

**discharge** Discharge occurs when the patient leaves the care of the facility to go home, for transfer to another health care facility, or by death. Also refers to the status of a patient.

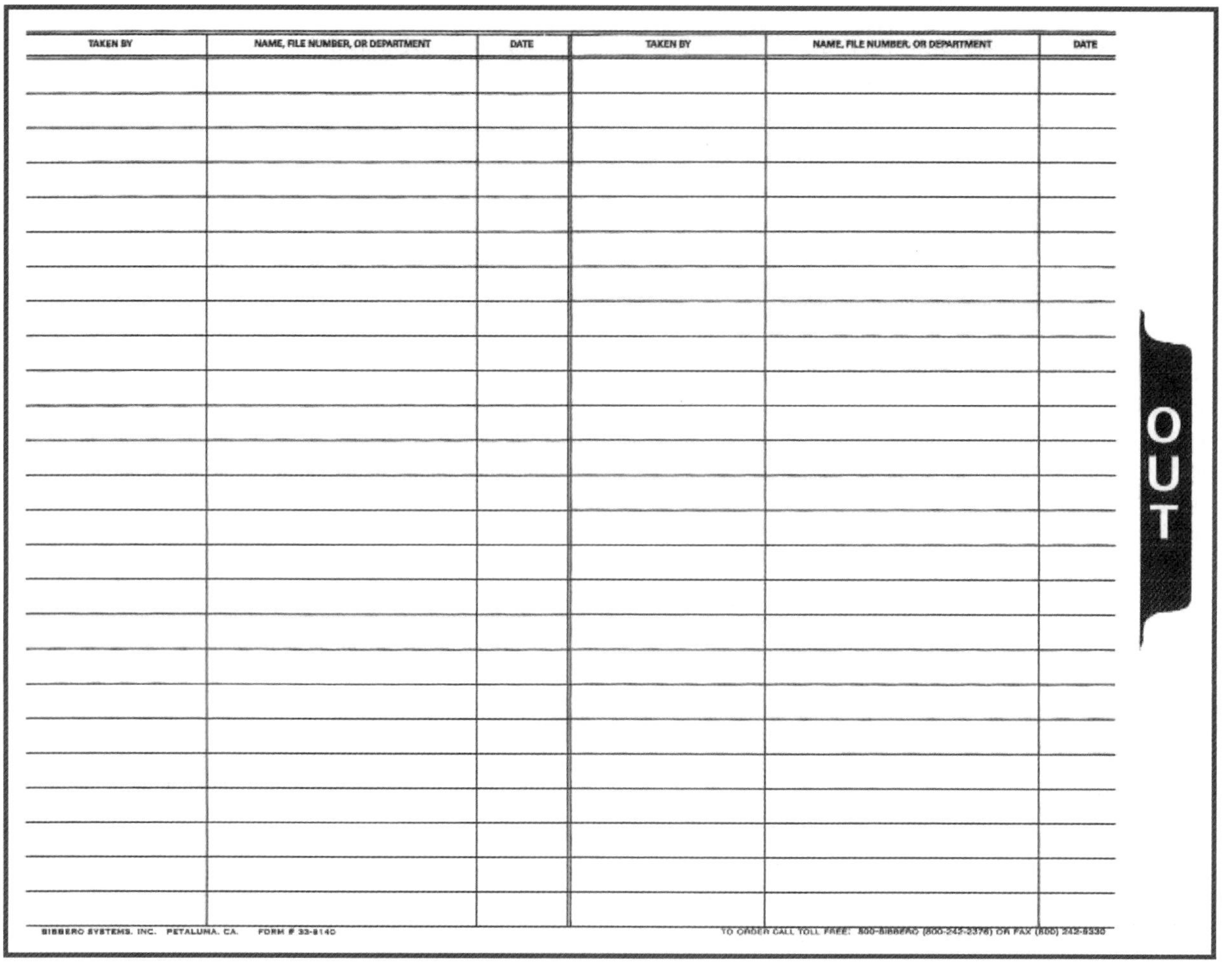

| TAKEN BY | NAME, FILE NUMBER, OR DEPARTMENT | DATE | TAKEN BY | NAME, FILE NUMBER, OR DEPARTMENT | DATE |
|----------|----------------------------------|------|----------|----------------------------------|------|
|  |  |  |  |  |  |

O
U
T

BIBBERO SYSTEMS, INC.   PETALUMA, CA.   FORM # 33-8140     TO ORDER CALL TOLL FREE:  800-BIBBERO (800-242-2376) OR FAX (800) 242-9330

Figure 9-16 The outguide identifies a record removed from its usual location. (Courtesy Bibbero Systems, Inc., Petaluma, CA.)

reference. The department may also require that the person requesting the records sign for them on pickup.

Returned records must be checked back into the department, which involves updating the chart locator system to note that the health record file has been returned. On a daily basis, records returned to the department must be signed in and placed back in their appropriate location. It is also very important to perform a regular (e.g., weekly) audit of the health records that are checked out to each location. For example, if 10 records are signed out to the clinic and, upon inspection of the clinic, all 10 records are not located, it is necessary to search for the missing records. Did they come back to the HIM department but not get checked in? Were the records transferred to a unit within the facility because the patient was admitted? Ensuring accurate tracking of patient records helps ensure and maintain the security of patient health records.

## Computerized Systems

Computerized chart locator systems can eliminate the need for physical outguides and cards, although some HIM departments use the manual chart locator system and the computer system simultaneously. In a computerized chart locator system, the new location to which the record is being "signed out" is entered into the computer system. Therefore if a chart is pulled from the permanent file location and sent to a clinic, the computerized chart locator system shows that the record is signed out to the clinic (Figure 9-17). Some physical files have bar codes that contain specific patient file identification information. This bar code can be used in a computerized chart locator system to facilitate accurate and

**bar code** The representation of data using parallel lines or other patterns in a way readable to a machine, such as an optical bar code scanner or a smartphone.

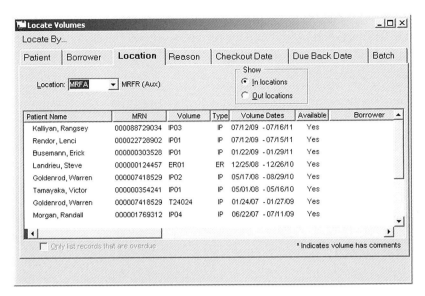

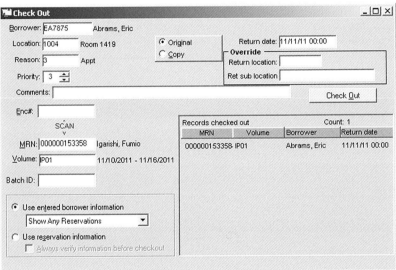

Figure 9-17 Chart locator screens. (Courtesy Meta Health Technology, a division of Streamline Health Solutions, Inc., Cincinnati, Ohio. Meta was acquired by Streamline Health Solutions, Inc. in August 2012.)

efficient processing (signing out of records). Scanning the bar code to accurately reflect the patient name and health record file eliminates the need for manual entry of this information. Ultimately it is very important that the chart locator system accurately reflect the current location of each patient record at all times.

A beneficial feature of some computerized chart locator systems is an automated prompt for the return of patient files. For example, patient files should leave the HIM department only when they are needed for continuity of patient care. The system prompt notifies the HIM staff of any files that were due back in the department but not yet signed in on the chart locator system. This prompt cues the clerk to locate the records.

The following scenario illustrates the computerized chart locator system: Mary Davidson has been a patient at the Diamonte facility several times over the past 5 years. In the course of her treatment, physicians have noted that Ms. Davidson is allergic to penicillin. On one particular evening in October, Mary is brought to the emergency department (ED) unconscious. Review of her personal belongings alerted health care workers to her name and DOB. The ED makes a routine call to the HIM department for her old records. The HIM department clerk enters "Mary Davidson" into the MPI system, and several patients with that name appear on the screen. Because the clerk has the DOB, she can easily check the MPI to find the correct patient file. With the MR# for the Mary Davidson in the

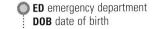

**ED** emergency department
**DOB** date of birth

ED, the clerk goes to the file room to look for the old record. She goes to the appropriate shelf in the terminal-digit order, but the record is not there. The clerk then returns to the computer to enter Ms. Davidson's medical record number in the chart locator system to see where the record is "signed out."

On doing so, the clerk learns that this record is signed out to the UR department for review. Knowing the routine of the facility, the clerk can go directly to the section of records set aside for the UR staff and retrieve Mary Davidson's record. The clerk then makes an entry into the chart locator system indicating that the record is being sent to the ED and that on its return to the HIM department it should be returned to the UR staff record section. Appropriate notes should also be made to tell the UR department that this record has been removed.

> **utilization review (UR)** The process of evaluating medical interventions against established criteria, on the basis of the patient's known or tentative diagnosis. Evaluation may take place before, during, or after the episode of care for different purposes.

---

### HIT-bit

#### PHONETIC SEARCH

*Phonetic searching* is the function in a computer system that queries the database for all names that sound like the name that has been entered. For example, all forms of the name Steven sound the same, even though they are spelled differently. With a phonetic feature, the computer can search for all sound-alike spellings of the name, such as Stephen, Stefan, Stephan, and Steven.

---

## EXERCISE 9-3

### Chart Locator Systems

1. A _____ is used to identify the location of records within a facility.
2. A manual chart locater system must use _____ to hold the place of the original record.
   a. spacers
   b. outguides
   c. indexers
   d. blank files
3. A manual chart locator system maintains more information about a charts location(s) than a computerized system.
   True
   False
4. Diamonte Hospital uses a computerized chart locator system. The ED has requested an old (paper) chart on Mr. Tom Jones. Prior to bringing the chart to the ED, the HIM clerk must:
   a. initial the chart.
   b. request verification from Mr. Jones' previous attending physician.
   c. sign the chart out of the HIM department to the ED.
   d. call the Diamonte attorney.
5. When Mr. Jones is discharged form the ED and his old (paper) chart is returned to the HIM department:
   a. the record must be signed back into the HIM department.
   b. the record must be initialed.
   c. the facility attorney must be contacted.
   d. the record should be shredded.

---

## INFORMATION SYSTEMS

These days everyone is familiar with computers, and HIM students will study this topic in great detail in a special course. However, in order for you to fully understand electronic storage of data, a brief a review of some computer terminology is required here.

Computers come in all shapes and sizes and are found in many products used in everyday life. In health care computers also range in size and storage capacity: from a small mobile wireless device the size of a watch battery to a desktop workstation to the mainframe and servers used to store and process all the information in a hospital. Increasingly,

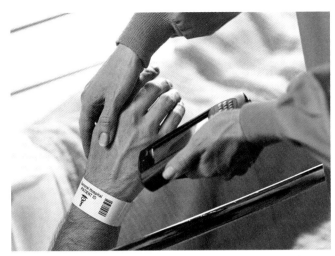

**Figure 9-18** A bar code scanner used on the nursing unit to scan a patient's wristband. (Courtesy Zebra Technologies Corporation, Lincolnshire, IL.)

physicians and other providers are using tablets and smartphones that run special applications allowing them to access and contribute to patient records in an EHR.

● **EHR** electronic health record

## Hardware and Software

The term *hardware* is used to describe all the physical parts that make up a computer. It includes all the wiring and circuit boards, the processor, main memory (RAM), and hard drive. *Hardware* also refers to more visible peripherals, which can be further classified into input, output, and storage devices. A mouse and keyboard are very common input peripherals, although health care providers use many other capture devices specific to health data collection. Workstations in the HIM department and in the nursing unit, for instance, may be equipped with bar code scanners (Figure 9-18). Common output peripherals are computer monitors and printers.

Software consists of the programs that allow the user to interact with a computer, along with all the applications a user runs to perform tasks. This includes the computer's operating system (e.g., Microsoft Windows or Mac OS X), an e-mail program, Web browser, and word processing and spreadsheet programs in addition to software unique to health care, like an EHR program.

## Storage

Computers use several different storage components to operate, and the functional capacities of these devices are growing larger as technology improves. The three types of storage are illustrated in Figure 9-19. Primary storage is housed on the motherboard of the computer, and put simply, the more capacity *(memory)* a computer has available, the faster it can operate. *Secondary storage* refers to a computer's hard drive, where many of its applications and files are stored. Offline storage includes optical drives (CD or DVD-ROM drives) and external hard drives, and examples of tertiary storage are zip disks and flash or thumb drives (Figure 9-20).

As stated previously, storage technology continues to advance, allowing more and more information to be stored in smaller and smaller spaces. Comparatively speaking, the amount of information that the computers used in today's health care environment can store is vast. The simple relationship described in Chapter 2, where 1 character = 1 byte, can lead to astonishing figures. A common DVD can store 4.7 gigabytes (GB), so that single **optical disk** could technically hold 4,707,319,808 bytes, or nearly 5 billion characters.

But addressing the question of how much paper health record information can be stored in kilobytes (KB), megabytes (MB), gigabytes (GB), terabytes (TB), and beyond is not exactly straightforward. The data contained in a health record is not just plain

● **optical disk** Electronic storage medium; a disk used to store digital data.

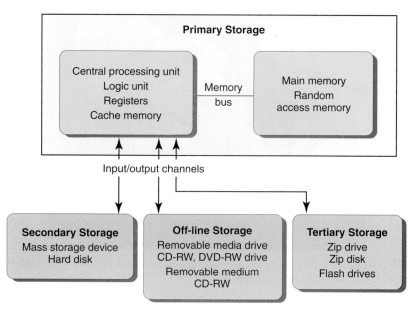

**Figure 9-19** Types of computer memory. CD-RW, rewriteable compact disk; DVD-RW, rewriteable digital video disk.

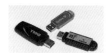

**Figure 9-20** Flash drives.

characters—it has formatting, images, and much other information hidden "behind the scenes." If the data were stored in simple text files, an inexpensive 1-GB flash drive might hold well over 500,000 pages of data; the same flash drive might only hold 50,000 pages if the information is in Microsoft Word files. Some types of diagnostic imaging can produce files so large that only a few images would fit on a 4.7-GB DVD. The illustration in Figure 9-21 converting shelf space to various types of digital storage assumes that about 22,000 pages of paper health records can be stored in 1 GB.

---

**HIT-bit** ·······················································

### THE PAPER EXPLOSION

Imagine that a busy clinic sees 75 patients each day and is open just 5 days a week.
    5 days × 75 patients = 375 records per week
    375 records per week × 52 weeks = 19,500 records annually
    If each record were only one sheet of paper, 19,500 records could amount to approximately four cases of paper. Medical records are typically more than one page long, and the paper generated in a single year can be substantial.

---

### RAID

Having the physical capacity to store the enormous volume of data needed for the various aspects of health care delivery is only part of the considerations surrounding digital storage technologies. Users of this information need to be able to access the data, and quickly. Consider an individual who wants to view a family photo on her laptop. Most people would be irritated if it took longer than 1 second to see the picture on the screen. Similarly, a neurosurgeon who needs to look at a patient's computed tomography (CT) scans (which can be very large files) must have relatively instant access to the images.

Today's EHR technology, in terms of both physical storage space and access to it, would not be possible with the use of magnetic tapes, an early solution to large data storage.

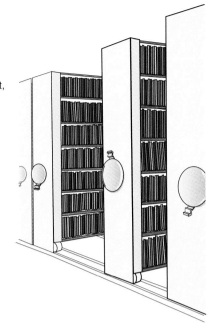

Computer storage

On the shelves pictured here (4 units, 7 shelves per unit, 36 inches wide), let's assume there are approximately 100,000 sheets of paper in the stored records.

Roughly 22,000 pages can be stored on 1 GB of memory space.

1 GB = 1000 MB

1 CD = 700 MB

1 DVD = 4.7 GB

As technology advances, memory devices improve size and capacities, allowing more information to be stored on progressively smaller devices.

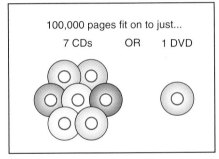

100,000 pages fit on to just...

7 CDs    OR    1 DVD

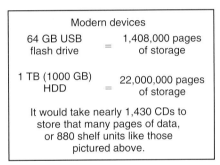

Modern devices

| 64 GB USB flash drive | = | 1,408,000 pages of storage |

| 1 TB (1000 GB) HDD | = | 22,000,000 pages of storage |

It would take nearly 1,430 CDs to store that many pages of data, or 880 shelf units like those pictured above.

**Figure 9-21** Digital storage technologies. CD, compact disk; DVD, digital video disk; GB, gigabyte; MB, megabyte; TB, terabyte.

Commonly, data is stored on **redundant arrays of independent disks** or **RAIDs**. Most RAIDs use magnetic hard drives, like the kind in a personal computer, although much larger. These drives are "stacked" together, splitting up and duplicating the data to enable larger capacities and faster access times.

With the development of high-speed networks, RAIDs and other storage devices are no longer limited to a single room—they can be spread out over large distances. This technology is called a **storage area network (SAN)**, which, thanks to special software, can provide data backup and faster retrieval.

## Scanned Imaging and Electronic Storage

Scanned document imaging saves a significant amount of space because it eliminates the need for paper storage (see Figure 9-21), but it has an additional benefit: Once printed pages are digitized, they can be burned to a CD, copied to a thumb drive, downloaded from an ftp (file transport protocol) site on a network, or viewed on virtually any computer connected to the network. This system has many advantages over the traditional paper record, which either followed the patient or was filed in the HIM department. With digitization, a patient's record can be accessed regardless of the user's location, and by multiple users at once. One of the more common and more cost-effective systems to accomplish scanning is called **COLD**, which stands for **computer output to laser disk**. This involves the reproduction of the original paper record into digitized pictures stored on optical disk. Like microfilm, COLD systems simply copy each printed page (front and back) of the

**redundant arrays of independent disks (RAIDs)** "Stacked" hard drives that split up and duplicate data to enable larger capacities and faster access.

**storage area network (SAN)** The use of RAIDs and other storage technologies over a network.

**ftp** file transport protocol

**document imaging** Scanning or faxing of printed papers into a computer system or optical disk system.
**computer output to laser disk (COLD)** Forms or reports generated from computer output transferred for storage on laser disk.

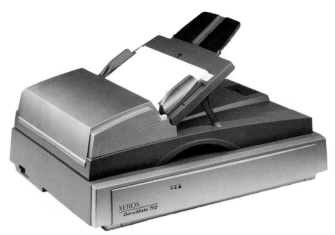

**Figure 9-22** A document scanner. (Courtesy Xerox Corporation, Norwalk, CT.)

**scanner** A machine, much like a copier, used to turn paper-based records into digital images for a computerized health record.

**MPI** master patient index

**electronic document management system (EDMS)** Computer software and hardware, typically scanners, that allow health record documents to be stored, retrieved, and shared.

**assembly** The reorganization of a paper record into a standard order.

**loose sheets** In a paper health record, documents that are not present when the patient is discharged. These documents must be accumulated and filed with the record at a later date.

**health information technology (HIT)** The specialty in the field of health information management that focuses on the day-to-day activities of health information management that support the collection, storage, retrieval, and reporting of health information.

**cloud computing** A computing architecture in which the resources, software, and application data are Internet based rather than existing on a local system.

**electronic health record (EHR)** A secure real-time, point-of-care, patient centric information resource for clinicians allowing access to patient information when and where needed and incorporating evidence-based decision support.

original health record. When the original pages of the patient health record are scanned into a computer system, the record may be saved on a disk similar to a DVD and made available on a network. The actual scanning process is analogous to sending a piece of paper through a copy machine. In this format, the **scanner** does not produce the image onto another piece of paper or plastic; instead, the image is digitally stored in a computer system or on optical disk and either printed out or viewed on a computer screen. Figure 9-22 is a scanner typically used in an HIM department.

Interestingly, this form of storage does not typically require a separate MPI system to locate the patient's health record. Patient identification by name or number is still a very important factor in the indexing of the patient information. The medical record number (or another unique number) is still used to name or identify the records; however, an EDMS is capable of searching for the patient's health information by using the index fields—that is, patient name, discharge date, or any other identifying data known to the system. It is important to note, however, that compared with a fully functional EHR, very few fields in a record scanned using a COLD system are indexed for searching and retrieval.

From a processing standpoint, assembly of the record using a scanner has an added advantage. If one page of the record was not scanned with the original record, it can be added later and remain identifiable by the system as a part of the patient's original record within the system. This system allows for the scanning and assembly of records before they are complete. Loose paper records, transcription, and sometimes signatures can be added at a later date.

Whether HIM professionals are storing scanned images of a paper record or dealing with the vast amounts of space needed to manage EHRs and digital imaging, issues of physical space and access are of concern when it comes to electronic records as well. Reliance on electronic data has grown as the cost of digital storage technologies and the bandwidth required to retrieve and exchange this information has become more affordable.

## Cloud Computing

*Cloud computing* has taken the idea of computer networking a step further. Put very simply, "the cloud" is the Internet. In conventional network computing, each user's software and processing is confined locally, either on his or her own terminal or on a local server. As described previously, users may connect to and access data from remote sources, but most of the applications and infrastructure are in-house. **Cloud computing** structures share many of those resources over the Internet. For example, rather than being loaded onto each computer in a hospital, the EHR software or application exists in the cloud, and each user accesses it using a Web browser. Practice Fusion (owned by the company of the same name in San Francisco, CA), the EHR software used in many illustrations in this text, is one example of a cloud-based EHR; the entire program—along with the data and the computer processing that makes the system work—is remote and accessed with a common web browser. No part of the EHR or any of the patient records it contains are on hard drives or computers in a physician's office. Alternatively, some cloud computing architectures are accessed through the use of very small applications or programs on each computer, tablet, or even mobile phone.

## EXERCISE 9-4
### Information Systems

1. A copier-like machine called a _____ is used to convert paper-based records into digital images for a computerized health care record.
2. The machine used to input a paper document into a computerized imaging system is called a:
   a. copier.
   b. indexer.
   c. mapper.
   d. scanner.
3. Images stored in a COLD system must be _____ for identification and future retrieval.
   a. copied
   b. indexed
   c. mapped
   d. e-mailed
4. Which of the following terms is used to describe the physical parts that make up a computer?
   a. Scanner
   b. Software
   c. Hardware
   d. RAM
5. Which of the following is an output peripheral?
   a. Keyboard
   b. Monitor
   c. Mouse
   d. RAM
6. Identify the input peripheral listed below:
   a. Monitor
   b. Printer
   c. Scanner
   d. RAM

7. Programs that allow the user to interact with a computer are known as:
   a. RAM.
   b. hardware.
   c. software.
   d. storage.
8. List the three types of computer storage discussed in this chapter.
9. Explain what an HIM manager would need to consider when looking to store paper files electronically.
10. Which of the following is used to provide data backup and faster retrieval over high-speed networks?
    a. RAM
    b. RAID
    c. SAN
    d. COLD
11. Identify two advantages of using scanned imaging.
12. Which of the following is a method of storage used with scanned (document) imaging?
    a. COLD
    b. RAID
    c. RAM
    d. SAN
13. Which of the following structures shares resources over the Internet?
    a. Software
    b. Cloud computing
    c. Hardware
    d. Off-line storage

## SECURITY OF HEALTH INFORMATION

Storage of health information requires methods to ensure its security. HIM professionals are considered custodians of patients' health information. They are responsible for ensuring that the information is complete, timely, accurate, and secure. HIM practitioners also ensure the physical security of health information. Security issues related to the storage of health records include damage of records by fire, water, theft, tampering, and destruction. Every HIM department has policies to safeguard records from these hazards. It is the specific responsibility of HIM practitioners and all designated employees to safeguard this information. Careful forethought and preparation for security of health records can prevent every HIM practitioner's worst nightmare.

## Disaster Planning

**The Joint Commission (TJC)** An organization that accredits and sets standards for acute care facilities, ambulatory care networks, long-term care facilities, and rehabilitation facilities, as well as certain specialty facilities, such as hospice and home care. Facilities maintaining TJC accreditation receive *deemed status* from the CMS.

**accreditation** Voluntary compliance with a set of standards developed by an independent agent, who periodically performs audits to ensure compliance.

Disaster planning is a method for planning and preparing to handle catastrophes and other emergencies that can adversely affect the normal performance of the health care environment. For example, a disaster can consist of a large number of patients requiring medical attention at the same time as a result of an explosion or a plane crash. In this situation, the increased number of patients needing treatment would necessitate implementation of a plan to handle their care and processing in a timely manner. All TJC-accredited facilities are required to maintain a disaster plan. Facilities must also educate HIM employees on the security procedures and make sure that they are prepared to follow procedure if a disaster occurs.

Security of health records is mandated by regulatory and accreditation agencies. HIM practitioners must protect all health information, including records; diagnosis, procedure, and physician indices; the MPI; computerized health information databases; radiographic films; and admission, discharge, and transfer logs.

### Fire Damage

Providing protection from fire for the health information environment can prevent irreversible damage to the facility's health records. Some of the systems and barriers that can assist in the protection from fire are chemical systems, sprinkler systems, fire walls, fire compartments, and fire extinguishers.

Chemical systems deplete the oxygen from the air in an area where a fire exists. File rooms and computer facilities may be equipped with this type of system. The chemical system is designed to sense fire and release a chemical that removes oxygen from the air in the room. Removing the oxygen smothers the fire to prevent further damage to files or facility.

Building structures such as fire walls or fire compartments are designed to contain a fire within a facility. Fire walls prevent a fire from moving in a parallel direction on a particular floor of the building. Health care facilities often feature double doors in the hallways, in which the doors are held open by magnets on each wall. When the fire alarm is triggered in a health care facility with fire walls, those double doors close to seal the fire and prevent it from spreading to other areas of the facility. A fire compartment is a structure in a building in which all sides of a room or area are protected by fire barriers. In other words, the walls, ceiling, and floor are all fire resistant. If a fire begins in a fire compartment, the compartment contains the fire; likewise, if the fire is outside the compartment, the contents within the compartment are protected from the fire. A fire compartment is the ideal solution to protect the permanent file area or a central computer system if a fire occurs in another part of the facility.

Sprinkler systems release water to extinguish fire when activated by heat or smoke. When a sprinkler system is used to safeguard files, it is important to have at least 18 inches of clearance between the top of the file space and the ceiling. Failure to keep these areas clear prevents the water sprinklers from extinguishing the fire at a lower level. In the event of a fire, sprinkler systems may extinguish the fire and cause minimal water damage to the facility's records.

All health care facilities are equipped with fire extinguishers. HIM employees must be familiar with the location of the nearest fire extinguisher. Employees must be able to operate the fire extinguishers in case of emergency. It is possible for a fire to begin in a very small trash can or near an electrical outlet. With use of a fire extinguisher, the fire can easily be controlled without activating a sprinkler system or chemical system.

### Water Damage

Water damage to health records, whether they are paper based or computerized, can occur because of flooding, storms, or fire control. A plan must be established to protect health information from water damage. For example, is the facility in an area where flooding is common? Some options for this scenario may be to relocate the file area to a higher floor of the facility, to elevate the file room a few feet, and, to have an emergency plan that can be activated to move records on low shelves to a higher location in the facility if the need arises. Health records maintained in file cabinets or on shelves that are closed or covered must also be considered for protection from flooding. Although damage to contents of file cabinets from a sprinkler system is usually minimal, sprinkler systems do cause damage to contents of open shelving units. The HIM professional should evaluate the health record environment and the potential for flood or water damage and should remember to protect computer terminals and to have a plan in case of emergency.

On a positive note, there are processes to assist in the restoration of paper health records that are damaged by water. If paper records are soaked with water or other fluid, acting quickly can restore and protect the information. Once the paper records dry, the opportunity to salvage them may be lost. Wet paper records may be salvaged, but records destroyed by fire are gone forever. Meeting with disaster recovery companies before disaster strikes provides information for the department that might not have been considered otherwise. The companies can supply references to other facilities that have used their services. Proactive conversations can be very useful to the facility in a disaster, because staff will know whom to contact, how long it will take for the records to arrive at the facility, and other helpful information to secure or preserve the health records.

## Theft and Tampering

The issues to consider when protecting health records from theft or tampering are the location of the health records, access to health records, and security. Health information, both paper and electronic form, must be protected from theft or tampering by parties both within and outside the facility. Within a facility, only authorized personnel should have access to patient health information, and they should have access only to the information that pertains to the completion of their job duties. Paper documents are secured by allowing release of an original record from the HIM department only if it is needed for the patient's treatment. The HIM department maintains appropriate measures to track the location of patient records. Other review of a patient's record must occur within the HIM department and is allowed only if the person reviewing the record is authorized to do so.

HIM professionals cannot follow every patient record checked out to every location in a facility. Therefore it is important to have policies and procedures in place to secure the information. This security may be achieved by (1) notifying others of the policies and procedures for security of information, (2) performing regular in-service training for facility employees to inform them of the rules governing health information, and (3) restricting the reasons for which a patient's health record is allowed to leave the department.

Additional security measures are as follows:
- After office hours, the HIM department should be closed and all access doors locked; only those people authorized to enter the department are allowed entrance. Anyone with

**Go To** Inservice training and policies are discussed under training and development, in Chapter 14 of this text.

a key to the area must be aware of all HIM policies and procedures regarding the appropriate use of health information.

- Areas may also be protected by a key code entry system. Access codes are assigned only to appropriate employees or physicians. After hours, an authorized physician can gain access to any incomplete health records with this code.
- A swipe badge security feature allows entry to the HIM department only with the appropriate access card, which is assigned to authorized physicians or employees.
- Computer passwords assigned to authorized users allow the facility to limit and monitor the people who access health information.
- Biometric technology, such as fingerprinting and retinal scanning, is also a means of limiting access to health records. With this technology, the system scans a person's fingerprint or retina to evaluate his or her authority to enter an area or gain access to a system.
- Cameras are another security feature found in health care facilities. In areas where there is greater need for security, cameras monitored by the facility's security personnel guard against unauthorized entry.

For computerized health information, a facility must secure records when transferring files from one system to another within or outside of the facility. For example, upgrading software or changing computers may require patient health information to be transferred from one information system to another. Copying of records from one system to another is acceptable; however, the HIM department must supervise this type of data transfer. Additionally, the department must validate that patient information is not deleted in the transfer. Failure to maintain complete patient information may affect future patient care. Likewise, an incomplete medical record may not be admissible in court as evidence in the event of litigation. An index of the old system should be maintained to verify the accuracy of the new system.

Electronic health information must be protected. Equipment should be secure, and precautions should be taken to prevent others from accessing the system. It is also important to ensure that the facility can update current systems and still retrieve information from legacy systems.

**litigation** The term used to indicate that a matter must be settled by the court and the process of engaging in legal proceedings.

**Go To** See Chapter 3 for a discussion of e-PHI.

---

### HIT-bit

#### ELECTRONIC HEALTH RECORD SECURITY

In a computer-based patient record environment, HIM file clerks are able to send a copy, a viewable image, of the patient's record while keeping the original in the computer system. Once a patient's record is in the system, it can be shared by many users simultaneously. HIM professionals should be aware of the security concerns in the computer environment. Patients' health records must be secure from potential for loss, computer tampering, deletion, and unauthorized access.

---

## Destruction of Health Information

There are circumstances in which it is appropriate to destroy health information. For example, records (stored on paper, microfilm, or electronic formats) may be destroyed at the completion of the retention period or when paper-based records have been successfully transferred to another medium, such as microfilm, CD, or optical disk. However, HIM employees must prevent negligent destruction. In a paper record environment, a common method of destroying health information is the shredding or incineration of the paper document. The destruction must occur in a confidential manner. It should be performed in the presence of a credentialed custodian of the HIM department or his or her delegate. Health information should never be left to be destroyed without the proper supervision. If a vendor is chosen for the destruction, the following questions should be answered: Do they use a third party for shredding? Is the third party compliant with HIPAA regulations? Is recycling an option? What is their procedure for destruction? How and when will written confirmation or a destruction certificate be obtained?

**custodian** The person entrusted with the responsibility for the confidentiality, privacy, and security of medical records.
**Health Insurance Portability and Accountability Act (HIPAA)** Public Law 104-191, federal legislation passed in 1996 that outlines the guidelines of managing patient information in terms of privacy, security, and confidentiality. The legislation also outlines penalties for noncompliance.

In the electronic record environment, destruction of health information may include entering a virus into the software system, destroying the equipment or software used to retrieve the health information, or otherwise removing the information from the system.

To prevent premature destruction of health information in the paper record environment, several measures must be taken. Employees should be aware of the appropriate content of the health record so that the valuable patient information is not inadvertently thrown out. Likewise, the employees should be aware of the **record retention schedule** for all materials in the HIM department. If the facility has chosen to store records in an alternative format, the finished product—microfilm, optical disks, or EHR files—must be reviewed to ensure that all of the information is intact before the original paper record is destroyed.

In an electronic record environment, a backup file of all health information in all systems must be completed daily. The backup copy allows information to be restored up to the time that the backup was created. This procedure is usually performed daily in health care facilities. The backup file copies the information from the systems in the facility. If the system crashes the next day, at least the facility will have all of the information necessary to restore the system to the previous day's business.

Electronic health information should be kept in an environment that supports the use of computers. The HIM department must maintain the computerized equipment so that it is free from harm by temperature, water, and other environmental effects. These considerations also apply to microfilm and optical disk storage. Microfilm and optical disks can be damaged by intense heat. Computers are affected by temperatures as well. Water can damage a computer and cause loss of function and information. Falling objects can damage computer equipment and disks, and liquids spilled on keyboards or hard drives can impair or destroy a system.

## Restoration of Information Lost Inadvertently

What can be done when health records are lost or destroyed inadvertently? It is important to have a plan of action. In an electronic record system, daily backups of the information in the system should allow full recovery of all patient information (prior to backup). In the event of inadvertent destruction of paper records, the only information that can be reproduced is the duplicate paper documents maintained by allied health departments within the facility. For example, the laboratory and radiology departments usually maintain duplicate copies of reports, the transcription department or service may be able to recover transcription of any dictated reports, and in some instances the billing office may maintain a file including patient information. As a last-resort effort, a facility may also find information in the attending physician's office. Often, the attending physician needs copies of patient information for follow-up care or to bill for services. Obtaining a copy of information sent to the physician can assist in the effort to recover this information.

## RECORD RETENTION

The length of time a record is kept by a facility is the record retention schedule. Health records must be maintained by a facility to support patient care; meet legal and regulatory requirements; achieve accreditation; allow research, education, and reimbursement; and support facility administration. The duration of record **retention** differs for the various types of records kept (e.g., laboratory data, radiology reports and films, fetal monitor strips, birth certificates, MPIs) and for different facilities and is defined by their respective accrediting agencies. Most states have laws mandating how long a facility must maintain health information. In the absence of state law, the facility must follow the federal requirements stipulated by the CMS, which is to save such records for 5 years. A facility should also consider extending retention time to allow for cases in which malpractice, patient age, or research activity requires review of the record.

---

**record retention schedule** The length of time that a record must be retained.

**optical disk** Electronic storage medium; a disk used to store digital data.

**Go To** Chapter 10 addresses the ways health records are used to generate facility statistics; Chapter 11 covers the use of health record data in research, education accreditation, and other applications; Chapter 12 discusses the use of health records in a compliance, legal, and regulatory environment.

**retention** The procedures governing the storage of records, including duration, location, security, and access.

**MPI** master patient index
**CMS** Centers for Medicare and Medicaid Services

## TABLE 9-8

### RETENTION SCHEDULE OF HEALTH CARE RECORDS

| TYPE OF HEALTH INFORMATION | RETENTION SCHEDULE |
|---|---|
| Acute care facility records | 10 years for adults |
|  | Age of majority + 10 years for minors (or statute of limitations) |
| Birth, death, surgical procedure registers | Permanent |
| radiographs | 5 years |
| Fetal monitor strips | Age of majority + 10 years |
| Master patient index (MPI) | Permanent |
| Diseases index | 10 years |
| Emergency department register/log | Permanent |
| Employee health records | 30 years |

Medicare Conditions of Participation (COP) require retention of records, films, and scans for at least 5 years. Each provider should develop a retention schedule for records in its facility.
Modified from AHIMA Practice Brief: Retention of Health Information. http://library.ahima.org/xpedio/groups/public/documents/ahima/bok1_049250.hcsp?dDocName=bok1_049250.

**American Health Information Management Association (AHIMA)** A professional organization supporting the health care industry by promoting high-quality information standards through a variety of activities, including but not limited to accreditation of schools, continuing education, professional development and educational publications, and legislative and regulatory advocacy.

The retention time for patient health records may be a specific number of years, or it can be counted from the date of the patient's last encounter. For example, assume that the retention schedule in a state is 10 years from the patient's last encounter and includes all previous records. Jane Ryan has an appendectomy at age 20, a broken ankle with repair at age 25, and treatment for a motor vehicle accident (MVA) at age 29, all at the same facility. Upon her admission for the ankle repair, the 10-year retention period for the appendectomy record starts over; it starts over again with the MVA admission. Jane's records are kept until a retention time of 10 years has lapsed from her last visit (when she is 39 years old, assuming no more admissions). However, if the retention schedule in the state does not include previous visits, then the appendectomy record can be destroyed when the retention period expires (when she is 30 years old). Refer to Table 9-8 for the retention schedule for health information suggested by the AHIMA.

## Retention Policy

Each HIM department must have a policy explaining how the medical records within the facility are stored. The policy describes which health records are maintained in the department, how each type of record is organized, the storage medium used, and the length of time each record is to be retained. The retention policy is very important to a facility with many records that may be stored in different locations. The policy must state that a record is maintained on every patient registered to the facility; must provide the retention schedule; must indicate how the records are identified, organized, or filed; must state their location; and must document alternative locations or media, if necessary.

## Facility Closure

What happens when a facility, physician's office, or clinic closes its operation? Where do the records go? In the event of a facility's closing, the retention schedule remains in effect. The facility must investigate the applicable laws to determine the best method for retaining the records. If the facility or practice is purchased, the records are managed by the new owner. However, if the practice or facility closes, the records must be maintained for the duration of the retention schedule in an appropriate, secure, confidential location.

The facility must notify its patients when it is closing. There are several excellent methods of informing patients of closure. One method is to run an advertisement in the local newspaper explaining the closure and what will happen to the patient records (Figure 9-23). Another method is to notify patients of the closure through letters or notices mailed

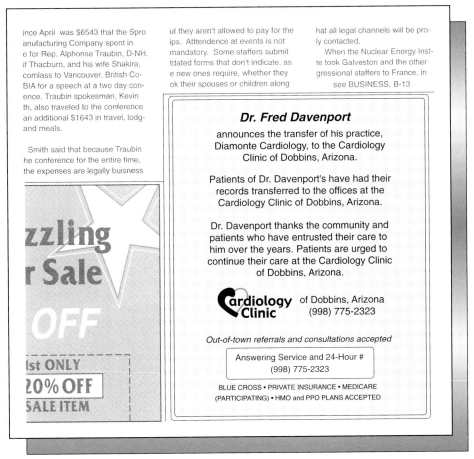

ince April  was $6543 that the Spro
anufacturing Company spent in
e for Rep. Alphonse Traubin, D-NH.
if Thacburn, and his wife Shakira,
comlass to Vancouver, British Co-
BIA for a speech at a two day con-
ence. Traubin spokesman, Kevin
th, also traveled to the conference
an additional $1643 in travel, lodg-
and meals.

Smith said that because Traubin
he conference for the entire time,
the expenses are legally buisness

ut they aren't allowed to pay for the
ips. Atttendence at events is not
mandatory.  Some staffers submit
tdated forms that don't indicate, as
e new ones require, whether they
ok their spouses or children along

hat all legal channels will be pro-
ly contacted.
When the Nuclear Energy Inst-
te took Galveston and the other
gressional staffers to France, in
see BUSINESS, B-13

**Dr. Fred Davenport**

announces the transfer of his practice,
Diamonte Cardiology, to the Cardiology
Clinic of Dobbins, Arizona.

Patients of Dr. Davenport's have had their
records transferred to the offices at the
Cardiology Clinic of Dobbins, Arizona.

Dr. Davenport thanks the community and
patients who have entrusted their care to
him over the years. Patients are urged to
continue their care at the Cardiology Clinic
of Dobbins, Arizona.

**Cardiology**   of Dobbins, Arizona
**Clinic**   (998) 775-2323

*Out-of-town referrals and consultations accepted*

Answering Service and 24-Hour #
(998) 775-2323

BLUE CROSS • PRIVATE INSURANCE • MEDICARE
(PARTICIPATING) • HMO and PPO PLANS ACCEPTED

Figure 9-23  Newspaper advertisement of facility closure.

directly to the patients' homes. It is also important to post similar notices in and around
the facility to notify patients of the closure. Because patient information is critical in the
continuity of care, it is important to maintain patient access to the records even after the
facility is closed. This goal may be accomplished by transferring the records to another
local facility or physician's office, as appropriate.

> **continuity of care** The broad range
> of health care services required
> by a patient during an illness or
> for an entire lifetime. May also
> refer to the continuity of care
> provided by a health care
> organization. Also called
> *continuum of care.*

## ■ EXERCISE 9-5
### Security of Health Information

1. To prepare for unexpected events such as a bomb threat, hurricane, or flood, a facility should routinely exercise which of the following policies?
   a. Confidentiality
   b. Release of information
   c. Disaster planning
   d. Code blue
2. Which of the following methods assist security of records on a computerized system?
   a. Microfilm
   b. Data dictionary
   c. Scanning
   d. Routine backups
3. Medical records should never be destroyed.
   True
   False
4. The length of time that a record must be retained is called the record _____ _____.

5. In the absence of state laws regarding retention of health care records, the CMS requires that records be maintained for:
   a. 10 years.
   b. 21 years.
   c. 30 years.
   d. 5 years.
6. List some of the ways water can be a threat to medical records.
7. List three methods used to protect records from fire.

*Match the terms on the left with their definitions on the right.*

| | |
|---|---|
| 8. ___ computer-based patient records | A. an alternative method for storing records |
| 9. ___ computerized records | B. a file identification system in which patients receive the same number for all admissions |
| 10. ___ serial | |
| 11. ___ unit | C. a file identification system in which the patient receives a new number for each subsequent admission |
| 12. ___ serial unit | |
| 13. ___ family unit | D. a file identification system that assigns the same number to an entire family, uniquely identifying each member with a modifier |
| 14. ___ index | |
| 15. ___ scanner | E. a file identification system in which the patient receives a new number for each subsequent admission; however, each previous admission is brought forward and filed with the most recent visit |
| 16. ___ retention schedule | |
| 17. ___ microfilm | |
| | F. a method of identifying patient records in a computer-based system |
| | G. the length of time required for maintenance of records |
| | H. a copier-like piece of equipment used to input paper records in a document imaging system |
| | I. a COLD system |
| | J. a system of patient health records that uses a database |

## SUGGESTED READING

American Health Information Management Association: Practice brief: protecting patient information after facility closure (updated): AHIMA Practice Brief. J AHIMA 70:3, 1999. http://library.ahima.org/xpedio/groups/public/documents/ahima/pub_bok2_000585.html.

American Health Information Management Association: Protecting patient information after a facility closure (updated). J AHIMA 2011. http://library.ahima.org/xpedio/groups/public/documents/ahima/bok1_049257.hcsp?dDocName=bok1_049257#BP4

Claeys T: Medical filing, ed 2, Albany, NY, 1997, Delmar.

Dooling J: Managing records between the EDMS and EHR, J AHIMA 82:38-39, 2011.

Huffman EK: Health information management, ed 10, Berwyn IL, 1994, Physicians' Record Company.

# CHAPTER ACTIVITIES

## CHAPTER SUMMARY

By maintaining health records that are accurate and organized, the HIM department provides a valuable service to the health care facility and the patient. Health records are vital to patient care and must be accessible, accurate, and complete. Maintenance of an organized storage area for paper health record files facilitates timely retrieval of records for all authorized users.

In a paper environment, in which numerical identification is used, the master patient index is the key tool to correlate the patient to his or her medical record number. Medical record (identification) numbers can be assigned with use of unit, serial, serial-unit, or family numbering systems. Filing methods use either the patient's name or the medical record number to organize the health record in the filing system. These filing methods are alphabetical, straight numerical, middle-digit, and terminal-digit order. The chart locator system allows the HIM department to keep track of the location of health records.

There are several different storage options for computerized health data, and technology continues to advance. Records that are maintained in an electronic system through scanning, or those in a fully functional EHR, must also be accurate and accessible.

HIM practitioners must consider the physical security issues of storing health records safely to prevent damage by fire, water, theft, tampering, destruction, and loss of confidentiality. HIM professionals must pay special attention to the storage details so that all authorized users in the facility have efficient and effective access to health information. Storage of health records is a function that many take for granted in the health care facility. This chapter is intended to stress the importance of this function and its impact on patient care and the health care facility.

## REVIEW QUESTIONS

1. Explain the importance of a master patient index.
2. Explain how an EMPI differs from an MPI.
3. Compare and contrast the different record identification systems.
4. Compare and contrast the various filing systems.
5. Explain a legacy system.
6. Describe a chart locator system.
7. Identify two input and two output peripherals and explain how they might be used in the HIM department or health care facility.
8. Name the three types of computer storage.
9. Identify the approximate storage capacity for a 1GB off-line flash drive.
10. Explain how RAID technology is helping health care facilities.
11. Explain when and how computer output to laser disk (COLD) systems are used.
12. Explain how cloud computing structures share resources.
13. Compare the following storage methods, listing the pros and cons of each: document imaging, onsite storage, offsite storage.
14. Explain why or when it is acceptable to destroy health information.
15. Identify and explain three reasons why health records must be retained by a health care facility.
16. Describe disaster planning and identify three specific events that an HIM professional should prepare to prevent.

## PROFESSIONAL PROFILE

### Enterprise MPI Supervisor

My name is Brett, and I am the Enterprise Supervisor for Diamonte's health care system. We have three acute care facilities located across our city along with a same-day surgery center, rehabilitation center, and a nursing home. Because there are limited health care resources in our area, many of our patients may receive care at any one of our facilities. This situation presents opportunities for our registration personnel to make errors when identifying whether or not a patient has a prior record in our MPI. Sometimes it is not a personnel error but rather the circumstances, such as emergency care, that cause erroneous entries. My job is to make sure the EMPI is accurate. Each day reports are generated to identify potential duplicate records in our EMPI. I am responsible for investigating each of these records to determine whether a correction must be made to fix an error. Sometimes the correction is simple; someone's name may be misspelled and all of the records are electronic and easily updated/corrected. On other occasions the error applies to a patient who has records in our legacy system and paper files in our offsite storage facility. Correcting these errors requires careful documentation and follow-up to be certain that every patient's record is available when needed for care and that future errors do not occur.

I started out at Diamonte as a patient registration clerk and transferred to the HIM department when I was almost finished with my associate degree in HIM. I worked in the scanning area for a while, and then I was asked to take on an MPI clean-up project. That went well and I was promoted to the corporate position last year.

### CAREER TIP

MPI maintenance is typically an HIM function. Although the research to determine whether a patient has multiple medical record numbers is often performed by clerical personnel, the actual combining of records in the system should be performed by, or authorized by, supervisory personnel. Knowledge of the data elements in the MPI and of the proper way to correct errors is essential. The clerical level of analysis can be an entry-level position even for someone with a few introductory HIM courses. There are consulting companies that specialize in this type of analysis, and additional education as well as management experience is often required for a professional to progress in the field.

## PATIENT CARE PERSPECTIVE

**Joseph**

I have been to Diamonte several times since we moved here 2 years ago. I have had blood tests and radiology here, plus I had a colonoscopy recently. I recently got a call from Brett at Diamonte, who noticed that I somehow had two medical record numbers. The information was mostly the same on both, but the Social Security numbers were slightly different and the insurance information was different. My company changed insurance plans last year, but we think the Social Security number was a clerical error. I faxed Brett the correct information after calling him back at the hospital. I really appreciate that they pay attention to these things.

## APPLICATION

### File System Conversion

Diamonte Hospital is preparing to convert its current filing system. The old system uses a six-digit medical record number for file identification, and the records are stored in straight numerical order on the file shelf. The new system will maintain the six-digit medical record number, but it will use terminal-digit filing because of the high volume of filing activity. The facility will also get rid of the compressible shelves and use open shelving.

Develop a plan for converting the straight numerical file system to terminal-digit filing. Remember that the medical record numbers will remain the same. The change will occur in the organization of the files on the shelves.

Determine how many shelf units and how much space will be needed to store the current records in an open-shelf system. Remember to allow for aisle space as necessary.

The current records of Diamonte occupy 3000 linear feet.

Open-shelf units contain eight shelves, and each unit is 38 inches wide (allowing for 36 inches of file space per shelf).

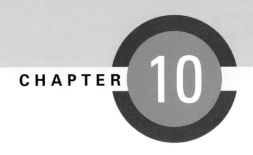

## CHAPTER 10

# STATISTICS

Nadinia Davis

## CHAPTER OUTLINE

ORGANIZED COLLECTION OF
  DATA
  Primary and Secondary Data
  Creation of a Database
  Data Review and Abstracting
  Data Quality Check
DATA RETRIEVAL
  Retrieval of Aggregate Data
  Retrieving Data
  Optimal Source of Data
  Indices
REPORTING OF DATA
  Reporting to Individual
    Departments
  Reporting to Outside Agencies

STATISTICAL ANALYSIS OF
  PATIENT INFORMATION
  Analysis and Interpretation
  Measures of Central Tendency
  Measures of Frequency
  Measures of Variance
PRESENTATION
  Line Graph
  Bar Graph
  Histogram
  Pie Chart
ROUTINE INSTITUTIONAL
  STATISTICS
  Admissions
  Discharges

Length of Stay
Average Length of Stay
Transfers
Census
Bed Occupancy Rate
Hospital Rates and
  Percentages
REGISTRIES
  Tumor or Cancer Registry
  Trauma Registry
  Other Registries
  Vital Statistics

## VOCABULARY

aggregate data
average length of stay
  (ALOS)
bar graph
bed control
census
central limit theorem
class intervals
discrete data
frequency distribution

histogram
index
inpatient service days
  (IPSDs)
Institutional Review Board
  (IRB)
length of stay (LOS)
line graph
mean
median

mode
normal curve
occupancy
outlier
percentage
pie chart
population
primary data
query
random selection

redact
registry
report
sample
secondary data
skewed
standard deviation
statistics
trend

## CHAPTER OBJECTIVES

*By the end of this chapter, the student should be able to:*

1. Distinguish between primary and secondary data.
2. Explain the criteria for creating a report from a
   database.
3. List and describe four examples of indices that can
   be queried from a patient database.
4. Calculate the length of stay for a patient, given the
   admission and discharge dates.

5. Retrieve appropriate data according to the request.
6. Identify the optimal source for retrieval of information.
7. Describe and state the uses for statistical tools.
8. Compute routine institutional statistics.
9. Prepare graphic representation of data appropriate to
   the data type.
10. List four examples of registries and their purposes.

**health record** Also called *record* or *medical record*. It contains all of the data collected for an individual patient.

**accreditation** Voluntary compliance with a set of standards developed by an independent agent, who periodically performs audits to ensure compliance.

**outcome** The result of a patient's treatment.

**performance improvement** Also known as *quality improvement (QI)* or *continuous quality improvement (CQI)*. Refers to the process by which a facility reviews its services or products to ensure quality.

**primary data** Data taken directly from the patient or the original source. The patient's health record contains primary data.

**treatment** A procedure, medication, or other measure designed to cure or alleviate the symptoms of disease.

In earlier chapters, the collection of health data for documentation in the health record was discussed. The health record is used to gather health data for storage in a physical location or database to facilitate retrieval for future use. Organizing specific data elements for each patient allows reporting of health information as it is mandated by law, accreditation, or policy or as needed by authorized users.

Important reasons to collect specific health data are statistical analysis, outcome analysis, and quality or performance improvement. Data analysis is a critical function in all health care facilities. To analyze data within one record or among multiple records, the health information management (HIM) professional must collect the data elements in the same way every time. An important function of the HIM department is the organized retrieval and reporting of these data. In previous chapters, the collection of health data was discussed in the context of providing proper patient care and following health care professional guidelines. The data were categorized into reports, such as the history and physical (H&P), laboratory reports, and nurses' notes. This chapter focuses on the importance of collecting specific data in an organized format—such as a data set for input to a database—so that the health information can be analyzed and reported as necessary. Basic analytical and reporting strategies are explored.

## ORGANIZED COLLECTION OF DATA

In order to be analyzed in a meaningful way, the data must first be collected appropriately. Appropriate collection of data is accomplished through the consistent use of forms and data screens to ensure timely, accurate, and valid data, as discussed in previous chapters. When one is using the data, it is important to understand the source of the data, including the most appropriate source for the purpose.

### Primary and Secondary Data

**Primary data** come from original sources, such as patient medical records. These are the data that are collected or generated by clinicians while they are treating a patient. The clinician is the original recorder/reporter of the data: the firsthand account of the patient's treatment. Examples of primary data are the history given by the patient to the nurse (Figure 10-1) and the patient's blood pressure or temperature reading as recorded by the monitor or the nurse. These data elements are documented in the patient's health record in a format that helps transform the raw data into usable information. Because the data are from the original patient record, they are considered primary data.

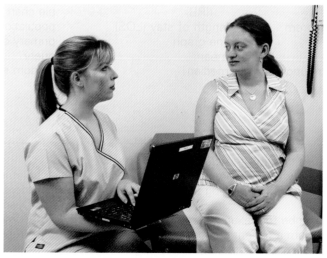

**Figure 10-1** Primary data are collected when the nurse talks to the patient to obtain her health history. (From Young: Kinn's The medical assistant, 11th ed, Philadelphia, 2011, Saunders, p 270.)

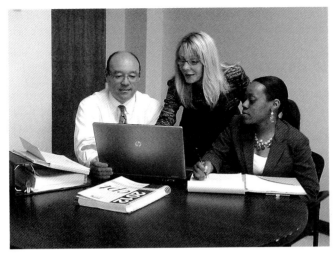

**Figure 10-2** As the HIM clerk reviews a health record and enters coded data into the abstract, she is creating secondary data.

Primary data are used when the identity of the patient is relevant to the user or the events recorded in the record are the focus of the review. For example, a physician who wants data for continuing patient care would be interested only in the patient-identifiable data from that specific patient's chart. A performance improvement team reviewer looking for compliance with protocols would probably need to review primary data.

**Secondary data** come from sources other than the original recorder/reporter of the data. Scholarly articles and aggregate (summarized) data are secondary sources. Census data and publicly available mortality data are examples of secondary health data. Abstracted data (data selected and reported from the health record) are secondary data and can be sorted and made available in a variety of formats. For example, a list of discharges sorted by physician is a physician index. The physician index is secondary data. Secondary data may be patient identifiable or may be **redacted** (patient identity removed) (Figure 10-2).

> ## HIT-bit
>
> ### DATA VERSUS INFORMATION
>
> Remember the difference between data and information: The data collected during patient care become health information only after careful organization and compilation. Data are raw elements. Information results from the interpretation of that data.

Hospital administrators and managers use both primary and secondary data for monitoring, tracking, and forecasting hospital and departmental activities, for example. Physicians may use such data for tracking volume and outcomes. Questions such as "How many?" "How often?" and "How well?" may be answered through analysis of the appropriate data.

For example, a physician might want a list of patients that she treated for a specific diagnosis or with a specified procedure, or to answer the question: *Which of my patients had a principal diagnosis of diabetes mellitus* or *On which of my patients did I perform surgery?* In these cases, the identity of the patients is relevant to the physician, and primary data would be accessed in order to provide the data. The report itself, however, is secondary data. The report might contain only a list of the patients and perhaps the relevant identification numbers. The report gives no insight into other issues that might be relevant to the cases.

A hospital administrator may want to know how many cases of a particular surgical type were performed during a period of time. Although the primary data would be used to produce the abstracted report, the patient-identifying information would not be relevant—it would be omitted from the report. If the report generated from the computer system contains patient identifiable data, such as name, such data would be redacted

---

**secondary data** Data taken from the primary source document for use elsewhere.

**aggregate data** A group of like data elements compiled to provide information about the group.

**abstracting** The recap of selected fields from a health record to create an informative summary. Also refers to the activity of identifying such fields and entering them into a computer system.

**redact** To remove patient-identifying information from a health record.

**Go To** See Chapter 2 for a discussion of the data dictionary.

**attending physician** The physician who is primarily responsible for coordinating the care of the patient in the hospital; it is usually the physician who ordered the patient's admission to the hospital.

**admission record** The demographic, financial, socioeconomic, and clinical data collected about a patient at registration. Also refers to the document in a paper record that contains these data.

**Uniform Bill (UB-04)** The standardized form used by hospitals for inpatient and outpatient billing to the CMS and other third party payers.

**query** To question the database for specific elements, information, or a report.

**report** The result of a query. A list from a database.

**payer** The individual or organization that is primarily responsible for the reimbursement for a particular health care service. Usually refers to the insurance company or third party.

**advance directive** A written document, like a living will, that specifies a patient's wishes for his/her care and dictates power of attorney, for the purpose of providing clear instructions in the event the patient is unable to do so.

**Medicare** Federally funded health care insurance plan for older adults and for certain categories of chronically ill patients.

**discrete data** Named and identifiable pieces of data that can be queried and reported in a meaningful way.

**ICD-10-CM** International Classification of Diseases, Tenth Revision—Clinical Modification. The U.S. clinical modification of the World Health Organization's disease classification system. Designated by HIPAA to represent diagnoses and reasons for health care encounters.

**ICD-10-PCS** International Classification of Diseases, Tenth Revision—Procedural Coding System. The U.S. code set designated by HIPAA to represent procedures performed in the inpatient setting.

**medical record number (MR#)** A unique number assigned to each patient in a health care system; this code will be used for the rest of the patient's encounters with that specific health system.

**abstract** A summary of the patient record.

**ambulatory care facility** An outpatient facility, such as an emergency department or physician's office, in which treatment is intended to occur within 1 calendar day.

**long-term care facility** A hospital that provides services to patients over an extended period; an average length of stay is in excess of 30 days. Facilities are characterized by the extent to which nursing care is provided.

**query** To question the database for specific elements, information, or a report.

**diagnosis related group (DRG)** A collection of health care descriptions organized into statistically similar categories.

(removed or blocked) from the report before the report was transmitted to the administrator. Such secondary reporting and analysis of patient data is the focus of this chapter.

## Creation of a Database

Because each data element is defined before it is collected, the database is a useful source of information. For example, "attending physician" is one of the data elements collected. One can collect this data element in the admission record by entering the identification number for the physician who matches the description of the attending physician (see Table 4-1). This information is reported on the Uniform Bill (UB-04) for each patient discharged. The collection of this data element on all patients in the database makes it possible to **query**, or ask, the database for information specific to the attending physician. For example, facilities should review a representative sample of records on all physicians on the medical staff at the facility when conducting studies of documentation and quality. To do so, the user must be able to run a **report** that lists records for each physician. The ability to query the database on the attending physician data element is therefore quite useful. In addition to documentation and quality studies, such a report might also be part of a review of physician practice patterns, including patient volume.

As noted previously, some data are required by the federal government and other payers. However, other data elements are collected only as specified by the facility. These types of data must be collected in the way in which they will be useful in the future. For example, in some cases, the type and frequency of consulting services, such as cardiology, and infectious disease, may influence the patient's outcomes and length of stay. To collect this type of data (if not already captured), as each patient record is abstracted, the HIM professional identifies consulting services and enters the corresponding physician identifiers into the abstract. Later, the user can access that information in the database in the way that he or she prefers. For example, the user might look at consulting services associated with a specific diagnosis or procedure or with a particular attending physician. Examples of additional data that might be captured are type of anesthesia, length of surgery, and consent details.

An example of other data that may be collected is advance directive acknowledgments. Facilities can include fields containing Yes or No to capture whether a patient has signed the advance directive acknowledgement statement or whether the patient has signed an Advance Beneficiary Notice (ABN), accepting responsibility for charges not payable by Medicare. Copies of the documents themselves would be on file, but their presence is not retrievable as a data field unless specifically captured. This Yes/No field is an example of a **discrete data** point: a named and identifiable piece of data that can be queried and reported in a meaningful way. ICD-10-CM/ICD-10-PCS codes and medical record number are also examples of discrete data.

Certain services provided to patients and supplies used to treat patients are not separately payable. However, hospital administration may wish to track such services and items for staff productivity or inventory control purposes. One way to do this is to enter charges to the patient's account that have no dollar amount associated with them. These data, then, would also be available for abstraction and analysis by authorized users.

## Data Review and Abstracting

When all required elements of the patient's data have been captured, the abstract is considered complete. All patient records must be abstracted as required to satisfy payer and facility guidelines for specific data. Each patient receiving services in a health care setting has an abstract. However, the abstract differs according to the setting (e.g., ambulatory care, long-term care). By collecting this data in the abstract, the facility is able to query the system (run reports) for information related to these topics.

Some of the typical queries of the abstract database are as follows:
- List of patients for a physician (Figure 10-3, *A*)
- List of patients by diagnosis, DRG, or procedure (Figure 10-3, *B*)
- List of patients by patient financial class (Figure 10-3, *C*)
- List of patients by age (Figure 10-3, *D*)

*Text continued on p. 297*

**Diamonte Hospital**
**Discharges by Physician**
**Discharge Date 2/19/2012**

**Attending Physician:**    Li, Xiaobo

| Admission | Discharge | LOS | Disch Disp | DOB | Age | Gender | Financial Class | Account | Pt Last Name | Pt First Name |
|---|---|---|---|---|---|---|---|---|---|---|
| 02/16/2012 | 02/19/2012 | 3 | 1 | 02/03/1944 | 68 | F | M | 203673 | Anderson | Judith |
| 02/11/2012 | 02/19/2012 | 8 | 3 | 01/03/1943 | 69 | M | C | 203489 | King | Robert |
| 02/18/2012 | 02/19/2012 | 1 | 1 | 09/10/1937 | 74 | M | C | 203741 | Hill | Paul |

A

**Diamonte Hospital**
**Disease Index**
**Discharge Date**

From 02/13/2012 through 02/20/2012

**Diagnoses**

| Z38.00 | Single liveborn, born in hospital, delivered without mention of Cesarean section |
|---|---|
| Z38.01 | Single liveborn, born in hospital, delivered by Cesarean section |
| Z38.30 | Twin birth, mate liveborn, born in hospital, delivered without mention of Cesarean section |
| Z38.31 | Twin birth, mate liveborn, born in hospital, delivered by Cesarean section |

| Principal Diagnosis | Secondary Diagnoses | | Principal Procedure | Secondary Procedure | Patient Last Name | Patient First Name | Admission | Discharge | LOS | Gender | MS-DRG | MR# |
|---|---|---|---|---|---|---|---|---|---|---|---|---|
| Z38.00 | Z23 | | 3E0134Z | | Johnson | Emma | 02/11/2012 | 02/13/2012 | 2 | F | 795 | 203290 |
| Z38.00 | Z23 | | 3E0134Z | | Williams | Mason | 02/11/2012 | 02/13/2012 | 2 | M | 795 | 203300 |
| Z38.00 | Z23 | | 3E0134Z | | Jones | Sophia | 02/12/2012 | 02/14/2012 | 2 | F | 795 | 203311 |
| Z38.00 | Z23 | | 3E0134Z | | Miller | Noah | 02/12/2012 | 02/14/2012 | 2 | M | 795 | 203314 |
| Z38.00 | Z23 | | 3E0134Z | | Rodriguez | Jackson | 02/13/2012 | 02/15/2012 | 2 | M | 795 | 203331 |
| Z38.00 | Z23 | | 3E0134Z | | Wilson | Ava | 02/13/2012 | 02/15/2012 | 2 | F | 795 | 203332 |
| Z38.00 | Z23 | | 3E0134Z | | Anderson | Ella | 02/14/2012 | 02/15/2012 | 1 | F | 795 | 203360 |
| Z38.00 | Z23 | | 3E0134Z | | Taylor | Ryan | 02/14/2012 | 02/16/2012 | 2 | M | 795 | 203365 |
| Z38.00 | Z23 | | 3E0134Z | | Hernandez | Michael | 02/15/2012 | 02/17/2012 | 2 | M | 795 | 203383 |
| Z38.00 | Z23 | | 3E0134Z | | Moore | Choe | 02/15/2012 | 02/20/2012 | 5 | F | 795 | 203396 |
| Z38.00 | P83.5 | Z23 | 3E0134Z | | Scott | Ethan | 02/17/2012 | 02/19/2012 | 2 | M | 794 | 203703 |
| Z38.00 | Z23 | | 3E0134Z | | Thompson | Sophia | 02/16/2012 | 02/18/2012 | 2 | F | 795 | 203437 |
| Z38.00 | Z23 | | 3E0134Z | | White | Wesley | 02/16/2012 | 02/18/2012 | 2 | M | 795 | 203440 |
| Z38.01 | Z23 | | 0VTTXZZ | 3E0134Z | Allen | Jayden | 02/15/2012 | 02/19/2012 | 4 | M | 795 | 203630 |
| Z38.01 | Z23 | | 3E0134Z | | Smith | Ethan | 02/11/2012 | 02/14/2012 | 3 | M | 795 | 203289 |
| Z38.01 | Z23 | | 3E0134Z | | Brown | Olivia | 02/12/2012 | 02/15/2012 | 3 | F | 795 | 203309 |
| Z38.01 | Z23 | | 3E0134Z | | Davis | Jacob | 02/13/2012 | 02/16/2012 | 3 | M | 795 | 203323 |
| Z38.01 | Z23 | | 3E0134Z | | Garcia | Aiden | 02/13/2012 | 02/17/2012 | 4 | M | 795 | 203327 |
| Z38.01 | Z23 | | 3E0134Z | | Martinez | Isabella | 02/14/2012 | 02/17/2012 | 3 | F | 795 | 203333 |
| Z38.01 | Z23 | | 3E0134Z | | Thomas | Lily | 02/15/2012 | 02/19/2012 | 4 | F | 795 | 203372 |
| Z38.01 | Z23 | | 3E0134Z | | Martin | Owen | 02/16/2012 | 02/19/2012 | 3 | M | 795 | 203416 |
| Z38.01 | Z23 | | 3E0134Z | | Jackson | Charlotte | 02/16/2012 | 02/20/2012 | 4 | F | 795 | 203431 |

B

**Figure 10-3** Queries to the abstract database: **A,** List of patients by physician. **B,** List of patients by diagnosis.

**Diamonte Hospital**
**Discharge Detail by Financial Class**
**Discharge Date 2/19/2012**

page 1
printed 2/20/2012

**Financial Class** B Blue Cross/Blue Shield
C Medicaid
G Managed Care
M Medicare
S Self-Pay

| Financial Class | Admission | Discharge | LOS | Disch Disp | DOB | Age | Gender | MS-DRG | Account |
|---|---|---|---|---|---|---|---|---|---|
| B | 02/15/2012 | 02/19/2012 | 4 | 1 | 02/15/2012 | 0 | M | 795 | 203630 |
| B | 02/17/2012 | 02/19/2012 | 2 | 1 | 12/03/1962 | 49 | M | 153 | 203700 |
| B | 02/16/2012 | 02/19/2012 | 3 | 1 | 02/03/1944 | 68 | F | 069 | 203673 |
| B | 02/13/2012 | 02/19/2012 | 6 | 1 | 08/21/1953 | 59 | F | 330 | 203505 |
| B | 02/17/2012 | 02/19/2012 | 2 | 1 | 05/08/1963 | 49 | F | 743 | 203698 |
| B | 02/16/2012 | 02/19/2012 | 3 | 1 | 03/28/1960 | 52 | F | 378 | 203659 |
| C | 02/16/2012 | 02/19/2012 | 3 | 1 | 07/13/1954 | 58 | M | 379 | 203677 |
| C | 02/11/2012 | 02/19/2012 | 8 | 3 | 01/03/1943 | 69 | M | 885 | 203489 |
| C | 02/18/2012 | 02/19/2012 | 1 | 1 | 12/31/1974 | 37 | F | 770 | 203778 |
| C | 02/13/2012 | 02/19/2012 | 6 | 1 | 01/15/1967 | 45 | F | 745 | 203546 |
| G | 02/17/2012 | 02/19/2012 | 2 | 1 | 03/11/1972 | 40 | F | 775 | 203688 |
| M | 02/15/2012 | 02/19/2012 | 4 | 1 | 06/21/1934 | 78 | M | 864 | 203621 |
| M | 02/13/2012 | 02/19/2012 | 6 | 1 | 12/24/1927 | 84 | M | 378 | 203508 |
| M | 02/18/2012 | 02/19/2012 | 1 | 3 | 02/23/1937 | 75 | F | 809 | 203787 |
| M | 02/16/2012 | 02/19/2012 | 3 | 1 | 06/30/1929 | 83 | M | 195 | 203684 |
| M | 02/19/2012 | 02/19/2012 | 0 | 1 | 11/04/1925 | 86 | F | 313 | 203793 |
| M | 02/18/2012 | 02/19/2012 | 1 | 1 | 11/06/1975 | 36 | F | 885 | 203754 |
| M | 02/11/2012 | 02/19/2012 | 8 | 3 | 04/07/1926 | 86 | F | 179 | 203493 |
| M | 02/18/2012 | 02/19/2012 | 1 | 1 | 09/10/1937 | 74 | M | 244 | 203741 |
| M | 02/11/2012 | 02/19/2012 | 8 | 3 | 08/19/1918 | 94 | F | 945 | 203496 |
| M | 02/14/2012 | 02/19/2012 | 5 | 1 | 08/09/1944 | 68 | M | 189 | 203601 |
| M | 02/12/2012 | 02/19/2012 | 7 | 1 | 11/30/1924 | 87 | F | 242 | 203503 |
| M | 02/13/2012 | 02/19/2012 | 6 | 3 | 08/30/1918 | 94 | M | 280 | 203583 |
| M | 02/13/2012 | 02/19/2012 | 6 | 3 | 01/26/1942 | 70 | F | 640 | 203561 |
| M | 02/16/2012 | 02/19/2012 | 3 | 1 | 12/27/1924 | 87 | F | 379 | 203644 |
| M | 02/13/2012 | 02/19/2012 | 6 | 3 | 03/23/1936 | 76 | F | 871 | 203559 |
| M | 02/15/2012 | 02/19/2012 | 4 | 3 | 09/02/1921 | 91 | M | 872 | 203623 |
| M | 02/13/2012 | 02/19/2012 | 6 | 3 | 12/12/1925 | 86 | M | 872 | 203592 |
| M | 02/14/2012 | 02/19/2012 | 5 | 3 | 11/14/1929 | 82 | F | 256 | 203613 |
| S | 02/15/2012 | 02/19/2012 | 4 | 1 | 07/30/1981 | 31 | F | 766 | 203614 |
| S | 02/17/2012 | 02/19/2012 | 2 | 1 | 02/17/2012 | 0 | M | 794 | 203703 |

**SUMMARY BY FINANCIAL CLASS**

| | | # of Pts | LOS | ALOS |
|---|---|---|---|---|
| B | Blue Cross / Blue Shield | 6 | 20 | 3.33 |
| C | Medicaid | 4 | 18 | 4.50 |
| G | Managed Care | 1 | 2 | 2.00 |
| M | Medicare | 18 | 80 | 4.44 |
| S | Self-Pay | 2 | 6 | 3.00 |

C

**Figure 10-3, cont'd** C, List of patients by financial class.

**Diamonte Hospital**
**Discharge Detail by Age**
**Discharge Date** 02/19/2012

| Newborn | 0 - 30 days | Newborn |
| Pediatric | 31 - 364 days | Infant |
| | 1 year - 16 years | Pediatric |
| Adults | 17 - 30 | |
| | 31 - 45 | |
| | 46 - 60 | |
| | 61 - 75 | |
| | over 75 | |

page 1
printed 2/20/2012

| Attending Physician Last Name | Attending Physician First Name | Admission | Discharge | Age | Gender | MS-DRG | PDx | Dx2 | Dx3 | PPx | Px2 | Px3 | Account | Pt Last Name | Pt First Name |
|---|---|---|---|---|---|---|---|---|---|---|---|---|---|---|---|
| **Newborn** | | | | | | | | | | | | | | | |
| Nelson | Kathleen | 02/17/2012 | 02/19/2012 | 0 | M | 794 | Z3800 | P835 | Z23 | 3E0134Z | | | 203703 | Scott | Ethan |
| Carter | Brent | 02/15/2012 | 02/19/2012 | 0 | M | 795 | Z3801 | Z23 | | 0VTTXZZ | 3E0134Z | | 203630 | Allen | Jayden |
| **Summary Newborns** | **Number of Patients** 2 | **Total Days** 6 | **ALOS** 3.00 | | | | | | | | | | | | |
| | | | | | | | | | | | | | | | |
| **Adults 31 - 45** | | | | | | | | | | | | | | | |
| Beard | Kristy | 02/15/2012 | 02/19/2012 | 31 | F | 766 | 0654 | O334xx0 | Z370 | 10D00Z1 | | | 203614 | Allen | Jessica |
| Hernandez | Antonio | 02/18/2012 | 02/19/2012 | 36 | F | 885 | F329 | R4585 | J45909 | | | | 203754 | Robinson | Jennifer |
| Perez | Catherine | 02/18/2012 | 02/19/2012 | 37 | F | 770 | O034 | | | 10D17ZZ | 10A07ZX | | 203778 | Martinez | Luz |
| Marks | Stacey | 02/17/2012 | 02/19/2012 | 40 | F | 775 | O702 | Z370 | | 0DQP0ZZ | 1097ZC | | 203688 | Scott | Donna |
| Shah | Lori | 02/13/2012 | 02/19/2012 | 45 | F | 745 | N898 | D500 | | 0UDB7ZZ | 30233N1 | 05HY33Z | 203546 | Thompson | Karen |
| **Summary Adults 31 - 45** | **Number of Patients** 5 | **Total Days** 14 | **ALOS** 2.80 | | | | | | | | | | | | |
| | | | | | | | | | | | | | | | |
| **Adults 46 - 60** | | | | | | | | | | | | | | | |
| Robert | Craig | 02/17/2012 | 02/19/2012 | 49 | F | 743 | D259 | D279 | N736 | 05HY33Z | 0UT00ZZ | 0DNW0ZZ | 203698 | Martin | Linda |
| Edwards | Gabriel | 02/17/2012 | 02/19/2012 | 49 | M | 153 | J101 | Z21 | F17200 | | | | 203700 | Hernandez | John |
| Thomas | Wendy | 02/16/2012 | 02/19/2012 | 52 | F | 378 | K921 | N390 | K862 | 0DJ08ZZ | | | 203659 | Harris | Susan |
| Donozo | Luis | 02/16/2012 | 02/19/2012 | 58 | M | 379 | K264 | R42 | I498 | 0DB68ZX | | 30233N1 | 203677 | Lopez | William |
| Marks | Stacey | 02/13/2012 | 02/19/2012 | 59 | F | 330 | K5660 | N321 | J9571 | 0DTN0ZZ | 0DQB0ZZ | 0DNW0ZZ | 203505 | Jackson | Carol |
| **Summary Adults 46 - 60** | **Number of Patients** 5 | **Total Days** 16 | **ALOS** 3.20 | | | | | | | | | | | | |

Figure 10-3, cont'd **D**, List of patients by age.

**Diamonte Hospital**
**Discharge Detail by Age**
**Discharge Date** 02/19/2012

### Adults 61 - 75

| | | | | | | | | | | | | | |
|---|---|---|---|---|---|---|---|---|---|---|---|---|---|
| Morgan | Randy | 02/14/2012 | M | 68 | 189 | J960 | J441 | F10980 | HZ2ZZZZ | | 203601 | Wright | John |
| Li | Xiaobo | 02/16/2012 | F | 68 | 069 | G459 | I480 | I69998 | | | 203673 | Anderson | Judith |
| Li | Xiaobo | 02/11/2012 | M | 69 | 885 | F323 | G20 | I8390 | | | 203489 | King | Robert |
| Phillips | Todd | 02/13/2012 | F | 70 | 640 | E8352 | N179 | E232 | | | 203561 | Taylor | Patricia |
| Li | Xiaobo | 02/18/2012 | M | 74 | 244 | I441 | I452 | E119 | Q2H63JZ | 0JH606Z | 203741 | Hill | Paul |
| Campbell | Jeremiah | 02/18/2012 | F | 75 | 809 | D590 | I425 | E119 | 30233N1 | | 203787 | Moore | Barbara |

| Summary Adults 61 - 75 | Number of Patients 6 | | | | Total Days 24 | ALOS 4.00 |
|---|---|---|---|---|---|---|

### Adults over 75

| | | | | | | | | | | | | | |
|---|---|---|---|---|---|---|---|---|---|---|---|---|---|
| Stewart | Dennis | 02/13/2012 | F | 76 | 871 | H7290 | N179 | J441 | | | 203559 | Miller | Frances |
| Baker | Sandra | 02/15/2012 | M | 78 | 864 | R509 | D469 | M069 | 30233N1 | | 203621 | Young | Richard |
| Turner | Derrick | 02/14/2012 | F | 82 | 256 | E1159 | I96 | E1042 | 0Y6P0Z0 | | 203613 | Wilson | Virginia |
| Edwards | Gabriel | 02/16/2012 | M | 83 | 195 | J189 | J449 | E119 | | | 203684 | Clark | Thomas |
| Beard | Kristy | 02/13/2012 | M | 84 | 378 | K2901 | D62 | I425 | 0W3P8ZZ | 30233N1 | 203508 | Hall | Frank |
| Kabob | Elias | 02/11/2012 | F | 86 | 179 | B59 | I509 | I10 | | | 203493 | Brown | Mildred |
| Turner | Derrick | 02/13/2012 | M | 86 | 872 | H61009 | J90 | T8584xA | | | 203592 | Walker | Joseph |
| Gonzalez | Jacqueline | 02/19/2012 | F | 86 | 313 | R0789 | I10 | K219 | | | 203793 | Jones | Ruth |
| Rigger | Marcus | 02/16/2012 | F | 87 | 379 | K921 | I129 | E119 | 0DJD8ZZ | | 203644 | Williams | Margaret |
| Parker | Philip | 02/12/2012 | F | 87 | 242 | I495 | N179 | E871 | 0JH606Z | 02H63JZ | 203503 | Johnson | Dorothy |
| Stewart | Frank | 02/15/2012 | M | 91 | 872 | H902 | I481 | A419 | | | 203623 | Lee | James |
| Parker | Philip | 02/13/2012 | M | 94 | 280 | I214 | J189 | I959 | 30233N1 | 02HK3JZ | 203583 | Lewis | William |
| Mitchell | Frank | 02/11/2012 | F | 94 | 945 | Z5189 | B370 | I509 | F07G7ZZ | F0821ZZ | 203496 | Smith | Helen |

| Summary Adults over 75 | Number of Patients 13 | | | | Total Days 66 | ALOS 5.08 |
|---|---|---|---|---|---|---|

### Summary

| | | Number of Patients | Total Days | ALOS |
|---|---|---|---|---|
| Newborn | 0 - 30 days | 2 | 6 | 3.00 |
| Adults and Children | | | | |
| Pediatric | 31 - 364 days | | | |
| | 1 year - 16 years | | | |
| Adults | 17 - 30 | | | |
| | 31 - 45 | 5 | 14 | 2.80 |
| | 46 - 60 | 5 | 16 | 3.20 |
| | 61 - 75 | 6 | 24 | 4.00 |
| | over 75 | 13 | 66 | 5.08 |
| | Total | 29 | 120 | 4.14 |

Figure 10-3, cont'd

D

## Data Quality Check

For maintenance of a functional database, abstracted data must be audited for quality: validity, accuracy, completeness, and timeliness, for example. To do so, an HIM professional other than the initial clerk, usually a supervisor, routinely audits the abstracts by pulling the patient health record, retrieving the abstract from the database, and verifying the data elements. In general, only a sample of the abstracts is reviewed. However, the supervisor must be sure to choose a random sample of abstracts that includes all of the employees' work. Errors are corrected, documented, analyzed, and tracked to improve the quality of the database. The quality of the data is extremely important because of the high volume of information that the database provides for the health care facility.

> **data validity** The quality that data reflect the known or acceptable range of values for the specific data.
>
> **data accuracy** The quality that data are correct.
>
> **completeness** The data quality of existence. If a required data element is missing, the record is not complete.
>
> **timeliness** The quality of data's being obtained, recorded, or reported within a predetermined time frame.

### HIT-bit

#### DATA ABSTRACT VERSUS ABSTRACTING DATA

In Chapter 5, the HIM function of completing the patient abstract by verifying and entering certain data fields was described. This function, called *abstracting*, originally described the transcription of these data fields into paper-based indices. With the advent of computerization, the abstractor entered the data onto a data collection form that was later entered into a computer system. Often, the data were maintained offsite. Printouts of the abstracted data were returned to the facility for proofreading and corrections, which were then returned to the offsite location for amendment and final reporting. In an electronic environment, the abstracting process consists largely of entering missing data, such as the diagnosis and procedure codes, consulting physicians, newborn weight, and perhaps the discharge disposition. Thus, although the activity itself has changed in nature somewhat, the name of the function has not.

Similarly named, the activity of querying and reporting of data from a database is, in effect, the extraction of the relevant data elements in order to create an abstract or subset of the available data.

The quality of the database enables performance improvement activities and appropriate decisions about the facility or about individual patients. Remember that data quality audits must be recorded for future comparison. It is important to document compliance or noncompliance with a set standard of quality for data. Over time, this information provides support for improvement efforts, indicates a need for improvement, or demonstrates quality. Discussion of database quality in the context of an electronic health record is continued in Chapter 11.

> **Go To** Chapter 11 details performance improvement activities and the role health information plays in the process.
>
> **performance improvement (PI)** Also known as *quality improvement (QI)* or *continuous quality improvement (CQI)*. Refers to the process by which a facility reviews its services or products to ensure quality.

### EXERCISE 10-1

#### Organized Collection of Data

1. What are primary data? Give an example.
2. What are secondary data? Give an example.

## DATA RETRIEVAL

Once a database exists, the data can be used for analysis or comparison. When health information is needed for utilization review, quality assurance, performance improvement, routine compilation, or patient care, the HIM department is asked to retrieve relevant data. With the right instructions on the type of information needed and its intended use, HIM personnel can provide high-quality health information on both individual patients and groups of patients. Compilation of health data for groups of patients is called aggregate data.

> **utilization review (UR)** The process of evaluating medical interventions against established criteria, on the basis of the patient's known or tentative diagnosis. Evaluation may take place before, during, or after the episode of care for different purposes.

| | A | B | C | D | E | F |
|---|---|---|---|---|---|---|
| 1 | | | | | | |
| 2 | MS-DRG | 291 - 293 | | | | |
| 3 | Discharges 2/1/2012 - 2/29/2012 | | | | | |
| 4 | | | | | | |
| 5 | | | | | | |
| 6 | | | | | | |
| 7 | MR# | Patient | D/C Date | LOS | Physician | MS-DRG |
| 8 | | | | | | |
| 9 | 056023 | Austin, Dallas | 02/27/2012 | 5 | Angel, M. | 291 |
| 10 | 197808 | Bixby, Helena | 02/12/2012 | 3 | Kabob, L. | 292 |
| 11 | 945780 | China, Dollie | 02/14/2012 | 6 | Chow, A | 291 |
| 12 | 348477 | Combeaus, Plato | 02/02/2012 | 4 | Thomas, B. | 293 |
| 13 | 403385 | Dimaro, Cheri | 02/28/2012 | 5 | Angel, M. | 293 |
| 14 | 471416 | Dondi, Mac | 02/04/2012 | 3 | Thomas, B. | 293 |
| 15 | 362156 | Foster, Dan | 02/22/2012 | 4 | Chow, A. | 291 |
| 16 | 483443 | Lates, Ricky | 02/10/2012 | 6 | Kabob, L. | 292 |
| 17 | 483441 | Smeadow, Shane | 02/01/2012 | 5 | Thomas, B. | 292 |
| 18 | 201801 | Titan, Tami | 02/14/2012 | 4 | Thomas, B. | 293 |

**Figure 10-4** List of patients with congestive heart failure shows aggregate data retrieval.

## Retrieval of Aggregate Data

**aggregate data** A group of like data elements compiled to provide information about the group.

**LOS** length of stay

**audit trail** A review of individual user access codes to determine who had access to patient health information and to ensure the access was deemed necessary for patient care.

**accounting of disclosures** The listing of the identity of those to whom certain protected health information has been disclosed.

**Institutional Review Board (IRB)** A committee within a facility charged with ensuring that research conducted within conforms to all applicable rules and regulations.

**Aggregate data** are a group of like data elements compiled to provide information about a group. For example, a collection of the length of stay (LOS) for all patients with the diagnosis of congestive heart failure (CHF) would be aggregate data, as shown in the report in Figure 10-4. Further review of the report shows that the LOS data element for each patient has been retrieved. This report can be analyzed to determine the average LOS and the most common LOS. Sorting by any single data element for each of these patients produces a meaningful list of aggregate data.

Requests for data come into the HIM department frequently. Most of these requests are routine and can be satisfied quickly. Others are more complex and may require some analysis. In either case, the HIM professional needs to record the request in detail, partly to evaluate whether the request can be granted and partly to clarify the exact requirements of the requester. The following details are helpful: the name and contact phone number of the person making the request, the date of the request as well as the date parameters for the information requested, the specific information requested, and the reason for the request. This information helps the person querying the database ensure that the most appropriate information is retrieved from the database and provides an audit trail for accounting of disclosures. The facility should have an administrative policy regarding who may obtain data and for what purposes. For example, residents may need to collect data on their own patients for educational purposes; however, a study involving other patients would require either faculty or possibly **Institutional Review Board (IRB)** approval. Similarly, Dr. Braun may request data on her own patients, but not on the patients of Dr. Wong.

Data requests should be formatted in order to ensure clarity and reduce the potential for error. Figure 10-5 illustrates a sample data request form. Note that the parameters for the report include the time period, the specific data elements requested, and the desired format of the output. In many cases, output format is determined by the system when predesigned reports are used. If it is possible to remove unnecessary data elements prior to delivering the report to the requestor, such removal should be done. For example, if patient identity is not required, then patient name and account references should be removed from the report. Most systems provide for custom report design, which may or may not be the responsibility of the HIM department. The ability to identify and extract data from a database is a useful skill that renders the user a more valuable member of the organization. Combined with an HIM professional's knowledge of the underlying data, particularly code sets, this is a desirable skill in his or her practice.

**Hospital name** _____

**Request for data**   Date requested _____ Date needed _____

**Requestor**

      Name _____

      Title _____

      Department _____

This data will be used for: _____

**Data specifications**

      Time period _____

      Patient type (check box)

          ☐ Inpatient

          ☐ Outpatient

          ☐ Both

      Additional parameters (Check all that apply.  If ALL are required, state ALL.)

          ☐ MS-DRG (specify) _____

          ☐ Diagnosis (specify) _____

          ☐ Procedure

              ○ ICD (specify) _____

              ○ CPT (specify) _____

          ☐ Physician

              ○ Attending (specify) _____

              ○ Surgeon (specify) _____

              ○ Consulting (specify) _____

          ☐ Other (specify) _____

**Output**

      Data Fields (List all required fields on the report) _____

      _____

      _____

      Media

          ☐ Word

          ☐ Excel

          ☐ Paper

**Delivery (Specify email address or location)** _____

Figure 10-5  A data request form.

## HIT-bit

### INSTITUTIONAL REVIEW BOARD

The Institutional Review Board (IRB) is a committee that is charged with ensuring that research conducted within the facility or by its employees and associates conforms to all applicable rules and regulations. The IRB is chiefly concerned with ethical issues, such as confidentiality and protection of the research subjects. However, other factors like the qualifications of the researchers to conduct a proposed project are also considered.

## Retrieving Data

The first step to retrieving appropriate useful information is to identify the population of interest. In health care a **population** can be defined as a group of people identified by a

**population** An entire group.

**medical record number (MR#)** A unique number assigned to each patient in a health care system; this code will be used for the rest of the patient's encounters with that specific health system.

**patient account number** A numerical identifier assigned to a specific encounter or health care service received by a patient; a new number will be assigned to each encounter, but the patient will retain the same medical record number.

**utilization review (UR)** The process of evaluating medical interventions against established criteria, on the basis of the patient's known or tentative diagnosis. Evaluation may take place before, during, or after the episode of care for different purposes.

**sample** A small group within a population.

**data dictionary** A list of details that describe each field in a database.

**demographic data** Identification: those elements that distinguish one patient from another, such as name, address, and birth date.

**nursing assessment** The nurse's evaluation of the patient.

**abstract** A summary of the patient record.

**query** To question the database for specific elements, information, or a report.

**HIM** health information management

**admitting diagnosis** The reason given by the physician for initiating the order for the patient to be placed into care in a hospital.

**face sheet** The first page in a paper record. Usually contains at least the demographic data and contains space for the physician to record and authenticate the discharge diagnoses and procedures. In many facilities, the admission record is also used as the face sheet.

**history and physical (H&P)** Health record documentation comprising the patient's history and physical examination; a formal, dictated copy must be included in the patient's health care record within 24 hours of admission for inpatient facilities.

particular characteristic or group of characteristics, such as race, age, gender, diagnosis, procedure, service, or financial class. From hospital data, one can also identify patients by date of admission, date of discharge, charge code, payer, or virtually any data element that is resident in the database. The population, then, consists of all patients with the characteristic under consideration. For example: *all inpatients discharged between January 1, 2012, and June 30, 2012, with a discharge status of 20 (expired)*.

The next step is to narrow the data request, if desired. Although some users may want to review all of the patients in the population, rarely will the user need all of the available data. Therefore the output of the data retrieval must be specified. In many systems, there are preformatted (a.k.a. "canned") reports that contain standard output that users would typically need: diagnoses, procedures, admission and discharge dates, gender, age, financial class, medical record number, patient account number, and patient name. Customized reports may also be available. For a customized report, it is important to be very specific as to the output desired. The user will get only what the user has specified. Therefore, if the attending physician's name is required, the user must ask for the attending physician's name to be included in the report. A common reason to request data is for surgical case review or utilization review. For these studies, the population of patients may be based on a diagnosis or the operation that was performed and includes the period under study.

Sometimes, the population is too large to be analyzed. This is often the case with coding audits. It is usually too expensive for auditors to review a population of 100% of the charts in a month, for example. Therefore a sample is generally chosen from the population. A **sample** is a small representation of the entire population.

## Optimal Source of Data

The next matter to discuss with regard to data retrieval is how to ascertain the optimal source of the data. In a well-constructed database, with unique data dictionary definitions, the computer program will have stored the data in only one place. Therefore the data will always be recorded at the best time by the best person, as defined in the data dictionary. For instance, the data dictionary probably specifies that the data element for a patient's name—and most other demographic data—will be recorded by the patient registration department when the patient arrives at the facility. Once the patient's name is recorded at registration, it is available in the system to populate electronic forms for all users. The name is not entered again and again by each user. Similarly, a nurse enters nursing assessments and notes—they are not entered by HIM personnel. The final diagnosis and procedure codes are stored in the system upon abstraction, and not a second time. For retrieval of a population report of all of the patients with a principal diagnosis of pneumonia, there is only one database where the patient's diagnosis is recorded: in the abstract. Thus writing a query or searching the database requires the user to understand the location of the data.

However, in a paper record, understanding the optimal source of data becomes critical. In many paper environments, the same information is recorded multiple times. The patient's admitting diagnosis, for example, is recorded on the face sheet by the admitting clerk; it is recorded on the nursing assessment by the nurse; and it is recorded on the admitting notes by the physician. What is the optimal, most reliable place to determine the patient's admitting diagnosis? It depends on the reason for the review. If one wants to learn why the patient thought he or she was admitted, the face sheet is probably the most important place to look. However, if one wants to know the physician's clinical reason for admitting the patient, the admitting note or the history and physical are better places to look.

Another example of how important it is to identify the optimal source of data is during a survey by The Joint Commission (TJC). TJC surveyors may ask to review specific records (e.g., records of patients who were restrained). This information is not normally identified in the patient abstract. From the HIM perspective, several different data elements in the database can indicate that a patient may have been restrained. In an electronic system, a special data field can be added to indicate (Yes or No) whether a patient was restrained. If a special data field does not exist, other information in the abstract may help identify patients who were restrained. For example, a certain diagnosis indicates that a patient may have required restraints (e.g., organic brain syndrome or delirium). Optimally, there are appropriate and timely orders, nursing notes describing the application, duration, and monitoring of the restraints, and a restraints log maintained on the nursing unit; still, the surveyors may want to obtain corroborating evidence or to search for missing documentation.

Trying to find the optimal source of data requires knowing the database and knowing how to query it and relate the data elements, as well as a bit of detective work. Sometimes one has to begin with known data and work backwards. For instance, if the chief financial officer wants to know how many fertility treatments were performed in the facility, the user would have to know the procedure codes for fertility treatments in order to query the system for all of those procedures. The result should be a list of patients, their health record numbers, and the fertility procedures performed. Another requestor may want a list of cases for MS-DRG 312 (Syncope and Collapse) and the total charges for each case. The HIM professional might have two canned reports: one that contains the DRG, but not the total charges; and another that contains the total charges, but not the DRG. If the requestor wants both, the professional has to look for a common field—usually the patient account number—and combine the two reports to get what the requestor wants. One common task of this nature is the insertion of an MS-DRG description into a report that contains only the MS-DRG itself. Figure 10-6 illustrates the latter example in which the VLOOKUP function in Excel is used.

## Indices

An **index** is a list that identifies specific data items within a frame of reference. The abstracting process has enabled facilities to create indices for diagnoses, procedures, and physicians. For example, the attending physician is systematically identified on each patient record during the abstract process. A listing of patients by attending physician creates what is called the physician index. Additional indices can be created if the data are captured in the system. Referring physician, primary care physician, and consulting physician are typically captured, and each surgical procedure has a performing physician's name attached to it. Therefore reporting lists of visits by physician relationship is possible. The database can also provide information about any group of patients according to the instructions given by the person requesting the information to HIM personnel and further refined by HIM personnel queries to the database. As with any other data, the quality of the data capture dictates the completeness and accuracy of such reporting.

It should be noted that physician attribution (the assignment to a case of a physician and the physician's relationship to the case) is a matter of some importance to the physicians themselves. Increasingly, payers are reviewing facility and physician claims together and assessing whether the billing is consistent. As such, if a physician submits a claim as an attending physician, but the facility has a different physician listed as attending, then the payer may question either or both claims. Physician attribution is also an important issue for recredentialing. A physician may have a minimum volume requirement in order to maintain privileges at a particular facility.

**The Joint Commission (TJC)** An organization that accredits and sets standards for acute care facilities, ambulatory care networks, long-term care facilities, and rehabilitation facilities, as well as certain specialty facilities, such as hospice and home care. Facilities maintaining TJC accreditation receive *deemed status* from the CMS.

**DRG** diagnosis related group

**index** A collection of patient data (or a database) specific to a diagnosis, procedure, physician, or action such as admission or discharge.
**abstracting** The activity of identifying data for specific fields and entering them into a computer system.

**payer** The individual or organization that is primarily responsible for the reimbursement for a particular health care service. Usually refers to the insurance company or third party.
**billing** The process of submitting health insurance claims or rendering invoices.

---

### HIT-bit

#### INDEX CARDS

Historically, manual indices were maintained on index cards or ledger books. HIM personnel recorded the patient's information on index cards according to the diagnosis, procedure, and attending physician. For example, each diagnosis would have an index card, and the HIM employee would record each patient with that diagnosis on the card. Therefore, if a list of all patients with a particular diagnosis were needed, the HIM employee would pull the appropriate diagnosis card.

**Report #1**

| | A | B | C | D | E | F | G | H | I |
|---|---|---|---|---|---|---|---|---|---|
| 1 | | | | | | | | | |
| 2 | | FY 2012 | | | | | | | |
| 3 | | Final | | | | | | | |
| 4 | | Rule | FY 2012 | | | | | | |
| 5 | | Post- | Final Rule | | | | | | |
| 6 | | Acute | Special | | | | | Geometric | Arithmetic |
| 7 | MS-DRG | DRG | Pay DRG | MDC | TYPE | MS-DRG Title | Weights | mean LOS | mean LOS |
| 8 | 291 | Yes | No | 05 | MED | HEART FAILURE & SHOCK W MCC | 1.5010 | 4.7 | 6.1 |
| 9 | 292 | Yes | No | 05 | MED | HEART FAILURE & SHOCK W CC | 1.0214 | 3.9 | 4.7 |
| 10 | 293 | Yes | No | 05 | MED | HEART FAILURE & SHOCK W/O CC/MCC | 0.6756 | 2.7 | 3.2 |

**Report #2**

| | A | B | C | D | E | F | G | H |
|---|---|---|---|---|---|---|---|---|
| 11 | MS-DRG 291 - 293 | | | | | | | |
| 12 | Discharges 02/01/2012 - 02/29/2012 | | | | | | | |
| 13 | | | | | | | | |
| 14 | MR# | Patient | D/C Date | LOS | Physician | MS-DRG | MS-DRG Description | |
| 15 | | | | | | | | |
| 16 | 056023 | Austin, Dallas | 02/27/2012 | 5 | Angel, M. | 291 | HEART FAILURE AND SHOCK W MCC | =VLOOKUP(F16,$A$8:$F$10,6,FALSE) |
| 17 | 197808 | Bixby, Helena | 02/12/2012 | 3 | Kabob, L. | 292 | HEART FAILURE AND SHOCK W CC | |
| 18 | 945780 | China, Dollie | 02/14/2012 | 6 | Chow, A | 291 | HEART FAILURE AND SHOCK W MCC | |
| 19 | 348477 | Combeaus, Plato | 02/02/2012 | 4 | Thomas, B. | 293 | HEART FAILURE AND SHOCK W/O CC/MCC | |
| 20 | 403385 | Dimaro, Cheri | 02/28/2012 | 5 | Angel, M. | 293 | HEART FAILURE AND SHOCK W/O CC/MCC | |
| 21 | 471416 | Dondi, Mac | 02/04/2012 | 3 | Thomas, B. | 293 | HEART FAILURE AND SHOCK W/O CC/MCC | |
| 22 | 362156 | Foster, Dan | 02/22/2012 | 4 | Chow, A. | 291 | HEART FAILURE AND SHOCK W MCC | |
| 23 | 483443 | Lates, Ricky | 02/10/2012 | 6 | Kabob, L. | 292 | HEART FAILURE AND SHOCK W CC | |
| 24 | 483441 | Smeadow, Shane | 02/01/2012 | 5 | Thomas, B. | 292 | HEART FAILURE AND SHOCK W CC | |
| 25 | 201801 | Titan, Tami | 02/14/2012 | 4 | Thomas, B. | 293 | HEART FAILURE AND SHOCK W/O CC/MCC | |

**Figure 10-6** The combination of two reports using the VLOOKUP function in Microsoft Excel. This example assumes that the two "reports" are on the same worksheet.

06/16/2012

**Diagnosis Index Discharges: 01/01/12 – 01/31/12**

| *Diagnosis Code* | *Description* | *Medical Record #* | *Admit Date* | *D/C Date* | *LOS* | *Physician* |
|---|---|---|---|---|---|---|
| O80 | Encounter for full-term uncomplicated delivery | 010111 | 12/30/2011 | 01/01/2012 | 2 | Oscar, D. |
| | | 125544 | 12/31/2011 | 01/01/2012 | 1 | Jons, J. |
| | | 098805 | 01/02/2012 | 01/04/2012 | 2 | Vida, E. |
| | | 112096 | 01/05/2012 | 01/06/2012 | 1 | Oscar, D. |
| | | 113095 | 01/09/2012 | 01/12/2012 | 3 | Jons, J. |

**Figure 10-7** Diagnosis index shown in a computerized format.

Indices may also be generated on the basis of the principal diagnosis or the principal procedure. Although indices were a very important tool in the retrospective analysis of patient data before computerization, the automation of data collection and on-demand printing make the necessity for routinely maintaining physical copies obsolete. However, in the event of a system conversion (abandoning an old system for a new one), care should be taken to preserve the historical data. Hospitals may be required by state regulation to retain the master patient index permanently, and abstracted data may logically be attached during the conversion.

Figure 10-7 shows a diagnosis index of diagnosis code O80 for discharges in January 2012 in computerized format.

**principal diagnosis** According to the UHDDS, the condition that, after study, is determined to be chiefly responsible for occasioning the admission of the patient to the hospital for care.

**principal procedure** According to the UHDDS, the procedure that was performed for definitive treatment, rather than one performed for diagnostic or exploratory purposes or was necessary to take care of a complication. If two procedures appear to meet this definition, then the one most related to the principal diagnosis should be selected as the principal procedure.

**master patient index (MPI)** A system containing a list of patients that have received care at the health care facility and their encounter information, often used to correlate the patient to the file identification.

### EXERCISE 10-2

**Data Retrieval**

1. What are aggregate data?
2. What is an index? Give an example.
3. What type of information could be obtained from indices?
4. How does one determine the optimal source of data?
5. What is the optimal source for the following data in an inpatient record?
   a. Medications that the patient has already received
   b. Possible diagnosis after 2 days in the hospital
   c. Patient's temperature

## REPORTING OF DATA

### Reporting to Individual Departments

Health data are used by various departments in the health care facility. The performance improvement department uses the database to retrieve specific cases and review the documentation found in the health records to determine compliance with accreditation standards, perform performance improvement studies, or study patient care outcomes. The finance department may use charge data to verify or prepare financial reports and budgets.

**accreditation** Voluntary compliance with a set of standards developed by an independent agent, who periodically performs audits to ensure compliance.

**performance improvement** Also known as quality improvement (QI) or continuous quality improvement (CQI). Refers to the process by which a facility reviews its services or products to ensure quality.

**outcome** The result of a patient's treatment.

**case management** The coordination of the patient's care and services, including reimbursement considerations.

**retrospective review** Review occurring after the act or event (i.e., after the patient is discharged).

**admission denial** Occurs when the payer or its designee (such as utilization review staff) will not reimburse the facility for treatment of the patient because the admission was deemed unnecessary.

**morbidity** A disease or illness.
**mortality** The frequency of death.

**CDC** Centers for Disease Control and Prevention

Case management may perform retrospective reviews to investigate admission denials. Infection control needs to identify and analyze reportable infectious disease cases. The HIM department has many customers for data, both internal and external.

## Reporting to Outside Agencies

Various agencies associated with health care facilities routinely require information. Some states gather information from facilities to create a state health information network. The information in the database is shared (without patient identifiers) so that facilities can compare themselves with other facilities. Organ procurement agencies may request information on deaths for a certain period to assess the facility's compliance with state regulations for organ procurement.

Certain statistics must be reported to the CDC so that disease prevalence, incidence, morbidity (illness), and mortality (death) can be studied. *Prevalence* is the portion of the population that has a particular disease or condition. *Incidence* is how many new cases of a particular disease or condition have been identified in a particular period in comparison with the population as a whole.

Regardless of the user for whom the report is being run, HIM department professionals charged with preparing the reports need to ensure that the data are gathered from the appropriate source.

## EXERCISE 10-3

### Reporting of Data

1. List two departments that use health databases. Why do they need the data?

## STATISTICAL ANALYSIS OF PATIENT INFORMATION

**LOS** length of stay
**ALOS** average length of stay

**diagnosis related group (DRG)** A collection of health care descriptions organized into statistically similar categories.

Determining which report to run is sometimes only the first step in providing information to a user. Once a report has been run, further review of that report may be necessary to provide truly useful information for decision making or interpretation. For example, refer to Figure 10-4, which was used to illustrate patient LOS in the aggregate data explanation. That report could be useful in determining average LOS (ALOS). Facilities typically review the ALOS for specific patient diagnoses. The facility's average is then compared with a national, corporate, or local average. This further analysis can determine whether a facility is within the expected LOS for that MS-DRG. The utilization review department analyzes patient LOS for each DRG and diagnosis. For an HIM professional to provide this information, he or she must run a report and then format it in an appropriate list or graph to represent the information for presentation.

All of the examples given here involve simple arithmetic, but they help the user answer important questions about the data. You may find it helpful to use a calculator or spreadsheet program to follow along and reproduce the example figures.

### Analysis and Interpretation

Once patient data have been collected and stored in a database, reports can be run and the data can be analyzed, interpreted, or presented with various tools. *Interpretation* is an explanation of the data within the context from which it was extracted. The simplest methods for analyzing data involve the statistical evaluations of mean, median, and mode. Exercise 10-4 contains a set of practice data that can be used to practice with the calculations discussed later. Keep in mind that the purpose of the calculations is to derive meaning from the data—in other words, to answer a specific question. Therefore the appropriate calculation must be selected that will provide the desired answer.

| MR # | Patient | D/C Date | LOS | Physician | Age |
|------|---------|----------|-----|-----------|-----|
| \multicolumn{6}{c}{**Report of CABG Patients**} | | | | | |
| \multicolumn{6}{c}{02/01/2012 - 02/29/2012} | | | | | |
| 560230 | Bianco, Helena | 02/07/2012 | 7 | Angelo, R. | 50 |
| 978081 | Chowski, Shane | 02/10/2012 | 8 | Kobob, L. | 53 |
| 045780 | Gombeaux, Glenn | 02/04/2012 | 12 | Chi, A. | 53 |
| 748473 | Phoster, Dodi | 02/12/2012 | 14 | Houmas, C. | 56 |
| 005338 | Sondi, Mac | 02/08/2012 | 8 | Angelo, R. | 59 |
| 671414 | Stephens, Henri | 02/14/2012 | 9 | Houmas, C. | 61 |
| 062150 | White, Jean | 02/20/2012 | 8 | Chi, A. | 62 |

Figure 10-8 A list of patients who underwent a coronary artery bypass graft (CABG) procedure can provide data to find the mean age of this group: Add all the ages in column 6, and divide by 7; the result, the mean age of this group, is 56 years.

## Measures of Central Tendency

One of the most common analyses performed on numerical data is the average. The term *average* generally refers to the arithmetic mean. *Average* answers the question: what does the typical case look like? The requestor may ask:

- What are the average total charges for patients in this DRG?
- What was the average length of stay for inpatients last month?
- What is the most common length of stay for patients with this diagnosis?

### Mean

The arithmetic **mean** describes what is commonly called the average of a group of numbers. Add the sum of the group of numbers, and divide the sum by the number of items in the group. The mean is used to compute a wide variety of averages: LOS, cost per case, or patient age. The question may be: what is the average age of patients receiving a coronary artery bypass graft (CABG)? To answer the question, calculate the arithmetic mean. Add the sum of the ages of the group of patients and then divide by the total number of patients in the group. Figure 10-8 provides a list of seven patients who had a CABG. To find the average age, add all of the ages (50, 53, 53, 56, 59, 61, 62 = 394), then divide by 7 (394/7 = 56.29, which rounds to 56). The average, or arithmetic mean, age of patients in this group is 56 years. Calculate this easily in Excel using the AVERAGE formula: = AVERAGE(cell range). Figure 10-9 provides an illustration.

The arithmetic mean is a useful and widely understood measure. However, it is sensitive to **outliers**: values that are very different from most of the other values in the sample or population. Going back to the example in Figure 10-8, assume that the youngest patient undergoing a coronary artery bypass graft (CABG) procedure was 20 years of age (rather than 50 years of age, Figure 10-10). In this case, the average is 52 years of age. There are no patients younger than 53 years of age in the group, except for the patient who is 20 years of age. Therefore the average of 52 years of age gives an incorrect impression of the patients undergoing CABG procedures. One way to help the user of the information to understand the underlying data is to calculate the median and report it along with the mean.

### Median

The **median** describes the midpoint of the data. The median is often used to help describe groups of data that contain values that are significantly different from the rest of the group.

**mean** The measure of central tendency that represents the arithmetic average of the observations.

**outlier** A patient whose length of stay or cost is far lower or higher than the average expected by the prospective payment system, notably the DRG.

**CABG** coronary artery bypass graft

**median** The measure of central tendency that represents the observation that is exactly halfway between the highest and lowest observations.

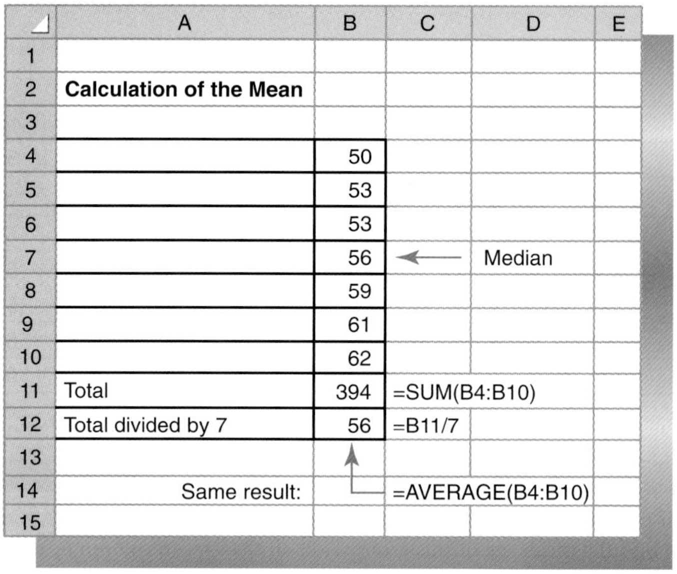

| ◢ | A | B | C | D | E |
|---|---|---|---|---|---|
| 1 | | | | | |
| 2 | **Calculation of the Mean** | | | | |
| 3 | | | | | |
| 4 | | 50 | | | |
| 5 | | 53 | | | |
| 6 | | 53 | | | |
| 7 | | 56 | ← | Median | |
| 8 | | 59 | | | |
| 9 | | 61 | | | |
| 10 | | 62 | | | |
| 11 | Total | 394 | =SUM(B4:B10) | | |
| 12 | Total divided by 7 | 56 | =B11/7 | | |
| 13 | | ↑ | | | |
| 14 | Same result: | | =AVERAGE(B4:B10) | | |
| 15 | | | | | |

**Figure 10-9** Using the AVERAGE function in Microsoft Excel.

## HIT-bit

### ROUNDING RULES

Calculations often result in more decimal places than is necessary or appropriate. For example, the average of 3, 5, 8, and 11 is 6.75: two decimal places more than the source numbers. Sometimes this many more decimal places is appropriate, such as in calculations of average length of stay. At other times, the additional decimal places reflect more detail than is needed.

To reduce the number of decimal places, one can truncate the number. To do so, just remove the unwanted digits. To truncate 6.75 to one decimal place leaves 6.7. However, truncating does not always result in appropriate accuracy. For statistical purposed, we round the numbers:

To round a number, identify the digit immediately to the right of the desired place. In this example, 5 is immediately to the right of 7. To round digits that are 5, 6, 7, 8, or 9, add 1 to the digit on the left. In our example, 6.75 rounds to 6.8. If we wanted only a whole number, 6.75 rounds to 7. This is called *rounding up* because the resulting rounded number is numerically higher than the original number.

To round digits that are 0, 1, 2, 3, or 4, merely truncate. The number 5.34 rounds to 5.3 or 5. This is called *rounding down,* because the resulting rounded number is numerically lower than the original number.

Unlike the mean, which is a formula calculation, the median describes the value in a particular location on a list.

To determine the median, arrange the data in numerical order from lowest to highest and then count toward the midpoint to obtain the median. Using the same group of data from Figure 10-8, first arrange the data in order: 50, 53, 53, 56, 59, 61, 62. Because there are seven numbers, it is easy to determine the midpoint. Which number is halfway between 1 and 7? The answer is 4. So beginning with the first patient's age (50), count to the fourth patient's age (56). The median age in this group of patients is 56 (the age of the patient in the middle of the list). In this group of patients, the mean and the median are the same. This means that the data are equally distributed on the two sides of the mean as well as the median: half of the observations are lower, and half of them are higher. If there is an

| ◢ | A | B | C | D | E | F |
|---|---|---|---|---|---|---|
| 1 | | | | | | |
| 2 | **Calculation of the Mean with Outlier** | | | | | |
| 3 | | | | | | |
| 4 | | 20 | | | | |
| 5 | | 53 | | | | |
| 6 | | 53 | | | | |
| 7 | | 56 | ← | Median | | |
| 8 | | 59 | | | | |
| 9 | | 61 | | | | |
| 10 | | 62 | | | | |
| 11 | Total | 364 | =SUM(B4:B10) | | | |
| 12 | Total divided by 7 | 52 | =B11/7 | | | |
| 13 | | | ↑ | | | |
| 14 | Same result: | | =AVERAGE(B4:B10) | | | |
| 15 | | | | | | |
| 16 | The outlier (20) drags the arithmetic mean to a value that does not represent the population. | | | | | |
| 17 | | | | | | |
| 18 | | | | | | |

**Figure 10-10** Calculation of the mean with outlier.

even number of observations, take the middle two and average them to determine the median. For example, the median of the series 50, 53, 56, and 58 is 54.5: $(53 + 56) \div 2$.

In the example in Figure 10-10, the mean is 52; however, the median is 56. Without looking at the data, you can tell that the data are unequally distributed around the mean because the middle observation is higher than the mean. In a small example such as this, these values hold no great significance. However, in a set of 300 observations, the data may be so unequally distributed that the mean must be adjusted to describe the data in a meaningful way.

### Adjusted Mean

One way to adjust the mean is to remove the highest and lowest observations. In a set of observations containing outliers (values that are very different from the rest of the observation values), this adjustment disregards the outliers and focuses on the observations that are most representative of the group under study. Try this with the Figure 10-10 example. Remove the observations 20 and 62. This results in a mean of 56 and a median of 56. When this group is being reported, the source of the calculations must be stated so that the user knows what was done with the data to make it meaningful. In a larger group of observations, removing the highest and lowest observations may have no impact if there are multiple outliers. In that case, remove a percentage of the highest and lowest observations. Up to 5% of the highest and 5% of the lowest is generally acceptable. In the absence of policies or conventions, it is up to the presenter (the analyzer of the data) to determine what percentage should be adjusted. However, a clear explanation of the adjustment must accompany the report. It may be useful to provide the report both with and without the adjustment so that the user can see exactly what impact the adjustment had on the reported data. Compare the two reports in Figure 10-11. Elimination of the three highest and lowest lengths of stay results in a mean and a distribution that are more accurately reflective of the most common observations.

### Geometric Mean

The problem with adjusting the mean is that valid cases are omitted from the report. This is problematic when all cases must be taken into consideration. The existence of outliers may be an important factor in the analysis, in which case they should not be ignored. If there are significant numbers of observations to be considered (usually more than 20), the

|  | A | B | C | D | E | F | G | H | I | J | K |
|---|---|---|---|---|---|---|---|---|---|---|---|
| 1 |  |  |  |  |  |  |  |  |  |  |  |
| 2 | REPORTING ADJUSTED MEANS |  |  |  |  |  |  |  |  |  |  |
| 3 |  |  |  |  |  |  |  |  |  |  |  |
| 4 | DATA: |  |  |  |  |  |  |  |  |  |  |
| 5 | Length of stay of 250 patients discharged in March 2012 |  |  |  |  |  |  |  |  |  |  |
| 6 |  |  |  |  |  |  |  |  |  |  |  |
| 7 | 1 | 2 | 3 | 3 | 3 | 4 | 4 | 5 | 5 | 6 |  |
| 8 | 1 | 2 | 3 | 3 | 3 | 4 | 4 | 5 | 5 | 6 |  |
| 9 | 1 | 2 | 3 | 3 | 4 | 4 | 4 | 5 | 5 | 6 |  |
| 10 | 1 | 2 | 3 | 3 | 4 | 4 | 4 | 5 | 5 | 6 |  |
| 11 | 1 | 2 | 3 | 3 | 4 | 4 | 4 | 5 | 5 | 6 |  |
| 12 | 1 | 2 | 3 | 3 | 4 | 4 | 4 | 5 | 5 | 6 |  |
| 13 | 1 | 2 | 3 | 3 | 4 | 4 | 4 | 5 | 5 | 6 |  |
| 14 | 1 | 2 | 3 | 3 | 4 | 4 | 4 | 5 | 5 | 6 |  |
| 15 | 1 | 2 | 3 | 3 | 4 | 4 | 4 | 5 | 5 | 6 |  |
| 16 | 1 | 2 | 3 | 3 | 4 | 4 | 4 | 5 | 5 | 7 |  |
| 17 | 1 | 2 | 3 | 3 | 4 | 4 | 4 | 5 | 5 | 7 |  |
| 18 | 1 | 2 | 3 | 3 | 4 | 4 | 4 | 5 | 5 | 7 |  |
| 19 | 1 | 2 | 3 | 3 | 4 | 4 | 4 | 5 | 5 | 7 |  |
| 20 | 1 | 2 | 3 | 3 | 4 | 4 | 4 | 5 | 5 | 7 |  |
| 21 | 1 | 2 | 3 | 3 | 4 | 4 | 4 | 5 | 5 | 7 |  |
| 22 | 1 | 2 | 3 | 3 | 4 | 4 | 4 | 5 | 5 | 7 |  |
| 23 | 1 | 2 | 3 | 3 | 4 | 4 | 4 | 5 | 5 | 7 |  |
| 24 | 1 | 2 | 3 | 3 | 4 | 4 | 5 | 5 | 5 | 7 |  |
| 25 | 1 | 2 | 3 | 3 | 4 | 4 | 5 | 5 | 5 | 7 |  |
| 26 | 1 | 2 | 3 | 3 | 4 | 4 | 5 | 5 | 6 | 8 |  |
| 27 | 1 | 3 | 3 | 3 | 4 | 4 | 5 | 5 | 6 | 8 |  |
| 28 | 1 | 3 | 3 | 3 | 4 | 4 | 5 | 5 | 6 | 8 |  |
| 29 | 1 | 3 | 3 | 3 | 4 | 4 | 5 | 5 | 6 | 10 |  |
| 30 | 1 | 3 | 3 | 3 | 4 | 4 | 5 | 5 | 6 | 125 |  |
| 31 | 1 | 3 | 3 | 3 | 4 | 4 | 5 | 5 | 6 | 250 |  |
| 32 |  |  |  |  |  |  |  |  |  |  |  |
| 33 | Mean = Total of all LOS / Number of patients |  |  |  |  |  |  |  |  |  |  |
| 34 | =SUM(A7:J31)/250 |  |  |  |  |  |  |  |  |  |  |
| 35 | OR |  |  |  |  |  |  |  |  |  |  |
| 36 | =AVERAGE(A7:J31) |  |  |  |  |  |  |  |  |  |  |
| 37 | Mean = 5.3 |  |  |  |  |  |  |  |  |  |  |
| 38 |  |  |  |  |  |  |  |  |  |  |  |
| 39 | Median = average of 125th and 126th value |  |  |  |  |  |  |  |  |  |  |
| 40 | =(E31+F7)/2 |  |  |  |  |  |  |  |  |  |  |
| 41 | OR |  |  |  |  |  |  |  |  |  |  |
| 42 | =MEDIAN(A7:J31) |  |  |  |  |  |  |  |  |  |  |
| 43 | Median = 4 |  |  |  |  |  |  |  |  |  |  |
| 44 |  |  |  |  |  |  |  |  |  |  |  |
| 45 |  |  |  |  |  |  |  |  |  |  |  |

To illustrate the calculation of the mean using a weighted frequency distribution, the FREQUENCY formula is used below. This is a three-step process.

1 List the categories in numerical order. In this case, all LOS values are listed.
2 Enter the frequency formula in the first Number of Patients cell (in this example, corresponding to the value 1).
3 Highlight the Number of Patients cells, including the one below the last LOS listed. Press F2, followed by Ctrl/Shift/Enter.

| FREQUENCY: | | | |
|---|---|---|---|
| LOS | Number of Patients | Total LOS | |
| 1 | 25 | 25 | |
| 2 | 20 | 40 | |
| 3 | 57 | 171 | |
| 4 | 65 | 260 | |
| 5 | 52 | 260 | |
| 6 | 15 | 90 | |
| 7 | 10 | 70 | |
| 8 | 3 | 24 | |
| 9 | 0 | 0 | |
| 10 | 1 | 10 | |
| 125 | 1 | 125 | |
| 250 | 1 | 250 | |
|  | 0 |  | |
|  | 250 | 1325 | 5.3 |

Mean = Total LOS / Total Number of Patients

Because there are 2 extreme outliers (1 patient with an LOS of 125 days and another with an LOS of 250 days), the mean can be adjusted to remove the top and bottom 1% - 2% of the cases. See how the mean approaches the median (4) below when the top and bottom 2 cases are removed.

| FREQUENCY: | | | |
|---|---|---|---|
| LOS | Number of Patients | Total LOS | |
| 1 | 23 | 23 | |
| 2 | 20 | 40 | |
| 3 | 57 | 171 | |
| 4 | 65 | 260 | |
| 5 | 52 | 260 | |
| 6 | 15 | 90 | |
| 7 | 10 | 70 | |
| 8 | 3 | 24 | |
| 9 | 0 | 0 | |
| 10 | 1 | 10 | |
| 125 | 0 | 0 | |
| 250 | 0 | 0 | |
|  | 0 |  | |
|  | 246 | 948 | 3.9 |

Mean = Total LOS / Total Number of Patients

While 5.3 is the actual mean, it is sometimes useful to calculate an adjusted mean and present BOTH means to illustrate the impact of extreme outliers on the group. One would not report ONLY the adjusted mean, because that would be misleading.

Figure 10-11 Reporting adjusted means data: length of stay of 253 patients discharged in March 2012.

| ⌐ | A | B | C |
|---|---|---|---|
| 1 | | | |
| 2 | **Calculation of the geometric mean** | | |
| 3 | | | |
| 4 | Discharges 2-9-2012 | | |
| 5 | Length of Stay | | |
| 6 | 25 | | |
| 7 | 64 | | |
| 8 | 5 | | |
| 9 | 5 | | |
| 10 | 4 | | |
| 11 | 5 | | |
| 12 | 8 | | |
| 13 | 6 | | |
| 14 | 4 | | |
| 15 | 5 | | |
| 16 | 2 | | |
| 17 | | | |
| 18 | 12.09 | =AVERAGE(A3:A13) | |
| 19 | 5 | =MEDIAN(A3:A13) | |
| 20 | 6.84 | =GEOMEAN(A3:A13) | |
| 21 | | | |

**Figure 10-12** Calculation of the geometric mean.

geometric mean may provide a more useful expression of the average than the arithmetic mean. CMS uses geometric mean length of stay (GMLOS or GLOS) to describe the ALOS of patients in individual MS-DRGs. The ALOS and GLOS are both listed, illustrating the impact of outliers in the population.

The geometric mean is calculated by multiplying the values times each other, then taking the nth root of the product. This calculation is best performed with more powerful statistical software than the Microsoft Excel program provides. However, Figure 10-12 gives a small example. Note that the arithmetic mean (12.09, which rounds to 12) in this example is not representative of the values in the group. The outliers 64 and 25 distort the arithmetic mean. The median is more representative of the group. The geometric mean (6.84, which rounds to 7) is more representative of the group than the arithmetic mean.

**CMS** Centers for Medicare and Medicaid Services

### Mode

**Mode** describes the number that occurs most often in a group of data. The mode is helpful in the study of the most common observation or observations. It answers questions such as, *What is the most common length of stay for normal newborns?* Unlike the mean and the median, which have a single value, there can be multiple modes in a group of data. In the list of CABG patients in Figure 10-8, the mode is 53. All of the other ages are observed only once. In a large group of observations, a mode with many observations may indicate a strong preference or tendency of the group. Because the mode is not a numerical calculation, it is possible that the group will have no mode. The lack of a mode is not inherently important.

**mode** The measure of central tendency that represents the most frequently occurring observation.

## Measures of Frequency

### Frequency Distribution

Another useful way to analyze data is to prepare a **frequency distribution**. It answers questions like: how many patients from each age category were admitted last month? A frequency distribution is a way of organizing data into mutually exclusive **class intervals** (groups, categories, or tiers that are meaningful to the user). In Figure 10-8, all of the patients are in their 50s and 60s: two class intervals that might be useful in identifying

**frequency distribution** The grouping of observations into a small number of categories.
**class intervals** Groups, categories, or tiers of the highest and lowest values that are meaningful to the user.

at-risk patients. Five patients are in their 50s; two are in their 60s. This gives us a frequency distribution as follows:

| Age | Number of Patients |
|---|---|
| 50 to 59 | 5 |
| 60 to 69 | 2 |

To construct a frequency distribution, organize the data into mutually exclusive equal groups or class intervals (so that no observation can belong in more than one group). All of the observations fit into one of the two groups. Notice that in this example, only two groups are necessary. The example data could also have been grouped as follows:

| Age | Number of Patients |
|---|---|
| 50 to 54 | 3 |
| 55 to 59 | 2 |
| 60 to 64 | 2 |
| 65 to 69 | 0 |

**Medicare** Federally funded health care insurance plan for older adults and for certain categories of chronically ill patients.

**third party payer** An entity that pays a provider for part or all of a patient's health care services; often the patient's insurance company.

This second grouping conveys the same data. The second grouping is more informative because it shows that the values are spread fairly evenly across the first three groups; however, there are no patients older than 65 years. Age is one of the criteria for Medicare eligibility. Therefore, if the potential third party payer is of interest in this set of patients, Medicare is less likely than other payers. Note that the groups have an equal number of possible values. Each group has five consecutive observation values. A frequency distribution should have the lowest number of groups or categories that can present the data informatively. When the number of groups or categories is too large, it is difficult for the user to digest the information.

## Percentages, Decimals, and Ratios

There are several common arithmetic ways to compare the relationship between two numerical values.

For this example, the question is: What is the relationship of male to female patients in the period?

Total patients in the period: 750, of which 500 are women and 250 are men.

*Ratios* show the two numbers as a fraction, typically reduced to its lowest common denominator. In this example, the ratio of women to men is 500/250, which can be expressed as 2/1 or 2:1. This gives the user a sense of the magnitude of the difference, but it is difficult to work with such a ratio or to compare it with another time period. For example, if the ratio in January is 500/250 and the ratio in February is 489:217, how do they compare?

To make the ratio easier to use, the ratio is converted to a decimal. 500 divided by 250 is 2.0; 489 divided by 217 is 2.25. So, the ratio of women to men increased from January to February by 0.25.

Often, the actual number of observations is confusing to the user. In that case, it is useful to also provide the **percentage** of observations. Presentation of the percentage standardizes the data so that unlike groups can be compared. To calculate a percentage, divide the number of observations in the category by the total number of observations, and multiply by 100. So in the previous example, the ratio in January was 2.0; the ratio in February was 2.25. The number of women in this case is 200% of the number of men in January, and 225% in February. Perhaps a more useful way to look at it is to express the numbers of women and men as percentages of the total number of patients and observe the changes in both figures (Table 10-1).

**percentage** Standardization of data so that unlike groups can be compared. Can be calculated by dividing the observations in the category by the total observations and multiplying by 100.

**TABLE 10-1**

**THE PERCENTAGES OF MEN AND WOMEN IN A FACILITY AND THE PERCENT CHANGE BETWEEN JANUARY AND FEBRUARY**

|  | JANUARY | | FEBRUARY | | |
|---|---|---|---|---|---|
|  | **NUMBER** | **PERCENT** | **NUMBER** | **PERCENT** | **CHANGE IN PERCENT** |
| Women | 500 | 66.7 | 489 | 69.3 | 2.6 |
| Men | 250 | 33.3 | 217 | 30.7 | −2.6 |
| *Total* | 750 |  | 706 |  |  |

**TABLE 10-2**

**COMPARING PAYER MIX**

|  | NUMBER OF DISCHARGES | |
|---|---|---|
| **PAYER** | **HOSPITAL A** | **HOSPITAL B** |
| Medicare | 5000 | 13229 |
| Medicaid | 2300 | 6032 |
| Blue Cross/Blue Shield | 1500 | 3975 |
| Commercial carriers | 950 | 2453 |
| Charity care | 500 | 1423 |
| Self-pay | 125 | 367 |
| Other payers | 90 | 325 |
| *Total discharges* | 10465 | 27804 |

|  | PERCENTAGE OF DISCHARGES | |
|---|---|---|
| **PAYER** | **HOSPITAL A** | **HOSPITAL B** |
| Medicare | 47.8% | 47.6% |
| Medicaid | 22% | 21.7% |
| Blue Cross/Blue Shield | 14.3% | 14.3% |
| Commercial carriers | 9.1% | 8.8% |
| Charity care | 4.8% | 5.1% |
| Self-pay | 1.2% | 1.3% |
| Other payers | 0.9% | 1.2% |
| *Total discharges* | 100% | 100% |

In the Figure 10-8 example, the percentages in each group are as follows:

| Age | Number of Patients | Calculation | Percentage |
|---|---|---|---|
| 50 to 54 | 3 | $\frac{3}{7} \times 100 =$ | 42.86 |
| 55 to 59 | 2 | $\frac{2}{7} \times 100 =$ | 28.57 |
| 60 to 64 | 2 | $\frac{2}{7} \times 100 =$ | 28.57 |
| 65 to 69 | 0 | $\frac{0}{7} \times 100 =$ | 0.00 |
| *Total* | 7 | — | 100.00 |

Percentages help the user compare observations in different time periods and when the group under study varies in size from the group to which it is being compared. For example, Table 10-2 compares the number of Medicare patients in Hospital A with the number in Hospital B. The actual numbers of patients are not comparable; however, the percentages show that the hospitals are very similar in the mix of payers.

## Measures of Variance

The difference between a benchmark or goal and the actual result or observation is a *variance*. If a facility expected 1000 admissions in May and there were 1200, then there is a variance of 200 admissions. The variance could be expressed as the number (200)

## TABLE 10-3

### COMMON SAMPLING METHODS

| | |
|---|---|
| Random | Selection is based on a list of random numbers. Items are sorted and numbered. The sample selection is made by matching the random number to the item number. If the items are unique, such as physician ID numbers, the random numbers can be matched to the items themselves. Selection can also be done with the use of computer software. |
| Systematic | Selection is made by choosing every nth item. Items are sorted in some logical order (by account number or discharge date, for example). If there are 100 items and 20 need to be reviewed, then select every 5th item, beginning with one of the first 5 on the list. The first item might be selected randomly by choosing the number out of a hat or asking someone to pick a number between 1 and 5. |
| Stratified | Before sample selection, the items are divided into segments to make sure that the segments are included in the analysis. For example, one might stratify cases by coder for a coding audit, by medical specialty for a documentation quality audit, or by month of discharge for ongoing record review. Once segmented, the individual items may be selected either randomly or systematically. |

or as a percentage (20%). Managers review and analyze these arithmetic variances in order to monitor results and take corrective action when results do not meet expectations. One routine review and analysis is financial: how much did the department spend on supplies compared with the amount that was budgeted (predicted and authorized in advance)?

Comparing one value against another is a simple arithmetic calculation; however, it is limited in application. Certainly, one could list all the variances noted in a given year and look at the **trend** (how the variances behave over time). Greater insight into the behavior of the observed values can be obtained by looking at the distribution of the values and their relationship to the arithmetic mean.

### Sampling a Population

Sometimes analysts are not able to analyze all of the values in a group. This might happen if the group is too large, such as all of the residents of Wyoming, or if the analysis is too time consuming, such as reviewing the coding of all inpatient records in a year. The entire group is called the population. If the population is too large to review completely, then the analyst will take a sample (subset) of the population. So if there are 1000 discharges in a month, the analyst may review 50 of the records.

In order for the analyst to make assumptions about the population using only a sample, the analyst must use a *random selection* of cases. In **random selection,** all cases have an equal chance of being selected and the cases are selected in no particular order or pattern. To select a random sample of 50 of the 1000 discharges, the analyst lists the discharges and numbers them (1 to 1000). A list of random numbers is selected, and each discharge that corresponds to a random number is selected for the sample. Other methods of sample selection may be used, depending on the needs of the analyst. The most common methods are described in Table 10-3.

### Normal Curve

The distribution of values in multiple samples may be very different from one group of observations to the next. So the observations of patient ages during one week may be very different from the observations of patient ages during another week. Neither group of observations may be truly representative of the distribution of ages in the entire patient population. However, if one takes the arithmetic mean of each of those groups and displays the frequency distribution of those means, that frequency distribution approaches symmetry. A picture of such a distribution is called the **normal curve.** In a normal curve, the observations are distributed evenly about the mean. The mean, median, and mode are equal. Note that the organization of the data is a frequency distribution of the values. This assumption of symmetry in the distribution of the means is called the **central limit theorem.** A set of observations that approaches a normal curve are illustrated in Figure 10-13.

**trend** The way in which a variance of values behaves over time.

**population** An entire group.
**sample** A small group within a population.
**random selection** In sampling of a population, a method that ensures that all cases have an equal chance of being selected and that the cases are selected in no particular order or pattern.

**frequency distribution** The grouping of observations into a small number of categories.
**normal curve** The symmetrical distribution of observations around a mean; usually in the shape of a bell.
**mean** The measure of central tendency that represents the arithmetic average of the observations.
**median** The measure of central tendency that represents the observation that is exactly halfway between the highest and lowest observations.
**mode** The measure of central tendency that represents the most frequently occurring observation.
**central limit theorem** The tendency of a large number of means to distribute symmetrically, approaching a normal distribution.

| | A | B | C | D | E | F | G | H | I | J | K |
|---|---|---|---|---|---|---|---|---|---|---|---|
| 1 | | | | | | | | | | | |
| 2 | | | | | | | | | | | |
| 3 | | | | | | | | | | | |
| 4 | **DATA:** | | | | | | | | | | |
| 5 | **Length of stay of 250 patients discharged in April 2012** | | | | | | | | | | |
| 6 | | | | | | | | | | | |
| 7 | 1 | 2 | 3 | 3 | 3 | 4 | 4 | 5 | 5 | 6 | |
| 8 | 1 | 2 | 3 | 3 | 3 | 4 | 4 | 5 | 5 | 6 | |
| 9 | 1 | 2 | 3 | 3 | 4 | 4 | 4 | 5 | 5 | 6 | |
| 10 | 1 | 2 | 3 | 3 | 4 | 4 | 4 | 5 | 5 | 6 | |
| 11 | 1 | 3 | 3 | 3 | 4 | 4 | 4 | 5 | 5 | 6 | |
| 12 | 1 | 3 | 3 | 3 | 4 | 4 | 4 | 5 | 5 | 6 | |
| 13 | 1 | 3 | 3 | 4 | 4 | 4 | 4 | 5 | 5 | 6 | |
| 14 | 1 | 3 | 3 | 4 | 4 | 4 | 4 | 5 | 5 | 6 | |
| 15 | 1 | 3 | 3 | 4 | 4 | 4 | 4 | 5 | 5 | 6 | |
| 16 | 2 | 3 | 3 | 4 | 4 | 4 | 4 | 5 | 5 | 6 | |
| 17 | 2 | 3 | 3 | 4 | 4 | 4 | 5 | 5 | 5 | 6 | |
| 18 | 2 | 3 | 3 | 4 | 4 | 4 | 5 | 5 | 5 | 6 | |
| 19 | 2 | 3 | 3 | 4 | 4 | 4 | 5 | 5 | 5 | 7 | |
| 20 | 2 | 3 | 3 | 4 | 4 | 4 | 5 | 5 | 5 | 7 | |
| 21 | 2 | 3 | 3 | 4 | 4 | 4 | 5 | 5 | 5 | 7 | |
| 22 | 2 | 3 | 3 | 4 | 4 | 4 | 5 | 5 | 5 | 7 | |
| 23 | 2 | 3 | 3 | 4 | 4 | 4 | 5 | 5 | 6 | 7 | |
| 24 | 2 | 3 | 3 | 4 | 4 | 4 | 5 | 5 | 6 | 7 | |
| 25 | 2 | 3 | 3 | 4 | 4 | 4 | 5 | 5 | 6 | 8 | |
| 26 | 2 | 3 | 3 | 4 | 4 | 4 | 5 | 5 | 6 | 8 | |
| 27 | 2 | 3 | 3 | 4 | 4 | 4 | 5 | 5 | 6 | 8 | |
| 28 | 2 | 3 | 3 | 4 | 4 | 4 | 5 | 5 | 6 | 8 | |
| 29 | 2 | 3 | 3 | 4 | 4 | 4 | 5 | 5 | 6 | 10 | |
| 30 | 2 | 3 | 3 | 4 | 4 | 4 | 5 | 5 | 6 | 12 | |
| 31 | 2 | 3 | 3 | 4 | 4 | 4 | 5 | 5 | 6 | 15 | |
| 32 | | | | | | | | | | | |
| 33 | Mean = Total of all LOS / Number of patients | | | | | | | | | | |
| 34 | =SUM(A7:J31)/250 | | | | | | | | | | |
| 35 | OR | | | | | | | | | | |
| 36 | =AVERAGE(A7:J31) | | | | | | | | | | |
| 37 | Mean = 4.144 | | | | | | | | | | |
| 38 | | | | | | | | | | | |
| 39 | | | | | | | | | | | |
| 40 | =STDEVP(A7:J31) | | | | | | | | | | |
| 41 | Standard Deviation = 1.66 | | | | | | | | | | |
| 42 | | | | | | | | | | | |
| 43 | | | | | | | | | | | |
| 44 | | | | | | | | | | | |
| 45 | | | | | | | | | | | |

| LOS | Frequency | % of Total Patients |
|---|---|---|
| 1 | 9 | 3.6% |
| 2 | 20 | 8.0% |
| 3 | 54 | 21.6% |
| 4 | 77 | 30.8% |
| 5 | 56 | 22.4% |
| 6 | 21 | 8.4% |
| 7 | 6 | 2.4% |
| 8 | 4 | 1.6% |
| 9 | 0 | 0.0% |
| 10 | 1 | 0.4% |
| 12 | 1 | 0.4% |
| 15 | 1 | 0.4% |
| | 0 | |
| TOTAL Patients | 250 | |

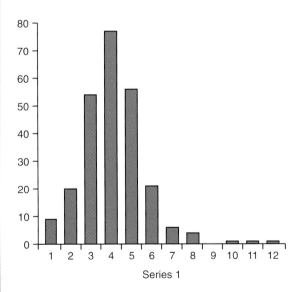

**Figure 10-13** The frequency distributions of these observations approaches a Normal Curve.

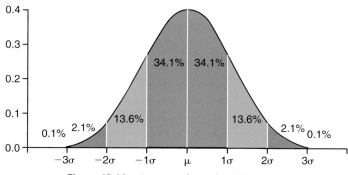

**Figure 10-14** Diagram of standard deviation.

**skewed** Frequency distributions that are not symmetrical, sometimes because of a small sample.

**coding** The assignment of alphanumerical values to a word, phrase, or other nonnumerical expression. In health care, coding is the assignment of numerical values to diagnosis and procedure descriptions.

**standard deviation** A measure of the average distance of observations from a mean.

**ALOS** average length of stay

### Skewedness

Frequency distributions that are not symmetrical are **skewed**. This skewedness might occur when a very small sample is taken and the observations do not truly reflect the population as a whole. For example, a review of coding using a sample of 5 cases out of 1000 may not yield results that are typical of the population. Nevertheless, a skewed distribution may truly represent the population. One would expect the ages of Medicare patients to be skewed, for example.

### Standard Deviation

Another commonly used measure of variance is the *standard deviation*. The **standard deviation** describes how closely the observations are distributed around the mean. The higher the standard deviation, the more loosely the observations are distributed. Figure 10-14 illustrates that 68.2% of observations falls within one standard deviation of the mean; an additional 27.2% (total 95.4%) falls within two standard deviations of the mean; and an additional 4.2% (total 99.6%) falls within three standard deviations of the mean. Note in Figure 10-14 that standard deviation is represented by the symbol $\sigma$ (lower case Greek sigma).

The standard deviation can be used to illustrate the extent to which an observation is different from the mean. This is useful for analyzing both clinical and financial data. For example, the ALOS of patients of a particular physician is 7 days, compared with the mean of 4 days for similar patients, varying greatly from the mean. It is not enough to say that the physician's patients on average stay 3 days longer than other patients, because there may be many physicians whose patients also stay 7 days. However, if the standard deviation of ALOS for these patients is 0.5, then an ALOS of 7 days is more than 3 standard deviations from the mean of 4 ($4 + 0.5\,\sigma + 0.5\,\sigma + 0.5\,\sigma = 5.5$): higher than 99.6% of all of the other physicians. The ALOS for these patients is tightly grouped from 2.5 to 5.5 days. In another example, if the total charges for a patient in MS-DRG 292 (Heart Failure and Shock with CC) are $65,000 and the mean for all patients in MS-DRG 292 is $50,000 with a standard deviation of $10,000, then the charges of $65,000 are only 1.5 $\sigma$ from the mean. In this case, 99.6% of the cases had total charges ranging from $20,000 to $80,000, a very loose distribution around the mean.

To calculate the standard deviation of a set of values, it is easiest to use a spreadsheet program. In Excel, for example, the formula for a sample standard deviation is: =stdev([range of values]), as illustrated in Figure 10-13.

## PRESENTATION

After analysis and interpretation, the data can be presented as information. To present data in a meaningful yet simple manner, the analyst uses tools to illustrate the information. Although there are many tools, the most common are bar graph, pie chart, and line graph. Table 10-4 explains how these presentation tools are used.

## TABLE 10-4

### PRESENTATION TOOLS AND THEIR USES

| PRESENTATION TOOL | CONSTRUCTION | PURPOSE |
| --- | --- | --- |
| Table | Column and rows. Construction depends on the items being compared. | Used to compare characteristics of items. Notice in this table that the items are listed in the first column and the two characteristics (construction and purpose) head the comparison columns. |
| Bar graph | Bars are drawn to represent the frequency of items in the specified categories of a variable. One axis represents the category. The other axis represents the frequency. | Used to compare categories with each other, the same category in different time periods, or both. |
| Line graph | The horizontal (x) axis represents the observation. The vertical (y) axis represents the value of the observation. A point is made that corresponds to each observation, and a line is drawn to connect the points. | Used to represent data over a period of time; information is plotted along the x and y axes. |
| Pie chart | In a circle, the percentage of each category is represented by a wedge of the circle that corresponds to the percentage of the circle. | Used to compare categories with one another in relation to the whole group. |
| Histogram | Like a bar graph, but the sides of the bars are touching. Horizontally, each bar represents a class interval. Vertically, the height of the bar represents the frequency of the class interval. | Used to illustrate a frequency distribution. |

## Line Graph

A **line graph** is best used to present observations over time. The vertical axis represents the value or number of observations. The horizontal axis in a line graph represents the time periods. Figure 10-15 provides an example of line graph construction. Note that the line graph is constructed by connecting the individual points that represent the observations.

Line graphs are also easy to read and interpret. Color presentation facilitates interpretation when multiple periods are superimposed on one another. For example, 3 years of data could be drawn on the same graph with each year represented by a different color. In black-and-white presentation, the line for each year could be drawn with different patterns; however, that is not as clear as using color.

Line graphs are also used to compare two variables. Figure 10-16 shows a line graph that compares LOS with age. Each patient is represented on the horizontal axis. The patients are presented in order of age. In this example, there is no relationship between two variables.

**line graph** A chart that represents observations over time or between variables by locating the intersection of the horizontal and vertical values and connecting the dots signifying the intersections.

**LOS** length of stay

## Bar Graph

A **bar graph** is used to present the frequencies of observations within specific categories. Each bar can represent the number of observations in a particular category. Bar graphs are also used to represent frequencies or values attached to specific events or causes. Bar graphs can be drawn either vertically or horizontally. In a vertical graph, the horizontal axis represents the categories, events, or causes. The vertical axis represents the value or number of observations, with the lowest value (often zero) at the bottom. Figure 10-17 provides an example of bar graph construction using the data from Table 10-2. Note that the bars for each category are separate from one another but the bars for subcategories can be adjacent. The values on the vertical axis are expressed in equal increments. Note that Excel uses the term *column* for a vertical graph and *bar* for the horizontal graph.

Bar graphs are easy to read and interpret. Color presentation also helps the user, particularly when there are subcategories. Bar graphs can also be used to present a portion of the data to highlight a specific point, such as top ten DRGs. Bar graphs are not particularly helpful when the data have a very wide range of values. For example, if one category has two occurrences and another has 30,000, the vertical axis might be difficult to draw in a meaningful way. Also, when there are many categories, including all of the appropriate descriptions can be difficult.

**bar graph** A chart that uses bars to represent the frequencies of items in the specified categories of a variable.

**diagnosis related groups (DRGs)** A collection of health care descriptions organized into statistically similar categories.

| | Number of discharges | |
|---|---|---|
| | Hospital A | Hospital B |
| 2008 | 7,846 | 32,451 |
| 2009 | 7,998 | 30,675 |
| 2010 | 8,432 | 31,246 |
| 2011 | 9,054 | 29,945 |
| 2012 | 9,578 | 28,435 |
| 2013 | 10,465 | 27,804 |

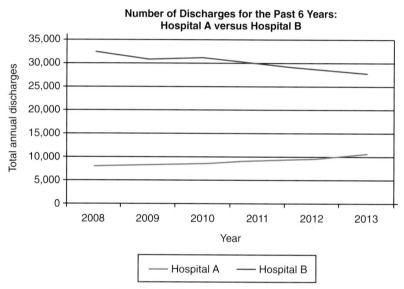

**Figure 10-15** Line graph construction.

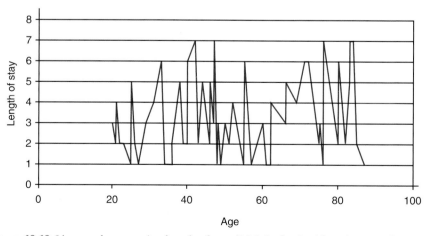

**Figure 10-16** Line graph comparing length of stay (LOS, in days) with patient age (in years).

Comparison of Hospital A and Hospital B by Payer

|  | Number of Discharges | |
| --- | --- | --- |
|  | Hospital A | Hospital B |
| Medicare | 5,000 | 13,229 |
| Medicaid | 2,300 | 6,032 |
| Blue Cross/Blue Shield | 1,500 | 3,975 |
| Commercial carriers | 950 | 2,453 |
| Charity care | 500 | 1,423 |
| Self-pay | 125 | 367 |
| Other payers | 90 | 325 |
| Total discharges | 10,465 | 27,804 |

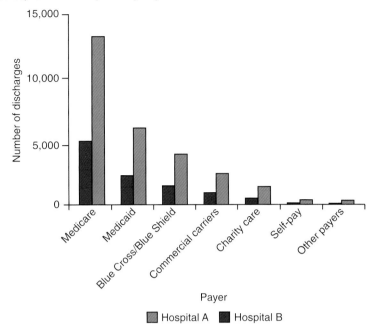

Comparison of Hospital A and Hospital B by Payer

|  | Percentage of Discharges | |
| --- | --- | --- |
| Payer | Hospital A | Hospital B |
| Medicare | 48% | 48% |
| Medicaid | 22% | 22% |
| Blue Cross/Blue Shield | 14% | 14% |
| Commercial carriers | 9% | 9% |
| Charity care | 5% | 5% |
| Self-pay | 1% | 1% |
| Other payers | 1% | 1% |
| Total | 100% | 100% |

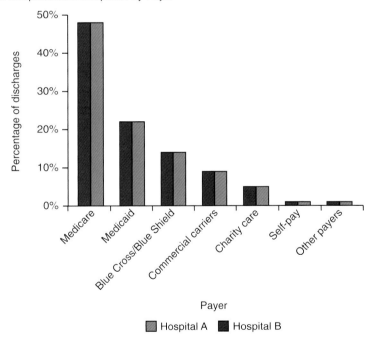

Figure 10-17  Bar graph construction using data from Table 10-2 to compare Hospital A and Hospital B by payer.

## Histogram

A **histogram** is a combination of a vertical bar graph whose sides are touching. Horizontally, each bar represents a class interval. Vertically, the height of the bar represents the frequency of the class interval. A line graph may be drawn to connect the midpoints of each class interval. Histograms are used only to draw frequency distributions of continuous data. Note that the bars are adjacent and a line approximates the curve created by the data (Figure 10-18).

**histogram** A modified bar graph representing continuous data. Each bar represents a class interval; the height of the bar represents the frequency of observations.

**class intervals** Groups, categories, or tiers of the highest and lowest values that are meaningful to the user.

**frequency distribution** The grouping of observations into a small number of categories.

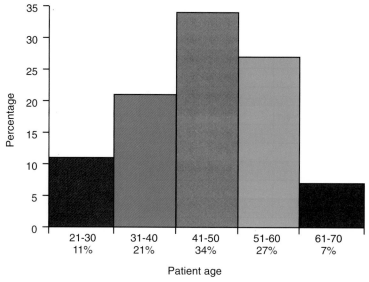

Figure 10-18 Histogram.

## Pie Chart

A **pie chart** is used to express the percentage of observations in each category of a variable. To use a pie chart, the analyst must convert the number of observations to a percentage. All of the observations (100%) must be included in the chart. Pie charts are drawn in a circle. Each "slice" of the circle or "pie" represents a category. The size of the slice corresponds to the percentage of observations. A complete circle is 360 degrees in circumference. To create an accurate drawing, multiply the percentages of observations by 360 to determine the number of degrees for the angle of the slice. To estimate the size of the slice, remember that a right angle is 90 degrees. Four 90-degree angles make a circle: 360 degrees. Therefore 25% of a circle is a quarter of the pie.

Pie charts have limited application and can be difficult to read if there are many categories. Because a pie chart represents 100% of the observations, all of the categories must be shown as a slice of the pie. If there are many small categories, it is sometimes useful to combine them in a meaningful way. However, pie charts can make a dramatic and easily understood statement. They are particularly useful when illustrating a variable with one or two dramatically large numbers of observations. Figure 10-19 shows the percentage of discharges, by payer, for Hospital C. Note that numerous payers who do not appear in the government and Blue Cross categories are combined together as "other payers."

Using a spreadsheet program, such as Microsoft Excel, to create graphs allows the user to experiment efficiently with the graph-making process and is best for professional-looking results.

**pie chart** A circular chart in which the frequency of observations is represented as a wedge of the circle.

**percentage** Standardization of data so that unlike groups can be compared. Can be calculated by dividing the observations in the category by the total observations and multiplying by 100.

## ▪ EXERCISE 10-4

### Statistical Analysis of Patient Information

*Use the table below showing the relationship between patient age (in years) and length of stay (LOS) to answer the following questions.*

| AGE | LOS | AGE | LOS | AGE | LOS | AGE | LOS |
|-----|-----|-----|-----|-----|-----|-----|-----|
| 20 | 3 | 34 | 1 | 49 | 1 | 71 | 6 |
| 21 | 2 | 36 | 1 | 50 | 3 | 72 | 6 |
| 21 | 4 | 36 | 2 | 51 | 2 | 73 | 5 |
| 22 | 2 | 38 | 5 | 52 | 4 | 75 | 2 |
| 22 | 2 | 39 | 2 | 55 | 1 | 75 | 3 |
| 23 | 2 | 40 | 2 | 55 | 6 | 76 | 1 |
| 25 | 1 | 40 | 6 | 57 | 1 | 76 | 7 |

|  | Hospital C | |
|---|---|---|
| Payer | Discharges | % of Total |
| Medicare | 4,500 | 43% |
| Medicaid | 2,250 | 21% |
| Blue Cross/Blue Shield | 1,625 | 15% |
| Commercial Carriers | 1,100 | 10% |
| Uncompensated Care | 650 | 6% |
| Self-Pay | 250 | 2% |
| Other Payers | 180 | 2% |
| Total | 10,555 | 100% |

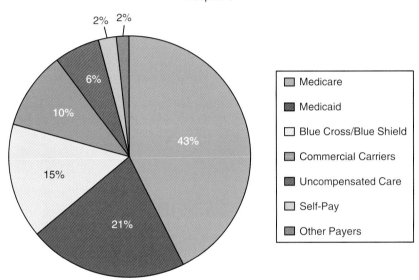

Figure 10-19  Pie chart construction using payer mix data.

## EXERCISE 10-4

### Statistical Analysis of Patient Information—cont'd

| AGE | LOS | AGE | LOS | AGE | LOS | AGE | LOS |
|---|---|---|---|---|---|---|---|
| 25 | 3 | 42 | 11 | 60 | 3 | 80 | 2 |
| 25 | 4 | 43 | 2 | 61 | 1 | 80 | 5 |
| 25 | 8 | 44 | 5 | 62 | 1 | 80 | 11 |
| 26 | 2 | 46 | 2 | 62 | 2 | 82 | 2 |
| 27 | 1 | 46 | 5 | 62 | 4 | 83 | 5 |
| 28 | 2 | 47 | 7 | 66 | 3 | 83 | 7 |
| 29 | 3 | 47 | 3 | 66 | 4 | 84 | 14 |
| 33 | 4 | 48 | 3 | 66 | 5 | 85 | 2 |
| 33 | 11 | 48 | 1 | 69 | 4 | 87 | 1 |

1. Calculate:
   a. mean age.
   b. mean length of stay.
   c. median age.
   d. mode of the length of stay.
2. Prepare a frequency distribution of the patients, by age.

| ADMISSIONS | | |
|---|---|---|
| Adults & children | 14,400 | Total number of adults and children admitted during the year |
| Newborns | 960 | Total number of babies born in the hospital during the year |
| | | |
| DISCHARGES (including deaths) | | |
| Adults & children | 14,545 | Total number of adults and children discharged during the year |
| Newborns | 950 | Total number of newborns discharged during the year |
| | | |
| INPATIENT SERVICE DAYS | | Number of days of service rendered by the hospital |
| Adults & children | 75,696 | to adults and children |
| Newborns | 1993 | to newborns |
| | | |
| TOTAL LENGTH OF STAY | | Sum of all the individual lengths of stay of |
| Adults & children | 72,107 | all adults and children discharged during the year |
| Newborns | 1974 | all newborns discharged during the year |
| | | |
| BED COUNT | | |
| Adults & children | 220 | Number of beds staffed, equipped, and available |
| Bassinets | 20 | Number of bassinets staffed, equipped, and available |
| | | |
| MORTALITY DATA | | Deaths (these numbers are included in Discharges, above) |
| Total adults & children | | |
| Under 48 hours | 20 | Total adult and child deaths within 48 hours of admission |
| Over 48 hours | 138 | Total adult and child deaths 48 hours after admission |
| Total newborns | | |
| Under 48 hours | 3 | Total newborn deaths within 48 hours of admission |
| Over 48 hours | 2 | Total newborn deaths 48 hours after admission |
| Anesthesia deaths | 1 | Number of patients who died after receiving anesthesia |
| | | |
| OPERATIONS | | |
| Number of patients operated on | 1200 | Number of patients on whom operations were performed |
| Surgical operations performed | 1312 | Number of individual surgical procedures performed |
| Anesthesia administered | 1200 | Number of individual administrations of anesthesia |
| Postoperative infections | 30 | Number of patients who developed infections as a result of their surgical procedures |
| | | |
| OTHER DATA | | |
| Nosocomial infections | 231 | Number of patients who developed infections in the hospital |
| Cesarean sections | 303 | Number of deliveries performed by cesarean section |
| Deliveries | 1304 | Number of women who gave birth in the hospital |

**Figure 10-20** Community Hospital's 2012 year-end statistics.

## ROUTINE INSTITUTIONAL STATISTICS

**statistics** Analysis, interpretation, and presentation of information in numerical or pictorial format derived from the numbers.

As discussed in Chapter 1, there are a number of ways to describe and distinguish among health care facilities. Analysis, interpretation, and presentation of data provide **statistics** that further identify a facility and its activities. Figure 10-20 contains a list of important statistics for Community Hospital for the year 2012.

### Admissions

Health care organizations always maintain statistics on the number of patients who are admitted to the facility. Review Figure 10-20 to identify the number of patients admitted to Community Hospital during 2012: 14,400 adults and children. The number of adults and children (14,400) does not include the number of newborn (NB) patients admitted (960). Unless otherwise specified, statistics for newborns are recorded separately from those of adults and children because the newborns are admitted to the facility for the purpose

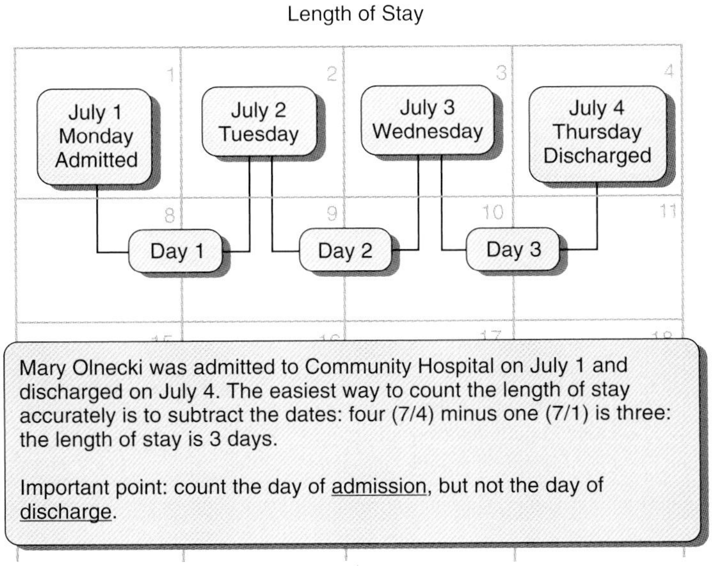

Length of Stay

> Mary Olnecki was admitted to Community Hospital on July 1 and discharged on July 4. The easiest way to count the length of stay accurately is to subtract the dates: four (7/4) minus one (7/1) is three: the length of stay is 3 days.
>
> Important point: count the day of <u>admission</u>, but not the day of <u>discharge</u>.

Figure 10-21  Calculation of length of stay within a calendar month.

of being born. Even though an NB may be ill, that is not the reason for his or her admission. A birth is an admission, and a health record is created for each NB at birth.

**⊘ NB** new born

## Discharges

Health care facilities also maintain statistics on the number of patients leaving the facility. The second item in Figure 10-20 is discharges. Once again, the NBs are listed separately from the adults and children. Note that the discharges include deaths, because death is, effectively, a discharge. Because the number of deaths is important for statistical purposes, they are also listed. The usual way a patient is discharged is by discharge order from the physician. Other ways include leaving against medical advice (AMA) and transfer to another facility. It should be noted that an individual who arrives at the facility already deceased (also known as dead on arrival or DOA) is not counted as an admission and is therefore not a discharge. The DOA may, however, be included in certain autopsy rates, if the autopsy is performed by a hospital pathologist.

**● discharge** Discharge occurs when the patient leaves the care of the facility to go home, for transfer to another health care facility, or by death. Also refers to the status of a patient.

**admission** The act of accepting a patient into care in a health care facility, including any nonambulatory care facility. Admission requires a physician's order.

## Length of Stay

The time that a patient spends in a facility is called the **length of stay (LOS)**. LOS is the measurement, in whole days, of the time between admission and discharge. Figure 10-21 illustrates how to calculate a patient's LOS. For example: A patient enters the facility on Monday, July 1, and is discharged on Thursday, July 4. The easiest way to calculate the LOS is to subtract the dates. Four minus one is three; therefore the LOS is 3 days.

It is important to note that when determining the LOS, one counts the day of admission but not the day of discharge. The times of admission and discharge are irrelevant to the calculation of inpatient LOS. In the previous example, the patient is considered to have stayed in the hospital on 3 days: July 1, July 2, and July 3. On July 4, the patient is no longer there. This is a fairly easy calculation when the patient enters and leaves the facility during the same month because one can just subtract the dates of the month.

LOS is more difficult to determine if the patient enters and leaves the facility in different months. For example, if the patient enters the hospital in July and leaves in August, three calculations are required:

*Step 1:* Calculate how many days the patient was there in July.
*Step 2:* Calculate how many days the patient was there in August.
*Step 3:* Add the Step 1 and Step 2 results to obtain the total days.

**● length of stay (LOS)** The duration of an inpatient visit, measured in whole days; the number of whole days between the inpatient's admission and discharge.

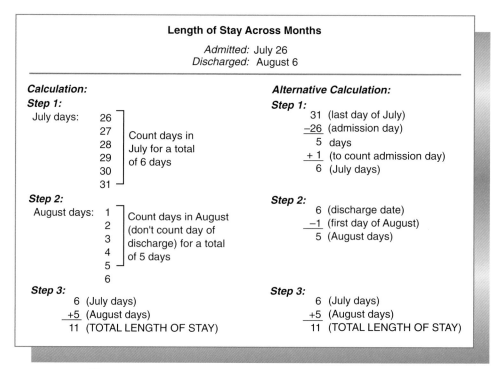

Figure 10-22 Calculation of length of stay across calendar months.

<table>
<tr><td colspan="2">**BOX 10-1**    **CALCULATION OF THE AVERAGE LENGTH OF STAY**</td></tr>
</table>

| Patient A: | 4 days |
|---|---|
| Patient B: | 2 days |
| Patient C: | 10 days |
| Patient D: | 32 days |
| Patient E: | 7 days |
| *Total:* | 55 days |

Average length of stay (ALOS): 55 days ÷ 5 patients = 11 days

Figure 10-22 gives an example of this calculation. The patient is admitted on July 26 and discharged on August 6.

*Step 1:* The patient is in the hospital in July for 6 days. Remember to count the day of admission.

*Step 2:* The stay in August is only 5 days because the day of discharge does not count.

*Step 3:* Add the 6 days in July to the 5 days in August.

*Result:* The LOS for this patient is 11 days.

It sometimes is necessary to calculate LOS manually. In an electronic environment, however, a spreadsheet program can calculate this type of information for you. In a spreadsheet program, such as Excel, it is easy to subtract the two dates and format the result as a number. Figure 10-23 shows the formula for subtracting two dates in Microsoft Excel.

## Average Length of Stay

LOS is very important in defining the type of facility and in analyzing its patient population. **Average length of stay (ALOS)** is calculated by adding up the LOSs for a group of patients and dividing by the number of patients in the group. Box 10-1 illustrates the ALOS of patients in an acute care facility using patients who were discharged in July as an example. In the example, the total LOS of all the patients combined is 55 days. Fifty-five days divided by five patients gives the average number of days, 11 days. This type of an average is called the arithmetic mean.

---

**average length of stay (ALOS)** The arithmetic mean of the lengths of stay of a group of inpatients.

**arithmetic mean** Also called the "average" or just "mean." Expresses the typical value in a set; computed by dividing the sum of the values in the set by the number of values in the set.

| ⌐ | A | B | C | D |
|---|---|---|---|---|
| 1 | | | | |
| 2 | | **Calculating Length of Stay Using Microsoft Excel** | | |
| 3 | | | | |
| 4 | | Admission Date | 9/15/12 | |
| 5 | | | | |
| 6 | | Discharge Date | 11/4/12 | |
| 7 | | | | |
| 8 | | Length of Stay | 50 | |
| 9 | | | | |
| 10 | | The formula in cell C6 is: | =C4-C2 | |
| 11 | | | | |

| ⌐ | A | B | C | D |
|---|---|---|---|---|
| 1 | Admit | Discharge | LOS | |
| 2 | 26-Jul | 6-Aug | 11 | |
| 3 | | | =B2-A2 | |
| 4 | | | | |

If you enter the formula without reformatting the cell the result will be 2/19/1900. This is because Microsoft Excel stores dates as numbers with 1/1/1900 as the first date in the series. By subtracting two dates, the result cell (C6) carries forward the date format. In order to show the actual number of days, be sure to format the cell (in this case, C6) as a Number.

To double-check the results:

Count 16 days in September (30 minus 15, plus 1)

31 days in October

3 days in November

Total: 50

Figure 10-23 Formula for subtracting two dates in Microsoft Excel to calculate LOS.

## HIT-bit

### NUMBER OF DAYS IN A MONTH

To calculate length of stay from one month to the next, it is important to know how many days there are in a month. Four months have 30 days: April, June, September, and November. February has 28 days, except in leap years (every 4 years), when it has 29 days. All of the other months have 31 days.

If you have trouble remembering how many days there are in a particular month, try creating a mnemonic. Using the first letters of each of the 30-day months, create a silly sentence that will help you associate them. You will want to use April and June in the sentence, because there are other months that begin with those letters. For example: "April and June are Not Summer" or "April's Sister is Not June." As a child, you may have learned the jingle "Thirty days hath September, April, June, and November; all the rest have 31, except February alone, which has 28 in time, and each leap year 29."

ALOS refers to the arithmetic mean of all the patients' LOSs within a certain period. Usually, ALOS is calculated monthly or annually or in some relevant period. ALOS might also be calculated by medical specialty, and it can even be calculated in terms of a specific physician's practice. These calculations are useful in determining whether a physician or a particular medical specialty conforms to the average in a particular hospital is higher or lower in terms of ALOS.

One of the characteristics of an acute care facility is that the ALOS of its patient population is less than 30 days. In reality, the ALOS of an acute care facility may be significantly less than that, depending on what type of patients it treats. For example, a community hospital with a large number of mothers and NBs, whose stay in the facility is generally 1

**ALOS** average length of stay
**NB** newborn

**acute care facility** A health care facility in which patients have an average length of stay less than 30 days and that has an emergency department, operating suite, and clinical departments to handle a broad range of diagnoses and treatments.

**Intrahospital Transfers**

|  | Unit A | Unit B | Total |
|---|---|---|---|
| 5/31/12 midnight census | 3 | 2 | 5 |
| Transfers in | +1 | +2 | +3 |
| Transfers out | −2 | −1 | −3 |
| 6/1/12 midnight census | 2 | 3 | 5 |

*Transfers between Units A and B have no impact on census*

Here is a table that reflects the same information:

|  | Unit A | Unit B | Total |
|---|---|---|---|
| 6/1/12 midnight census | 3 | 2 | 5 |
| Admissions | +2 | 0 | +2 |
| Discharges | −2 | −1 | −3 |
| 6/2/12 midnight census | 3 | 1 | 4 |

**Figure 10-24** Intrahospital transfers.

## TABLE 10-5

### TRANSFERS AFFECTING THE CENSUS ON THREE DIFFERENT NURSING UNITS

|  | PATIENT CARE UNITS | | | |
|---|---|---|---|---|
|  | UNIT A | UNIT B | UNIT C | TOTAL |
| Beginning | 4 | 6 | 8 | 18 |
| Admissions | +2 | +3 | +1 | +6 |
| Discharges | −1 | −2 | 0 | −3 |
| Unit transfers | +1 | +1 | −2 | 0 |
| Ending | 6 | 8 | 7 | 21 |

to 3 days, will tend to have a very low ALOS—perhaps only 4 or 5 days. On the other hand, a trauma center hospital with a large number of patients with serious trauma, burns, and transplants might have an ALOS closer to 12 or 13 days.

## Transfers

Patients can be transferred from one unit to another inside a facility, or they can be discharged and transferred to another facility (Figure 10-24). When a patient is transferred internally, there is no impact on the overall census or on the total admissions or discharges for the day. However, the transfer does affect the census on the nursing units from which the patient was transferred and to which the patient was transferred.

In the Table 10-5 example, two patients from Unit C were transferred: one to Unit A and one to Unit B. This did not affect the total number of patients in the hospital; it only affected the number of patients on the individual units.

A patient may be transferred to another facility upon discharge. Refer to Table 5-5 for a list of possible discharge dispositions.

Discharge disposition is a discrete data point that can be queried for reporting purposes. It might answer these questions: How many patients with CHF were discharged to home? How many septicemia patients expired?

**CHF** congestive heart failure

<table>
<tr><td colspan="2">BOX 10-2   CENSUS</td><td></td></tr>
</table>

| | TOTAL |
|---|---|
| 6/1/2013 midnight census | 5 |
| Admissions | +2 |
| Discharges | −3 |
| 6/2/13 midnight census | 4 |

Because the number of discharges (decrease) was more than the number of admissions (increase), the inpatient census decreased.

## HIT-bit

### TRANSFER DATA

The transfer of a patient to another facility requires the transfer of sufficient information to support effective continuity of care. A special transfer form is used, and copies of all or part of the health record may accompany the patient. The receiving hospital (the hospital to which the patient is transferred) counts the patient as an admission. *Interhospital transfer* describes this movement of a patient from one facility to another. *Intrahospital transfer* reflects movement of a patient between nursing units and therefore has no overall impact on census. Figure 10-24 shows the transfer of patients between two nursing units on May 31, 2012.

## Census

The total number of patients in the hospital at any given time is called the **census**. The term census describes both the physical activity of counting (or confirming a computer-generated list of) the patients as well as the resultant total. Admissions increase the census; discharges decrease the census (Box 10-2). For statistical purposes, the census is taken at the same time every day, usually but not always at midnight, so that the facility can compare the census from day to day over time. This census number is also called the midnight census. For practical purposes, a computer database allows the patient registration department to view the census at any time.

Hospital administrators like to review the census by nursing unit, wing, or floor. This view enables administrators to identify underutilized areas for planning purposes. It also allows nursing managers to plan and control staffing. The impact of the two admissions and three discharges on the census taken between June 1 and June 2, 2012, is detailed by nursing unit in Table 10-5 and by patient in Box 10-2.

**census** The actual number of inpatients in a facility at a point in time, for comparative purposes, usually midnight.

## HIT-bit

### TRACKING PATIENTS INHOUSE

Historically, the admissions department used a chart to keep track of all of the rooms in the facility. The chart was called a bed board and provided a method for the facility to keep track of which patient rooms were vacant or occupied. If a room was occupied, the admissions clerk would put on the chart the name(s) of the patient(s) in that room and mark the room occupied. Today, this procedure has been automated; however, some hospitals have maintained the manual bed-board system as a backup.

Newborn beds are called *bassinets* and are located in a part of the unit called the *nursery*.

The patient access (registration) department is generally responsible for assigning a patient to a bed within a particular room. The function of assigning the bed is often called **bed control**. Manual tracking of patient admissions, discharges, and transfers between

**bed control** The function of assigning beds in an acute care facility.

**TABLE 10-6**

**NUMBER OF PATIENTS WHO RECEIVED SERVICES DETAILED BY PATIENT**

|  | INPATIENTS | TOTAL |
|---|---|---|
| 6/1/11 midnight census | M. Brown | 5 |
|  | S. Crevecoeur |  |
|  | F. Perez |  |
|  | P. Smith |  |
|  | R. Wooley |  |
| Admissions | C. Estevez | 2 |
|  | B. Mooney |  |
| Discharges | S. Crevecoeur | 3 |
|  | C. Estevez |  |
|  | B. Mooney |  |
| 6/2/11 midnight census | M. Brown | 4 |
|  | F. Perez |  |
|  | P. Smith |  |
|  | R. Wooley |  |

units can be very cumbersome and time consuming. Further, manual tracking systems are not available outside the bed control office. Therefore many facilities employ electronic bed control systems that can be accessed by nursing, housekeeping, and administration as well as the bed control staff.

A census does not measure all of the services provided by the hospital. What about the patient who is admitted at 10:40 AM and dies before midnight? That patient would not be present for the counting of the midnight census. The facility counts these patients in the service days for the facility called **inpatient service days (IPSDs)**. IPSDs are calculated by adding the admissions to the previous day's census, subtracting the discharges, then adding the patients who were admitted and discharged on the same day.

**inpatient service day (IPSD)** A measure of the use of hospital services, representing the care provided to one inpatient during a 24-hour period.

---

**HIT-bit**

**CALCULATING DAYS OF SERVICE**

In counting days of service, as in length of stay, we count the day of admission but not the day of discharge. This makes sense because if the hospital counted the day of discharge as well, it would conceivably charge twice for the same bed on the same day. The same principle allows the facility to count 1 day of service for a patient who is admitted and discharged on the same day.

---

The census report in Box 10-2 does not indicate how many patients received services on June 2, 2012. Table 10-6 shows the admission and discharge detailed by patient. The two patients who were admitted on June 2 were also discharged the same day. Table 10-7 analyzes the service days received by those patients. From this analysis, 6 days of service (IPSDs) were actually rendered by the hospital.

The census need not be analyzed patient by patient to calculate IPSDs. One can obtain the total number of patients admitted and discharged on the same day from census reports (Table 10-8). Once IPSDs have been calculated, the data can be added, averaged, graphed, and trended over time. The census is also a means to calculate occupancy, as mentioned, because it includes all patients who were admitted and discharged the same day. Because the census counts only patients in beds at a point in time, calculating IPSDs is a better measure of the use of hospital facilities. Figure 10-25 illustrates all the IPSD concepts discussed so far.

At the end of 2011, there were 325 patients in Community Hospital. At the end of 2012, the adults and children census was 180 (Figure 10-26). There were 145 fewer adults and children in the hospital at the end of the year 2012 than there were at the beginning. How

**IPSD** inpatient service day

## Census Statistics

| A&C = Adults and children | NICU = Neonatal ICU | D/C = Discharges |
| N/B = Newborn | Adm. = Admissions | IPSD = Inpatient service days |

| | Adults & Children | | | Newborns | | |
| | UNIT A | UNIT B | TOTAL A&C | N/B nursery | NICU | TOTAL N/B |
|---|---|---|---|---|---|---|
| 6/1/12 midnight census | 15 | 17 | 32 | 3 | 1 | 4 |
| Admissions/births | +4 | +2 | +6 | 2 | 0 | 2 |
| Discharges/deaths | −5 | −4 | −9 | 0 | 0 | 0 |
| Transfers in | +2 | +1 | +3 | 0 | +1 | +1 |
| Transfers out | −1 | −2 | −3 | −1 | 0 | −1 |
| 6/2/12 midnight census | 15 | 14 | 29 | 4 | 2 | 6 |
| Adm. & D/C 6/2/12 | +2 | +1 | +3 | 0 | 0 | 0 |
| 6/2/12 IPSD | 17 | 15 | 32 | 4 | 2 | 6 |

*Sometimes these reports are generated from the main system. If the report from the main system is not in the desired format, it can sometimes be downloaded to a computerized spreadsheet program for reformatting or alternative presentation, such as a graph. Any report that is prepared on a spreadsheet should be spot-checked for accuracy potential errors.*

Figure 10-25 Census statistics.

## The Fiscal Year

| QUARTER | Month | # of Days | Admissions | Discharges | Census | |
|---|---|---|---|---|---|---|
| | | | | | 325 | 12/31/11 |
| I | January | 31 | 1125 | 1148 | 302 | |
| | February | 29 | 1543 | 1555 | 290 | |
| | March | 31 | 1445 | 1430 | 305 | |
| II | April | 30 | 1406 | 1398 | 313 | |
| | May | 31 | 1242 | 1247 | 308 | |
| | June | 30 | 1004 | 994 | 318 | |
| III | July | 31 | 1254 | 1248 | 324 | |
| | August | 31 | 1145 | 1148 | 321 | |
| | September | 30 | 1212 | 1224 | 309 | |
| IV | October | 31 | 1478 | 1502 | 285 | |
| | November | 30 | 1567 | 1598 | 254 | |
| | December | 31 | 1229 | 1303 | 180 | |
| Total | | **366** | **15,650** | **15,795** | | **12/31/12** |

*2012 was a leap year. In non-leap years, February has 28 days, for a total of 365 days in the year.*

Figure 10-26 The fiscal year.

**TABLE 10-7**

**ANALYSIS OF PATIENTS WHO RECEIVED A DAY OF SERVICE ON JUNE 2, 2012**

| INPATIENTS | ANALYSIS | 6/2 DAY OF SERVICE |
|---|---|---|
| M. Brown | Inpatient on 6/1 and 6/2 | 1 |
| S. Crevecoeur | Discharged 6/2 | 0 |
| C. Estevez | Admitted and discharged 6/2 | 1 |
| B. Mooney | Admitted and discharged 6/2 | 1 |
| F. Perez | Inpatient on 6/1 and 6/2 | 1 |
| P. Smith | Inpatient on 6/1 and 6/2 | 1 |
| R. Wooley | Inpatient on 6/1 and 6/2 | 1 |
| *Total days of service* | | 6 |

**TABLE 10-8**

**INPATIENT SERVICE DAYS CALCULATED FROM CENSUS**

| | TOTAL |
|---|---|
| 6/1/12 midnight census | 5 |
| Admissions | +2 |
| Discharges | −3 |
| 6/2/12 midnight census | 4 |
| Patients admitted and discharged on 6/2 | +2 |
| 6/2/12 inpatient service days | 6 |

did that happen? Look at the admissions and discharges. There were more discharges than admissions during the year: 145, to be exact.

Understanding the relationship among the statistics helps us to use these data effectively. For example, Figure 10-20 shows that 14,545 adults and children were discharged in 2012. The total LOS for all of those patients combined was 72,107 days. Therefore the ALOS for adults and children in 2012 was 4.96 days (72,107 ÷ 14,545 = 4.96).

All health care facilities keep track of their statistics according to the fiscal year, which is a 12-month reporting period. A facility's reporting period can be the calendar year (January 1 through December 31), or July 1 through June 30, or October 1 through September 30. Figure 10-26 is organized into fiscal periods. To understand this concept, think of how a year is organized into days, weeks, and months. Hospital statistics are calculated by the relevant fiscal period. In addition to days, weeks, and months, data can be grouped into months or quarters. Each quarter represents 3 months, or approximately one fourth of the year.

## Bed Occupancy Rate

**occupancy** In a hospital, the percentage of available beds that have been used over time.

**licensed beds** The maximum number of beds that a facility is legally permitted to have, as approved by state licensure.

**bed count** The actual number of beds that a hospital has staffed, equipped, and otherwise made available for occupancy by patients for each specific operating day.

**Occupancy** refers to the number of inpatient beds used by patients in a particular period. It is typically expressed as a percentage. As noted previously, the use of beds is measured by IPSD. So, if a hospital has 150 licensed beds and the IPSD for yesterday was 75, then yesterday's occupancy was 50%: (75 ÷ 150) × 100. Calculating occupancy with IPSD takes into consideration patients who are admitted and discharged on the same day.

Occupancy over a period of more than 1 day is calculated by dividing the number of days that patients used beds (total IPSDs) by the number of beds available (bed count × the number of days in the period). Bed count is different from licensed beds. Licensed beds are the number of beds permitted for the hospital according to the hospital's license from the state. Bed count is the number of beds that are actually staffed and available for patients at any time. A hospital may be licensed for 250 beds but have only 200 of them staffed and set up. Although the licensed beds cannot change without permission from the state, the bed count may change frequently. So the denominator of the occupancy equation needs to take into consideration how many days the hospital maintained bed count at various levels.

> **BOX 10-3    RATES AND PERCENTAGES**
>
> **RATE**
>
> $$\frac{67 \text{ female patients}}{134 \text{ total patients}} = \frac{1}{2}$$
>
> Half of the patients are female.
>
> **PERCENTAGE**
>
> $$\frac{67 \text{ female patients}}{134 \text{ total patients}} = 0.50 \ (\times 100) = 50\%$$
>
> Fifty percent of patients are female.

> **BOX 10-4    HEALTH CARE STATISTICS FORMULAS**
>
> **AVERAGE INPATIENT SERVICE DAYS (IPSDs)**
>
> $$\frac{\text{Total IPSDs for a period (excluding newborns)}}{\text{Total number of days in the period}}$$
>
> **AVERAGE NEWBORN INPATIENT SERVICE DAYS**
>
> $$\frac{\text{Total newborn IPSDs for a period}}{\text{Total number of days in the period}}$$
>
> **AVERAGE LENGTH OF STAY (ALOS)**
>
> $$\frac{\text{Total LOS (discharge days)}}{\text{Total discharges (including deaths)}}$$
>
> **BED OCCUPANCY RATE**
>
> $$\frac{\text{Total IPSDs for a period}}{\text{Total bed count days in the period}} \times 100$$
>
> (Calculated as bed count × number of days in the period.)
>
> **NEWBORN BASSINET OCCUPANCY RATIO FORMULA**
>
> $$\frac{\text{Total newborn IPSDs for a period}}{\text{Total newborn bassinet count} \times \text{number of days in the period}} \times 100$$
>
> **OTHER RATES FORMULA**
>
> $$\frac{\text{Number of times something occurred}}{\text{Number of time something could have occurred}} \times 100$$

## Hospital Rates and Percentages

There are many ways to look at hospital statistics. The general rule is to look at the number of times something occurred in comparison with (divided by) the number of times it could have occurred. This basic calculation provides a rate of occurrence. Multiplied by 100, the rate of occurrence is expressed as a percentage. Box 10-3 provides an example of rates versus percentages.

For example, it might be necessary to know the percentage of hospital patients who acquired nosocomial infections. Figure 10-20 shows that there were 231 occurrences of nosocomial infections at Community Hospital in 2012. Because 15,495 (14,545 + 950) patients were treated (discharged), 15,495 is the number of possible occurrences of nosocomial infections. The percentage of nosocomial infections is 1.5%.

The key to understanding hospital rates and percentages is understanding the underlying data and how those data elements relate to one another. Some of the most common types of calculations are shown in Box 10-4.

Thus there are many ways to report data. The way in which they are reported depends on the needs of the user. It is important for the HIM professional to understand the needs of the user to help identify the data for meaningful reporting and presentation.

**nosocomial infections** Hospital-acquired infections.

## EXERCISE 10-5

### Routine Institutional Statistics

*Use information in the table below to answer the following questions.*
*First Quarter Data, Diamonte Hospital, 10/1/12-12/31/12*

| | | |
|---|---|---|
| Admissions | Adults and children | 9218 |
| | Newborns | 290 |
| Discharges (including deaths) | Adults and children | 9014 |
| | Newborns | 303 |
| Inpatient service days | Adults and children | 35,421 |
| | Newborns | 432 |
| Total lengths of stay | Adults and children | 32,542 |
| | Newborns | 608 |
| Bed count | Adults and children | 450 |
| | Newborns | 30 |
| Mortality data | Total adults and children: | |
| | <48 hours | 12 |
| | ≥48 hours | 132 |
| | Total newborns: | |
| | <48 hours | 2 |
| | ≥48 hours | 1 |
| | Anesthesia deaths | 1 |
| | Fetal deaths: | |
| | Early | 3 |
| | Intermediate and late | 9 |
| | Maternal deaths | 1 |
| | Postoperative deaths: | |
| | <10 days | 45 |
| | ≥10 days | 5 |
| Operations | Number of patients operated on | 836 |
| | Surgical operations performed | 889 |
| | Anesthesia administered | 856 |
| | Postoperative infections | 12 |
| Miscellaneous | Cesarean sections | 69 |
| | Deliveries | 349 |
| | Nosocomial infections | 13 |
| | Consultations | 2756 |

1. What is the hospital's fiscal year?
2. Calculate the following:
   a. Average inpatient service days
   b. Average newborn inpatient service days
   c. Average length of stay
   d. Bed occupancy
   e. Consultation rate
   f. Nosocomial infection rate

## REGISTRIES

**registry** A database of health information specific to disease, diagnosis, or implant used to improve the care provided to patients with that disease, diagnosis, or implant.

A **registry** is a collection of data specific to a disease, diagnosis, or procedure, the purpose of which is to study or improve patient care. Unlike an index, which lists all occurrences of a particular field, such as diagnosis or procedure, a registry is compiled of cases that conform to strict guidelines as defined by the registry (case finding) and the identification and reporting of very specific data related to the case. Common registries are the Tumor or Cancer Registry, Trauma Registry, AIDS Registry, Birth Defect Registry, and Implant Registry. The data are collected specific to the diagnosis, disease, or implant so that users can compare, analyze, or study the groups of patients. A registry is typically maintained by an agency external to the facility or provider and characteristically requires active follow-up of the reported cases.

## Tumor or Cancer Registry

The study of the causes and treatments of cancers is of importance to individuals and also as a public health issue. Many cancers, such as some types of lung cancer, are thought to be of environmental origin; others seem to have a genetic component. It is only by analyzing data collected from cancer patients that researchers can begin to identify the actual causes with the hope of finding preventive measures and effective treatments.

State-based cancer registries are data systems that collect, manage, and analyze data about cancer cases and cancer deaths. In each state, medical facilities (including hospitals, physicians' offices, therapeutic radiation facilities, freestanding surgical centers, and pathology laboratories) report these data to a central cancer registry.

Established by Congress through the Cancer Registries Amendment Act in 1992, and administered by the Centers for Disease Control and Prevention (CDC), the National Program of Cancer Registries (NPCR) collects data on the occurrence of cancer; the type, extent, and location of the cancer; and the type of initial treatment.

Before NPCR was established, 10 states had no registry, and most states with registries lacked the resources and legislative support they needed to gather complete data. Today, NPCR supports central cancer registries in 45 states, the District of Columbia, Puerto Rico, and the U.S. Pacific Island Jurisdictions. These data represent 96% of the U.S. population. Together, NPCR and the National Cancer Institute's Surveillance, Epidemiology, and End Results (SEER) Program collect data for the entire U.S. population. (*National Program of Cancer Registries: About the Program*, 2011)

Detailed data collection includes demographic data (name, address, identification number) and clinical data (diagnoses, procedures, pathology). Pathology data include grading (classifying the growth of the tumor) and staging (describing whether the tumor has spread and how far). Many providers complete the basic registry reporting; however, a certified cancer registry also requires patient follow-up.

Individuals who specialize in collecting data for this registry may become Certified Tumor Registrars (CTRs) through the National Cancer Registry Association (http://www.ncra-usa.org/certification).

## Trauma Registry

Researchers can identify trauma (injury) victims by the ICD-10-CM codes associated with the external cause of morbidity and the injury itself. Because these codes are collected and reported on the UB-04 and through various data sets such as UHDDS, they are available in the providers' and payers' databases as well as through state and federal databases. However, for study of the severity of the injury and the effectiveness of specific treatments, a trauma registry provides more data.

In 2006, the National Trauma Data Bank (2007) released "the National Trauma Data Standard (formerly National Trauma Registry) data dictionary, developed in collaboration with HRSA, state trauma managers, trauma registry vendors, and other stakeholders in the trauma community." (U.S. Department of Health and Human Services, 2012). Trauma registry data includes traumatic injuries, such as head injuries and burns, of patients receiving care as well as injury data related to patients who died before care could be rendered.

The American Trauma Society (ATS) offers a certification process for Certified Specialist Trauma Registry (CSTR; http://www.amtrauma.org/index.html).

## Other Registries

Birth defects and transplants are examples of other entities for which registries may be maintained. Varying degrees of detail are collected. Birth defects may not be detected at

**ICD-10-CM** International Classification of Diseases, Tenth Revision—Clinical Modification. A code set used for diagnosis of disease.

**morbidity** A disease or illness.

**Uniform Bill (UB-04)** The standardized form used by hospitals for inpatient and outpatient billing to CMS and other third party payers.

**Uniform Hospital Discharge Data Set (UHDDS)** The mandated data set for hospital inpatients.

**payer** The individual or organization that is primarily responsible for the reimbursement for a particular health care service. Usually refers to the insurance company or third party.

birth, and later reporting may be acceptable. Transplant registries match potential donors with recipients and follow those patients after the transplant.

## Vital Statistics

Vital statistics refers to the number of births, deaths, and marriages and to statistics on health and disease. In the health care facility, specific information regarding patient births and deaths is reported to the state's Department of Vital Statistics, also known as Vital Records. Newborns must be registered with the Department of Vital Statistics within a specific time frame after birth. Within the health care facility, the HIM department is sometimes responsible for recording newborns' demographics, parents, and clinical information to submit to Vital Records.

Death certificates must also be submitted to the state's department of vital records after a patient's death. The death certificate records the patient's demographic information and the cause and place of death. In some states, this information is initiated by the nursing staff and completed by the funeral home; in others, the HIM staff may be required to participate in the submission of this information to the department of vital statistics.

Birth and death certificate data are increasingly collected electronically at the point of care. Paper submissions, where applicable, are collected at the point of care and submitted at the municipal level. The local registrar submits that data to the state, which in turn submits the data through the National Vital Statistics System to the National Center for Health Statistics (NCHS), a component of the Centers for Disease Control and Prevention. Standards for data collection and reporting are developed by the NCHS. Appendix A contains the example birth, death, and fetal death forms published in 1989. State forms vary depending on specific additional data the state wishes to collect (Tolson et al, 1991).

**vital statistics** Public health data collected through birth certificates, death certificates, and other data-gathering tools.

**point-of-care documentation** Clinical data recorded at the time the treatment is delivered to the patient.

**National Center for Health Statistics (NCHS)** A division of the CDC that collects and analyzes vital statistics. Acts as one of the ICD-10-CM Cooperating Parties.

**Go To** Appendix A or the Evolve site for sample birth and death certificate forms.

## EXERCISE 10-6

### Registries

1. What is a registry?
2. What is the difference between a registry and an index?
3. List and describe four registries.

## WORKS CITED

National Trauma Data Bank: History of the New Data Standard. http://www.ntdsdictionary.org/index.html. Published 2007.

Tolson GC, Barnes JM, Gay GA, Kowaleski JL: The 1989 revision of the U.S. standard certificates and reports. National Center for Health Statistics. Vital Health Stat 4(28), 1991. http://www.cdc.gov/nchs/data/series/sr_04/sr04_028.pdf.

U.S. Department of Health and Human Services, Centers for Disease Control and Prevention, National Program of Cancer Registries (NCRPs): About the Program. Published 2012. http://www.cdc.gov/cancer/npcr/about.htm.

## CHAPTER ACTIVITIES

### CHAPTER SUMMARY

Health information must be collected in a systematic, defined format. The database created by this systematic collection is then a source of information for departments within the organization as well as agencies external to the facility.

The data can be analyzed, interpreted, and presented to appropriate users through the use of the statistical tools, including: arithmetic mean, median, and mode, geometric mean, and standard deviation, as well as bar graphs, pie charts, and line graphs. The analysis of a facility's data is also referred to as the *facility's statistics*, which describes the services and activities of the facility.

An important use of health information databases is the identification of cases to report to registries, such as cancer registry and trauma registry.

## REVIEW QUESTIONS

1. Explain the different between primary and secondary data. Give an example of each.
2. List individual departments and outside agencies to which a provider might report information.
3. List four statistical tools and explain their use.
4. What is the formula for computing the average length of stay?
5. The following patients were discharged from pediatrics for the week 7/15/12 to 7/20/12:

| Patient Name | Admission Date | Discharge Date |
|---|---|---|
| Groot | 7/13/12 | 7/15/12 |
| Smith | 7/12/12 | 7/15/12 |
| Brown | 7/11/12 | 7/16/12 |
| Kowalski | 7/10/12 | 7/20/12 |
| Zhong | 7/09/12 | 7/19/12 |
| Frank | 6/29/12 | 7/18/12 |

What is the average length of stay of these patients?
6. How do percentages facilitate data analysis?
7. Why are census data important? How is census calculated?

## PROFESSIONAL PROFILE

### Clinical Data Analyst

My name is Maggie, and I am the clinical data analyst at Diamonte. I am responsible for overseeing the quality of the data contained in the health information management (HIM) database.

I am the contact person for all matters concerning the HIM database. In this role, I process all requests for reports from the HIM database. When quality management, administration, physician, or case management staff members need information from our database, they come to me. I make sure I know the following:

• What information they want
• Why they need it
• The time frame for the information
• When they need the report

This information helps me run the correct report so that employees may use the information as necessary in their presentation, decision making, or investigation. Sometimes, the users have a question, but they don't really know how to answer it.

I find this part of my job very rewarding. I enjoy receiving a request that people think is impossible because I know that our HIM database contains the information that they need. Providing those reports is really exciting.

## PATIENT CARE PERSPECTIVE

**Dr. Lewis**

Our group is considering adding another physician and we wanted to confirm the gap in the group. We think we need a pulmonologist, because our own records show a high level of referrals, but we don't have enough data to make that decision. I called Maggie at Diamonte and obtained a report on all patients admitted by physicians in our group as well as our patients who were treated by hospitalists. I asked for a spreadsheet that listed each patient for the past 2 years, the first 5 diagnoses, the first 5 procedures, and the ID for the attending physician and the PCP of record. With that data, we were able to determine that we admit enough patients with respiratory problems; however, they were mostly covered by the hospitalists. So we are looking for a pulmonologist who is comfortable working with hospitalists.

## APPLICATION

### Making Data Informative

Health information professionals are commonly asked to analyze data for presentation. The presentation may be a simple table or report, or it may include graphs.

1. Using the Internet, locate a database of patient information for query of a diagnosis related group assigned by your instructor. Prepare a report with a graph for presentation to your instructor.
2. Using the coronary artery bypass graft report in Figure 10-14, prepare a presentation for your instructor demonstrating the average length of stay for the patients of each physician.

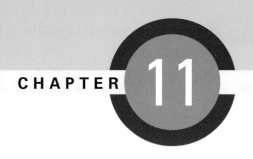

**CHAPTER**

# QUALITY AND USES OF HEALTH INFORMATION

Melissa LaCour

335

## CHAPTER OBJECTIVES

*By the end of this chapter, the student should be able to:*

1. Discuss the various ways health information is used by a health care facility.
2. Discuss the various ways health information is used by those outside of the health care facility.
3. Understand the intent of various health care regulations and standards.
4. Review health records for documentation of compliance with accreditation standards.
5. Explain how health information is monitored to ensure quality.
6. Explain performance improvement.
7. Identify performance improvement tools.
8. Explain the purpose of various data-gathering tools.
9. Explain how health information is used by specific committees in the health care organization.

This text so far has discussed the obvious reason(s) to document health information: patient care. And yet, timely, accurate, and complete health information is essential for many other reasons. This chapter explores the methods used to evaluate and ensure data quality as well as how quality health information is used for reimbursement, litigation, accreditation, marketing, research, education, and performance improvement.

Many of the uses of health information have already been discussed in this text. The information that follows may seem repetitious, but an understanding of the many different ways health information is used is essential to HIM professionals. Although each and every use of health data is important, the measurement of quality, discussed in the second part of this chapter, cannot be understated.

## USES OF HEALTH INFORMATION

The uses of health information can be classified as internal to the health care facility or external. Here is a list of some internal health care facility uses:

- To improve patient care
- To support and collect reimbursement
- To support and prove compliance for licensing, accreditation, and certification
- To support the administration of the facility
- To provide evidence in litigation
- To educate future health care professionals

Agencies outside the health care facility (external) use health information for the following reasons:

- To study the mortality rates and the prevalence and incidence of morbidity
- To support litigation
- To develop community awareness of health care issues
- To influence national policy on health care issues through legislation
- To educate patients and health care professionals
- To develop health care products

The aforementioned uses are the most obvious, but they may not include every possible use of health information.

## IMPROVING PATIENT CARE

Health information is used to improve the quality of care provided to patients. Many people have been in a health care facility and thought that a few things could have been improved. For instance, did the patient have to wait too long to see the physician? Was communication among the health care professionals inadequate? There may have even been an impression that no one knew exactly what was going on.

Historically, health information management (HIM) professionals have reviewed the documentation of patient health care after the patient is discharged to determine whether patients received appropriate care. Review of the patient's record after discharge is called

---

**health information** Organized data that have been collected about a patient or a group of patients. Sometimes used synonymously with the term health data.

**HIM** health information management

**discharge** Discharge occurs when the patient leaves the care of the facility to go home, for transfer to another health care facility, or by death. Also refers to the status of a patient.

retrospective review; this method of review analyzes how, when, and where the patient received care. Retrospective reviews provide statistical information to support decisions that will improve care for future patients. Although retrospective reviews can be effective in improving future care, they cannot change or improve the outcome for patients who have already been discharged. The alternative to retrospective review is concurrent review. **Concurrent review** of patient health information provides timely information that is used to support decisions made while the patient is still in the hospital. Concurrent information provides an opportunity to change or improve the patient's outcome. This process is discussed in greater detail later in this chapter, in the section about health information in quality activities.

## SUPPORT AND COLLECTION OF REIMBURSEMENT

Reimbursement refers to the amount of money that the health care facility receives from the party responsible for paying the bill. Health care, although personal in service, has evolved into a large and sometimes very impersonal industry. All health care providers have a vested interest in their financial operations. As with any other business, a health care provider offers a service or product and then charges a fee for that service or product. The provider may obtain reimbursement from for example—the patient, an insurance company, a managed care organization, or the state or federal government.

The patient's health record, which contains documentation of all of the patient's care, supports the charges for services and supplies. The health record contains documentation of the type of product or service, the date and time at which the service was provided, and the individual who provided the service to the patient.

HIM coding personnel review the patient's health record to identify the correct diagnoses and procedures and then assign the appropriate ICD-10-CM/PCS and HCPCS/CPT codes. These codes are documented on the UB-04 or the CMS-1500 form; they tell the payer why the patient received health care (the diagnosis) and whether any procedures were performed that affect reimbursement. Accurate coding requires a thorough analysis of the complete health record. Inaccurate coding causes the facility to submit false claims for reimbursement. From a compliance perspective, submission of false claims is a crime punishable by law; therefore HIM coders are educated in the review of records and the appropriate assignment of codes for reimbursement. Revenue cycle management (RCM) ensures timely, accurate submission of patient bills for payment.

### HIT-bit

#### REIMBURSEMENT FOR HEALTH CARE

Several people may be involved in reimbursement for health care. The patient can pay for health care services out of pocket or through an insurance plan. Paying out of pocket involves a transaction between two people, or parties. If the patient chooses to pay with insurance, a third party is introduced. The insurance company becomes a third party payer. In health care, a *payer* is the person or party responsible for the bill.

## LICENSURE, ACCREDITATION, AND CERTIFICATION

Health care facilities must have a license to operate. Licensure of a health care facility is performed by the state in which the facility is located. Among the many requirements necessary to receive a license, the facility must maintain documentation (a health record) on all patients.

As discussed in Chapter 1, health care facilities that provide care to Medicare and Medicaid patients receive reimbursement from the federal government. The Centers for Medicare and Medicaid Services (CMS) oversees the federal responsibilities of the Medicare and Medicaid programs. For a facility to receive reimbursement from the federal

**retrospective review** Review occurring after the act or event (i.e., after the patient is discharged).

**concurrent review** Review occurring during the act or event (i.e., a chart review during the patient's stay in the facility).

**managed care** A type of insurer (payer) focused on reducing health care costs, controlling expensive care, and improving the quality of patient care provided.

**Go To** Review reimbursement and the revenue cycle in Chapter 7.

**coding** The assignment of alphanumerical values to a word, phrase, or other nonnumerical expression. In health care, coding is the assignment of numerical values to diagnosis and procedure descriptions.

**revenue cycle management (RCM)** All the activities that connect the services being rendered to a patient with the provider's reimbursement for those services.

**Uniform Bill (UB-04)** The standardized form used by hospitals for inpatient and outpatient billing to the CMS and other third party payers.

**analysis** The review of a record to evaluate its completeness, accuracy, or compliance with predetermined standards or other criteria.

**claim** The application to an insurance company for reimbursement of services rendered.

**ICD-10-CM/PCS** International Classification of Diseases, Tenth Revision—Clinical Modification/Procedural Coding System

**HCPCS/CPT** Healthcare Common Procedure Coding System/Current Procedural Terminology

**CMS-1500** Centers for Medicare and Medicaid Services 1500 form

**licensure** The mandatory government approval required for performing specified activities. In health care, the state approval required for providing health care services.

**Conditions of Participation (COP)**
The terms under which a facility is eligible to receive reimbursement from Medicare.

**certification** Approval by an outside agency, such as the federal or state government, indicating that the health care facility has met a set of predetermined standards.

**TJC** The Joint Commission
**CARF** Commission on Accreditation of Rehabilitation Facilities
**NIAHO** National Integrated Accreditation for Healthcare Organizations
**AOA** American Osteopathic Association

**accreditation** Voluntary compliance with a set of standards developed by an independent agent, who periodically performs audits to ensure compliance.

**deemed status** The Medicare provision that an approved accreditation is sufficient to satisfy the compliance audit element of the Conditions of Participation.

**operative report** The surgeon's formal report of surgical procedure(s) performed. Often dictated and transcribed into a formal report.

**DD** date dictated
**DT** date transcribed

government, it must be certified under Medicare's Conditions of Participation (COP). The COP are the CMS rules and regulations (standards) that govern the Medicare program. **Certification** under the COP, performed by the state, attests that a health care facility has met the CMS standards.

Accreditation is another means by which some health care facilities may be approved to serve state-funded and federally funded patients. Accreditation, like certification, recognizes that a facility has met a predetermined set of standards. However, accreditation is voluntary. Facilities are not mandated to attain accreditation, but they may be motivated by third party payer requirements for reimbursement and the perception that accreditation indicates a certain quality of care necessary to compete in the marketplace. Accreditation is performed by organizations such as TJC, CARF, NIAHO, and the AOA. In some health care settings, a successful survey by TJC and some other accreditation agencies results in assignment of deemed status by the CMS, by which TJC accreditation is accepted in lieu of the Medicare COP certification.

What does any of this have to do with health information? Licensure, certification, and accreditation require that a facility prove compliance with regulations or standards. Much of the proof necessary to validate certification and accreditation standards is found in a review of the patient records. The certification or accreditation survey of the records reveals the quality of care delivered to patients within a facility. The survey record review is coordinated to determine whether the facility is providing care within the established guidelines. For example, TJC requires that an operative report be completed immediately after surgery. In cases in which the physician chooses to dictate the operative report, an operative note should be made part of the patient's chart and should include information pertinent to the operation that a health care professional might need to know in the absence of the detailed operative report. In a check for compliance with this standard, a sample of surgery records would be pulled for review. The surveyor, HIM personnel, or others would review the record to determine the date and time of surgery. The date and time of the surgery are used for comparison with the dates on which the operative report was dictated and transcribed, both of which are indicated on the operative report in Figure 11-1.

---

## HIT-bit

### TRANSCRIPTION REPORT DATA

A transcriptionist records on each operative report both the date on which the report was dictated by the physician and the date on which it was transcribed, along with the transcriptionist's initials. This information is found at the end of each transcribed report.

---

At the end of the report, the transcriptionist's initials, the date dictated (DD), and date transcribed (DT) are indicated in the mm/dd/yyyy format shown. This information identifies who the transcriptionist was, when the report was dictated, and when it was transcribed. In an electronic health record (EHR), time stamps are inherent in the process of record entries, including the signature on the dictation. If speech recognition technology is used, the timing of the interaction is also automatically recorded.

## ADMINISTRATION

*Administration* is the common term used to describe the management of the health care facility. In management of health care, the services that are provided must be evaluated. Managers want to be certain that they are providing health care services in an efficient and effective manner. The administrators responsible for a facility are concerned with personnel and financial and clinical operations of the health care facility. Health information is used in administrative aspects to support reimbursement, make decisions regarding services, and analyze the quality of patient care.

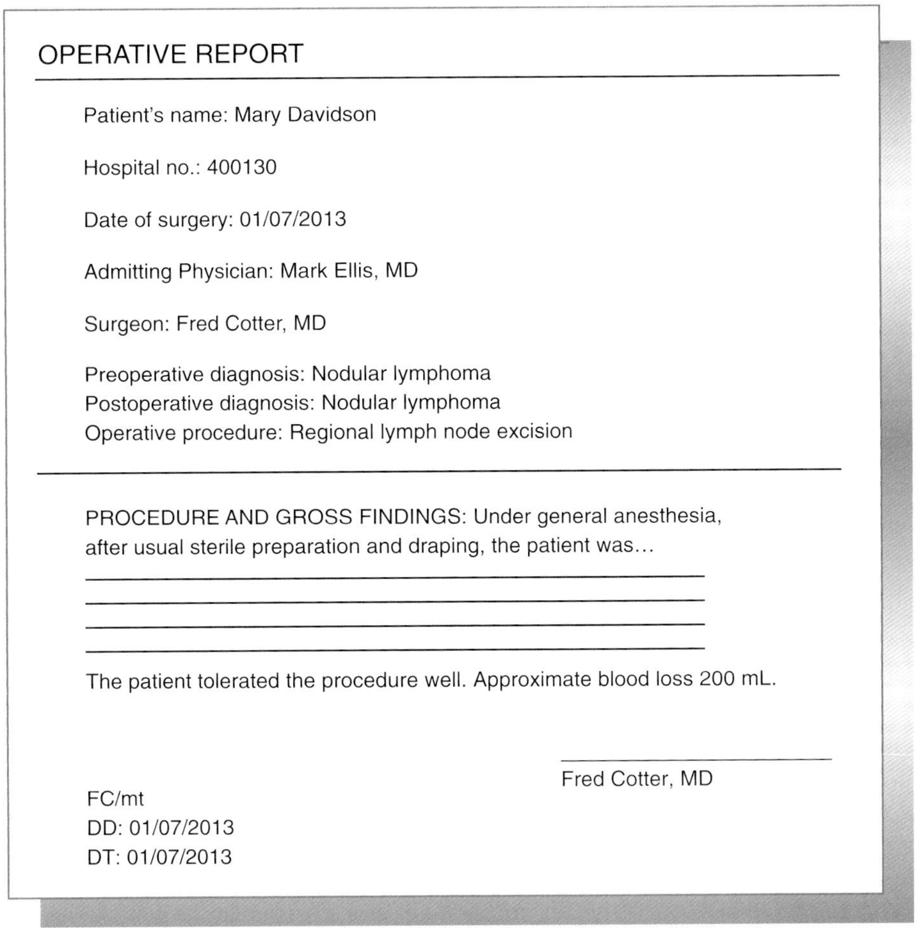

---

## OPERATIVE REPORT

Patient's name: Mary Davidson

Hospital no.: 400130

Date of surgery: 01/07/2013

Admitting Physician: Mark Ellis, MD

Surgeon: Fred Cotter, MD

Preoperative diagnosis: Nodular lymphoma
Postoperative diagnosis: Nodular lymphoma
Operative procedure: Regional lymph node excision

---

PROCEDURE AND GROSS FINDINGS: Under general anesthesia, after usual sterile preparation and draping, the patient was...

The patient tolerated the procedure well. Approximate blood loss 200 mL.

Fred Cotter, MD

FC/mt
DD: 01/07/2013
DT: 01/07/2013

**Figure 11-1** Operative report with date dictated (DD) and date transcribed (DT).

The administrators of the facility rely on the review of health information to make decisions regarding the management of the facility. For example, review of health information may indicate that improper coding, which affects reimbursement, caused a significant decrease in revenue or that patients who receive physical therapy soon after heart surgery recover in a shorter time. Health information is also used to make decisions about the health care services offered, to formulate policies, and to design an organizational structure.

Administrators also use health information to negotiate and evaluate contracts with managed care companies or other vendors, such as surgical supply companies and laundry services. For surgical supply companies and laundry services, the facility uses statistics from its database to negotiate terms of a contract. The statistics help the facility determine the proper quantities of supplies to purchase.

**statistics** Analysis, interpretation, and presentation of information in numerical or pictorial format derived from the numbers.

## PREVALENCE AND INCIDENCE OF MORTALITY AND MORBIDITY

Health care facilities are required to report statistics on communicable and infectious diseases to agencies of the federal government, as discussed in Chapter 10. The agencies use this information to aid in the prevention and treatment of these diseases. As you read about this use of health information, it is important to understand some statistical terms. **Prevalence** is the extent to which something occurs—that is, the number of existing cases. **Incidence** is the rate of occurrence—that is, the number of new cases. Prevalence and incidence are very similar terms, but they differ in that incidence captures only new cases of a disease, and prevalence captures all existing cases of the disease. By studying the

**prevalence** Rate of incidence of an occurrence, disease, or diagnosis or the number of existing cases.
**incidence** Number of occurrences of a particular event, disease, or diagnosis or the number of new cases of a disease.

**mortality rate** The frequency of death.

**morbidity rate** The rate of disease that can complicate a condition for which the patient is seeking health care services; or, the prevalence of a particular disease within a population.

**Department of Human and Health Services (DHHS)** The U.S. agency with regulatory oversight of American health care, which also provides health services to certain populations through several operating divisions.

**Centers for Disease Control and Prevention (CDC)** A federal agency that collects health information to provide research for the improvement of public health.

**Health Insurance Portability and Accountability Act (HIPAA)** Public Law 104-191, passed in 1996, that outlines the guidelines of managing patient information in terms of privacy, security, and confidentiality. The legislation also outlines penalties for noncompliance.

**protected health information (PHI)** Individually identifiable health information that is transmitted or maintained in any form or medium by covered entities or their business associates.

**Go To** Review HIPAA's role in creating transaction code sets in Chapter 6.

**American Recovery and Reinvestment Act (ARRA)** Also called the "stimulus bill," 2009 federal legislation providing many stimulus opportunities in different areas. The portion of the law that finds and sets mandates for health information technology is called the HITECH (Health Information Technology for Economic and Clinical Health) Act.

**meaningful use** A set of measures to gauge the level of health information technology used by a provider and required, in certain stages, in order to receive financial incentives from CMS.

**CMS** Centers for Medicare and Medicaid Services

number of cases and the speed at which a disease is spreading in a given population, the government can target areas for prevention and treatment.

The other statistics that are reported as a result of the review of health information are mortality rates and morbidity rates. **Mortality rates** indicate the frequency of death. **Morbidity rates** convey the prevalence and incidence of disease or sickness. Federal agencies monitor, study, and determine the impact of diseases on American public health. Morbidity rates may also refer to statistics used within the hospital to study the frequency of certain complications, such as infection rates.

Within the U.S. government, the Department of Health and Human Services (DHHS) is responsible for overseeing many agencies that have an impact on health care. The mission of the Centers for Disease Control and Prevention (CDC) is "to promote health and quality of life by preventing and controlling disease, injury, and disability" (Centers for Disease Control and Prevention, 2010). The agencies of the CDC use health information to study diseases and support their mission. The centers, institutes, and offices in the CDC are responsible for a wide variety of health issues, including minority health, human immunodeficiency virus, sexually transmitted diseases, tuberculosis prevention, occupational safety and health, chronic disease prevention and health promotion, infectious diseases, and genetics.

## NATIONAL POLICY AND LEGISLATION

Federal and state governments use health information when making decisions related to health care. Sometimes their decisions have an impact only on Medicare and Medicaid beneficiaries; at other times, their decisions influence the legislation that governs other areas of health care. For example, the Health Insurance Portability and Accountability Act (HIPAA) of 1996 affects health plans, health care clearinghouses, and providers. This legislation affects many aspects of health care, including the portability of health insurance, privacy and security of health information, and the standardization of electronic transfer of health information. Among many things HIPAA made universal are the following:

- The term *protected health information (PHI)*, the individually identifiable health information specific to a patient
- The practice of providing a "notice of privacy practice" or privacy notice to all patients receiving health care, making them aware of how their health information could and would be used by the health care provider
- National standards for electronic health information transactions supporting interoperability of software products to exchange or share health information

In February 2009, President Barack Obama signed Public Law 111-5, known publically as the American Recovery and Reinvestment Act (ARRA). Although the law was intended to do as the title suggests—provide funding to an ailing economy—it also provided stimulus money for various projects, including health information technology (HIT). The section of this law that dealt specifically with HIT is known as the Health Information Technology for Economic and Clinical Health (HITECH) Act. This act promoted many things related to health information but was specifically intended to promote implementation of the electronic health record (EHR). To ensure implementation of the EHR, the government provided incentives for providers who not only implemented an EHR but also provided proof of "meaningful use" of the product in the health care delivered to its patients. For the benefit of Americans the HITECH act defined "meaningful use" and required that certified EHR technology be used in meaningful, connected, and measurable ways.

In other aspects of federal regulation, health information is used to determine the type of coverage that Medicare or Medicaid patients receive. Specifically, the CMS (and other agencies) reviews the history of care provided to its beneficiaries and determines the cost and quality of that care to make decisions and enact legislation. These decisions and the legislation affect future coverage, reimbursement, and availability of services for Medicare and Medicaid beneficiaries.

SURGEON GENERAL'S WARNING:
Smoking by pregnant women may
result in fetal injury, premature
birth, and low birth weight.

Figure 11-2 Surgeon general's warning on tobacco for pregnant women.

Health care policy is another method the federal government uses to influence health care. The U. S. Surgeon General is an advisor, spokesperson, and leader for many health issues that affect the United States public. For example, a familiar influence of the U.S. Surgeon General is the warnings on tobacco and alcohol products manufactured in the United States (Figure 11-2).

How did the Surgeon General's office decide that this warning was necessary? The incidence and prevalence of certain diseases, combined with research requiring review of health information, indicate that tobacco and alcohol products can cause harm to society. The warning statements are one way the government has tried to affect how and when people use these products. The Surgeon General also works to educate the public and advise the President about disease prevention and health promotion in the United States.

In order to facilitate the aggregate data collection necessary to make such public health decisions, HITECH legislation requires that providers use EHR technology to collect and report data on certain diseases and treatments. Box 11-1 lists core set and additional clinical quality measures (CQMs) that are monitored in order to improve public health decision making.

## DEVELOPMENT OF COMMUNITY AWARENESS OF HEALTH CARE ISSUES

For many diseases in our society, people have organized into groups to promote awareness, raise money for research, and increase prevention. Special lapel ribbons are worn to promote awareness of a particular disease. Breast cancer and acquired immunodeficiency syndrome (AIDS) awareness groups are quite common. These groups use widely known symbols (i.e., the pink and red ribbons, respectively) to promote public education. Since such groups have become involved in health care, more people are educated about the prevention, detection, and treatment of various diseases. These groups use health information, research, and statistics to inform the public. Health information in this case may relate to different populations' exposure to a disease. Health information about the prevention, cause, and treatment of a particular disease can improve the recognition of the disease in a population. For many diseases, a diagnosis at an early stage is easier to treat, and the patient's prognosis is better.

## LITIGATION

**Litigation** is the process by which a disputed matter is settled in court. During litigation, health information is used to support a plaintiff's or a defendant's case. Health records can support or validate a claim of physician malpractice. However, the opposite can be proved if there is complete and accurate documentation showing that the physician was not at fault. The health record, when admissible in court, provides evidence of the events that are alleged in a lawsuit.

Standards of care, expert testimony, and research are other sources of health information that may be used as evidence in a trial. Standards of care provide information about the typical method of providing services to a patient with a particular diagnosis. Expert testimony in health care gives the jury information or an explanation that helps them

**aggregate data** A group of like data elements compiled to provide information about the group.

**Health Information Technology for Economic and Clinical Health (HITECH) Act** A subset of the American Recovery and Reinvestment Act (2009) legislation providing federal funding and mandates for the use of technology in health care.

**electronic health record (EHR)** A secure real-time, point-of-care, patient centric information resource for clinicians allowing access of patient information when and where needed and incorporating evidence-based decision support.

**litigation** The term used to indicate that a matter must be settled by the court and the process of engaging in legal proceedings.

**Go To** Chapter 12 provides more information about the use of health information in litigation.

**MEANINGFUL USE: CLINICAL QUALITY MEASURES**

**PHYSICIANS MUST REPORT PATIENT CARE DATA ON THE FOLLOWING CORE SET OF CLINICAL QUALITY MEASURES (CQMs)**

- Hypertension: Blood Pressure Measurement
- Preventive Care and Screening Measure Pair: (a) Tobacco Use Assessment, (b) Tobacco Cessation Intervention
- Adult Weight Screening and Follow-up

*or*

- Weight Assessment and Counseling for Children and Adolescents
- Preventive Care and Screening: Influenza Immunization for Patients 50 Years Old or Older
- Childhood Immunization Status

**PHYSICIANS MUST CHOOSE THREE ADDITIONAL MEASURES TO REPORT FROM THIS LIST**

1. Diabetes: Hemoglobin A1c Poor Control
2. Diabetes: Low Density Lipoprotein (LDL) Management and Control
3. Diabetes: Blood Pressure Management
4. Heart Failure (HF): Angiotensin-Converting Enzyme (ACE) Inhibitor or Angiotensin Receptor Blocker (ARB) Therapy for Left Ventricular Systolic Dysfunction (LVSD)
5. Coronary Artery Disease (CAD): Beta-Blocker Therapy for CAD Patients with Prior Myocardial Infarction (MI)
6. Pneumonia Vaccination Status for Older Adults
7. Breast Cancer Screening
8. Colorectal Cancer Screening
9. Coronary Artery Disease (CAD): Oral Antiplatelet Therapy Prescribed for Patients with CAD
10. Heart Failure (HF): Beta-Blocker Therapy for Left Ventricular Systolic Dysfunction (LVSD)
11. Anti-Depressant Medication Management: (a) Effective Acute Phase Treatment, (b) Effective Continuation Phase Treatment
12. Primary Open Angle Glaucoma (POAG): Optic Nerve Evaluation
13. Diabetic Retinopathy: Documentation of Presence or Absence of Macular Edema and Level of Severity of Retinopathy
14. Diabetic Retinopathy: Communication with the Physician Managing Ongoing Diabetes Care
15. Asthma Pharmacologic Therapy
16. Asthma Assessment
17. Appropriate Testing for Children with Pharyngitis
18. Oncology Breast Cancer: Hormonal Therapy for Stage IC-IIIC Estrogen Receptor/Progesterone Receptor (ER/PR) Positive Breast Cancer
19. Oncology Colon Cancer: Chemotherapy for Stage III Colon Cancer Patients
20. Prostate Cancer: Avoidance of Overuse of Bone Scan for Staging Low Risk Prostate Cancer Patients
21. Smoking and Tobacco Use Cessation, Medical Assistance: (a) Advising Smokers and Tobacco Users to Quit, (b) Discussing Smoking and Tobacco Use Cessation Medications, (c) Discussing Smoking and Tobacco Use Cessation Strategies
22. Diabetes: Eye Exam
23. Diabetes: Urine Screening
24. Diabetes: Foot Exam
25. Coronary Artery Disease (CAD): Drug Therapy for Lowering LDL (Low-Density Lipoprotein) Cholesterol
26. Heart Failure (HF): Warfarin Therapy Patients with Atrial Fibrillation
27. Ischemic Vascular Disease (IVD): Blood Pressure Management
28. Ischemic Vascular Disease (IVD): Use of Aspirin or Another Antithrombotic
29. Initiation and Engagement of Alcohol and Other Drug Dependence Treatment: (a) Initiation, (b) Engagement
30. Prenatal Care: Screening for Human Immunodeficiency Virus (HIV)
31. Prenatal Care: Anti-D Immune Globulin
32. Controlling High Blood Pressure
33. Cervical Cancer Screening
34. *Chlamydia* Screening for Women
35. Use of Appropriate Medications for Asthma
36. Low Back Pain: Use of Imaging Studies
37. Ischemic Vascular Disease (IVD): Complete Lipid Panel and LDL Control
38. Diabetes: Hemoglobin A1c Control (<8.0%)

Adapted from Centers for Medicare and Medicaid Services: Medicare EHR Incentive Program: Attestation User Guide, version 4. https://www.cms.gov/Regulations-and-Guidance/Legislation/EHRIncentivePrograms/downloads//EP_Attestation_User_Guide.pdf. Published 2012.

understand the highly technical language used in the health care profession. Research information furnishes information that the judge or jury can use to make decisions as well. Health information, whether specific to a patient or a disease, is helpful in litigation that involves a person's health or injury.

## EDUCATION

Health information is used in the education of health care professionals and patients. For example, physicians, nurses, physical therapists, and pharmacists need health information for instruction and examples as they learn how to perform their duties. The documentation of past occurrences provides an excellent opportunity to show others how to handle patient care in the future. Medical institutions use case studies of patients to teach new students about a disease process. Health care professionals are required to earn continuing education credits in their fields to keep their credentials current and to comply with professional standards. These professionals perform case studies on new and intriguing cases or present new technology for the education of their peers.

Likewise, health information is presented to patients and the community to inform them of the prevention, causes, incidence, and treatment for many diseases. This use of health information involves research, statistics, and information on new technology for treatment or prevention of disease.

**incidence** Number of occurrences of a particular event, disease, or diagnosis or the number of new cases of a disease.

## RESEARCH

**Research** is the systematic investigation into a matter to obtain or increase knowledge. Health-related research requires a tremendous amount of investigation of health information. In the health care profession, documentation from previous patient care, combined with the scientific process, allows physicians and other researchers to improve, develop, or change patient care and technology. The intention, of course, is to affect health care by giving patients the treatment they need to live longer, healthier, happier lives.

Researchers review the health information from past or present patient health care. They retrieve data specific to their topic and analyze them to look for trends or suggested ways to enhance a treatment, disease, or diagnosis. They can analyze a patient's response to medication or treatment, a prognosis, and the stages of a disease process—that is, the way in which the disease develops. Health information is documented during the course of the research. Although the health information may not be reported in the traditional form of a health record, it must be organized and stored in a manner that facilitates its retrieval and reference at a later date.

**research** The systematic investigation into a matter to find fact.

### HIT-bit

**RESEARCH**

Pharmaceutical companies perform a great deal of research on medications before receiving approval to market them to the consumer. This research involves clinical trials in which patients with a known diagnosis or predisposition are given the medication or a placebo or routine treatment. While receiving the medication, the patients are monitored to determine the impact of the medication on their condition. In later clinical trials, the new medication is administered to a wider group for more extensive study. Results of this monitoring are reported in the patients' health records.

## MANAGED CARE

Managed care is the coordination of health care benefits by an insurance company to control access and emphasize preventive care. Managed care organizations use health information internally and in their relationship with health care providers. A managed care organization chooses to use a health care provider's services on the basis of an analysis of the provider's performance. The managed care organization requires the health care facility to provide information about its services, performance, patient length of stay (LOS), outcomes, and so on. The managed care organization uses this information to determine whether to include the facility as a provider for the organization's beneficiaries.

This data gathering is part of the contract negotiation and evaluation. Before entering into a managed care contract, the managed care organization and the health care provider exchange a great deal of health information. While the facility is providing this information to the managed care organization, it also begins evaluating its own data to determine its

**managed care** A type of insurer (payer) focused on reducing health care costs, controlling expensive care, and improving the quality of patient care provided.
**outcome** The result of a patient's treatment.

**LOS** length of stay

**National Committee for Quality Assurance (NCQA)** A nonprofit entity focusing on quality in health care delivery that accredits managed care organizations.

**accreditation** Voluntary compliance with a set of standards developed by an independent agent, who periodically performs audits to ensure compliance.

**Healthcare Effectiveness Data and Information Set (HEDIS)** A performance measure data set published by health insurance companies that employers use to establish healthcare contracts on behalf of their employees.

**marketing** Promoting products or services in the hope that the consumer chooses them over the products or services of a competitor.

**dialysis** The extracorporeal elimination of waste products from bodily fluids (e.g., blood).

**Go To** Review Chapter 10 for more detail on the statistical analysis of health information.

**LOS** length of stay

ability to provide health care to this group of beneficiaries. With this information, the facility can determine whether the contract is viable.

## The National Committee for Quality Assurance

Managed care organizations can also be accredited by the National Committee for Quality Assurance (NCQA). The NCQA requires that managed care organizations comply with clinical and administrative performance standards, including a requirement for health records. Therefore the use of health information within a managed care organization has an impact not only on the benefits of the group members but also on the accreditation of the organization.

The National Committee for Quality Assurance (NCQA) was founded in 1990. It is a nonprofit entity focusing on quality in health care delivery by accrediting managed care organizations. Partnering with employers, third-party payers, providers, and consumers (patients), the NCQA has issued a special data set called **HEDIS, the Healthcare Effectiveness Data and Information Set**. With standard measures of coverages, health insurance companies and employers can use HEDIS to negotiate group plans for employees.

## MARKETING

**Marketing** is the promotion of products and services in the hope that the consumer chooses them over the products and services of a competitor. Health information can be used for marketing. Many health care facilities are in business to make a profit. Regardless of their status, for-profit or not-for-profit, they must raise enough funds to sustain their business. Facilities routinely involve themselves in situations that allow them to compare their business with that of the competition. They analyze market share and compare usage and cost of particular services and information about patient LOS. In other words, they analyze statistical information obtained from health care information databases to determine whether there is a need for new treatment or technology in the community. Perhaps a study reveals that the facility has a significant share of the maternity market. There are methods that the facility can use to promote other services to patients who have used its maternity services. Facilities also analyze trends that show a need for a specific type of health care, such as dialysis care, midwifery, sports medicine, or laser surgery.

The marketing department also uses a successful survey by an accreditation agency as a way to promote the facility in the community. Because the accreditation recognizes compliance with set standards, an accredited facility is perceived as better than one that is not accredited.

Table 11-1 reviews all of the uses of health information mentioned in the previous sections.

### TABLE 11-1

#### USES OF HEALTH INFORMATION

| USE | EXAMPLE/EXPLANATION |
|---|---|
| Improvement in patient care | The health care facility uses the documentation in the health record to determine patient care. |
| Support and collection of reimbursement | Documentation of health care is used to support and collect reimbursement for services rendered to patients. |
| Licensing, accreditation, and certifications | Health information must be maintained as a requirement of licensure. Likewise, it supports compliance with certification requirements and accreditation standards. |
| Administration | Health information is used to make decisions regarding the delivery of health care services. |
| Prevalence and incidence of morbidity and mortality | Statistics are reports to aid in the prevention and treatment of certain diseases. |
| National policy and legislation | Research and statistics are references to establish policy and legislation related to health care (i.e., Medicare and Medicaid). |

**TABLE 11-1**

**USES OF HEALTH INFORMATION—cont'd**

| USE | EXAMPLE/EXPLANATION |
|---|---|
| Development of community awareness of health care issues | Research and literature are used to educate the public regarding health care issues (e.g., cancer awareness programs). |
| Litigation | Health information is used to support or prove a fact in a lawsuit. |
| Education | Health information is used to educate patients, clinicians, allied health professionals, and the public. |
| Research | Health information is used to support and document health care research. |
| Managed care | A managed care organization evaluates health information (statistics) to determine whether to include a facility in its plan. Also, managed care organizations use health information to analyze services provided to their beneficiaries. |
| Marketing | Analysis of health information provides statistical information that the marketing department can use to promote the facility within a community. |

## EXERCISE 11-1

### Uses of Health Information

1. Can you think of another use for health information besides those listed in this chapter?
2. Each month the tumor registry personnel are required to report the _____ of breast cancer for the facility. They report this statistic by determining the number of new cases of breast cancer for the month.
3. The method of reviewing patient information during hospitalization is known as _____.
4. Successful completion of a Medicare Conditions of Participation survey results in _____ for the health care facility.
5. Health information may be used in _____to support the plaintiff's claim.
6. _____ refers to death within a population.
7. Health information may be analyzed to support a _____ campaign to promote the facility within its community.
8. The number of existing cancer cases reported by the tumor registry is known as _____.
9. _____ refers to disease within a population.
10. The monies collected by the health care facility from the payer are known as _____.
11. Physicians may perform _____ to determine the cause or best treatment for a particular disease.
12. The postdischarge review of the record is known as _____.
13. Certification may be obtained by complying with which one of the following?
    a. COP
    b. MPI
    c. Medicaid billing regulations
    d. TJC

## THE QUALITY OF HEALTH CARE

The quality of health care data has been a running theme throughout this text. It is essential to note that high-quality data are used to monitor, verify, and improve patient care, reduce inefficiencies, and lower costs.

Some people define *quality* as "something that is excellent," on the basis of a personal definition, whereas others may judge quality by the outcome of the service (success, dead, alive). The level of quality is determined by the expectations of the customer evaluating the product or service. Thus the most important concept of quality is measurement.

Customers of any product or service judge its quality. In health care, there are many customers—patients, physicians, insurance companies, attorneys, accreditation agencies, and employees, to name a few. Therefore a discussion of quality management in health care can focus on many different areas of service. Patients determine quality according to their perception of the services and care they receive. Physicians perceive the facility through the eyes of their patients, their office staff, and their professional and personal interactions with employees in the facility. Insurance companies perceive the quality of a

**outcome** The result of a patient's treatment.

**HIM** health information management

**risk management** The coordination of efforts within a facility to prevent and control inadvertent occurrences.

**case management** The coordination of the patient's care and services, including reimbursement considerations.

**The Joint Commission (TJC)** An organization that accredits and sets standards for acute care facilities, ambulatory care networks, long-term care facilities, and rehabilitation facilities, as well as certain specialty facilities, such as hospice and home care. Facilities maintaining TJC accreditation receive *deemed status* from CMS.

**Go To** Chapter 5 to review examples of preventive, detective, and corrective controls.

**preventive controls** Procedures, processes, or structures that are designed to minimize errors at the point of data collection.

**detective controls** Procedures, processes, or structures that are designed to find errors after they have been made.

**corrective controls** Procedures, processes, or structures that are designed to fix errors when they are detected. Because errors cannot always be fixed, corrective controls also include the initiation of investigation into future error prevention or detection.

facility through the cost and outcome of the services provided to their beneficiaries. Employees may perceive the facility's quality through the competence of the staff and support from the administration. Accreditation agencies perceive quality in terms of the facility's compliance with set standards. The facility itself measures quality on the basis of its priorities, market share, and customer feedback. These are only a few examples of how a facility's quality is assessed, but it is certain that a health care facility is judged or assessed from many different perspectives. However it assesses quality, the facility must use a formal method for measuring, documenting, and improving quality.

---

## HIT-bit

### QUALITY IN THE EYES OF A PATIENT AS A CUSTOMER—CUSTOMER SERVICE

Quality is perceived through the eyes of the patient according to the patient's priorities. For some patients, a prolonged life far outweighs the pain caused by a medical procedure. For example, a patient who suffers from persistent heart attacks requires bypass surgery to correct his heart dynamics and improve his chances for a longer life. The patient experiences tremendous pain from the surgery; however, if he no longer has heart attacks after the operation, his condition is improved. The patient is probably pleased with the outcome despite the intense pain that he experienced during recovery from the procedure. Therefore quality was not determined by the amount of pain experienced by the patient.

For another patient, the health care experience may end with a healthy new baby. However, during the course of the patient's stay, the nurses and employees of the facility were rude, uncooperative, and of little help to the new mother. Although the experience ended well, this patient perceived the quality as poor because of her interaction with the staff.

Note that each circumstance is different, but in each case the quality of the service is determined by the customer.

---

Health care facilities have a quality management department, usually staffed by HIM and nursing professionals, to monitor and assess quality. It is the primary responsibility of this department to educate those in the health care facility about the quality management and performance improvement process and to monitor the assessment of quality for the facility. This department monitors the facility's compliance with accreditation standards by performing a significant number of record reviews, participating in and often coordinating medical staff and facility committees, and oversees performance (quality) improvement. This department also works closely with the HIM, risk management, and case management functions to coordinate efforts to improve quality. The department is also ultimately responsible for coordinating the duties associated with on-site accreditation surveys, such as those conducted by TJC.

A discussion of quality should always begin with a review of the founding quality theories. The next section provides a simple explanation of three quality theories (though there are many others) and the use of health information in quality activities.

## QUALITY MANAGEMENT THEORIES

Customer expectation and accreditation standards prompted the development of methods to prevent, detect, or correct flaws in a product or service to improve the quality. These methods are referred to as preventive controls, detective controls, or corrective controls, respectively.

To understand why these quality management methods are important, you will find it helpful to know something about those who are credited with the founding theories: Deming, Juran, and Crosby. Their theories contain very similar and yet sometimes contradictory rules for managing quality. Although these writers did not become famous working with the health care industry, each has influenced the way the health care industry monitors quality. Therefore it would be correct to say they have inadvertently influenced the necessity to use health information to monitor quality and, in doing so, have promoted the improvement of the quality of health information.

## Deming

Of the three quality management pioneers, W. Edwards Deming was the first and is perhaps the most widely known. Deming established his reputation when the Japanese used his philosophy to rebuild their industry after World War II. As consumers increasingly chose products that were made in Japan, American industry realized the value of adopting a quality management philosophy.

Deming's philosophy is process oriented, with an emphasis on how a task is performed or a product is produced. A product that does not meet company standards must be identified before it is completed. If the problem is noted after the production is completed, the company may not be able to correct it. However, if a company inspects the process as the product is being developed, problems are more likely to be addressed and corrected before it is too late. Deming developed 14 principles to implement a successful quality management program and identified seven "deadly diseases" that would harm a quality management program. Deming's quality principles (consolidated by Rudman, 1997) are as follows:

- Change plus innovation equals stability and organizational survival.
- Organizations have a responsibility to provide employees with appropriate education and resources.
- Organizations must foster employee empowerment and pride in work.
- Organizations should emphasize process and eliminate benchmark standards and performance evaluation.
- Quality is emphasized constantly.

## Juran

Another pivotal approach to quality management is Joseph M. Juran's "quality trilogy." According to Juran, every quality management program should have a strong yet balanced infrastructure of quality planning, control, and improvement. He also defined a successful program as one that is acceptable to the entire organization; the program should be as important to the employees as it is to the administrators. Finally, Juran emphasized the value of documentation and data in the quality management program.

## Crosby

Philip Crosby is best known for the term *zero defects*. The Crosby quality management philosophy requires education of the entire organization. Education of the entire organization requires that everyone—staff employees, supervisors, managers, and administrators—learn about the program and be motivated to participate.

For a health care facility to effectively improve the quality of its care and services, it needs to adopt some method or philosophy similar to the three mentioned here. The idea of checking the quality of health care provided in the United States is not new. Quality, however, is a major focus for the health care industry.

### ▪ EXERCISE 11-2
#### Quality Management Theories

1. What is quality? Take a moment to define quality, and then discuss your thoughts with another person. Is that person's perception of quality the same as yours?
2. According to Juran's quality management philosophy, a quality management program should have a strong and balanced infrastructure of quality:
   a. planning, doing, and acting.
   b. planning, control, and improvement.
   c. management philosophy.
   d. with zero defects.

3. Your health care facility is embarking on a new quality effort. For weeks now, administrators, managers, and supervisors have been involved in meetings and training to ensure that everyone in the organization has a clear understanding of the new quality initiative message. The board has announced that this new effort will involve everyone in the organization. At the very core of this initiative is the motto "zero defects." This organization is being guided by the philosophy of which of the following thinkers?
    a. Deming
    b. Juran
    c. Crosby
    d. Shewhart

4. Which of the following philosophies emphasizes detecting problems before a product or process is completed?
    a. Deming
    b. Juran
    c. Crosby
    d. Shewhart

5. Diamonte Hospital is committed to their continuous quality improvement (CQI) philosophy. They currently have several performance improvement (PI) teams organized to address the processes associated with the delivery of patient care. This facility is most likely being guided by the theories of which of the following philosophers?
    a. Deming
    b. Juran
    c. Crosby
    d. Shewhart

## HISTORY AND EVOLUTION OF QUALITY IN HEALTH CARE

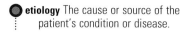 **etiology** The cause or source of the patient's condition or disease.

In the eighteenth century, hospitals had a high incidence of deadly epidemics—owing to the lack of knowledge of disease etiology and infection control—and relatively high death rates. The poor received health care in hospitals, which were often administered by charitable organizations, mostly churches. The wealthy were usually visited in their homes. The concept of quality in health care can be traced to the late nineteenth century, when hospitals finally became known as places where people could go to get well, because of advances in the knowledge of disease and infection control. During this time, two important associations were founded: the American Medical Association (AMA) and the American Hospital Association (AHA). These two associations worked diligently to promote high-quality health care through standardized medical education and hospital functions. Figure 11-3 presents a time line of the evolution of quality in health care.

### HIT-bit

**AMERICAN MEDICAL ASSOCIATION AND AMERICAN HOSPITAL ASSOCIATION**

The American Medical Association (AMA) was founded in 1847.

The American Hospital Association began as the Association of Hospital Superintendents in 1899. In 1910 the name was changed to the AHA (http://www.aha.org/about/history.html).

These associations remain prestigious members of the health care industry. Their missions still guide improvement—whether focusing on the education of physicians or the physical health care facilities. Their activities and priorities seek public health excellence.

### Medical Education

Before the existence of formal medical education, physicians were trained through an apprenticeship. By the early twentieth century, many medical institutions existed to educate physicians. But the education of these physicians was not standardized. Each institution could decide which courses were required to obtain a medical degree. For this reason, the

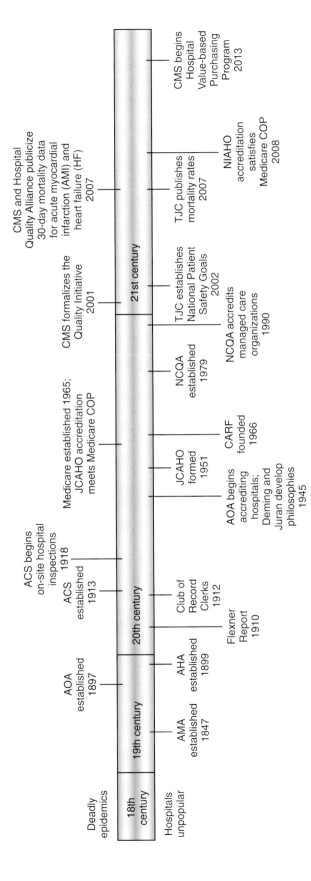

**Figure 11-3** Timeline of the evolution of quality in health care. ACS, American College of Surgeons; AHA, American Hospital Association; AMA, American Medical Association; AOA, American Osteopathic Association; CARF, Commission on Accreditation of Rehabilitation Facilities; CMS, Centers for Medicare and Medicaid Services; COP, Conditions of Participation; JCAHO, Joint Commission on Accreditation of Healthcare Organizations; NCQA, National Committee for Quality Assurance; NIAHO, National Integrated Accreditation for Healthcare Organizations; THC, The Joint Commission.

**AMA** American Medical Association

**accreditation** Voluntary compliance with a set of standards developed by an independent agent, who periodically performs audits to ensure compliance.

**American College of Surgeons (ACS)** A national professional organization that supports surgeons, to encourage higher quality of care for surgical patients.

**health record** Also called *record* or *medical record*. Contains all of the data collected for an individual patient.

health care profession increased in size and number of physicians, but the quality of patient care was not improving. Although having more physicians seemed like a good solution to an ailing population, the facts suggested that more needed to be done to improve the quality of health care. Medical institutions needed a standardized mechanism to guide the training of physicians.

Abraham Flexner studied the quality of medical education in the United States. His report in 1910 documented critical issues and discrepancies in medical education. The findings in the Flexner Report prompted the closing of many training institutions, revisions of the required curriculum in those that remained, and implementation by the AMA of a mechanism for accreditation of medical education institutions. It also led to a validation of competency for medical professionals.

## Standardization and Accreditation

During this period, most patients encountered health care in hospitals for surgical intervention. Not long after the Flexner report, in 1913 the **American College of Surgeons (ACS)** was founded as an association of surgeons "to improve the quality of care for the surgical patient by setting high standards for surgical education and practice" (American College of Surgeons, 2012). The ACS assumed responsibility for reviewing the quality of health care provided to patients in hospitals. Its efforts to analyze quality involved review of information from patient health records, which revealed insufficient documentation of patient care.

In an attempt to standardize contents of the patient health record so that future reviews could provide useful information, the ACS developed the Hospital Standardization Program. This program established standards, or rules, by which the ACS would survey hospitals to assess quality of care. The first survey after the establishment of the Hospital Standardization Program revealed that only 13% of the hospitals surveyed (with 100 beds or more) met the standards. The ACS then determined that for a facility to be considered a hospital it must meet a set of minimum standards. These minimum standards required health records to be maintained in a timely, accurate fashion and specified the minimum content or required documentation for a health record (Box 11-2).

### HIT-bit

**"IF IT ISN'T DOCUMENTED, IT DIDN'T HAPPEN"**

The proof is in the documentation. The old saying, "If it isn't documented, it didn't happen," had an effect on the history of health care. The lack of documentation prohibited the effective study of quality to improve health care.

### BOX 11-2 MEDICAL RECORD SPECIFICATIONS—MINIMUM STANDARDS

A complete case record should be developed, consisting of the following information:
- Patient identification data
- Complaint
- Personal and family history
- History of current illness
- Physical examination
- Special examinations (consultations, radiography, clinical laboratory)
- Provisional or working diagnosis
- Medical and surgical treatments
- Progress notes
- Gross and microscopic findings
- Final diagnosis
- Condition on discharge
- Follow-up
- Autopsy findings in the event of death

By the 1950s, the ACS was overwhelmed by the demand of hospitals for surveys. The establishment of the Joint Commission on the Accreditation of Hospitals (JCAH) was a collaborative effort supported by the AMA, AHA, and ACS. The JCAH was established to relieve the ACS of the responsibility of surveying hospitals. Over time, JCAH accreditation became popular in nonacute health care settings, and in 1987 the organization was renamed the Joint Commission on Accreditation of Healthcare Organizations (JCAHO), now called The Joint Commission (TJC).

## Accreditation Agencies

Accreditation is a common indicator of quality and compliance with predetermined standards in today's health care industry. TJC is no longer the only accreditation agency. In 2008, the CMS approved accreditation by the **National Integrated Accreditation for Healthcare Organizations (NIAHO)** for acute care facilities. NIAHO is a subsidiary of Det Norske Veritas (DNV), a Norwegian foundation that specializes in risk management. DNV focuses on the maritime, energy, food and beverage, and health care industries. NIAHO hospital accreditation is based on the CMS's Conditions of Participation (COP). Surveys are conducted annually and are focused on education and performance improvement. Acute care facilities that maintain accreditation from either TJC or the NIAHO receive "deemed status" from the CMS, meaning they satisfy the compliance audit portion of the Conditions of Participation and are therefore able to receive reimbursement from Medicare and Medicaid.

Other examples of accreditation bodies are the Commission on Accreditation of Rehabilitation Facilities (CARF), which accredits rehabilitation facilities; the American Osteopathic Association (AOA); Healthcare Facilities Accreditation Program (HFAP); the Accreditation Association for Ambulatory Health Care, which accredits ambulatory care facilities; and the NCQA, which accredits managed care organizations.

---

## HIT-bit

### HISTORY OF THE AMERICAN HEALTH INFORMATION MANAGEMENT ASSOCIATION

The history of the American Health Information Management Association (AHIMA) can be traced back to the Club of Record Clerks, which was organized in 1912 by a small group of women known as medical record librarians. The group officially initiated the Association of Record Librarians of North America (ARLNA), which included members from both the United States and Canada. The first president of this organization was Grace Whiting Myers. Eventually, the members from Canada and the United States separated, and the U.S. organization became known as the American Association of Medical Record Librarians (AAMRL). In 1970 the association changed its name to the American Medical Record Association (AMRA). AMRA conferred the following credentials: Accredited Record Technician (ART) and Registered Record Administrator (RRA). Over the next 20 years, the roles and responsibilities of the ART and the RRA reflected more diverse areas. By 1991 the association voted to change the name of the AMRA to the American Health Information Management Association (AHIMA). Since that time, the credentials have also changed from ART to Registered Health Information Technician (RHIT) and from RRA to Registered Health Information Administrator (RHIA). The change from medical records to health information was motivated by the changes in the health care environment and in the responsibilities of the association's members. HIM professionals hold positions in various roles, health care settings, and associated areas, such as hospitals, alternative health care settings, consulting, accreditation agencies, managed care companies, case management, quality management, insurance agencies, and attorneys' offices.

AHIMA is a membership organization with offices in Chicago and Washington, D.C.

---

**ACS** American College of Surgeons
**AMA** American Medical Association
**AHA** American Hospital Association

**The Joint Commission (TJC)** An organization that accredits and sets standards for acute care facilities, ambulatory care networks, long-term care facilities, and rehabilitation facilities, as well as certain specialty facilities, such as hospice and home care. Facilities maintaining TJC accreditation receive *deemed status* from the CMS.

**National Integrated Accreditation for Healthcare Organizations (NIAHO)** A compliance and accreditation entity partnered with CMS to ensure quality and standards in acute care settings. Facilities maintaining NIAHO accreditation receive *deemed status* from the CMS.
**risk management** The coordination of efforts within a facility to prevent and control inadvertent occurrences.
**Conditions of Participation (COP)** The terms under which a facility is eligible to receive reimbursement from Medicare.
**performance improvement (PI)** Also known as *quality improvement (QI)* or *continuous quality improvement (CQI)*. Refers to the process by which a facility reviews its services or products to ensure quality.

**Commission on Accreditation of Rehabilitation Facilities (CARF)** An organization that accredits behavioral health and rehabilitation facilities.

**NCQA** National Committee for Quality Assurance

**Go To** In Chapter 1, Table 1-8 provides a list of major accreditation agencies.

## ORYX

The evaluation and assurance of quality has always been central to TJC's accreditation of health care facilities. But periodic on-site surveys can only present a "snapshot" of a

**ORYX** A data set collection tool used by TJC to measure the quality of patient care in hospitals.

**outcome** The result of a patient's treatment.

**National Patient Safety Goals** Guidance created by TJC to recommend patient safety measures in accredited facilities.

**mortality rate** The frequency of death.

**CMS** Centers for Medicare and Medicaid Services

**certification** Approval by an outside agency, such as the federal or state government, indicating that the health care facility has met a set of predetermined standards.

**reimbursement** The amount of money that the health care facility receives from the party responsible for paying the bill.

facility's performance. Efforts to integrate a more continuous view of a health care organization's performance into TJC's accreditation process resulted in the ORYX initiative, introduced in 1997. Under ORYX, hospitals, long-term care facilities, behavioral health facilities, and home health organizations transmit data to TJC on a number of performance measures relating to patient care and outcomes. These core measure sets (which ask for data on acute myocardial infarction [AMI], children's asthma care, heart failure, pneumonia, stroke, and substance abuse, to name a few) are intended to standardize comparison, using data that the facility has already collected. Analysis of the hospital's performance using more current data allows the facility to react to the most current data, taking steps toward improvement.

### Patient Safety Goals

TJC continued to promote quality by establishing **National Patient Safety Goals** for health care facilities in 2002. These goals were established to help TJC facilities focus on issues directly related to patient safety. TJC created an advisory group of knowledgeable patient safety experts to help them identify the goals; these experts included physicians, nurses, pharmacists, risk managers, and clinical engineers. The patient safety goals provide guidance or recommend procedures on issues like accurate patient identification, communication among health care providers, medicine safety, health care–associated infections, reduction of patient falls, and risk assessment to ensure patient safety.

### Quality Check

In 2004 TJC also began an outcomes measurement program designed to hold health care facilities publicly accountable by publishing mortality rates for specific diseases so that consumers would have this information available when choosing a health care provider. The first publicly published outcomes for core measures were of mortality rates for acute myocardial infarctions (AMIs) and heart failure, followed by pneumonia in 2008. Making this information available to patients was such a success that the CMS now also reports data for hospitals on the 30-day readmission rates for patients with these conditions as well as for the in-hospital adverse events.

Information is made available to the public through a Web site called QualityCheck.org. This Web site provides information to consumers about the accreditation and certification of health care facilities. It offers free reports of a hospital's performance measures, National Patient Safety Goal compliance, National Quality Improvement Goal performance, patient satisfaction data, and special quality awards received by the facility; it identifies facilities that have been certified for disease-specific care and health care staffing.

## Medicare and Medicaid's Hospital Quality Initiative

When the federal government began paying for health care, the quality and cost of care for the beneficiaries became the government's concern. Thus the federal government began performing reviews of the actual care received by Medicare patients through audits of patient health records. Reviewers travelled to health care facilities and looked at the health record documentation to be certain that Medicare patients were receiving appropriate care. If the documentation did not comply with the Medicare regulations and reflect high-quality care, the facility was cited and its administrators had to explain why the services did not meet minimal standards; in some cases, a return of reimbursements was required.

In the twenty-first century, the health care industry is heavily regulated and surveyed for compliance with standards and quality. In 2001 the CMS formalized the Quality Initiative, which uses surveys and quality measures to make information about the care received at hospitals more transparent. Hospitals that can compare the quality of care they deliver with that of other hospitals and a public who can view costs and ratings of facilities create strong incentives to improve.

### Value-Based Purchasing

Always looking for ways to motivate hospitals to improve, the CMS began a new plan in 2013 called the Hospital Value-Based Purchasing Program. According to the CMS

(2012a), the program is designed to reimburse acute care hospitals a value-based incentive, "based either on how well the hospitals perform on certain quality measures or how much the hospitals' performance improves on certain quality measures from their performance during a baseline period." As with other improvement plans, a hospital must establish a baseline of data in order to measure improvement. In other words, the facility will collect data on specific performance measures, and then its improvement will be based on bettering those measures in future years. This type of plan requires that a hospital establish performance improvement plans or programs, discussed later in this chapter.

## Quality Improvement Organizations

CMS reviews are performed by a **Quality Improvement Organization (QIO)**, a private team of health care professionals contracting with the CMS to inspect the quality of health care delivery and to address beneficiaries' concerns about the care they have received from providers. QIOs use that information to improve overall quality. There is one QIO for each state, each U.S. territory, and the District of Colombia (for a total of 53 nationwide); these are largely not-for-profit organizations, whose 3-year contracts with the CMS are called the statement (or scope) of work (SOW) (CMS, 2012c).

Formerly called peer review organizations (PROs), QIOs are administered under CMS's **Health Care Quality Improvement Program (HCQIP)**. As stated on QualityNet (2012), CMS's news Web site, "QIOs work with consumers, physicians, hospitals, and other caregivers to refine care delivery systems to make sure patients get the right care at the right time, particularly among underserved populations. The program also safeguards the integrity of the Medicare trust fund by ensuring payment is made only for medically necessary services and investigates beneficiary complaints about quality of care."

To that end, QIOs review the aggregate and secondary data reported by facilities and perform onsite reviews of hospitals and other providers, examining health records and outcomes and conducting specific case reviews, during which they look for anomalies that may result in poor patient care. For example, a Medicare beneficiary (or an individual on his or her behalf) may file a claim if the beneficiary felt he or she was discharged from a hospital too early. In that instance, a QIO review of the case is mandatory: The state's QIO will examine the health record, including admission date, admitting diagnosis, and treatments provided, to determine whether the patient's discharge was appropriate and whether he or she was "medically stable" at the time of discharge. Reviewers in the QIO are trained to identify certain criteria and to refer the matter to a physician within the QIO to decide whether the discharge was appropriate. These sorts of cases may also be flagged if an individual is readmitted to a facility within a certain time, usually 30 days.

In other cases, QIOs analyze secondary data to look for trends that might indicate inefficiencies, or even fraud, both of which consume resources unnecessarily. A QIO review is prompted if a hospital requests an adjustment to a higher-weighted diagnosis related group (DRG), for example, which may indicate an abuse of CMS reimbursement. But a QIO may also initiate a review on the basis of larger patterns displayed by a particular provider over time; these patterns include the following (CMS, 2012b):

- Inappropriate, unreasonable, or medically unnecessary care (including setting of care issues)
- Incorrect DRG assignment
- Inappropriate transfers
- Premature discharges
- Insufficient, poor documentation, or patterns of failing to provide medical records

The goal of all these reviews is to improve the quality of health care while reducing costs. QIOs look for ways to improve the delivery of care by interacting directly with providers, reviewing health records, examining patient outcomes, and finding trends that might provide opportunities for improvement. The HCQIP oversees individual QIOs in the Quality Improvement Organization Program, collecting data for overall quality improvement. With this information, this organization sets national focal points for all QIOs in the scope of work, reviewing clinical topics that suggest disparity in care. The 8th

---

**Quality Improvement Organization (QIO)** An organization that contracts with payers, specifically Medicare and Medicaid, to review care and reimbursement issues.

**Health Care Quality Improvement Program (HCQIP)** A quality initiative established by the Balanced Budget Act (1997) that administers various review processes in order to identify and improve care outcomes for Medicare beneficiaries.

**outcome** The result of a patient's treatment.

**admitting diagnosis** The reason given by the physician for initiating the order for the patient to be placed into care in a hospital.

**discharge** Discharge occurs when the patient leaves the care of the facility to go home, for transfer to another health care facility, or by death. Also refers to the status of a patient.

**diagnosis related groups (DRGs)** A collection of health care descriptions organized into statistically similar categories.

**CMS** Centers for Medicare and Medicaid Services

**HCQIP** Health Care Quality Improvement Program

**SOW** statement of work

**random selection** In sampling of a population, a method that ensures that all cases have equal chances of being selected and that the cases are selected in no particular order or pattern.

**coding** The assignment of alphanumerical values to a word, phrase, or other nonnumerical expression. In health care, coding is the assignment of numerical values to diagnosis and procedure descriptions.

**billing** The process of submitting health insurance claims or rendering invoices.

**claim** The application to an insurance company for reimbursement of services rendered.

**Medicare Administrative Contractor (MAC)** Regional, private contractor who processes reimbursement claims for the CMS.

**Medicaid Integrity Contractor (MIC)** A contractor who works with CMS to identify fraud and waste through claims audits and other data collection activities.

**performance improvement (PI)** Also known as *quality improvement (QI)* or *continuous quality improvement (CQI)*. Refers to the process by which a facility reviews its services or products to ensure quality.

**recovery audit contractors (RACs)** Entities contracting with the CMS that audit providers, using DRG assignment and other data to identify overpayments and underpayments.

**revenue cycle** The groups of processes that identify, record, and report the financial transactions that result from the facility's clinical relationship with a patient.

**retrospective review** Review occurring after the act or event (i.e., after the provider received payment).

**algorithm** A procedure (set of instructions) for accomplishing a task.

**CMS** Centers for Medicare and Medicaid Services

and 9th SOWs (2005-2008 and 2009-2011) looked for specific treatments that have shown efficacy on the basis of public health data in a variety of provider settings. Over time, acute myocardial infarctions (heart attacks), pneumonia, breast cancer, diabetes, heart failure, and end-stage renal disease have all been clinical topics of focus. The aims of the 10th SOW (2011-2014) include reducing readmissions, hospital-acquired conditions, and promoting immunizations and screenings.

### Hospital Compare

The CMS also monitors quality from the standpoint of the patient by administering the Hospital Consumer Assessment of Healthcare Providers and Systems (HCAHPS) survey. Feedback from a random selection of discharged patients is compiled on the basis of questions about their experiences at the facility. Patients are asked to rate their communication with clinicians and other hospital staff, the cleanliness and quietness of the hospital, as well as to give overall ratings.

With the implementation of a standardized survey on a national level, hospitals have a means to compare their performance with that of other facilities and to set goals to improve the quality of their delivery. Furthermore, because the results of surveys are made public, at http://hospitalcompare.hhs.gov, potential patients as consumers of health care can view ratings for each hospital and use that information to choose their providers. This availability provides strong incentives for hospitals to improve the quality of their services.

### Programs to Combat Fraud

As discussed in Chapter 7, errors in coding and billing can lead to denial of reimbursement. Third party payers conduct numerous audits for a variety of quality attributes, particularly billing and the quality of the documentation that supports billing. The CMS conducts audits of Medicare and Medicaid claims through several contractors: Medicare Administrative Contractors (MAC) and **Medicaid Integrity Contractors (MICs)**.

Some of these audits are conducted for benchmarking and provider performance evaluation and improvement. The Program for Evaluating Payment Patterns Electronic Report (PEPPER) and Comprehensive Error Rate Testing (CERT) are examples of such audits.

PEPPER provides hospitals with a Microsoft Excel report that can be used by the health care facility to perform internal audits on medical claims. The report trends data for the facility as well as offers comparison with other hospitals, helping the health care facility identify the types of bills that are susceptible to errors, "over-coding" (adding codes not reflected in the documentation), "under-coding," (failing to add codes that are appropriate based on the documentation), and questionable medical necessity admissions. With this information, hospitals can initiate internal review of health records in association with coding and billing to ensure accuracy. These internal reviews often give the hospital information that promotes quality improvement in areas like physician documentation, medical coding, and patient care.

The CERT program uses a random sampling of Medicare claims to measure errors associated with payments in the Medicare fee-for-service (FFS) program. The process includes review of health records with the associated claim to determine whether they are in compliance with the CMS coverage, coding, and billing rules. Noncompliance results in the sending of letters to the health care provider the note the errors and overpayment or underpayment as appropriate. The health care facility can use notices from this program to identify internal areas of focus for performance improvement.

Other audits are specifically designed to target potential bill errors, fraud, and abuse. MICs and Medicaid recovery audit contractors (RACs) are examples of contractors whose audits are focused on identifying and correcting billing errors. Until recently, audits were entirely retrospective, conducted sometimes years after the dates of service and completion of the revenue cycle. In 2011 the CMS raised awareness among providers that prepayment audits were in development. Unlike a retrospective audit (review), which can recoup payment from the provider, a prepayment audit prevents the erroneous payment from taking place. Prepayment audits are driven by data-mining algorithms: software programs that compare data elements and produce exception reports of potential errors. So instead of relying on detective and corrective controls to recoup payments, CMS is developing and implementing more sophisticated preventive controls over billing errors. Changes to these programs occur frequently; therefore the details are best obtained from the CMS Web site (www.cms.gov).

---

## HIT-bit

### FRAUD

*Fraud* is the wilful intention to deceive for personal gain. The term fraud is used to describe such a false claim. False claims that are not the result of wilful intent are termed abuse. In either case, the payer is wrongfully billed. The facility should have a compliance plan in place to ensure that the coding of health information and the billing comply with federal, state, and coding guideline requirements.

---

## ▪ EXERCISE 11-3
### History and Evolution of Health Care Quality

1. Which association was the first to recognize a need for quality in health care and was organized for the purpose of promoting it?
2. What was the name of the first program (set of standards) designed to measure quality in a health care setting?
3. Voluntary accreditation attained by successfully undergoing a survey according to the standards set forth in the comprehensive accreditation manual for hospitals is given by which of the following organizations?
   a. MCOP
   b. CMS
   c. Medicare
   d. TJC
4. Which of the following groups was the predecessor of TJC?
   a. Hospital Standardization
   b. AHIMA
   c. NCQA
   d. ACS
5. The _____ preceded TJC in the survey of hospitals in comparison with set standards.
6. Which of the following is *NOT* a National Patient Safety Goal?
   a. Patient identification
   b. Acute myocardial infarction
   c. Communication among health care providers
   d. Reduce falls
7. List the first two core measures established by CMS.

---

## MONITORING THE QUALITY OF HEALTH INFORMATION

Health records are among the primary documents used by health care facilities to evaluate compliance with the standards set by the accreditation or certification agencies. In brief, health information documentation is analyzed to review the quality of patient care, and this analysis of documentation helps the facility recognize opportunities to improve its performance. This analysis of quality should occur both concurrently (while the patient is in the facility) and retrospectively (after the patient has been discharged).

The HIM department is responsible for monitoring the quality of health information. Each function in the HIM department exists to ensure quality in the documentation; the department, led by a credentialed HIM professional, coordinates review of HIM functions to ensure that the health information is timely, complete, accurate, and valid. The director of HIM must manage the department functions in a manner that promotes useful and accurate information. The director and other personnel ensure quality by reviewing the functions of the HIM department and by developing standards and review processes to monitor competency and compliance with these standards.

**acute care facility** A health care facility in which patients have an average length of stay less than 30 days and that has an emergency department, operating suite, and clinical departments to handle a broad range of diagnoses and treatments.

**history and physical (H&P)** Health record documentation comprising the patient's history and physical examination; a formal, dictated copy must be included in the patient's health care record within 24 hours of admission for inpatient facilities.

**progress notes** The physician's record of each interaction with the patient.

**physician's orders** The physician's directions regarding the patient's care. Also refers to the data collection device on which these elements are captured.

**discharge summary** The recap of an inpatient stay, usually dictated by the attending physician and transcribed into a formal report.

**Go To** See Chapter 4 for the contents of a complete health record.

**face sheet** The first page in a paper record. Usually contains at least the demographic data and contains space for the physician to record and authenticate the discharge diagnoses and procedures. In many facilities, the admission record is also used as the face sheet.

**consent** An agreement or permission to receive health care services.

**anesthesia report** An anesthesiologist's documentation of patient evaluations before, during, and after surgery, including the specifics of the administration of anesthesia.

## Data Quality Characteristics

The value of data quality cannot be overemphasized. As the health care industry moves to an electronic health record, the individual fields are subject to tighter quality review and scrutiny than in a paper record. Recall that in paper records, variation in documentation styles is supported by free text fields that are often converted to menu selections or shorter narrative blocks. As such, it is critical that those who create, document, and review the data share an understanding of the scope and nature of the data to be collected. To that end, AHIMA recently updated its data quality management model (AHIMA, 2012). The key characteristics therein of quality data are discussed here.

### Timely Health Information

Timeliness of health information relates to documentation of an event close to the time it occurred. Health information should be documented as events occur, treatment is performed, or results are noticed. Delaying documentation could cause information to be omitted. Reports must be dictated and typed in a timely manner.

The following are examples of timeliness:

- In the physician's office, the patient documents the history before seeing the physician, and the physical examination is completed during the office visit.
- In an acute care facility, the history and physical (H&P) must be on the record within 24 hours of the patient's admission to the facility, and progress notes must be documented daily. Physician's orders must be dated and timed. A discharge summary should be recorded when the patient is discharged and no later than 30 days after discharge.

### Complete Health Information

Completeness (comprehensiveness) of health information requires that the health record contain all pertinent documents with all of the appropriate documentation—that is, face sheet, H&P, consent forms, progress notes, anesthesia record, operative report, recovery room record, discharge notes, nursing documentation, and so on. Incomplete records can jeopardize patient care, impair correct reimbursement, and skew data used for administrative purposes. Review of health records to ensure that each record is complete is called *quantitative analysis*. Concurrent review of records by clinical areas to ensure completeness is an important quality control activity. Comprehensiveness also refers to the compilation of the record from all sources in which it is collected. If multiple systems are involved, then all systems must be accessed to obtain the complete record.

### Accurate Health Information

Accuracy of health information requires that the documentation reflect the event as it really happened, including all pertinent details and relevant facts. Review of health records for pertinent documentation involves examination of the content of each document. All of the pages in the health record must be for the same patient and also for the same visit. In the electronic record, the validity of specific fields can be checked at the time of data entry. For health information to be valid, the data or information documented must be of an acceptable or allowable predetermined value or within a specified parameter. This requirement particularly pertains to the documentation of clinical services provided to the patient. For example, there are predetermined accepted values for blood pressure and temperature.

### Accessibility

In a paper environment, accessibility has traditionally meant that the record is available promptly, as needed, and is securely protected during processing, transportation, and long-term storage from inappropriate viewing and use. The electronic record can improve the speed with which users can obtain patient data as well as download and manipulate it. However, the assignment of access rights can be complicated. Data must be provided, as needed, but only to those with a legal right to obtain it.

## Data Consistency

Every time data is collected, it must be collected the same way, according to the specifications of the field. For example, if the facility collects birth weight in grams, then all birth weights must be collected and recorded in grams. If the software into which it is collected converts the grams to pounds and ounces for some reporting purpose, the conversion formula must be correct. If the facility uses case mix index to estimate reimbursement and track efficiency, the data should be normalized to MS-DRGs for weighting purposes.

## Data Currency

Data are useful only if they reflect the values that pertain to the period under review. For example, representation of 2012 data in ICD-10-CM or PCS format may be useful for gap analysis or planning purposes; however, communication with payers in that format is not current. Similarly, once a diagnosis code has been updated, the prior year's code is not current and should not be used.

## Data Definition

As discussed in Chapter 2, the fields used to compile a patient record must be clearly defined. A data dictionary codifies this effort and provides a reference point for data collection device creators as well as users to understand exactly what a field represents and how to collect and record that data.

## Data Granularity

**Granularity** refers to the level of detail with which data is collected, recorded, or calculated. For example, the individual length of stay for a patient is measured in whole days. However, the average length of stay for multiple patients is generally represented with one or more decimal places, such as 4.1 days or 4.13 days. To an administrator using average length of stay for control purposes, a movement from 4.13 to 4.14 days could be significant.

## Data Precision

For both data collection and reporting purposes, the use of the data drives the precision with which it is represented. For example, it is not useful for billing purposes to know merely that the patient is a resident of a particular state, the exact street address, city, and zip code are also required. However, for analysis of a facility's catchment area, the zip code or county may be the level of precision required.

## Data Relevancy

Relevancy has two components; should the data be collected at all and, if so, is it being collected in a way that is meaningful in light of the purpose for collecting it? Collection of data should take place only if there is a reason for collecting it that is meaningful in context. For example, hair color has no relevance as a data item to collect regarding a patient entering the hospital for an appendectomy. However, it is a critical data element in reporting to security an individual behaving suspiciously in or around the facility. On the other hand, race is a field that is required to be collected per the Uniform Hospital Discharge Data Set (UHDDS). National Uniform Billing Committee (NUBC) has very specific categories for collecting the field defined as race. Collecting race as "black" or "white" would not be relevant for this purpose.

## Quality Assurance

Several aspects of monitoring quality involve ensuring that the employees in the HIM department are performing their functions appropriately and that the functions work correctly to promote the employees' productivity. Assembly, analysis, coding, abstracting, completion of records, filing/archiving, release of information, and transcription or document creation all must happen within specified time frames to enhance the timeliness,

---

**case mix index** The arithmetic average (mean) of the relative weights of all health care cases in a given period.

**diagnosis related groups (DRGs)** A collection of health care descriptions organized into statistically similar categories.

**field** A collection or series of related characters. A field may contain a word, a group of words, a number, or a code, for example.

**data dictionary** A list of details that describe each field in a database.

**granularity** The level of detail with which data is collected, recorded, or calculated.

**Uniform Hospital Discharge Data Set (UHDDS)** The mandated data set for hospital inpatients.

**NUBC** National Uniform Billing Committee

**assembly** The reorganization of a paper record into a standard order.

**analysis** The review of a record to evaluate its completeness, accuracy, or compliance with predetermined standards or other criteria.

**coding** The assignment of alphanumerical values to a word, phrase, or other nonnumerical expression. In health care, coding is the assignment of numerical values to diagnosis and procedure descriptions.

**abstracting** The recap of selected fields from a health record to create an informative summary. Also refers to the activity of identifying such fields and entering them into a computer system.

**release of information (ROI)** The term used to describe the HIM department function that provides disclosure of patient health information.

**quality assurance (QA)** A method for reviewing health care functions to determine their compliance with predetermined standards that requires action to correct noncompliance and then follow-up review to ascertain whether the correction was effective.

**QA** quality assurance

**TJC** The Joint Commission

completion, accuracy, and validity of the record. The monitoring of these functions is called quality assessment or **quality assurance (QA)**. QA monitoring ensures that HIM functions are working effectively within the department's standards. QA is a retrospective analysis, performed at the end of a patient's visit or after discharge.

## Quality Assurance in the Health Information Management Department

HIM department managers set the standards for performance of HIM functions. Taking into consideration all of the regulations governing health records, HIM professionals determine for their facility the appropriate level of quality and productivity for each function. For example, let us assume that the HIM professional at a particular facility determined that assembly and analysis should occur within 24 hours of the patient's discharge and that the records should be assembled correctly 100% of the time (Table 11-2). This standard required that patient records be checked to ensure that the function was happening according to the standard. Plainly stated: Were records being assembled within 24 hours of discharge (every day) and were they assembled correctly 100% of the time? A supervisor would monitor assembly on a daily basis to monitoring compliance with this standard. The results of the review would be documented for review by the HIM director. If the review revealed that the records were not being assembled correctly 100% of the time or not being assembled within the 24-hour time frame, then action was taken to correct the problem. The same process was applied to the other standards set for HIM functions; reviews were performed, compliance was noted, and any problems were actively addressed to prevent recurrence. QA reviews of coding ensured that the coding staff was accurately coding all records in a timely fashion. In a QA review of the release of information function, the HIM supervisor reviewed several requests to ensure that the release occurred in a timely fashion and that the facility's procedure for release of information was followed.

Today, the evaluation and monitoring of HIM functions remain important. TJC continues to require that facilities monitor the quality of their functions. The focus, however, is on quality improvement.

### HIT-bit

**QUALITY ASSURANCE VERSUS PERFORMANCE IMPROVEMENT**

The 1984 TJC standards outlined specific instructions requiring each department in the health care facility to develop a monitoring and evaluation program. By requiring the participation of all staff and departments in the facility, TJC planned to move health care facilities from retrospective QA to performance improvement.

## TABLE 11-2

### QUALITY MONITORS FOR HEALTH INFORMATION MANAGEMENT FUNCTIONS

| HIM FUNCTION | STANDARD (EXAMPLE) | HOW THE FUNCTION IS AUDITED |
|---|---|---|
| Assembly | Health records are assembled within 24 hours of discharge with 100% accuracy. | Supervisor reviews a sample of records monthly to check accuracy. |
| Analysis | Health records are analyzed (quantitative) within 24 hours of discharge with 100% accuracy. | Supervisor reviews a sample of records monthly to check accuracy. |
| Coding | All records are coded within 48 hours of discharge with 100% accuracy. | Supervisor reviews a sample of records monthly to check accuracy. |
| Abstracting | Health information is correctly abstracted on all patient records within 72 hours of discharge. | Supervisor reviews a sample of records monthly to check accuracy. |
| Filing | Health records are filed in correct filing order 100% of the time. | Supervisor reviews a section of the file area monthly to check accuracy. |
| Release of information | Requests for information are processed according to law and hospital policy within 48 hours of the request, 100% of the time. | Supervisor reviews a sample of requests monthly to check accuracy. |

# Performance Improvement

**Performance improvement (PI)**, also known as *quality improvement* (QI), refers to the process by which a facility reviews its services or products to ensure quality. It is no longer acceptable to simply meet a standard; the facility should always seek to improve its performance. PI can focus on one task or job in the facility or focus on a process that involves more than one department. This makes PI a hospital-wide function that occurs *interdepartmentally* and *intradepartmentally*. The prefix *inter-* means "between" or "among," therefore **interdepartmental** means "between departments." The prefix *intra-* means "within," therefore **intradepartmental** means "within a department." It can be multidisciplinary, involving employees to represent each area of the health care facility. Employees participate in teams to reach a solution to improve a process. All employees are encouraged to improve their work, surroundings, efforts, processes, and products. The philosophy of PI is that by improving the process, the outcome—patient care—will ultimately be improved.

> ## HIT-bit
>
> ### INTERDEPARTMENTAL OR INTRADEPARTMENTAL
>
> To help you remember the difference, think about interstate highways, which you would use to go between the states. You would have an interdepartmental meeting between departments. Since the prefix *intra-* means "within" (e.g., intravenous injections, which are delivered into, or within, the blood vessels), an intradepartmental meeting would be one within a department.

The PI process begins with a formal policy on or statement of how the facility will conduct and document improvement efforts. The organization-wide PI process is directed by a committee, either the medical executive committee (MEC) (discussed later in this chapter) or another committee established strictly for this purpose. All departments are required to improve processes both internally and in their relationships with other departments. Most facilities choose a model designed by a QI philosopher. The model not only helps the facility document the PI process to support accreditation and certification standards but also provides a measure for the facility to monitor its efforts internally. Multidisciplinary teams use the chosen model to accomplish PI.

Several PI models provide structures for a health care facility to follow. Ultimately, one model is chosen, and the entire organization uses this model to facilitate and document PI.

### Plan, Do, Check, and Act Method

A popular method for monitoring and improving performance is the Plan, Do, Check, and Act method, also called the PDCA method, which was developed by Walter Shewhart.

The PDCA method is easy to understand and follow, making it one of the most widely used models (Figure 11-4). The *Plan* phase consists of data collection and analysis to propose a solution for the identified problem. The *Do*, or implementation, phase tests the proposed solution. The *Check* phase monitors the effectiveness of the solution over time. The *Act* phase formalizes the changes that have proved effective in the Do and Check stages.

The key point to remember is that a process is being improved. The area of concentration is the process itself, and not any one individual's job performance. For a process to be improved, all persons who are involved in the process must be part of the team. For example, an interdepartmental PI team has employees representing each department involved in a process that affects them. An intradepartmental PI team works to improve a process within a department; for example, the HIM department could organize a team to improve the effectiveness of the postdischarge query process. Box 11-3 shows a PI example applying the PDCA method to this process.

**performance improvement (PI)** Also known as *quality improvement (QI)* or *continuous quality improvement (CQI)*. Refers to the process by which a facility reviews its services or products to ensure quality.

**interdepartmental** A relationship between two or more departments (e.g., HIM and the business office).

**intradepartmental** Occurrence or relationship within a department (e.g., assembly and analysis within HIM).

**outcome** The result of a patient's treatment.

**PI** performance improvement

**PDCA Method**

| | | In this stage you: |
|---|---|---|
| **P** | Plan | • Coordinate a team<br>• Investigate the problem; gather data<br>• Discuss potential solutions<br>• Decide on a plan of action |
| **D** | Do | **Here's where you test the plan of action:**<br>• Educate employees on the new process<br>• Pilot the new process |
| **C** | Check | **During the Pilot be sure to:**<br>• Monitor the new process during the pilot<br>• Did the plan of action work the way the team intended?<br>• Make necessary adjustments and continue the pilot |
| **A** | Act | **Once you are certain that the process is an improvement:**<br>• Change the policy<br>• Educate and train all affected employees<br>• Implement the new process |

**Figure 11-4** PDCA method.

---

**BOX 11-3  APPLYING PDCA TO PHYSICIAN QUERIES**

*Problem*: Queries of physician for accurate information are required for coding/billing; billing can be delayed.

*HIM Team*: Coders, analysts, clinical documentation improvement (CDI) specialist

**PLAN**: First review delayed bills, identify physician culprits, examine specific diagnoses and procedures that are problematic, review process for communicating with physicians. Brainstorm how to get physicians to answer queries.

**DO**: Implement changes necessary to resolve problems identified in planning phase.

**CHECK**: Review coding and billing delay data to determine impact of the changes; if positive impact, proceed to ACT, if not go back to PLAN part of the process.

**ACT**: Institutionalize the new procedures into policy and practice.

---

**advance directive** A written document, such as a living will, that specifies a patient's wishes for his or her care and dictates power of attorney, for the purpose of providing clear instructions in the event the patient is unable to do so.

Consider another example: A facility is required by state law to inform its patients about advance directives. State laws regarding advance directives vary dramatically. In our example, the state assigns the responsibility of advance directives, patients' rights, and health care options to the hospital. The law does not require the patient to have an advance directive or to make any decisions immediately; it simply states that the patient must be made aware of his or her rights. To prove compliance with this state law, the facility requires the patient to sign an advance directive acknowledgment form at the time of admission. This acknowledgment form, signed by the patient and the admitting clerk, serves as proof that the patient was given the advance directive information.

In some instances the health care facility may need to improve the method and accuracy by which it provides this information to its patients. To improve the collection of the acknowledgment form for advance directives, all persons involved in the advance directive collection process should be a part of the team, including the patient. The customer's perspective must be considered to truly evaluate the quality of a process or product, Figure 11-5 describes additional members of a hypothetical advance directive PI team.

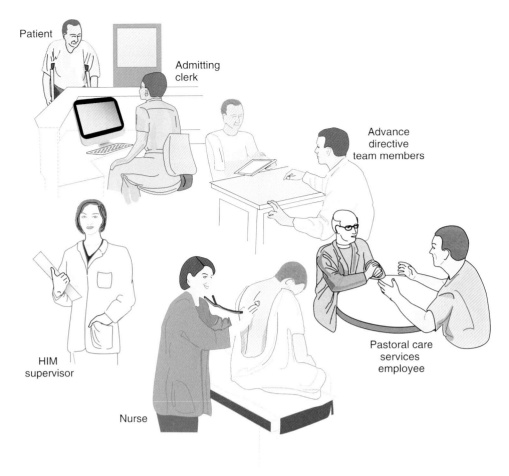

**Figure 11-5** Advance directive team members.

---

**PATIENT SELF-DETERMINATION ACT OF 1990**

The Patient Self-Determination Act of 1990 promotes public awareness of patients' rights, health care options, and advance directives. An *advance directive* is a living will or durable medical power of attorney that allows a patient to inform health care professionals of his or her wishes if the patient becomes incapable of doing so.

---

Here is one example of how it may currently happen in the health care facility. During the admission process the patient is presented with the question: "Do you have an advance directive?" If the answer is yes, the patient is asked to provide a copy of the living will or medical power of attorney for the hospital to keep on file. If the answer is no, the patient is given additional information about making an advance directive. The employees in the social services department provide information if the patient has any questions regarding the advance directive. Therefore the social service representative must be knowledgeable of both the content of the advance directive and the patient's concerns and other related issues. An advance directive is often an end-of-life determination. Pastoral care services assist the patient and family members with spiritual and emotional concerns. Their representation on the team may provide additional insight regarding other concerns affecting the patient or family during consideration of the advance directive statements. The nurse, being very involved in the patient care process and communicating often with the patient, is also an important member of the PI team. From the HIM department, a quantitative analysis employee should be represented because of his or her knowledge of the record review process. To be effective, all people who are a part of this process must be included on the PI team—patient, admitting clerk, social services, pastoral care, HIM.

**power of attorney** The legal document that identifies someone as the legal representative to make decisions for the patient when the patient is unable to do so.

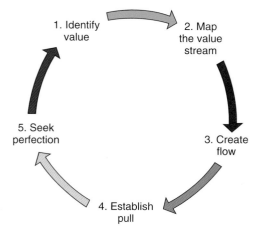

1. Identify the value in the process or product being improved.
2. Identify every step in the process or product creation and eliminate unnecessary steps that do not add value.
3. Align all of the necessary or required steps into a tightly aligned process or smooth flow.
4. Let customers "pull" the process (i.e., watch the customer's demand and respond to it).
5. Repeat these steps until perfection, a process with no waste.

**Figure 11-6** Steps for implementing lean techniques. (Modified from Lean Enterprise Institute: Principles of lean. http://www.lean.org/WhatsLean/Principles.cfm. Accessed April 19, 2012. Illustration Copyright © 2012, Lean Enterprise Institute (www.lean.org). Used with permission.)

### Lean

With roots in efforts started by Henry Ford in 1913 on the Model T automotive assembly line, and advanced by Kiichiro Toyoda, Taiichi Ohno, and others at Toyota in the 1930s, lean is also a PI process that began in manufacturing but has found application in health care settings (Lean Enterprise Institute, 2012). A somewhat less formal model than PDCA, lean or "lean thinking" seeks to create value—which may be defined in this context as anything the customer would pay for—by reducing waste and wasteful activities. Lean thinking looks for ways to accomplish a task with less work, reducing inefficiencies and thereby improving the process. Because lean accepts that there are always ways to improve, it is a philosophy of continuous improvement. That is, lean philosophy embraces a culture in which individuals in the organization are constantly looking for ways to improve the way things are done. This continuous improvement is expected of everyone in the organization, not just managers or policy makers. Figure 11-6 illustrates the implementation of lean, although you should note its circular pattern: improvement is not a one-time instance, it is continuous.

The lean PI philosophy can be adopted by health care facilities to improve many processes, including admission and discharge processes, patient scheduling and movement between departments for treatment, clinical processes, coding and billing, and emergency room wait time.

### Six Sigma

Another PI method, originally developed by Motorola in 1986 but made famous by General Electric in 1995, is called Six Sigma. As explained on the Web site www. isixsigma.com, "Six Sigma is a disciplined, data-driven approach and methodology for eliminating defects (driving toward six standard deviations between the mean and the nearest specification limit) in any process—from manufacturing to transactional and from product to service" (iSixSigma, 2012). Whereas lean thinking philosophy can be thought of as a less structured approach used by an entire organization, Six Sigma is a highly regimented approach to PI, driven by specially trained individuals ("Black Belts" and "Green Belts") who guide others through a strict problem-solving method. Health care facilities may choose to adopt this method of PI, establishing an organization philosophy to systematically strive for quality using a PI approach based on statistical data representing performance. Six Sigma uses

**PDCA** plan, do, check, act

| DMAIC (pronounced "duh-may-ick") | DMADV (pronounced "duh-mad-vee") Also called DFSS – Design for Six Sigma |
|---|---|
| Used to improve existing process | Used to create a new process or product |
| **Define** the problem specifically | **Define** design goals |
| **Measure** the current process (collect data) | **Measure** and identify characteristics that are Critical To Quality (CTQ) |
| **Analyze** and investigate cause and effect relationships | **Analyze** for development and design |
| **Improve** the current process, pilot potential solutions | **Design** details |
| **Control** establish systems to monitor and maintain control of the new process | **Verify** the design, set up pilots |

**Figure 11-7** Two approaches for Six Sigma.

different approaches to quality according to whether the facility is improving a current process or product (DMAIC), or creating a new process or product (DMADV). The basic steps for each approach are listed in Figure 11-7.

## Benchmarking

**Benchmarking** is a PI technique used by one facility to compare performance of its processes with the same process at another facility with noted superior performance; sometimes this method is used internally to compare current performance with a previous exemplary performance. By reviewing a process that is effective in another facility, the HIM department may discover methods or processes that would improve its own facility. Some processes are better served by throwing out the old model (the way things have always been done) and starting with a clean slate. The benchmarking technique can provide the facility with new and better methods for accomplishing the same tasks. Benchmarking internally, against previous performance, allows the facility to compare previous practices to current ones. Box 11-4 lists examples of common processes facilities use for benchmarking.

**benchmarking** An improvement technique that compares one facility's process with that of another facility that has been noted to have superior performance.

**PI** performance improvement

## EXERCISE 11-4
### Monitoring the Quality of Health Information

1. What type of quality monitoring does TJC require health care facilities to perform?
2. In the popular PDCA performance improvement method, which step of the process involves monitoring the effectiveness of the solution over a period of time?
   a. Plan
   b. Do
   c. Check
   d. Act
2. Which of the following abbreviations is used to describe the continuous improvement of processes within a facility?
   a. QA
   b. QM
   c. PI/QI
   d. UM
3. In addition to PDCA methods, list two other PI methods that are popular among health care facilities.
4. To improve quality according to a standard, a health care facility may use _____, comparing its performance to that of a similar facility.
5. Retrospective review of the product of a service is _____.
6. The alternative to quality assurance, _____, is an ongoing effort to improve processes within the health care facility.

| BOX 11-4 | EXAMPLES OF BENCHMARKS IN AN ACUTE CARE SETTING |
|---|---|

Internal benchmarks:
- Days in accounts receivable (A/R) versus previous periods
- Discharged, not final billed (DNFB)
- Release of information (ROI) compliance

External benchmarks:
- Average length of stay (ALOS)
- Case mix index (CMI)
- Operating margins
- Program for Evaluating Payment Patterns Electronic Report (PEPPER) reports

## ORGANIZATION AND PRESENTATION OF DATA

To effectively communicate the information obtained from PI activities, it is necessary to understand how to organize and present the data in a brief but effective informative format. The information is commonly presented in a meeting.

### Meetings

Meetings are an important method for bringing people together to improve performance. Meetings can be used to gather information or impart information. Meetings are used to inform the attendees of the purpose of a presentation. Everyone gets the same message at the same time. Meetings can be used to gather information about the process from the people who are involved, educate other members of the team, and keep the team focused on the goal of improving the process.

The facilitator plays an important role in the PI team meeting. The facilitator is the person who keeps the team focused on the goal (e.g., improvement in the collection of patient advance directives). During improvement efforts, it is common for a team to get sidetracked by equally pressing issues that need to be corrected. A facilitator makes sure that the team does not deviate too far off course. Such deviation could impair the team's ability to accomplish its goal.

### HIT-bit

**MEETING ROLES**

A few people in the meeting play key roles to ensure that the meeting is organized and orderly:

*Leader:* The leader is responsible for organizing the meeting and motivating the participants toward the goal.

*Facilitator:* The facilitator keeps the meeting on track, making sure that it is proceeding as necessary to accomplish the goal. The facilitator is not necessarily a member of the meeting or team but is there to ensure that the meeting progresses.

*Recorder:* The recorder acts as a secretary, taking minutes of the meeting and documenting the necessary proceedings of the meeting. The events of a meeting should be recorded and documented in the minutes of the meeting, which help the team track its progress and stay focused on the goal. The recorder's responsibilities should also include taking attendance, noting each member who is present and absent. Minutes keep the team aware of any unresolved issues. Meeting agendas and minutes are discussed in more detail in Chapter 14.

*Timekeeper:* The timekeeper is responsible for keeping the team on schedule, making sure that the meeting starts and ends on time, and so on.

**TABLE 11-3**

**TOOLS AND TECHNIQUES FOR THE PRESENTATION OF DATA**

| TOOLS AND TECHNIQUES | PRIMARY FUNCTION | BENEFITS |
|---|---|---|
| Flowchart | Displays the process | Facilitates understanding of the process<br>Identifies stakeholders<br>Clarifies potential gaps and system breakdowns |
| Run chart | Displays performance over time | Increases understanding of the problem<br>Identifies changes over time |
| Control chart | Displays how predictable the process is over time | Identifies change in the process as a result of intentional or unintentional changes in the process<br>Identifies opportunities for improvement |
| Pie chart | Displays the percentage each variable contributes to the whole | Identifies variables affecting process<br>Increases understanding of the problem |
| Bar chart | Compares categories of data during a single point in time | Increases understanding of the problem<br>Identifies differences in variables<br>Compares performance with known standards |
| Pareto chart | Identifies the most frequent trend within a data set | Identifies principal variables affecting the process<br>Identifies opportunities for improvement |
| Cause-and-effect (fishbone) chart | Displays multiple causes of a problem | Identifies root causes<br>Identifies variables affecting the process<br>Identifies opportunities for improvement<br>Plans for change |
| Scatter diagram | Displays relationship between two variables | Increases understanding of the relationship between multiple variables |
| Brainstorming | Rapidly generates multiple ideas | Promotes stakeholder buy-in<br>Increases understanding of the problem<br>Identifies variables affecting the process |
| Multivoting | Consolidates ideas | Achieves consensus among stakeholders<br>Prioritizes improvement strategies |
| Nominal group technique | Rapidly generates multiple ideas and prioritizes them | Identifies the problem<br>Achieves consensus among stakeholders<br>Prioritizes improvement strategies<br>Plans for change |
| Root cause analysis | Identifies the cause of the problem | Increases understanding of the problem<br>Identifies multicause variables affecting the process<br>Identifies opportunities to improve<br>Plans for change |
| Force field analysis | Identifies driving and restraining forces that impact proposed change | Identifies and lists variables affecting process<br>Plans for change |
| Consensus | Generates agreement among stakeholders | Increases understanding of the problem<br>Reduces resistance to change<br>Plans for change |

From Hamric, AB: Advanced practice nursing. Adapted from Powell SK: Advanced case management: outcomes and beyond, Philadelphia, 2000, Lippincott. Used with permission.

## Performance Improvement Tools

Many tools facilitate the use of data in the PI process. There are tools to gather information and to organize or present the information in a useful manner. Data-gathering tools help the team explore or at least acknowledge issues surrounding the process of concern. Organization and presentation tools make a statement about the information that is gathered. Two data-gathering tools, brainstorming and surveys, are discussed here, as well as several organization and presentation tools: bar graphs, line graphs, pie charts, decision matrices, and flowcharts. Table 11-3 contains a comprehensive list of presentation tools and techniques.

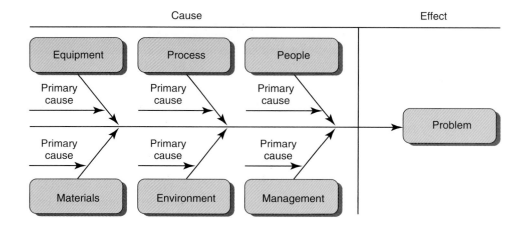

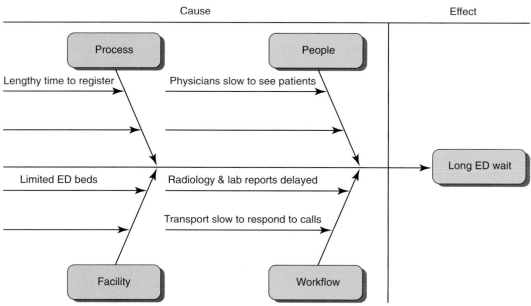

**Figure 11-8** This fishbone chart (*top*) was used during a brainstorming session to organize the possible causes of longer emergency department (ED) wait times (*bottom*).

**brainstorming** A data-gathering quality improvement tool used to generate information related to a topic.

**ED** emergency department

## Data-Gathering Tools

**Brainstorming** is a method in which a group of people discuss ideas, solutions, or related issues on a topic or situation. It is a data-gathering tool used to identify as many aspects, events, or issues surrounding a topic as possible. This process encourages the involvement of everyone in the group. All ideas are accepted, no matter how insignificant they may appear. When brainstorming, the group should have a topic and a place to write down the ideas mentioned by the group. To begin the process, the team's facilitator explains that this tool is used to gather all ideas related to the issue—regardless of how unusual they may seem.

For example, a PI team is organized to reduce the length of time that a patient waits to receive treatment in the ED. At the team's first meeting, the members brainstorm all of the possible factors that could have an impact on the patient's wait in the ED. The team members are encouraged to mention anything that could affect the patient's wait time. Note that at this stage the members do not need to prove that the factors they mention actually affect the patient's wait time. Brainstorming is simply a data-gathering tool; many organization tools can be used to narrow improvement efforts, such as a fishbone chart (Figure 11-8).

## HIT-bit

### BRAINSTORMING RULES

Collect as many ideas as possible from all participants, with no criticisms or judgments made while ideas are being generated.

1. All ideas are welcome, no matter how silly or far out they seem. Be creative. The more ideas, the better, because at this point no one knows what might work.
2. Absolutely no discussion takes place during the brainstorming activity. Talking about the ideas will take place *after* brainstorming session is complete.
3. Do not criticize or judge. Don't even groan, frown, or laugh. All ideas are equally valid at this point.
4. Do build on others' ideas.
5. Do write all ideas on a flip chart or board so the whole group can easily see them.
6. Set a time limit (e.g., 30 minutes) for the brainstorming session.

From Maricopa Community Colleges, Maricopa Center for Learning and Instruction: Studio 1151: Brainstorming. http://www.mcli.dist.maricopa.edu/authoring/studio/guidebook/brain.html. Published 2001.

## TABLE 11-4

### SURVEY QUESTIONS

| OPEN QUESTION | LIMITED ANSWER QUESTION |
|---|---|
| How would you describe your visit to our emergency department? | Choose one of the following to describe the emergency department during your recent visit:<br>a. Very clean<br>b. Adequately clean<br>c. Unclean<br>d. Very dirty |
| How long did you wait in the emergency department before being seen by a physician? | How long did you wait in the emergency department before being seen by a physician?<br>a. Less than 1 hour<br>b. 1 to 2 hours<br>c. 2 to 3 hours<br>d. Longer than 3 hours |

A **survey** is set of questions designed to gather information about a specific topic or issue. A survey can be used routinely to gather information from a group, or it can be designed as part of a PI team's efforts. For example, many facilities conduct a survey of patients after a visit to the facility. The data collectors want to find out how the patient perceived the service. This type of survey can be used to measure patient satisfaction. When significant dissatisfaction is observed, the facility may organize a PI team to address the issue. In the previously mentioned emergency department example, the PI team could develop a survey to ask patients why they think it took so long to receive treatment. The questions on a survey can be open ended, which means that the response areas are blank. With open-ended questions, patients are free to answer the question in their own words. However, this method of questioning may not provide enough information to determine how much improvement is necessary. Table 11-4 provides an example of the same survey question asked in two different ways.

### Data Organization and Presentation Tools

Data organization and presentation tools are used to communicate information quickly to another person or group. Because PI is a team effort, it is important to organize information and display it so that the group can interpret or understand it. Such tools include graphs, tables, and charts. A **graph** is an illustration of data. A **table** organizes data in rows and columns. These visual tools can be quite persuasive, and positive information can be emphasized just as easily as negative information. Consider the following example: The number of cigarette-smoking freshmen on a college campus declined 40% between 2009

**survey** A data-gathering tool for capturing the responses to queries. May be administered verbally or by written questionnaire. Also refers to the activity of querying, as in "taking a survey."

**graph** An illustration of data.
**table** A chart organized in rows and columns to organize data.

| Year | 2009 | 2010 | 2011 | 2012 | 2013 | |
|---|---|---|---|---|---|---|
| # of freshmen who smoke | 1299 | 1157 | 885 | 588 | 462 | |
| *Total # of freshmen* | 2095 | 2103 | 2099 | 2100 | 2098 | |
| % of freshmen who smoke | 62% | 55% | 42% | 28% | 22% | |
| Total # of smokers on campus | 3247 | 3264 | 3254 | 3272 | 3269 | |

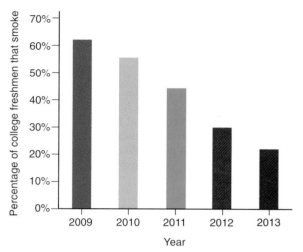

**Figure 11-9** Bar graph showing percentages of college freshmen who smoked cigarettes, 2009 to 2013.

**prevalence** Rate of incidence of an occurrence, disease, or diagnosis or the number of existing cases.

**incidence** Number of occurrences of a particular event, disease, or diagnosis or the number of new cases of a disease.

and 2013. However, overall smoking prevalence on the campus was virtually unchanged during that time. We can take the positive data—the decrease in the number of freshmen who smoked from 2009 to 2013—and plot it on a graph to show a positive trend in smoking cessation (Figure 11-9).

However, the same statement can also provide a negative picture because the overall number of people smoking on the campus remains about the same. The same statement could be graphed in two different ways: The positive graph shows that the number of freshmen who smoke has decreased, and the negative graph shows that the total percentage of people who smoke remains unchanged.

### Bar and Line Graphs

Bar and line graphs, also known as charts, relate information along the horizontal (*x* axis) and the vertical (*y* axis). In a bar graph, data is displayed for discrete data elements, one axis being used to represent the group or indicator, and the other axis used to plot the data for the group. For example, Figure 11-9 is a bar graph showing the categories (2009, 2010, 2011, 2012, 2013) along the *x* axis that represent the years in which freshmen smoking was measured. The data plotted along the *y* axis indicate the percentage of freshmen who smoke for each year. Changing the bar graph to a line graph provides an illustration of the data points across a continuum and may display a percentage of people smoking over the course of the 5-year period. In Figure 11-10, the bars have been replaced with points that are connected by lines. Line graphs are used to plot data over time. This line graph is an easy way to depict the trend of the same data as they are measured continuously, month to month or year to year.

Note the labels and headings used in Figures 11-9 to 11-11. The headings describe the graph or chart, giving the reader an idea of what information is included. On bar and line graphs, the labels on the axes identify what is being measured and how it is being measured. On the pie chart, a key might be used to indicate which color is associated with each group. The following is a list of reminders for creating graphs:

- Include information about the time frame of the data or the date on which the data were collected.
- Make sure the graph is legible, especially when presenting the information on an overhead projector to a large group.
- Choose the best graph for the data that is presented—for example, percentages relate well on a pie chart, but the total of the percentages must equal 100% for the pie chart to be accurate.
- Be prepared to explain the graph if questioned by the audience.
- Software programs such as Microsoft Excel can simplify the creation of the aforementioned graphs, tables, and charts. These programs make it very easy to turn data into an easy-to-read presentation tool.

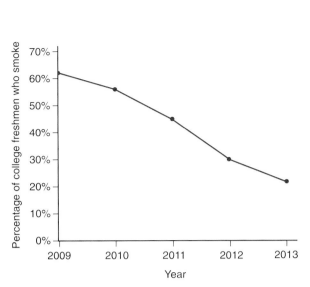

Figure 11-10  Line graph of same data in Figure 11-9.

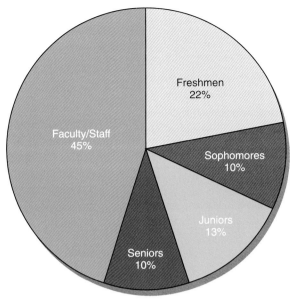

Figure 11-11  Pie chart of the percentages of different populations on campus who smoke.

## TABLE 11-5

### DECISION MATRIX

|  | FRESHMAN | SOPHOMORES | JUNIORS | SENIORS | FACULTY-STAFF | TOTAL |
|---|---|---|---|---|---|---|
| Commercials | 2 | 2 | 2 | 2 | 1 | 9 |
| Smoking areas | 3 | 3 | 3 | 3 | 3 | 15 |
| Peer pressure | 3 | 3 | 2 | 2 | 1 | 11 |

### Pie Chart

A pie chart is a graphical illustration of information as it relates to a whole. For example, a pie chart can be used to illustrate the percentages of different populations on campus who smoke. When considering this type of chart, imagine a pie, the pieces of which represent percentages. If the pie is cut into even slices, all of the pieces are equal. However, when the size of each piece represents the various smoking populations on campus, we can easily determine which group smokes the most because the sizes vary (see Figure 11-11).

### Decision Matrix

A **decision matrix** can help a group organize information. This tool is used when the PI team must narrow its focus or choose among several categories or issues. For example, if a PI team is organized to decrease smoking on the college campus, the members may begin by brainstorming to determine all the issues that influence a person's decision to smoke. Once the team has identified the factors on campus that influence this decision, the team must decide which influential factors they can change. A decision matrix can be used to analyze which of the factors would cause a decrease in the number of smokers if removed. Table 11-5 shows a decision matrix in which each group of smokers is analyzed to determine which issue has the greatest influence on that group's decision to smoke.

First, note that the first row of the table identifies the groups of smokers and the first column identifies the issues that may influence a person's decision to smoke. To complete the decision matrix, the PI team analyzes each group according to the influences that the team identified. Team members can write their comments in the squares, or they can assign a value—in this case, 1 for least likely to influence the person to smoke, 2 for moderate influence, and 3 for most likely to influence the person to smoke. The final column on the

**pie chart** A circular chart in which the frequency of observations is represented as a wedge of the circle.

**decision matrix** A quality improvement tool used to narrow focus or choose between two or more related possible decisions.
**brainstorming** A data-gathering quality improvement tool used to generate information related to a topic.

right is a total, or decision, column. The influence with the highest rating or the influence that occurred in each of the categories would be the team's target. In this case, the first, and by far easiest, way to decrease smoking on campus would be to eliminate some of the smoking areas.

*Flowchart*

> **advance directive** A written document, such as a living will, that specifies a patient's wishes for his or her care and dictates power of attorney, for the purpose of providing clear instructions in the event the patient is unable to do so.

A *flowchart* is a tool used to organize the steps involved in a process. Because the PI team is interdisciplinary, some of the team members may not understand the process they are intended to improve. The flowchart provides an illustration of how the process works within the facility. For an example, refer to the advance directive process shown in Figure 11-5. Figure 11-12 is a flowchart of the advance directive process showing how the facility informs the patient about the advance directive and how the health care professional obtains the patient's signature on the acknowledgment form. Flowcharts help the team streamline a process and eliminate unnecessary steps. Flowcharts utilize standard symbols that are defined by ANSI (American National Standards Institute) so that flowcharts created adhere to standardized symbols for universal understanding.

## EXERCISE 11-5

### Organization and Presentation of Data

1. Which graph would you use to show that the overall percentage of people smoking on campus has remained unchanged?
2. _____ is a PI technique used to solicit participation and information from an entire group.
3. A supervisor and her team of employees are confronted with two solutions to a problem. Each solution involves time, money, and space. Which quality management tool might the supervisor use to help her and her team choose a solution?

## HEALTH CARE FACILITY COMMITTEES

*Committees* are formal organizational tools that facilities use to conduct business. The committee structure of the health care facility is outlined in the medical staff bylaws, rules, and regulations. Some committees are required by accreditation agencies. Although all health care facilities have committees, the roles and functions of committees in the facilities vary. Examples of committees within a health care facility are medical staff departments, infection control, safety, surgical case review, pharmacy and therapeutics, and HIM. The following discussion briefly explains how these committees use health information.

### Medical Staff Committees

The medical staff of a health care facility is a self-governed group of physicians divided into departments on the basis of their practices, such as the department of medicine, department of surgery, department of obstetrics, and department of pediatrics. The medical staff structure is directed by an elected group of physicians; such positions include chief or president of the medical staff, the president-elect (incoming chief of staff), and a chairperson for each department. Each medical staff department has a committee meeting in which business directly related to that field of medicine is discussed. The committee reviews patient cases, determines appropriate documentation, and discusses standards of care, as necessary. The medical staff departments also use statistics acquired from health information to make decisions regarding physician membership, privileges, and compliance with accreditation standards.

> **TJC** The Joint Commission

Accreditation by TJC requires that a facility review specific cases of patient care in the areas of surgery, medication usage, and blood and tissue usage. For example, the department of surgery performs surgical case review as an accreditation requirement. The facility reviews statistics related to operations and the health records of surgical cases with

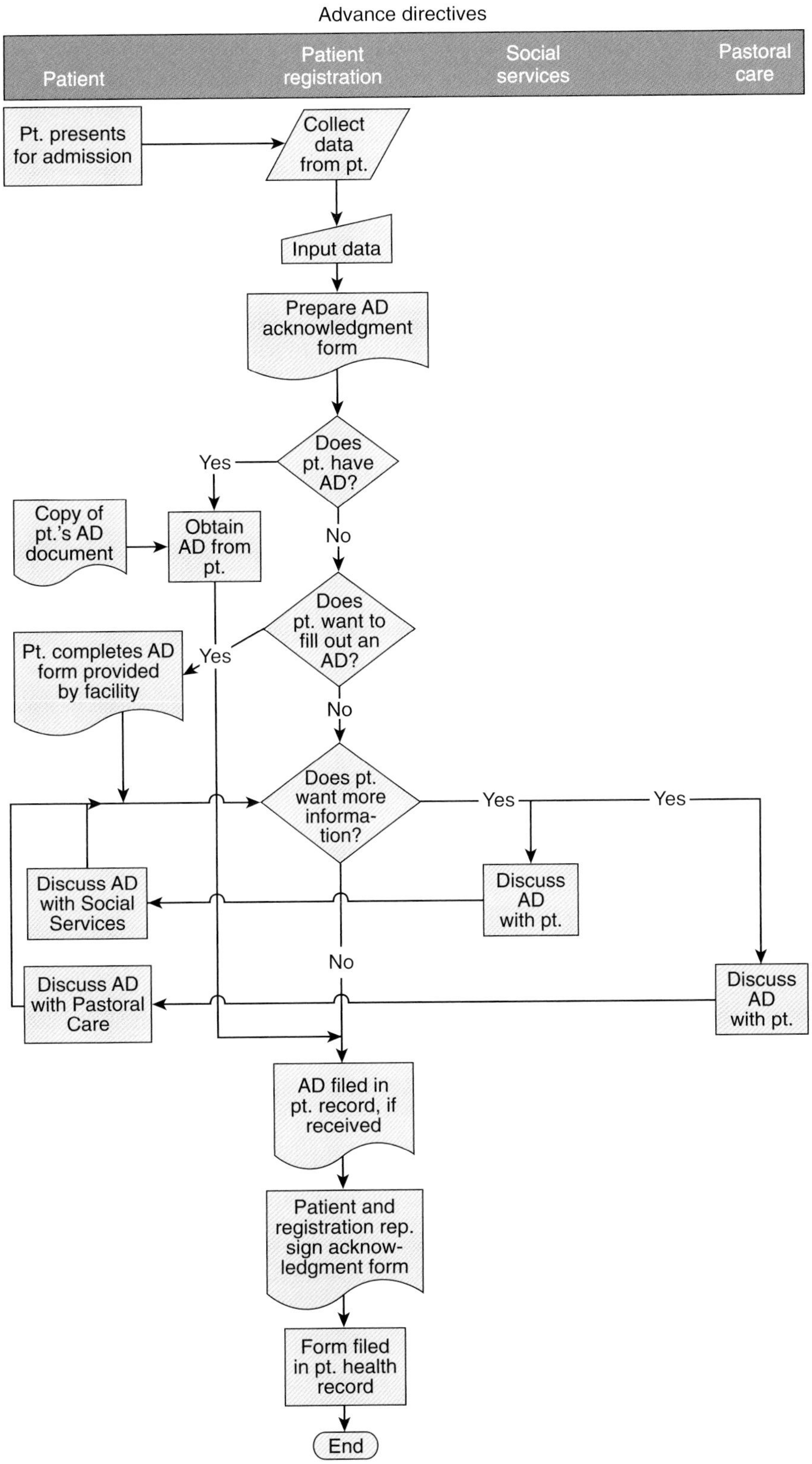

**Figure 11-12** Flowchart of the advance directive process showing how the facility informs the patient *(pt.)* about the advance directive *(AD)* and how the health care professional obtains the patient's signature on the acknowledgement form. Rep., representative.

unexpected outcomes (e.g., a patient who goes into cardiac arrest during an appendectomy or a case in which the wrong operation was performed). Medication usage is typically reviewed by the pharmacy and therapeutics (P&T) committee. The P&T committee is composed of members of the medical staff, with representatives from nursing, administration, and the pharmacy also represented. The committee reviews medications administered to patients, specifically targeting any adverse reactions that a patient has had as a result of medication. The P&T committee also oversees the hospital formulary, which is a listing of the drugs used and approved within the facility. Blood usage is also a review that requires participation from the medical staff. This review analyzes the appropriate protocol, method, and effects for patients receiving blood transfusions (or blood products).

The business and decisions of the departments of the medical staff are reported to the medical executive committee (MEC) for action, recommendation, or correspondence to the governing board. The "med exec committee," as it is commonly called, acts as a liaison to the governing board of the facility. This committee is composed of the chief of staff and elected positions, with a representative from each of the medical staff departments.

**● MEC** medical executive committee

## Health Information Management Committee

The HIM committee, commonly referred to as the medical record committee, serves as a consultant to the director of the HIM department. The HIM committee is typically responsible for reviewing the documentation in patient health records, reviewing and advising forms development, and assisting in compliance with accreditation standards. Some facilities have expanded the HIM committee into a more global quality committee, with the HIM committee reporting specific metrics at least quarterly. Many important health information issues can be addressed by this committee. Box 11-5 is a sample agenda for an HIM committee; the committee can review the findings of the record review teams, the percentage of delinquent medical records, and QA and PI activities. Members of the HIM committee include the director of HIM, physicians from each department of the medical staff, nursing staff, and quality management personnel.

**● QA** quality assurance
**PI** performance improvement

## Infection Control Committee

The infection control committee is organized to analyze the rate of infection of the patients within a facility. This committee meets regularly to determine whether patients are entering the facility with infections that can harm the staff or other patients or whether patients are acquiring infections within the facility, nosocomial infections, that affect their care, treatment, and LOS.

The infection control committee is also involved in preventing and investigating infections. Members of the infection control committee include physicians, nurses, quality management personnel, and HIM personnel. To evaluate infection control rates within a facility, the committee must analyze information from patient health records.

**● LOS** length of stay
**HIM** health information management

---

**BOX 11-5** | **AGENDA FOR HEALTH INFORMATION MANAGEMENT COMMITTEE**

**HIM COMMITTEE MEETING**
October 19, 2014
  Agenda:
    I. Call to order
    II. Review of minutes
    III. Old business
    IV. Record review
    V. New business
    VI. Reports
    VII. Delinquent record count
    VIII. Quality audit of HIM functions
    IX. Adjourn
    *Next meeting:* November 16, 2014

## Safety Committee

The safety committee is organized to assist the safety officer, who is responsible for providing a program to create a safe environment for patients, visitors, the community, and staff. Health care facilities must adhere to numerous requirements from the U.S. Occupational Safety and Health Administration (OSHA), TJC, state licensing boards, and federal agencies. The safety committee evaluates the information presented by the safety officer, ensures safety of the environment, and performs disaster planning. Occasionally, the safety committee also reviews the incident reports of cases related to the facility's environment. Members of the safety committee are appointed and may include clinical and nonclinical employees.

## EXERCISE 11-7
### Health Care Facility Committees

1. Which of the following is the committee often responsible for reviewing health care records according to accreditation standards, checking physician record completion statistics, and acting as the consultant to the director of health information management?
   a. HIM committee
   b. Safety committee
   c. Infection control committee
   d. P&T committee
2. Infections acquired by patients while they are in the hospital are known as:
   a. nosocomial infections.
   b. comorbidities.
   c. secondary infections.
   d. opportunistic infections.
3. Which of the following committees acts a liaison to the governing board of the facility?
   a. Surgical case review
   b. P&T committee
   c. Medical executive committee
   d. Credentials committee
4. Which of the following medical staff committees reviews medication usage?
   a. Surgical case review
   b. P&T committee
   c. Medical executive committee
   d. Credentials committee

## HEALTH INFORMATION IN QUALITY ACTIVITIES

Review/analysis of health records provides useful information to committees, physicians, administrators, and outside organizations. Quality analysis of health records involves two processes: quantitative analysis and qualitative analysis. The focus in this chapter is on qualitative analysis. Typically, these two reviews are performed separately, but they can occur simultaneously.

## Quantitative Analysis

To evaluate the quality of patient care, the health record must be complete—meaning that all of the information must be included in the record. Analysis of the record to ensure that the documentation is complete is called **quantitative analysis**. An example of quantitative analysis is the review of an inpatient record for an H&P and discharge summary. Likewise, the operative reports, laboratory reports, radiology reports, and notes must be present and authenticated by the health care professional who wrote the notes, reports, or information.

**quantitative analysis** The process of reviewing a health record to ensure that the record is complete according to organization policies and procedures for a complete medical record.

**discharge summary** The recap of an inpatient stay, usually dictated by the attending physician and transcribed into a formal report.

**authenticate** To assume responsibility for data collection or the activities described by the data collection by signature, mark, code, password, or other means of identification.

**H&P** history and physical

**qualitative analysis** Review of the actual content of the health record to ensure that the information is correct as it pertains to the patient's care.

**data accuracy** The quality that data are correct.

**timeliness** The quality of data's being obtained, recorded, or reported within a predetermined time frame.

Quantitative analysis includes review of the record for the authentication or signatures. This analysis is performed on every health record.

## Qualitative Analysis

**Qualitative analysis** is the review of the health record for accuracy and timeliness of contents. The information must be correct and appropriate as it pertains to the patient's care. In qualitative analysis, the patient's diagnoses, procedures, and treatment are analyzed. Qualitative analysis checks the validity of health information and the timeliness of data entries. A detailed review of the actual documentation in the record is performed to assess whether the clinically pertinent information has been recorded. Figure 11-13 provides an

**GENERIC RECORD REVIEW FORM**

MR#_____ Attending physician: _____

Admit date: _____ Discharge date: _____

DRG: _____ Procedure: _____ Reviewer: _____ Review date: _____

| CRITERIA | Y | N | N/A |
|---|---|---|---|
| Advance directive acknowledgment form signed by patient | | | |
| Patients with advance directives have copy on the health record | | | |
| H&P documented within 24 hours of admission (and prior to surgery) | | | |
| H&P contains: Chief complaint | | | |
| Medical history | | | |
| Family history | | | |
| Psychological status | | | |
| Social status | | | |
| Review of systems | | | |
| Physical examination | | | |
| Plan | | | |
| Initial nursing assessment documented within 24 hours of admission | | | |
| Discharge planning addressed | | | |
| All entries dated and authenticated | | | |
| Goals and treatment plans documented | | | |
| Progress notes documented daily | | | |
| Surgery/procedure performed | | | |
| Informed consent documented in the health record | | | |
| Preanesthesia assessment documented | | | |
| Immediately prior to procedure patient is reassesed for anesthesia | | | |
| Postoperative monitoring of the patient | | | |
| Postoperative monitoring includes: Physiologic status | | | |
| Mental status | | | |
| IV fluids | | | |
| Meds | | | |
| Unusual events | | | |
| Operative report is documented immediately following the procedure | | | |
| Operative report includes: Procedure | | | |
| Findings | | | |
| Specimen(s) removed | | | |
| Postop Dx | | | |
| Surgical progress note documented immediately following procedure | | | |
| Discharge summary signed and documented within 30 days of discharge | | | |
| Discharge summary includes documentation of: Diet | | | |
| Meds | | | |
| Follow-up | | | |
| Activity | | | |
| Diagnosis | | | |

**Figure 11-13** Generic record review form. H&P, history and physical; IV, intravenous; Meds, medications; Postop Dx, postoperative diagnosis.

example of a generic (qualitative analysis) record review form that looks for basic information about the timeliness, completeness, accuracy, and validity of the health record.

The reviewer will use this generic form to determine whether the health record meets the minimum requirements set by the TJC. Notice that the form captures information about the timeliness of the H&P: whether it was completed within 24 hours of admission. It also captures information about the content of the document: whether it contains the chief complaint, history of present illness, family history, mental status, and so on. This information is required by TJC. When TJC representatives survey a health care facility, they review the health records to see whether this information is a part of the H&P. The record must be monitored before the survey to ensure that the information is present.

Ideally, a qualitative review should be performed on every health record. However, because it takes a significant amount of time to perform qualitative analysis on paper records, a determination is made about which records to review. Accreditation agencies set the guidelines for this type of record review. Typically, qualitative analysis should be performed at least quarterly. The records chosen for review should represent a sample—usually 30 records or 5% of the monthly average (whichever is greater). Record review may be based on the categories of medical staff in the facility or on specific diagnoses, procedures performed, problems identified in previous audits, or payer denials. To prevent a biased result, records must be reviewed for each physician on staff.

### Record Review

The quantitative and qualitative review functions performed by HIM professionals to ensure quality of documentation in patient health records are also known as *record review*. The record review is required by TJC standards to be performed quarterly by a multidisciplinary team of health care professionals who are involved in patient care. HIM professionals read and understand the TJC guidelines and then coordinate the review of the patient records at the facility. The HIM professional typically is responsible for ensuring that the documentation in these records complies with the standards set by the TJC. Much of the record review that occurs now is concurrent because of a methodology that TJC uses during the facility survey called tracer methodology.

### Tracer Methodology

The TJC **tracer methodology** follows, or traces, a current patient's stay in the health care facility. At the beginning of TJC survey, the surveyors request a current patient census for the facility. From that census, the surveyors choose the charts that they will review during the survey. These charts are reviewed concurrently during the survey of those patients who are currently in the facility. From the review of these inhouse charts, the surveyors determine which physicians they will review, which staff members they will interview, and which policies and procedures they will review. The goal is to evaluate how health care is being performed in "real time." In previous TJC surveys, the management team sat in a meeting and answered all of the surveyor's questions on policy and procedures, were able to choose (with some restrictions) the charts that the surveyors would review, and could sometimes even select the physicians who were involved. With the tracer methodology, the surveyors interview the staff members who are involved in patient care and ask them questions about policies and procedures. This is also how the surveyors determine which physicians will be reviewed in the credentialing portion of the survey and which employee files to review in human resources. This process shows whether all of the facility employees know the policies and procedures, rather than just the managers. In essence, the whole survey process revolves around the review of the concurrent health records of the facility during the survey. Therefore the concurrent review of health records is more important today than it was in previous years. The facility should have in place a process for regularly performing this type of record review before the TJC survey takes place.

### Value of Record Review

Qualitative analysis of health information serves several purposes. The most important reason to perform this review is to evaluate the quality of patient care. On review of a sample of patients with a diagnosis of pneumonia, for example, it may be found that a

---

**completeness** The data quality of existence. If a required data element is missing, the record is not complete.

**data validity** The quality that data reflect the known or acceptable range of values for the specific data.

**TJC** The Joint Commission

**H&P** history and physical

**chief complaint** The main reason a patient has sought treatment.

**accreditation** Voluntary compliance with a set of standards developed by an independent agent, who periodically performs audits to ensure compliance.

**tracer methodology** TJC method of onsite review of open records in which the surveyors follow the actual path of documentation from start to finish.

**census** The actual number of inpatients in a facility at a point in time, for comparative purposes, usually midnight.

**concurrent review** Review occurring during the act or event (i.e., a chart review during the patient's stay in the facility).

**qualitative analysis** Review of the actual content of the health record to ensure that the information is correct as it pertains to the patient's care.

**outcome** The result of a patient's treatment.

**reimbursement** The amount of money that the health care facility receives from the party responsible for paying the bill.

**case management** The coordination of the patient's care and services, including reimbursement considerations.

**electronic health record (EHR)** A secure real-time, point-of-care, patient centric information resource for clinicians allowing access to patient information when and where needed and incorporating evidence-based decision support.

**concurrent analysis** Any type of record analysis performed during the patient's stay (i.e., after admission but before discharge).

**continuity of care** The broad range of health care services required by a patient during an illness or for an entire lifetime. May also refer to the continuity of care provided by a health care organization. Also called *continuum of care*.

**clinical decision-making system (CDS)** A computer application that compares two or more items of patient data in order to advise clinicians on the treatment of that specific patient.

**physician's orders** The physician's directions regarding the patient's care. Also refers to the data collection device on which these elements are captured.

**clinical pathway** A predetermined standard of treatment for a particular disease, diagnosis, or procedure designed to facilitate the patient's progress through the health care encounter.

**evidence-based medicine** Health care delivery that uses clinical research to make decisions in patient care.

sputum culture was ordered in 50% of the cases. Additionally, the culture was obtained immediately after a diagnosis of pneumonia was suspected. The general treatment for pneumonia is to start the patient on some type of antibiotic. However, if the sputum culture reveals a gram-negative specimen, normal antibiotics will not resolve the patient's pneumonia. The patient must be put on a more specific medicine. Early detection of the organism facilitates prompt medication and, ideally, a shorter period of recovery. The facility uses this information to educate the physicians and the clinical staff. The information shows the difference in patient outcome between those who received appropriate care and those who did not. The information can also show the effect of the treatment on cost of health care or reimbursement.

These analyses—qualitative analysis and record review—are essential to the accreditation of the health care facility. Accreditation bodies expect facilities to continuously monitor and analyze their compliance with predetermined standards. The quarterly review of health information to determine this compliance can prevent a facility from failing an accreditation survey. If detected early, noncompliance with standards can be corrected before a survey.

### Record Review Team

It is important to formalize record review practices as a policy identifying who is responsible for performing the record reviews. Multidisciplinary or interdisciplinary teams are organized for this function. Health care professionals who document information in the patient health record meet at least quarterly to review records against the standards. Record review teams include physicians, nurses, physical therapists, occupational therapists, radiologists, laboratory workers, dietitians, case managers, and pharmacists. Members of the record review team are challenged to determine whether a record is in compliance with TJC standards. Record review requires team members to know where and by whom health information is documented. In the multidisciplinary team record review, health care professionals who document information in the health record learn the importance of the documentation. For example, a nurse reviewing records to measure compliance with patient education standards may realize that the documentation in the records does not support that patient education is actually being accomplished. This problem may not have been identified and corrected without the record review.

The results of the record reviews must be communicated to the medical staff committee or a quality care review committee that understands the importance of health information and the effect it has on the quality of patient care as well as on facility accreditation.

### Electronic Health Record and Performance Improvement

The electronic health record (EHR) also requires quantitative and qualitative analysis. The EHR is only as good as the information that is entered. It is important that analysis of the health information remain a key function. However, it is expected that quantitative and qualitative analyses will occur concurrently in the EHR. Concurrent analysis provides information in a timely manner that can have an impact on patient care. The electronic system allows an organization to evaluate key health data elements across the continuity of care in a report rather than having to retrieve individual charts; this automation helps ensure that required data elements are completed appropriately, often initiating PI.

One quality aspect of the EHR is the clinical decision-making system (CDS). Computers can be programmed to recognize data as information. This feature allows the computer to determine or prompt the next course of action. In some cases, the computer analyzes each course of action. For example, in the pneumonia scenario, when pneumonia is entered as a suspected diagnosis, the computer searches for a physician's order to obtain a sputum culture. In addition, the computer recognizes the laboratory results of the sputum culture and is able to suggest the next course of action to the attending physician. This automation is discussed in more detail in Chapter 3.

## Clinical Pathways

A **clinical pathway** is the "multidisciplinary plan of best clinical practice" for a specific diagnosis (OpenClinical, 2012). The plan can come from best practices and evidence-based documents, or the organization can, after studying or reviewing a significant number of health records for patients with a particular diagnosis, develop a guide or plan for patients with that diagnosis. By doing so, a facility can streamline the patient's stay in the hospital, coordinate multidisciplinary care, and ideally eliminate any unnecessary time spent in the facility or at a particular level of care. The goal is to provide high-quality patient care in an efficient and effective manner. It is important to note that this does not mean that all patients will be treated the same. If the patient's condition warrants a change from the clinical pathway, appropriate treatment is rendered, and ideally, the patient's condition improves. Often, when clinical pathways are utilized, practitioners document only exceptions to the pathway, so daily documentation for standards of care many not be necessary.

## Utilization Review

**Utilization review (UR)** is the function or department that ensures appropriate, efficient, and effective health care for patients. It also monitors patient outcomes and compares physician activities.

"Appropriate" may also refer to what is covered by the patient's insurance plan. A health insurance plan may require a specific test before approving a specific treatment or procedure. The expectation is that the test will provide definitive information regarding the necessity of the treatment or procedure. For example, before approving arthroscopy of the knee, an insurance company may require magnetic resonance imaging (MRI). In the past, the physician had sole responsibility for determining the procedures and treatments that a patient would or would not receive. Today, such decisions may be heavily influenced by the third party paying the bill.

CMS and other payers have established efforts to reduce the number of short inpatient LOSs, as these can be costly and may not be medically necessary. When a physician in the emergency department, for example, makes a diagnosis of pneumonia, the DRG for pneumonia is sent to the payer either while the patient is still in the ED or shortly after admission. During the evaluation process, use of nationally accepted screening criteria such as InterQual or Milliman provides standards for determining medical necessity, using weights of **severity of illness (SI)** and **intensity of service (IS)** for the specific diagnosis to determine the appropriate LOS for the patient, and the amount the insurer will reimburse. Given all the factors of a particular weighted DRG, the payer may determine that the patient should have an inpatient stay of 3 days. Because the hospital will not receive payment for an LOS longer than that, UR staff may have to request a recertification of the patient on the basis of changes in his or her condition to justify a longer LOS—or risk receiving a payment that does not cover the cost of services.

Payers study historical patient treatment by analyzing patient health records to identify "best practices," or a specific plan of treatment to identify the best standard of care. The QIOs who contract with Medicare closely monitor diagnosis data and hospital statistics to limit the potential for overpayment, in situations like short LOSs. For this reason, UR staff work to help physicians move patients through the system efficiently, providing guidance on the screening criteria for admitting diagnoses and the working DRG used during inpatient stay. This is not to say that physicians do not order tests that payers do not approve. Nor does it imply that payers overrule physician orders. However, there is significant controversy over the influence of payers in medical decision making.

## Case Management

**Case management** is the coordination of the patient's care within the facility. Case management is performed by health care professionals, typically nurses or BCSWs within the facility, as well as by the payers who send their employees into the facility to oversee or coordinate care. The health care professional coordinating the care is called a *case manager*. Case management in practice is multidisciplinary. The coordinator interacts with all the health care professionals involved in the patient's care. With such a team, the expectation is that the communication among the disciplines (e.g., physical therapy, occupational therapy, nursing, medical) will facilitate appropriate, effective, and efficient health care for the patient.

**utilization review (UR)** The process of evaluating medical interventions against established criteria, on the basis of the patient's known or tentative diagnosis. Evaluation may take place before, during, or after the episode of care for different purposes.

**diagnosis related groups (DRGs)** A collection of health care descriptions organized into statistically similar categories.
**severity of illness (SI)** In utilization review, a type of criteria based on the patient's condition used to screen patients for the appropriate care setting.
**intensity of service (IS)** In utilization review, a type of criteria consisting primarily of monitoring and diagnostic assessments that must be met in order to qualify a patient for inpatient admission.

**Go To** Refer to Chapter 7 to review the role of SI in reimbursement.

**QIO** Quality Improvement Organization

**admitting diagnosis** The reason given by the physician for initiating the order for the patient to be placed into care in a hospital.
**working DRG** The concurrent diagnosis related group (DRG). The DRG that reflects the patient's current diagnosis and procedures while still an inpatient.

**case management** The coordination of the patient's care and services, including reimbursement considerations.

**BCSW** board-certified social worker

Typically, the case manager is the employee assigned to review the patient's care, interact with the health care team, and ensure that the services provided are covered by the patient's insurance. The case manager is assigned to the patient when the patient is admitted to the facility. Review of the patient's health information to determine the plan of care happens concurrently. Case management also involves multidisciplinary meetings of health care professionals to coordinate the patient's plan of care and continually update each discipline on the patient's progress.

The team members in this multidisciplinary effort may include, but are not limited to, physicians, nurses, physical therapists, occupational therapists, respiratory therapists, speech therapists, HIM coders, and patients (in some settings). Each person on the team attends the case management meeting to discuss the development or progress of the patient's care. The case manager is also concerned with planning for the patient's discharge, making sure that the patient's status is reviewed for appropriate placement in the next health care facility or that care is received via home health or follow-up in the physician's office. Each team meeting is documented and becomes a part of the patient's health record. When necessary, the plan of care is also updated.

## Risk Management

**Risk management (RM)** is the coordination of efforts within a facility to prevent and control **potentially compensable events (PCEs)**. A PCE is any event that could cause a financial loss or lead to litigation. Risk management is a TJC requirement and often one of the stipulations required by the insurance company that provides insurance coverage to the health care facility. Depending on the size and type of facility, the RM department may contain an attorney who is an employee of the facility, or RM may simply be the responsibility of one of the leaders in the facility's administration. This department monitors PCEs, leads or is involved in the safety committee, and works to ensure a safe environment for patients and employees through training, education, and facility improvements.

> **patient care plan** The formal directions for treatment of the patient, which involves many different individuals, including the patient. It may be as simple as instructions to "take two aspirins and drink plenty of fluids," or it may be a multiple-page document with delegation of responsibilities. Care plans may also be developed by discipline, such as nursing.

> **risk management (RM)** The coordination of efforts within a facility to prevent and control inadvertent occurrences.
> **potentially compensable event (PCE)** An event that could cause the facility a financial loss or lead to litigation.

> **TJC** The Joint Commission

---

### HIT-bit

#### SEQUESTERED FILE

The HIM department maintains a sequestered file for all cases that are identified as potentially compensable events (PCEs) or that are currently involved in litigation against the facility. This file is kept in a locked cabinet that contains the health records. Access to the file is generally limited to the department director. Records released from the file must not leave the department and can be reviewed only under direct supervision.

---

The health record serves as evidence of patient-related events that occur within the facility. The patient health record includes documentation of the facts of an incident as they are related to the care of the patient. For example, if a patient falls out of the bed during his or her stay in the health care facility, the documentation in the patient's record would indicate the time and date of the occurrence. It would also document the position of the patient's bed, use of side rails, and other pertinent information, such as the patient's diagnosis, medications administered, and instructions given to the patient before the incident.

This type of documentation in the health record is different from the occurrence, or incident, report completed when there is an inadvertent occurrence (Figure 11-14). An *incident report* is an administrative discovery tool used by the facility to obtain information about the incident. The incident report is not a part of the patient's health record, nor is it mentioned in any documentation.

Incident reports should be completed immediately by the employee or employees most closely associated with the incident. The incident report is used to perform an investigation

---

**Incident Report**

**Do Not File in Medical Records**

*Confidential and privileged health care quality improvement information prepared in anticipation of litigation*

Name: _____  Employee ☐ Patient ☐ Visitor ☐

Attending physician: _____
MR # _____  SS # _____
D.O.B. __/__/__  Sex: M[ ]  F[ ]
Admission date: __/__/__
Primary diagnosis: _____

Facility name: _____
_____
Site (if applicable) _____
City _____
Facility ID# _____
State _____
Phone # _____

---

**SECTION I: General Information**

**General Identification (circle one):**
001 Inpatient
002 Outpatient
003 Nonpatient
004 Equipment only

**Location (circle one):**
005 Bathroom/toilet
006 Beauty shop
007 Cafeteria/dining room
008 Corridor/hall
009 During transport
010 Emergency department
011 Exterior grounds
012 ICU/SCU/CCU
013 Labor/delivery/birthing
014 Nursery
015 Outpatient clinic
016 Patient room
017 Radiology
018 Recovery room
019 Recreation area
020 Rehab
021 Shower room
022 Surgical suite
023 Treatment/exam room

**Treatment Rendered (circle one):**
024 Emergency room
025 First aid
026 None
026 Transfer to other facility
027 X-ray

---

**SECTION II: Nature of Incident**  (Circle all that apply):

001 Adverse outcome after surgery or anesthetic
002 Anaphylactic shock
003 Anoxic event
004 Apgar score of 5 or less
005 Aspiration
006 Assault or altercation/combative event
007 Blood or IV variance

008 Blood/body fluid exposure
009 Code/arrest
010 Damage/loss of organ
011 Death
012 Dental-related complication
013 Dissatisfaction/noncompliance*
014 Equipment operation*
015 Fall with injury*
016 Fall without injury*

017 Handling of and/or exposure to hazardous waste
018 Informed consent issue
019 Injury to other
020 Injury to self
021 Loss of limb
022 Loss of vision
023 Medication variance*
024 Needle puncture/sharp injury

025 Paralysis
026 Patient-to-patient altercation
027 Perinatal complication*
028 Poisoning
029 Suspected nonstaff-to-patient abuse
030 Suspected staff-to-patient abuse
031 Thermal burn
032 Treatment/procedure issue
033 Ulcer: nosocomial stage III/IV

*\* Complete appropriate area in Section III*

---

**SECTION III: Type of Incident**

**If death, circle all that apply:**
001 After medical equipment failure
002 After power equipment failure or damage
003 During surgery or postanesthesia
004 Within 24 hours of admission to facility
005 Within 1 week of fall in facility
006 Within 24 hours of medication error

**Blood/IV Variance Issues (circle all that apply):**
007 Additive
008 Administration consent
009 Contraindications/allergies
010 Equipment malfunction
011 Infusion rate
012 Labeling issue
013 Reaction
014 Solution/blood type
015 Transcription
016 Patient identification
017 Allergic/adverse reaction
018 Infiltration
019 Phlebitis

**Dissatisfaction/Noncompliance (circle all that apply):**
020 AMA
021 Elopement
022 Irate or angry (either family or patient)
023 Left without service
024 Noncompliant patient
025 Refused prescribed treatment

**Falls (circle all that apply):†**
001 Assisted fall
002 Found on floor
003 From bed
004 From chair
005 From commode/toilet
006 From exam table
007 From stretcher
008 From wheelchair
009 Patient states—unwitnessed
010 Unassisted fall
011 While ambulating
012 Witnessed fall

† For any marks in this field, Section V must be completed

**Medication Variance Issues (circle all that apply):**
013 Contraindication/allergies
014 Delay in dispensing
015 Incorrect dose
016 Expired drug
017 Medication identification
018 Narcotic log variance
019 Not ordered
020 Ordered, not given
021 Patient identification
022 Reaction
023 Route
024 Rx incorrectly dispensed
025 Time of dose
026 Transcription

**Figure 11-14** Incident report. AMA, (patient left hospital) against medical advice; CCU, cardiac care unit; ICU, intensive care unit; Rx, medication (prescribed); SCU, surgical care unit.

---

into the facts surrounding the incident. Facts discovered immediately after the incident can significantly affect the facility's ability to defend, comprehend, or determine the cause of the incident or the liability of the parties in an incident. Examples of inadvertent occurrences are listed in Box 11-6.

Occasionally, events are not recognized as incidents during the patient's stay. Review of documentation by HIM staff members may identify a PCE. As a result, health information is used in risk management to gather facts surrounding an occurrence; support the claim, should it require litigation; or provide information to prevent a future occurrence.

> **BOX 11-6**   **EXAMPLES OF INADVERTENT OCCURRENCES**
>
> - An employee falls in the hallway on a slippery floor, injuring his knee.
> - A visitor entering the elevator is struck by the door as it closes.
> - A missing patient is found on the roof of the health care facility.
> - A patient falls out of bed; assessment of the patient found on the floor of the room reveals a broken arm.
> - A nurse injures her back during transport of a large, uncooperative patient.

## EXERCISE 11-8

### Health Information in Quality Activities

1. Specify the number of records that would be reviewed at the following facilities using the rule of 5% or 30 discharges (whichever is greater):
   a. Hospital A has 1200 discharges each month.
   b. Hospital B has 400 discharges each month.
   c. Hospital C has 150 discharges each month.
2. Health records contain demographic, socioeconomic, financial, and clinical data. If one of the TJC standards requires that the health record contain personal identification information for each patient, where could this information be found in the health record?
3. What would you need to do if an employee reports that he or she fell while on a nursing unit, injuring his or her left knee?
4. A predetermined course of treatment for a patient with a particular diagnosis is known as a(n) _____.
5. A method used to effectively manage patients during their hospitalization is known as _____.
6. Thorough review of the patient's health information to determine pertinence, appropriateness, or compliance with standards is _____.
7. The _____ process would be initiated after a patient fall from the bed to gather information and coordinate the claim.
8. Ensuring appropriate, efficient, and effective patient care is a process of _____.
9. Which of the following is an important process in the determination of the facility's compliance with documentation standards?
   a. Physician profile review
   b. Record review
   c. Mediation review
   d. PDCA

## WORKS CITED

AHIMA: Data Quality Management Model. Appendix A: Data Quality Management Model Domains and Characteristics. AHIMA 83(7):68–71, 2012.

American College of Surgeons: What Is the American College of Surgeons? http://www.facs.org/about/corppro.html. Published 2012.

Centers for Disease Control and Prevention: Vision, Mission, Core Values, and Pledge. http://www.cdc.gov/about/organization/mission.htm. Published 2010.

Centers for Medicare and Medicaid Services (CMS): Hospital Quality Initiative. https://www.cms.gov/Medicare/Quality-Initiatives-Patient-Assessment-Instruments/HospitalQualityInits/index.html?redirect=/HospitalQualityInits/20_OutcomeMeasures.asp. Accessed May 10, 2012a.

Centers for Medicare and Medicaid Services (CMS): Quality Improvement Organization Manual, revision 2, Chapter 4: Case Review. https://www.cms.gov/manuals/downloads/qio110c04.pdf. Published 2003. Accessed April 3, 2012b.

Centers for Medicare and Medicaid Services (CMS): Quality Improvement Organizations. https://www.cms.gov/QualityImprovementOrgs. Accessed April 3, 2012c.

iSixSigma: What is Six Sigma? http://www.isixsigma.com/new-to-six-sigma/getting-started/what-six-sigma/. Accessed May 8, 2012.

Lean Enterprise Institute: A brief history of lean. http://www.lean.org/WhatsLean/History.cfm. Published 2009. Accessed April 19, 2012.

OpenClinical: Clinical Pathways. http://www.openclinical.org/clinicalpathways.html. Published 2012.

QualityNet: QIO Directory. http://www.qualitynet.org/dcs/ContentServer?c=Page&pagename=Qnet Public%2FPage%2FQnetTier2&cid=1144767874793. Accessed April 3, 2012.

Rudman WJ: Performance improvement in health information sciences, Philadelphia, 1997, Saunders.

## SUGGESTED READING

de Koning H, Verver JP, van den Heuvel J, et al: Lean Six Sigma in healthcare. J Healthc Qual 28:4–11, 2006.

The Juran Institute: Juran Health Care. http://www.juran.com/industries_health_care_index.html.

PEPPER (Program for Evaluating Payment Patterns Electronic Report): Welcome to PEPPER resources. http://www.pepperresources.org.

Womack JP, Jones DT: Lean thinking: banish waste and create wealth in your corporation, New York, 2003, Simon & Schuster.

Womack JP, Roos D, Jones DT: The machine that changed the world: the story of lean production, 1991, New York, HarperCollins.

# CHAPTER ACTIVITIES

## CHAPTER SUMMARY

Health information is widely accepted as an important part of the health care industry, and people take for granted that it will be timely, complete, accurate, and valid. As specifically noted in this chapter, the uses of health information are not limited to the internal needs of a health care facility. Patient health information is valuable to many outside the facility. Notably, this chapter reflects the importance of continued efforts to ensure high-quality health information so that it may be used effectively to make decisions about patient care, to establish compliance with standards, and to improve patient care. Having standardized information for all patients, as first required by ACS minimum standards, is important. With standardized information, health care professionals are able to compare one patient's care with another's and determine the quality of each. Standardized information allows for similar information to be shared as well as compared.

With ongoing performance improvement initiatives like National Patient Safety Goals and outcomes measures, the health care record and health information provide the data needed for reporting as well as compliance. Likewise, PI efforts often rely on documentation in patient records to investigate, monitor, and ensure quality.

Ensuring that health information is of high quality allows others to use this vital information for the benefit of patients, communities, payers, and providers.

## REVIEW QUESTIONS

1. List and describe five *internal* health care facility uses of health information.
2. List and describe three *external* uses of health information (external: outside of the health care facility.)
3. Briefly explain the philosophies of Deming, Juran, and Crosby.
4. List three National Patient Safety goals and explain why they are targeted.
5. List two outcome measures publically reported by the CMS.
6. Explain how health information is used to measure the quality of patient care.
7. Explain the PDCA method for performance improvement.
8. Describe the lean performance improvement process.
9. Identify the Six Sigma steps for improvement of an established process.
10. Explain how health information is monitored in the HIM department to ensure quality.

11. List and explain the tools used for data gathering.
12. List and explain the tools used for data organization and presentation.
13. Identify three committees in a health care facility and how they use health information.
14. Explain the structure of the medical staff committee in a health care facility.
15. Explain the purpose and composition of the HIM committee in a health care facility.
16. Explain the differences and similarities among risk management, utilization management, and case management.

## CAREER TIP

Ongoing record review is a TJC requirement, and HIM credentialed professionals are logical leaders for record review and quality auditing. Preparation for this challenge includes a thorough understanding of TJC standards, including the interrelationship among the standards: Provision of Care and Record of Care, for example. Monthly review of TJC's newsletter, *Perspectives,* and annual, thorough review of the standards that affect HIM practice are essential.

## PROFESSIONAL PROFILE

### Assistant Director, HIM

My name is Kim, and I am the assistant director of the health information management (HIM) department. I am responsible for coordinating review of health records (ongoing record review) to ensure compliance with The Joint Commission standards. Record review is performed on a monthly basis at Diamonte. According to standards, my staff and I review 50 records each month. I make sure that all of the records are pulled before the meeting and prepare enough forms for review of the 50 records. During the multidisciplinary review meeting, I help the team members when they have a problem interpreting a standard or locating information in the health record. After all 50 records have been reviewed, I collect the forms and tabulate the scores to determine the compliance with each standard. I then present the results of this review to the HIM committee for recommendation and action, as necessary. If the committee suggests a corrective action to improve compliance with a standard, I coordinate that effort. After the implementation of the corrective action, I report back to the HIM committee to show whether compliance has been achieved.

## PATIENT CARE PERSPECTIVE

### Dr. Lewis's Partner, Dr. Milque

I sit on the ongoing record review committee. It is a very interesting process. At first, I thought it was a waste of time to look at these records and that the regulators were just making us jump through hoops. However, now that I have seen for myself the problems that users of the records have when documentation is missing or inaccurate, I have become an advocate of record review. I recently addressed the medical staff on the importance of completing records as soon as possible after discharge. In this electronic environment, 30 days is much too long to wait for a completed record.

## APPLICATION

### Record Review

Members of the record review team perform a mock record review. Use the health record forms provided on the Evolve site and the generic record review form (see Figure 11-13) to identify where the information on the record review form should be located in the patient's record.

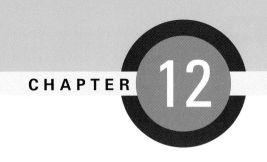

CHAPTER 12

# CONFIDENTIALITY AND COMPLIANCE

Kathleen Frawley

## CHAPTER OUTLINE

## VOCABULARY

access
accounting of disclosures
advance directive
amendment
business associate
business record rule
certification
competency
compliance
Conditions of Admission
confidential
  communications
confidentiality
consent
correspondence
court order
covered entity

custodian
defendant
designated record set
disclosure
discovery
emancipation
exceptions
Federal Drug and Alcohol
  Abuse Regulations
hearsay rule
Health Insurance Portability
  and Accountability Act
  (HIPAA)
informed consent
jurisdiction
liability
litigation

malpractice
minimum necessary
negligence
Notice of Privacy Practices
outsourcing
permitted disclosure
personal health record
physician-patient privilege
plaintiff
power of attorney
preemption
privacy
privacy officer
prospective consent
protected health
  information (PHI)
public priority exception

release of information
required disclosure
restriction
retention
retrospective consent
right to complain
right to revoke
security
statute
subpoena
subpoena ad testificandum
subpoena duces tecum
The Joint Commission
  (TJC)
tort
use
verification

## CHAPTER OBJECTIVES

*By the end of this chapter, the student should be able to:*

1. Distinguish among privacy, confidentiality, and security.
2. Explain the foundation for privacy regulation.
3. List and describe the federal laws and regulations governing patient privacy and confidentiality.
4. Explain the components of the HIPAA privacy regulations.
5. Understand how HITECH legislation has changed HIPAA regulations.
6. List and describe the types of subpoenas.

7. Define *jurisdiction*.
8. Prepare information for copying, photocopy it, and send it out.
9. Differentiate between release of patient information with and without consent.
10. Develop and implement departmental policies and procedures regarding release of information to patients.
11. Develop and implement departmental policies and procedures regarding release of information to care providers.
12. Understand accreditation and its importance.

**release of information (ROI)** The term used to describe the HIM department function that provides disclosure of patient health information.

**Health Insurance Portability and Accountability Act (HIPAA)** Public Law 104-191, federal legislation passed in 1996 that outlines the guidelines of managing patient information in terms of privacy, security, and confidentiality. The legislation also outlines penalties for noncompliance.

**Health Information Technology for Economic and Clinical Health (HITECH) Act** A subset of the American Recovery and Reinvestment Act (2009) legislation providing federal funding and mandates for the use of technology in health care.

**HIM** health information management

**confidentiality** Discretion regarding the disclosure of information.
**privacy** The right of an individual to control access to medical information.
**security** The administrative, physical, and technological safeguards used to protect patient health information.

**physician-patient privilege** The legal foundation that private communication between a physician and a patient is confidential. Only the patient has the right to give up this privilege.
**diagnosis** The name of the patient's condition or illness.
**treatment** A procedure, medication, or other measure designed to cure or alleviate the symptoms of disease.

**minimum necessary** A rule requiring health providers to disclose only the minimum amount of information necessary to accomplish a task.

The topic of confidentiality was introduced in Chapter 5 with regard to the function of release of information. This chapter focuses on the release of information (ROI) and confidentiality as it relates to the actions of health care workers and outside parties. It includes an overview of the federal **Health Insurance Portability and Accountability Act (HIPAA)** Privacy Regulations, its expansion following the passage of the Health Information Technology for Economic and Clinical Health (HITECH) Act, regarding patient rights, as well as uses and disclosures of health information. The importance of confidentiality, the rules critical to ensuring the confidentiality of a health record, and problems that can occur when requests for release of health information are received are also discussed. The function of release of information is primarily the responsibility of the health information management (HIM) department but may occur at other locations in the continuity of health care and by a number of other individuals also involved at various junctures.

## CONFIDENTIALITY

### Definition

Although the terms *privacy* and *confidentiality* are often used synonymously, they have different meanings. **Confidentiality** implies the use of discretion in the disclosure of information. In very simple terms, it is like keeping a secret. When a patient is receiving medical care, no matter what the facility, no matter whom the provider, that information is confidential—it is secret. It may not be released to a person who is not authorized to receive it. **Privacy** is the right of the individual to control access to that information. **Security** is the administrative, physical, and technological safeguards used to protect information.

### Legal Foundation

The foundation for confidentiality is **physician-patient privilege**. This concept refers to communication between the patient and his or her physician. To promote complete and honest communication between the physician and patient, such communication cannot be disclosed to other parties without authorization. Although the facility owns the physical or electronic record, the patient owns the information in the record. Only the patient can waive the right to keep that communication confidential. Although the concept of physician-patient privilege varies from state to state, this privilege generally prevents confidential communications between physicians and patients related to diagnosis and treatment from being disclosed in court.

### Scope

The scope of confidentiality is very broad. It includes not only the confidentiality of the written or electronic record but also spoken information. There are some basic guidelines that a health care professional can follow when working in a health care facility. First, health care professionals should never discuss information about patients in a public place, such as the cafeteria, elevators, and hallways, because others may be able to hear their conversations.

If it becomes necessary to discuss a patient in a public place, minimum necessary patient identifiers should be used—that is, the patient should be discussed only by diagnosis or in some manner that prevents others from being able to identify the patient. However, care should be taken even in this regard. For example, discussing a patient by room number can violate the patient's privacy if the conversation is overheard by someone who knows what room the patient is in (e.g., a family member). This may seem like common sense, but it is one of the most common violations of a patient's right to confidentiality.

All employees should sign a confidentiality agreement when they are hired. Annual re-signing of that document, along with in-service training in the necessity for understanding and complying with the facility's confidentiality policies and procedures, is recommended. Figure 12-1 is a sample confidentiality agreement.

A second issue in confidentiality is the physical maintenance of the patient's health record. Physical documents should be kept in a binder or folder at all times. Binders or folders containing a specific patient's documents should be identified only with the patient's name, medical record number, and room number (if applicable). No matter how the record is maintained, the outside of the folder or binder should not contain any diagnostic information or anything of significance that could be read by a casual passerby. On the nursing unit, only the bed number should be visible on the patient's binder. An important exception to this rule is a warning about allergies. Patient allergies should be clearly noted on the front of the binder. Employees are often tempted to mark the binder with clinically significant information, such as "HIV Positive." Such sensitive information should not be

> **health record** Also called *record* or *medical record*. It contains all of the data collected for an individual patient.
>
> **medical record number (MR#)** A unique number assigned to each patient in a health care system; this code will be used for the rest of the patient's encounters with that specific health system.

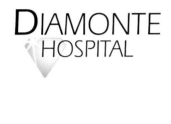

CONFIDENTIALITY AGREEMENT

I, _____ , understand that I have a legal and ethical duty to maintain the confidentiality of the private health information of all patients treated at this facility. During the course of my employment or assignment at Diamonte Hospital, I will have access to confidential patient information.

I understand that I am obligated by state law, federal law, and Diamonte Hospital to protect and safeguard the confidentiality of all patient data and/or health information. I agree that I will not disclose any patient information to any person, except that which is necessary in the course of my employment or assignment, even after my term of employment or assignment ends.

I understand that violation of this agreement may result in punitive legal action and disciplinary action, including termination of my employment or assignment.

_____        _____
Signature of Employee/Student/Volunteer        Date

_____        _____
Signature of Witness        Date

**Figure 12-1** Confidentiality agreement.

visible. Some facilities place color-coded stickers or other symbols on the outside of the binder to circumvent this rule; however, these symbols should not be easily recognizable by the casual observer.

Confidentiality procedures extend to the hallways and to the patient's room itself. Even health care professionals do not have a right to access a patient's record unless they are actually working with the patient. The patient's actual diagnoses, procedures, and appointments should not be displayed where the casual observer can see them. This is a common failing in facilities where multiple individuals need to know the activities of a patient. For example, in an inpatient rehabilitation facility, patients do not generally remain in their rooms. They are transported to other parts of the facility for various therapies, or they may be taken out of the facility for a procedure. The temptation is to post the patient's schedule and other details in a common area where all health care providers can see it. To protect the patient's privacy, however, such postings should be confined to restricted areas.

Certain special considerations apply to technology in the facility. Computer screens should be placed so that they are not in public view. A health care professional accessing a patient's record at a computer terminal may be called away temporarily. It is very important for the person to log off the computer before leaving so that patient information is not visible to anyone who is not authorized to view it. Computer systems should always provide an automatic log-off after a certain period of idle time. A typical screen saver is not sufficient for the purpose of protecting patient information. The entire record should be logged off and made inaccessible without a specific user name and password. Passwords should not be shared among caregivers, even for reasons of efficiency. Passwords should not be written near computers or anywhere that unauthorized users could obtain them.

## Legislation

A **statute** is a law that has been passed by the legislative branch of government. Legislation dealing with confidentiality and health information varies at the state level. Federal regulations, discussed in the following section, must also be followed.

Each state has licensure requirements for health care facilities. Generally, states also have regulations regarding medical records. Health care facilities must comply with these regulations in order to maintain their facility license. A facility often has to follow federal laws, federal regulations, state laws, and state regulations. The Health Insurance Portability and Accountability Act (HIPAA) clarifies that when the privacy regulations conflict with state law, the regulation or law that gives the patient more rights or is more restrictive should prevail. This is called **preemption.** Therefore practices vary from state to state, and HIM professionals must become familiar with applicable state laws and licensure rules and regulations as well as federal laws and regulations.

**statute** A law that has been passed by the legislative branch of government.

**licensure** The mandatory government approval required for performing specified activities. In health care, the state approval required for providing health care services.

**preemption** The legal principle supporting the HIPAA stipulation that when the privacy regulations conflict with state law, the regulation or law that gives the patient more rights or is more restrictive should prevail.

## ▪ EXERCISE 12-1

### Confidentiality

1. What is the difference between privacy and confidentiality?
2. What is the legal foundation for confidentiality?

## HEALTH INSURANCE PORTABILITY AND ACCOUNTABILITY ACT

**Medicare** Federally funded health care insurance plan for older adults and for certain categories of chronically ill patients.

**Medicaid** A federally mandated, state-funded program providing access to health care for the poor and the medically indigent.

Public Law 104-191 is the legal reference for the Health Insurance Portability and Accountability Act of 1996, commonly known as HIPAA. Title II contains the Administrative Simplification Section. Within Title II are major categories dealing with health information: Electronic Transactions and Code Sets, Unique Identifiers, the Privacy Rule, and the Security Rule. The purpose of Title II is to improve the Medicare and Medicaid programs and to improve the efficiency and effectiveness of health information systems by establishing a common set of standards and requirements for handling electronic information.

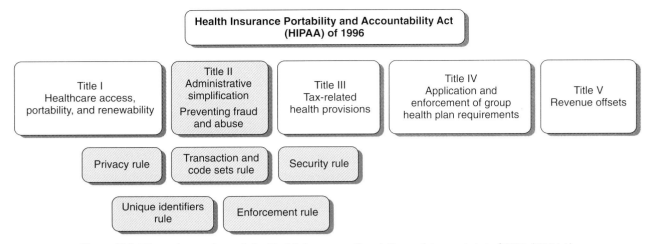

Figure 12-2 The major sections of the Health Insurance Portability and Account Act of 1996 (HIPAA).

The HIPAA Privacy Regulations address the use and disclosure of protected health information in any format: verbal, written, or electronic. The HIPAA Security Regulations address administrative, physical, and technical safeguards to protect health information that is collected, maintained, used, or transmitted electronically.

Health care providers, health care plans, and health care clearinghouses must comply with the HIPAA privacy and security regulations if they participate in federally funded programs. HITECH provisions have expanded this legislation to include any organization that obtains and manages health information. These groups are known as **covered entities**. Business associates must also comply. **Business associates** are those contracted vendors that use confidential health information to perform a service on behalf of the covered entity. Figure 12-2 illustrates the major sections of HIPAA.

**Go To** Review HIPAA's *transaction code sets* in Chapter 6.

**Go To** The importance and impact of HITECH is discussed in Chapter 3.

**covered entity** Under HIPAA and HITECH provisions, any organization that collects and manages health information.
**business associates** Under HIPAA, a contracted vendor that uses confidential health information to perform a service on behalf of a covered entity.

### HIT-bit

#### EXAMPLES OF BUSINESS ASSOCIATES

Typical business associates of the health information department are an outsourced medical transcription company, the release-of-information vendor, legal counsel representing the health care facility, reimbursement consultants, and the microfilm/imaging/storage vendor. They are not members of the facility's workforce, but they use or disclose health information to perform a function or activity on behalf of the health care facility.

## Privacy Regulations

This chapter focuses on the Privacy Rule because health information professionals play key roles in assisting health care facilities with HIPAA privacy compliance. The rule introduces the role of **privacy officer**, appointed by the facility to handle privacy compliance. Facilities must also designate a person to handle any complaints, though the privacy officer usually handles this role as well. Health care facilities have been required to be in compliance with HIPAA's Privacy Rule since 2003.

**privacy officer** The designated official in the health care organization who oversees privacy compliance and handles complaints.

## Protected Health Information

The Privacy Rule addresses the uses and disclosures of **protected health information** (**PHI**). PHI is individually identifiable health information that is transmitted or maintained in any form or medium by covered entities or their business associates. This includes oral, written, and electronic information. Some examples of PHI are name, address, telephone number, fax number, e-mail address, Social Security number, medical record number,

**protected health information (PHI)** Individually identifiable health information that is transmitted or maintained in any form or medium by covered entities or their business associates.

health plan number, account number, driver's license number, license plate number, URL, Internet service provider address, biometric identifiers (e.g., fingerprints), photos, and all relevant dates (e.g., dates of birth, admission, and discharge). These data items could identify a person, thereby violating his or her right to privacy.

## Uses and Disclosures

Health information is used to treat patients. When a physician reviews a test result, it is a **use** of PHI. A **disclosure** occurs when PHI is given to someone. For example, an insurance company is given a copy of an emergency department record to verify that the patient's condition was indeed an emergency, as defined in the patient's health insurance policy. This disclosure may be necessary to obtain reimbursement from the insurer.

> ### HIT-bit
>
> #### PRIVACY AND SECURITY CREDENTIALS
>
> Many health information professionals serve as privacy officers for their facilities. AHIMA offers a special credential: CHPS (Certified in Healthcare Privacy and Security).

PHI cannot be used or disclosed unless the Privacy Rule requires or permits it to be used or disclosed. There are two types of **required disclosures**: disclosures to the patient, and disclosures to the Secretary of the Department of Health and Human Services for compliance auditing purposes. There are also several **permitted disclosures** outlined in the Privacy Rule. All disclosures that are specifically authorized by the patient are permitted. Disclosures for treatment purposes, payment of the patient's bill, or health care operations such as risk management are all permitted and do not need to be authorized by the patient. Disclosures for research purposes are permitted under specific conditions.

Uses and disclosures of PHI without patient authorization are also permitted for certain public priorities. These are considered **exceptions**. Covered entities must comply with the conditions in the exceptions. The following are some exceptions:

- As required by law
- For public health activities
- About victims of abuse, neglect, or domestic violence
- For health oversight activities
- For judicial and administrative proceedings
- For law enforcement
- About decedents (to coroners, medical examiners, funeral directors)
- To facilitate cadaver organ donation and transplants
- For certain research
- To avert a serious threat to health or safety
- For specialized government functions (e.g., military, veterans' groups, national security, protective services, State Department, correctional facilities)
- For workers' compensation (as authorized by law)

> ### HIT-bit
>
> #### USES FOR HEALTH CARE OPERATIONS
>
> Some examples of health care operations are risk management, infection control, quality improvement, legal counsel, and case management. For example, an infection control nurse is allowed to review the medical records of a patient with an infectious disease without authorization in order to investigate the outbreak, keep statistics, and prevent the spread of a disease to other patients.

---

**use** The employment of protected health information for a purpose.

**disclosure** When patient health information is given to someone.

**reimbursement** The amount of money that the health care facility receives from the party responsible for paying the bill.

**required disclosure** A disclosure to the patient and to the Secretary of the Department of Health and Human Services for compliance auditing purposes.

**compliance** Meeting standards. Also the development, implementation, and enforcement of policies and procedures that ensure that standards are met.

**permitted disclosure** Disclosure authorized by the patient, or allowed for treatment, payment, or health care operations.

**risk management** The coordination of efforts within a facility to prevent and control inadvertent occurrences.

**exceptions** In HIPAA, uses and disclosures of protected health information for certain public priorities without patient authorization.

**workers' compensation** An employer's coverage of an employee's medical expenses due to a work-related injury or illness.

## Notice of Privacy Practices

Covered entities are required to establish policies and procedures addressing HIPAA privacy issues. One of the most important policies is the **Notice of Privacy Practices**. This document summarizes the facility's privacy policies and explains how the facility may use or disclose patient health information. The notice must be written in clear and simple language and provide examples. Contact information, such as telephone number, for the privacy officer/complaint designee must be included in the notice. Facilities must also obtain a signed acknowledgment from the patient that the notice was received.

## Patient Rights

The Privacy Rule gives patients certain rights, including the right to receive a notice of the privacy practices. In some situations, patients may request a higher level of privacy. In this case, they have the right to ask for additional **restrictions** on the use of their PHI or additional limitations on the amount of PHI disclosed. For example, a patient may ask that the facility not allow her next-door neighbor, a nurse who would normally have access to the record for patient care, to have access to her PHI. Facility administrators must decide whether they can comply with the patient's request. They do not have to honor such a request. For example, the facility may be small, with a limited nursing staff, and the next-door neighbor may need to be involved in the patient's care due to a staffing shortage. A common restriction (called an *opt-out* in HIPAA) is a patient's request to be removed from the patient directory. In other words, individuals calling the facility would not be told that the patient is there, and calls would not be forwarded to the patient. The patient may also ask for **confidential communications**. For example, the patient may ask that the bill be mailed to another address instead of the home address.

Patients have the right of access to their health information. **Access** refers to the ability to learn the contents of a health record by reading it or obtaining a copy. There are many reasons that patients would want access to their record. Many patients are now keeping their own **personal health records (PHRs)**. The purpose of a personal health record is to document the patient's history and provide information for continuing patient care. The American Health Information Management Association (AHIMA) and the American Medical Association (AMA) are both encouraging patients to track their own health information.

The patient is generally required to sign an authorization form or a request-for-access form to obtain or read copies of his or her health information. State laws and regulations vary regarding **retention**, but many facilities do destroy old records after the required retention period has passed. If a patient's appendectomy took place 30 years ago, the paper record may no longer exist. Therefore it is in the patient's best interest to maintain a personal file of health information.

The only legitimate reason to deny access to a patient is if the patient's health care provider decides that the information in the record would be harmful to the patient. This is an unusual circumstance that pertains primarily to behavioral health cases. If knowledge of the information in the record would be harmful to the patient, the provider must document reasons for the refusal of access. Health care providers must also follow a formal appeals process if access is denied. Figure 12-3 illustrates the flow of the decision-making process with regard to access requests.

The HIPAA Privacy Regulations require health care providers to define their **designated record set** to respond to an individual's right to request access, request amendment, and request restriction to his or her PHI. The designated record set must include the legal medical records, the billing records of the patient, and any other information with which a decision was made that affects the patient. Patients have full access to the designated record set. Access by others is discussed later in this chapter.

Patients may not always agree with the information in their designated record set. The HIPAA privacy regulations give every patient the right to request an **amendment** of his or her health information. When a patient asks to amend health information, he or she should be given an amendment/correction request form to complete. It is generally given to the privacy officer for review and response to the patient within 60 days. If the facility cannot

**HIPAA** Health Insurance Portability and Accountability Act

**Notice of Privacy Practices** A notice, written in clear and simple language, summarizing a facility's privacy policies and the conditions for use or disclosure of patient health information.

**PHI** protected health information

**restriction** Under HIPAA's Privacy Rule, the right of patients to limit the use of their protected health information.

**confidential communications** The sharing of patient health information protected from disclosure in court, such as patient/physician. Also refers to transmission of information so as to minimize the risk of inadvertent disclosure, such as patient requesting mailing to an alternative address.

**access** The ability to learn the contents of a record by obtaining it or having the contents revealed.

**personal health record (PHR)** A patient's own copy of health information documenting the patient's health care history and providing information on continuing patient care.

**American Health Information Management Association (AHIMA)** A professional organization supporting the health care industry by promoting high-quality information standards through a variety of activities, including but not limited to accreditation of schools, continuing education, professional development and educational publications, and legislative and regulatory advocacy.

**retention** The procedures governing the storage of records, including duration, location, security, and access.

**designated record set** A specific portion of the patient's health information, consisting of medical records, reimbursement and payer information, and other information used to make health care decisions, all of which may be accessed by the patient under HIPAA provisions.

**amendment** A change to the original document.

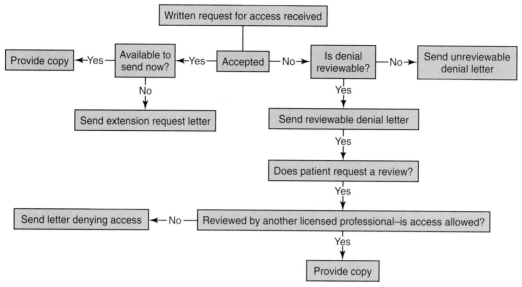

**Figure 12-3** The flow of the decision-making process with regard to access requests.

respond within 60 days, one 30-day extension is allowed. However, the patient must be informed in writing that there is a delay and given an expected date of response. The amendment can be denied if any of the following applies:

- The information was not created by the facility.
- The information is not part of the designated record set.
- The information is not available for access.
- The information is accurate and complete.

Patients are also given the **right to revoke** authorization to disclose their PHI. For example, a patient may authorize his or her attorney to receive a copy of his or her medical record and later change attorneys. The patient would be allowed to revoke the original authorization to Attorney A and authorize a new disclosure to Attorney B.

Facilities are also required to give patients an **accounting of disclosures** upon request. This accounting is basically a list indicating who received information about the patient as well as when, why, and how the disclosure was made. Some disclosures do not require this accounting. Disclosures for treatment, payment, some health care operations, and patient-authorized disclosures do not require accounting. Most facilities track all disclosures, even those for which accounting is not required, because thorough documentation is a good practice. HIPAA requires health care facilities to keep all documentation with regard to an accounting of disclosures for 6 years. However, under the HITECH provisions of the American Recovery and Reinvestment Act (ARRA), if a covered entity uses or maintains an electronic health record (EHR), the HIPAA exception for tracking and documenting disclosures for treatment, payment, and health care operations no longer applies if that disclosure is made through an EHR. In this situation, patients have the right to receive an accounting of disclosures made by the covered entity during the 3 years prior to the date on which the accounting is requested.

**right to revoke** The right to withdraw consent or approval for a previously approved action or request.

**accounting of disclosures** The listing of the identity of those to which certain protected health information has been disclosed.

**American Recovery and Reinvestment Act (ARRA)** Also called the "stimulus bill." 2009 federal legislation providing many stimulus opportunities in different areas. The portion of the law that finds and sets mandates for health information technology is called the HITECH (Health Information Technology for Economic and Clinical Health) Act.

**electronic health record (EHR)** A secure, real-time, point-of-care, patient centric information resource for clinicians allowing access to patient information when and where needed and incorporating evidence-based decision support.

## HIT-bit

### REQUEST FOR AMENDMENT

Usually, the privacy officer contacts the physician or health care professional whose documentation the patient is contesting. This professional reviews the request and decides whether to correct the information. If the professional stands by the information as being correct, the patient is notified that his or her request is denied because the information is accurate and complete. If the patient disagrees with the denial, he or she must be given the opportunity to provide a statement of disagreement. The patient may request that all future releases include a copy of the request for amendment, the facility's denial letter, and the disagreement statement.

Finally, patients have a **right to complain**. They must be given the ability to discuss their concerns about privacy violations with a staff member and ultimately with the U.S. Department of Health and Human Services (DHHS). The Office of Civil Rights has been given DHHS authority to investigate complaints, enforce the privacy rule, and impose penalties for HIPAA violations. Penalties may be civil or criminal and may involve fines and imprisonment depending on the circumstances.

## HITECH Expansion of HIPAA

Health care delivery has changed significantly since HIPAA was enacted in 1996. The increased use of technology for the storage, sharing, and retrieval of health information has raised new concerns over the confidentiality and use of PHI. Chapter 3 introduced the American Recovery and Reinvestment Act (ARRA), which President Obama signed into law on February 17, 2009. Within this legislation is the Health Information Technology for Economic and Clinical Health (HITECH) Act provisions, which sought to fund and direct the future of health information technology. In response to new issues surrounding privacy, the HITECH Act has also strengthened and revised the HIPAA Privacy and Security regulations.

Under the HITECH Act, business associates of covered entities are required to comply with the administrative, physical, and technical safeguard requirements of the HIPAA Security regulations. New types of business associates have been identified. It is important to note that under HITECH provisions, business associates face the same civil and criminal penalties as covered entities. Health information exchanges, regional health information organizations, and e-prescribing gateways that provide data transmission of protected health information (PHI) to a covered entity and that require routine access to protected health information are now included as health care business associates.

There are other key provisions in the HITECH Act. Its passage created a Chief Privacy Officer under the Office of the National Coordinator for Health Information Technology (ONC), charged with advising the ONC on issues related to privacy. Restrictions are further established on the sale of health information. New conditions are established for the use of health information for marketing and fundraising functions. Personal health records (PHRs) with noncovered entities are now protected.

Patients are provided with the right to request restrictions on disclosures of their health information. Covered entities must comply with a requested restriction if the disclosure is to a health plan for the purposes of payment or health care operations. Under HIPAA, patients have had the right to review their protected health information, though electronic records were typically printed out and presented in paper form. The HITECH Act mandates that covered entities maintaining electronic health records are required to provide an electronic copy of an individual's protected health information, either to that individual or to the physician or entity of the patient's choice.

HIPAA maintained exceptions for disclosures of health information for treatment, payment, and health care operations. That is, a patient who requested an accounting of the disclosures of her record might not see disclosures of her PHI for these uses. Under HITECH, however, these exceptions do not apply if the disclosure was made through the EHR, and in an account of disclosures these must now be included. This is a major change, considering the incentives and mandates the HITECH Act has placed on providers to implement EHR. The patient's right to an accounting for disclosures from an EHR, however, applies to only 3 years prior to the date on which the accounting is requested, rather than the 6 years permitted under HIPAA. For example, the patient is treated at a hospital that has an electronic medical record. Under HITECH provisions, the patient can request an accounting of disclosure. Because the hospital has an EHR, only 3 years of information must be provided.

The HITECH Act requires covered entities, when using or disclosing protected health information or requesting protected health information from another covered entity, to limit the information disclosed to a limited data set. If more information is needed, it must be the **minimum necessary**.

**right to complain** The patient's right to discuss his or her concerns about privacy violations.

**HITECH** Health Information Technology for Economic and Clinical Health Act

**business associate** Under HIPAA, a contracted vendor that uses confidential health information to perform a service on behalf of a covered entity.

**protected health information (PHI)** Individually identifiable health information that is transmitted or maintained in any form or medium by covered entities or their business associates.

**Office of the National Coordinator for Health Information Technology (ONC)** An executive division of the U.S. Department of Health and Human Services that coordinates and promotes the national implementation of technology in health care.

**disclosure** When patient health information is given to someone.

**covered entity** Under HIPAA and HITECH provisions, any organization that collects and manages health information.

**minimum necessary** A rule requiring health providers to disclose only the minimum amount of information necessary to accomplish a task.

**business associate** Under HIPAA, a contracted vendor that uses confidential health information to perform a service on behalf of a covered entity.

**DHHS** Department of Health and Human Services

Patients must be notified when there is a breach of unsecured protected health information. This requirement applies to covered entities, business associates, personal health record vendors, and companies that service personal health records. Notifications must be made without unreasonable delay and in no case later than 60 calendar days after the discovery of the breach. Covered entities are required to provide notice of a breach to individuals in writing, by first class mail, sent to the last known address of the individual (or to the next of kin if the individual is deceased). In cases in which there is insufficient information to provide the written notice, a substitute form of notice must be provided. This could be a posting on the covered entity's Web site or in major print or broadcast media.

If the breach involves more than 500 patients, notification must also be made to prominent media outlets. Notice must also be provided to the Secretary of Health and Human Services. If the breach involves fewer than 500 patients, the covered entity may maintain a log of these breaches and submit it annually. If the breach involves more than 500 patients, the notice to the Secretary must occur at the same time notice is given to the patient. The Secretary publishes a list on the DHHS Web site of each covered entity involved in a breach of unsecured protected health information involving more than 500 patients.

---

## HIT-bit

### BREACH NOTIFICATION

Under the definition of *breach*, it is important to note that there are three exceptions: (1) any unintentional acquisition of, access to, or use of protected health information by a workforce member; (2) any inadvertent disclosure by a person who is authorized to access protected health information; and (3) a disclosure of protected health information in which a covered entity and business associate has a good faith belief that an unauthorized person to whom the disclosure was made would not reasonably have been able to retain such information. For example, you are walking down the hall delivering records to the nursing units. You overhear the nursing staff discussing a patient. This would be considered an incidental disclosure and not a breach.

---

The following information must be provided in the breach notification:
- A brief description of what happened, including the date of the breach and the date of the discovery of the breach, if known
- A description of the types of unsecured protected health information that was involved in the breach (such as full name, social security number, date of birth, home address, account number)
- The steps individuals should take to protect themselves from potential harm resulting from the breach
- A brief description of what the covered entity involved is doing to investigate the breach, mitigate losses, and protect against any further breaches
- Contact procedures for individuals to ask questions or learn additional information, which must include a toll-free telephone number and an e-mail, Web site, or postal address.

## EXERCISE 12-2

### HIPAA

1. Describe HIPAA. Why is it important?
2. What is PHI?
3. What is a covered entity?
4. What is a business associate?
5. When a breach of the protected health information of more than _____ patients occurs, covered entities must notify the media and the Secretary of the Department of Health and Human Services.

**⋮ ACCESS**

Despite the need for privacy, there are legitimate reasons for various parties to have access to a patient's PHI. These reasons include the following: treatment (continuing patient care), payment (reimbursement), and health care operations. In addition, the patient may wish to provide access to third parties, such as lawyers.

## Continuing Patient Care

Confidentiality presents some interesting issues for continuity of patient care. The attending physician and direct care providers involved with the patient should have full access to the patient's health information in order to treat the patient. However, what if a physician wishes to review his neighbor's medical record? Should he be given access simply because he is a physician? No. The health care professional must have direct patient involvement or a specific "need to know" in order to obtain the patient's information. Any other access to a patient's record requires specific patient authorization. An example of inappropriate access is a facility employee looking at a family member's medical record without the patient's permission. This misuse of access would be a confidentiality violation. Electronic records systems should provide audit trails indicating who accessed what patient information so that compliance with confidentiality can be documented and violations identified.

It is important to convey to employees of the HIM department and the facility in general that inappropriate access to a record is illegal and will lead to disciplinary measures. The HIPAA Security Regulations discussed earlier in this chapter have a section dealing with workforce security and termination procedures if someone violates the rules. Dismissal of employees who inappropriately access health records is not excessively harsh; it is common.

Health care professionals outside the facility in which the patient was originally treated may also need certain health information. HIPAA's Privacy Regulations allow the use and disclosure of health information for continuing patient care, without specific patient authorization. However, it is common practice to ask for authorizations or at least written requests from outside health care providers because thorough documentation is required for accreditation and certification.

## Reimbursement

Another reason to disclose health information is for reimbursement purposes. In the current health care environment, various payers may need to review the record. HIPAA's Privacy Regulations allow the use and disclosure of health information for payment purposes without authorization. However, it is common practice to have patients sign a **Conditions of Admission** form upon admission to a hospital; this form includes authorization for the release of health information to the party who is financially responsible. This type of authorization constitutes **prospective consent**. In other words, the patient is authorizing the release of information *before* that information has been generated.

Although this authorization is not required—because HIPAA allows release of health information for payment purposes without authorization—it is a common practice because it informs patients that their health information may be disclosed in order for the bill to be paid. In addition, the Notice of Privacy Practices informs the patient that his or her health information may be disclosed for reimbursement purposes.

In most other cases, such as third party release of information for legal purposes, *retrospective consent* is necessary. **Retrospective consent** means that the patient authorizes the use or disclosure of health information *after* care has been rendered.

## Health Care Operations

HIPAA's Privacy Regulations also allow the use and disclosure of health information for health care operations purposes without authorization. Health care operations include functions such as risk management, infection control, case management, and quality

---

**continuity of care** The broad range of health care services required by a patient during an illness or for an entire lifetime. May also refer to the continuity of care provided by a health care organization. Also called *continuum of care.*

**attending physician** The physician who is primarily responsible for coordinating the care of the patient in the hospital; it is usually the physician who ordered the patient's admission to the hospital.

**audit trail** A review of individual user access codes to determine who had access to patient health information and to ensure that the access was deemed necessary for patient care.

**reimbursement** The amount of money that the health care facility receives from the party responsible for paying the bill.

**Conditions of Admission** The legal agreement between the health care facility and a patient (or the patient's legal agent) to perform routine services. May also include the statement of the patient's financial responsibility and prospective consent for release of information and examination and disposal of tissue.

**prospective consent** Permission given prior to having knowledge of the event to which the permission applies. For example, a permission to release information before the information is gathered (i.e., before admission).

**Notice of Privacy Practices** A notice, written in clear and simple language, summarizing a facility's privacy policies and the conditions for use or disclosure of patient health information.

**retrospective consent** Permission given after the event to which the permission applies. For example, permission to release information after the information is gathered (i.e., after discharge).

**minimum necessary** A rule requiring health providers to disclose only the minimum amount of information necessary to accomplish a task.

**litigation** The term used to indicate that a matter must be settled by the court and the process of engaging in legal proceedings.
**plaintiff** The party who initiates litigation.
**defendant** The party or parties against whom the plaintiff has initiated litigation.

**Go To** See the section on negligence and malpractice later in this chapter.

**discovery** The process of investigating the circumstances surrounding a lawsuit.
**certification** The custodian's authentication that the copies of medical records used in litigation are true and complete.
**custodian** The person entrusted with the responsibility for the confidentiality, privacy, and security of medical records.

**HIM** health information management

**business record rule** An exception to the hearsay rule. Allows health records to be admitted as evidence in legal proceedings because they are kept in the normal course of business, are recorded concurrently with the events that they describe, and are recorded by individuals who are in a position to know the facts of the events that are described.

improvement. However, under the HITECH provisions of ARRA, the information disclosed should be a limited data set. If more information is needed, it must be the minimum necessary. Under the minimum necessary standard, covered entities must make reasonable efforts to limit the patient-identifiable information they disclose to the least amount necessary.

## Litigation

Litigation is an area of disclosure in which authorization to release information is required (unless it is to the health care provider's attorney for defense—this is an operations purpose). **Litigation** is the process by which one party sues another in a court of law. Litigation often results when a patient has been injured, either accidentally or intentionally. The party who is suing is the **plaintiff**. The party who is being sued is the **defendant**.

The legal aspects of health information and health care in general are too broad to discuss in this book. However, a general understanding of how a trial works is helpful knowledge for the HIM professional. Most lawsuits that require disclosure of medical records are based on some injury to the patient. A shopper slips and falls in the grocery store, spraining her back, and sues the store. A pedestrian is hit by a car, breaks a leg, and sues the driver of the car. A physician amputates the wrong foot, and the patient sues the physician and the hospital.

The plaintiffs in these cases file a complaint with the court that states the issues, the reason they chose that particular court, and what outcome they desire. In the grocery store example, the plaintiff may file a complaint in a state court stating that the grocery store's floor was wet and posed a hazard, which was the cause of the accident. The complaint is filed in that court because the store is located in that state and the plaintiff lives in that state. The plaintiff wants the court to agree that the store was at fault and to order the store to pay for the plaintiff's medical care and loss of income. The steps in this type of litigation are listed and defined in Box 12-1.

There are two steps in the aforementioned lawsuit in which health records may be required. The first step is during the **discovery** process. During discovery, the lawyers may want a copy of the documentation of the plaintiff's treatment to verify the extent and timing of the injuries as well as the nature, extent, and cost of care. The record may be needed again in court during the trial if it is used as evidence. During both of these steps, a certified or notarized copy of the original record is usually required. **Certification** is the process whereby the official custodian of the medical records certifies that the copies are true and complete copies of the original records. The **custodian**, usually the HIM director, is the official keeper of the medical records and may be called to testify.

The certification and use of health records as evidence in court is based on the **business record rule**. The business record rule states that health records may be accepted as evidence in the following instances:

---

**BOX 12-1** | **STEPS IN LITIGATION**

1. Prelitigation medical review panel or tribunal (does not apply in all states for medical malpractice claims)
2. Filing of the lawsuit in the appropriate state or federal court
3. Discovery: various techniques (e.g., depositions, interrogatories, requests for production of documents and things, admissions of fact, independent medical examinations) are used to discover pertinent information relating to the facts and issues of the case
4. Pretrial settlement hearing
5. Mediation before trial
6. Trial by judge or jury
7. Appeal of the decision or judgment

From Aiken TD: Legal and ethical issues in health occupations, Philadelphia, 2008, Saunders, p. 221.

> **BOX 12-2  COMMON ELEMENTS OF A VALID SUBPOENA**
>
> - Name of the court where the lawsuit is brought
> - Names of the parties to the lawsuit
> - Docket number of the case
> - Date, time, and place of the requested appearance
> - Specific documents to be produced, if a subpoena duces tecum is involved
> - Name and telephone number of the attorney who requested the subpoena
> - Signature, stamp, or seal of the official empowered to issue the subpoena
> - Witness fees, where provided by law
>
> From McWay D: Legal aspects of health information management, Albany, NY, 1996, Delmar.

- They are kept in the normal course of business.
- They are recorded by individuals who are in a position to be knowledgeable of the events that are being recorded.
- They are documented contemporaneously with those events.

The business record rule is an exception to the **hearsay rule**, which prohibits second-hand accounts of events. If the hearsay rule applied to health records, then a nurse's documentation of a patient's statements or a physician's subjective notes would not be admissible evidence (i.e., it would not be allowed to be presented in court).

The choice of a court in which to file the complaint is primarily a matter of **jurisdiction**. Jurisdiction means that the court has authority over the issue, the person, or both. There are courts of limited jurisdiction, such as traffic court, which may decide only certain types of cases. Other courts have general jurisdiction, such as state courts, and they may decide a wide variety of cases. In general, these courts have jurisdiction over citizens of the states in which they operate. There are also federal courts, whose jurisdiction extends to issues regarding federal statutes, regulations, and treaties; events that occur on federal land; and legal actions between citizens of different states.

There are several different avenues through which access to the record can be obtained during litigation. First, the patient can sign an authorization to release the information to either the patient's lawyer or the defendant's lawyer. It is presumed that when a patient institutes litigation and uses the medical condition as a foundation for the litigation, he or she is waiving the right to confidentiality.

Another avenue of approach is through the *subpoena* process. A **subpoena** is a direction from an officer of the court. The direction may be to testify (**subpoena ad testificandum**) or to provide documentation (**subpoena duces tecum**; Figure 12-4). The HIM department may receive a subpoena from the patient's lawyer or from the defendant's lawyer. A subpoena is valid for access to health records only if the subpoena itself is valid and the court through which the subpoena is issued has jurisdiction over the party to whom the subpoena is addressed. Box 12-2 lists the common elements of a valid subpoena.

The HIPAA Privacy Regulations state that a covered entity may disclose protected health information in the course of any judicial or administrative proceeding in response to the following:

- A court order, but only the protected health information expressly authorized for release by the order
- Subpoena duces tecum, provided that the covered entity:
  - receives a written statement and accompanying documents from the party seeking the information that reasonable efforts have been made to ensure that the individual who is the subject of the information has been notified of the request or that reasonable efforts have been made to secure a qualified protective order for the information
  - makes reasonable efforts to limit the protected health information used or disclosed to the minimum necessary to respond to the request

The requirement to provide sufficient notice to the individual is met when a party provides a written statement and accompanying documentation that demonstrates the following:

---

**exceptions** In HIPAA, uses and disclosures of protected health information for certain public priorities without patient authorization.

**hearsay rule** The court rule that prohibits most testimony regarding events by parties who were not directly involved in the event.

**subjective** In the SOAP format of medical decision making, the patient's description of the symptoms or other complaints.

**jurisdiction** The authority of a court to decide certain cases. May be based on geography, money, or type of case.

**confidentiality** Discretion regarding the disclosure of information.

**subpoena** A direction from an officer of the court.

**subpoena ad testificandum** A direction from an officer of the court to provide testimony.

**subpoena duces tecum** A direction from an officer of the court to provide documents.

**covered entity** Under HIPAA and HITECH provisions, any organization that collects and manages health information.

AO 88 (rev. 07/10) Subpoena to appear and testify at a hearing or trial in a civil action

# UNITED STATES DISTRICT COURT
### for the

|  |  |  |
|---|---|---|
| _____ | ) | |
| *Plaintiff* | ) | Civil Action No. |
| *v.* | ) | |
| _____ | ) | |
| *Defendant* | ) | |

### SUBPOENA TO APPEAR AND TESTIFY
### AT A HEARING OR TRIAL IN A CIVIL ACTION

**TO:**

**YOU ARE COMMANDED** to appear in the United States district court at the time, date, and place set forth below to testify at a hearing or trial in this civil action. When you arrive, you must remain at the court until the judge or a court officer allows you to leave.

| Place: | Courtroom No.: |
|---|---|
| | Date and Time: |

You must also bring with you the following documents, electronically stored information, or objects *(blank if not applicable)*:

The provisions of Fed. R. Civ. P. 45(c), relating to your protection as a person subject to a subpoena, and Fed. R. Civ. P. 45 (d) and (e), relating to your duty to respond to this subpoena and the potential consequences of not doing so, are attached.

Date: _____

*CLERK OF COURT*

OR

_____          _____
*Signature of Clerk or Deputy Clerk*                    *Attorney's signature*

The name, address, e-mail, and telephone number of the attorney representing *(name of party)* _____ _____ , who issues or requests this subpoena, are:

**Figure 12-4** Sample subpoena to testify in a civil case.

- A good faith attempt was made to notify the individual.
- The notice included sufficient information to permit the individual to raise an objection with the court.
- The time for the individual to raise objections has lapsed, no objection was filed or objections have been resolved by the court, and the disclosure is consistent with the resolution.

AO 88 (rev. 07/10) Subpoena to appear and testify at a hearing or trial in a civil action (page 2)

Civil Action No.

### PROOF OF SERVICE
*(This section should not be filed with the court unless required by Fed. R. Civ. P. 45.)*

This subpoena for *(name of individual and title, if any)* _____
was received by me on *(date)* _____.

☐ I served the subpoena by delivering a copy to the named person as follows: _____

_____

_____ on *(date)* _____ ; or

☐ I returned the subpoena unexecuted because: _____

_____ .

Unless the subpoena was issued on behalf of the United States, or one of its officers or agents, I have also tendered
to the witness fees for one day's attendance, and the mileage allowed by law, in the amount of
$ _____ .

My fees are $ _____ for travel and $ _____ for services, for a total of $ _____ .

I declare under penalty of perjury that this information is true.

Date: _____          _____
                                                *Server's signature*

                               _____
                                                *Printed name and title*

                               _____
                                                *Server's address*

Additional information regarding attempted service, etc:

**Figure 12-4, cont'd**

---

A qualified protective order is an order of a court that prohibits the parties from using or disclosing the PHI for any purpose other than the litigation or proceeding for which such information was requested and requires the return to the covered entity or destruction of the PHI (including any copies) at the end of the litigation or proceeding.

A **court order** is the direction of a judge who has made a decision that an order to produce the records is necessary. Again, the issue of jurisdiction arises. For example, if an older patient's children seek to declare the patient legally incompetent (unable to make decisions about his or her affairs), the judge may issue a court order to obtain the patient's health records. Box 12-3 gives the components of a valid court order authorizing disclosure.

**PHI** protected health information

**court order** The direction of a judge who has made a decision that an order to produce information (on the record) is necessary.

**disclosure** When patient health information is given to someone.

> **BOX 12-3  COMPONENTS OF A VALID COURT ORDER AUTHORIZING DISCLOSURE**
>
> - Name of the court issuing the order authorizing disclosure
> - Names of the parties to the lawsuit
> - Docket number of the case
> - Limitations for disclosure of only those components of the patient's records that are essential to fulfill the objective of the order
> - Limitations on disclosure to those persons whose need for information is the basis of the order
> - Any other limitations on disclosure that serve to protect the patient, the physician-patient relationship, and/or the treatment given, such as sealing the court proceeding from public scrutiny
>
> From McWay D: Legal aspects of health information management, Albany, NY, 1996, Delmar.

### Negligence, Medical Malpractice, and Liability

Some types of litigation concern the delivery of patient care itself. A lawsuit may be filed when there is harm to the patient, even if the damage is unintentional. When a surgeon amputates the wrong foot it is a clear example of harm or damage to the patient, though there are other cases. Invasion of privacy and breach of contract—especially when it concerns patient confidentiality—are common types of claims of which HIM professionals in particular must be aware. Again, many books are devoted solely to the complexities of health care and the law, but it is important to introduce several key concepts.

*Negligence* comes from a Latin word meaning "to neglect." In the case of the shopper who slipped and fell at the grocery store, the supermarket may have been negligent if the floor had been recently mopped, and it *neglected* to warn customers with "Caution - Wet Floor" signs. The type of harm (or **tort** in legal terminology) this caused was not intentional, but reasonable care may have prevented the accident. **Negligence** therefore refers to a wrong against an individual caused by a failure to be careful, or a failure to foresee the potential for harm.

*Malpractice* revolves around the concept of negligence. When a patient seeks treatment from a physician, the physician and patient enter an agreement in which the physician is obligated to use his or her skills to treat the patient with care, and at a standard of professional competence. **Malpractice** occurs when a health care provider incurs harm to a patient because of a failure to practice reasonable standards of care. Most instances of medical malpractice involve medical error, such as misdiagnosis of a patient's condition, or a surgeon who inadvertently leaves an instrument in a patient during an operation. Malpractice may also refer to intentional wrongdoing, though the majority of medical malpractice claims result from negligence on the part of the provider.

A legal **liability** is the responsibility for harm or damage caused by one's actions—or inactions. A physician who has amputated a patient's left foot instead of his right foot is probably liable for the harm caused to the patient. Employers are also liable for the actions of their employees and can be sued under the doctrine of vicarious liability (respondent *superior*). However, many physicians are not employees of the hospital, and, as independent practitioners, vicarious liability excludes hospitals themselves from the actions of non-employee physicians. This situation changed after the 1965 case, *Darling v. Charleston Community Memorial Hospital*. In *Darling*, a physician fit a football player's broken leg with a cast that was too tight. Nurses employed by the hospital alerted the physician of the boy's worsening condition over the next several days, but the treating physician failed to take appropriate action, and eventually the leg had to be amputated. The boy's parents sued the hospital, and the court found that the hospital failed to monitor the quality of care being delivered within. After the Charleston case, hospitals could be sued directly under "corporate negligence."

---

**tort** Harm, damage, or wrongdoing that entitles the injured party to compensation.

**negligence** Carelessness or lack of foresight that leads to harm or damage.

**malpractice** In health care, harm to a patient caused by a failure to practice within the standards of professional competence.

**liability** The legal responsibility for wrongdoing.

## EXERCISE 12-3

### Access

1. What is jurisdiction?
2. What is the hearsay rule? How does it affect cases involving health records?
3. What are the components of the business record rule?
4. Explain the difference between retrospective consent and prospective consent. Why is the difference important?
5. Over what events or circumstances does a federal court have jurisdiction?
6. Number the steps in a civil lawsuit in their correct order:
   _____ Appeal
   _____ Complaint
   _____ Discovery
   _____ Pretrial conference
   _____ Satisfying the judgment
   _____ Trial
7. The legal term for harm or damages suffered by an individual is _____.
8. How has the doctrine of corporate negligence affected hospitals?

## CONSENT

In health care, **consent** refers to the patient's agreement to allow something to occur. Consents underlie virtually all of a patient's contacts with health care professionals. Consents may be either implied or expressed. When a patient makes an appointment with a physician to get a flu shot, consent to have the shot is implied because the patient showed up for the appointment. Express consent, however, would involve signing a consent form to take the shot.

### Informed Consent

For a patient to give consent, the patient must be of legal age, competent, and provided with sufficient information to make a reasonable decision about the issue to which he or she is consenting.

*Legal age* generally refers to having achieved the statutory age, which is determined by state law. Statutory age is usually 18 years. There are some exceptions, such as emancipated minors and minors receiving psychiatric treatment, chemical dependency counseling, or prenatal care. State laws outline the conditions in which minors are given **emancipation** (i.e., consideration as an adult even though they are younger than the statutory age). A common reason for emancipation is marriage.

**Competency** is the patient's ability to make reasonable decisions. A patient is competent if a court has not declared the individual incompetent and the patient is capable of understanding the alternatives and consequences of his or her decision. A patient who has been declared incompetent by a court has a guardian who can consent on behalf of the patient. This guardian is given a health care **power of attorney**. In general, a patient is assumed to be competent unless there is evidence to the contrary. When a patient's competence is in doubt, the patient's physician and hospital attorney should be contacted for guidance.

**Informed consent** requires an explanation of the process, procedure, risks, or other activity to which the patient is consenting. Sufficient information must be provided to the patient so that he or she can make an informed decision about the matter. Documentation of this informed consent is required before health care can be rendered.

### Admission

For admission to a health care facility or a visit to a physician's office, the patient is asked to sign a document consenting to medical treatment. This type of consent is very general and covers routine procedures, such as physical examinations and medical therapies,

**consent** An agreement or permission to receive health care services.

**emancipation** Consideration of a patient as an adult even though the patient is younger than the statutory age.

**competency** The ability to successfully complete a task or skill.

**power of attorney** The legal document that identifies someone as the legal representative to make decisions for the patient when the patient is unable to do so.

**informed consent** A permission given by a competent individual, of legal age, with full knowledge or understanding of the risks, potential benefits, and potential consequences of the permission.

**admission** The act of accepting a patient into care in a health care facility, including any nonambulatory care facility. Admission requires a physician's order.

Community Hospital
555 Street Drive
Town, NJ 07999
(973) 555-5555

554879
Green, John
44 Avenue Street
Town, NJ 07999

Dr. Ramundo

**Admission Consent**

1. I understand that I am suffering from a condition requiring diagnosis and medical and/or surgical treatment. I voluntarily consent to such medical treatment deemed necessary or advisable by my treating physician, his associates, or assistants, in the treatment and care rendered to me, while a patient in Community Hospital. I also give permission for the services of any consulting physician that my attending physician deems necessary in his/her treatment of me.
2. I authorize Community Hospital, its medical and surgical staff, and its medical and other employees to furnish the appropriate hospital service and care deemed necessary by my condition.
3. I am aware that the practice of medicine and surgery is not an exact science and I acknowledge that no guarantees have been made to me as to the results of any diagnosis, treatment, or hospital care that I may receive at Community Hospital.
4. I authorize the transfer of medical information to any federal, state, or local government institution, or any agency, nursing home, or extended care facility to which I may be transferred or from which I may require assistance.
5. I certify that the information given by me regarding my health insurance is current and accurate, to the best of my knowledge. I authorize the release of any information needed to act on obtaining reimbursement from the parties so named. I understand that I am responsible for any health insurance deductibles or copayments and I do hereby agree to pay all bills rendered by Community Hospital for my hospital, medical, and nursing care that are not covered by these parties.
6. I authorize Community Hospital to retain, preserve, and use for scientific or teaching purposes, or dispose of at their convenience, any specimens or tissues taken from my body and any x-rays, photographs, or similar data taken during my hospitalization.
7. This form has been fully explained to me and I certify that I understand its contents.

_____     _____
Witness                                              Date

_____     _____
Interpreter                                          Date

_____     _____
Signature of patient, agent, or legal guardian      Date

**Figure 12-5** Sample of Conditions of Admission to a hospital.

**inpatient** An individual who is admitted to a hospital with the intention of staying overnight.

**Conditions of Admission** The legal agreement between the health care facility and a patient (or the patient's legal agent) to perform routine services. May also include the statement of the patient's financial responsibility and prospective consent for release of information and examination and disposal of tissue.

**advance directive** A written document, such as a living will, that specifies a patient's wishes for his or her care and dictates power of attorney, for the purpose of providing clear instructions in the event the patient is unable to do so.

nutrition counseling, and prescribing medications. In an inpatient facility, this consent is usually called the Conditions of Admission (Figure 12-5). The Conditions of Admission form generally also includes permission for the facility to use patient information for education, research, and reimbursement.

Under the Patient Self-Determination Act, all health care providers that receive Medicare or Medicaid funding are required to inform patients of their legal right to accept or refuse treatment and the right to formulate advance directives. An **advance directive** is defined as a written document such as a living will or durable power of attorney for health care.

## Medical Procedures

The Conditions of Admission form includes only routine procedures and administrative issues. For invasive procedures, such as surgery, a specific consent is required. Anesthesia delivery and human immunodeficiency virus (HIV) testing are examples of other procedures that require specific consent. These consents are intended, in part, to document the extent to which procedures have been explained to patients, including the known risks of the procedures. Figure 12-6 shows a consent for surgery form.

## Community Hospital
555 Street Drive
Town, NJ 07999
(973) 555-5555

| Consent to Operation or Other Procedure(s) |
|---|

554879
Green, John
44 Avenue Street
Town, NJ 07999

Dr. Ramundo

1.  I understand that _____ is proposed to be performed by _____ and/or his/her associates and whomever may be designated as assistants.

2.  I understand that the nature and purpose of the operation or procedure is to _____
    _____
    _____

3.  I understand that possible alternative methods of treatment are _____
    _____
    _____

4.  I understand that the risks and possible complications of this operation or procedure are _____
    _____

5.  I am aware that the practice of medicine and surgery is not an exact science and I acknowledge that no guarantees have been made to me as to the result of this procedure.

6.  I consent to the examination and disposition by hospital authorities of any tissue or parts which may be removed during the course of this operation or procedure.

7.  I understand the nature of the proposed operation or procedure(s), the risks and possible complications involved, and the expected results, as described above, and hereby request that such operation or procedure(s) be performed.

8.  I realize that an operation or procedure requires numerous assistants, technicians, nurses, and other personnel and I give my consent to care by such personnel before, during, and after the operation or procedure to be performed.

9.  I also consent to videotaping or photographing of the operation or procedure for scientific or teaching purposes.

_____  _____
Witness (may not be a member of operating team)    Date

_____  _____
Interpreter                                        Date

_____  _____
Signature of patient, agent, or legal guardian     Date

I have discussed with the above patient the nature of the proposed operation or procedure(s), the risks and possible complications involved, and the expected results, as described above.

_____
Signature of counseling physician

**Figure 12-6** Sample of consent for surgery.

## EXERCISE 12-4

### Consent

1. Permission to perform a medical procedure generally requires the patient's _____.
2. A 16-year-old patient presents in the emergency department for treatment of stomach pain. She is conscious, alert, and oriented. Who is the appropriate individual to sign the consent for treatment?
3. What are the elements of a valid authorization for release of information?
4. A permission that is given after the event to which the permission applies is _____.

## RELEASE OF INFORMATION

**release of information (ROI)** The term used to describe the HIM department function that provides disclosure of patient health information.
**correspondence** Mailing or letters exchanged between parties.
**outsourcing** Refers to services that are provided by external organizations or individuals who are not employees of the facility for which the services are being provided.

**DHHS** Department of Health and Human Services

**disclosure** When patient health information is given to someone.
**exceptions** In HIPAA, uses and disclosures of protected health information for certain public priorities without patient authorization.

**physician-patient privilege** The legal foundation that private communication between a physician and a patient is confidential. Only the patient has the right to give up this privilege.

In both paper-based and electronic environments, portions of the record must sometimes be disclosed. Duplication may be accomplished by photocopying the paper record, printing a copy from a computer or microfilm printer, or transmitting the information electronically, such as by faxing it from an electronic system. In practice, the duplicate is generally provided in paper format, regardless of how it is stored or maintained. The function of disclosing health information in the HIM department is often called **release of information** (ROI) or **correspondence**. This function is often **outsourced** (i.e., performed by outside contractors instead of facility personnel).

### Required Disclosures

HIPAA's Privacy Rule discusses two types of required disclosures:
- To the individual who is the subject of the information
- To the secretary of the DHHS for purposes of determining compliance

### Permitted Disclosures

All other disclosures are permitted. The following are permitted disclosures:
- To the individual or his personal representative
- For treatment, payment, or health care operations
- For public priority purposes (exceptions)
- As authorized by the patient

### Authorized Disclosures

The patient may authorize the release of his or her information to anyone. Remember that only the patient (or his or her personal representative) can waive the physician-patient privilege. Documentation of the patient's consent to release information is accomplished by completion of an authorization form. As with consents for medical procedures, the concept of informed consent applies. The patient must know in advance the nature and purpose of the consent for disclosure. Therefore consents for release of information should be retrospective. In other words, the patient cannot be fully informed about what is being released until after the information has been generated.

### HIT-bit

#### PERSONAL REPRESENTATIVE

A *personal representative* is an individual who is authorized to act on behalf of the patient. For example, a parent is generally a personal representative of his or her minor child. This title would also apply to a legal guardian or person acting "in loco parentis" of a minor child. In addition, if state law gives a person authority to act on behalf of a deceased individual (usually the executor, administrator, spouse, or next of kin), then that person would be considered a personal representative.

Technically, it is not necessary for a patient to complete a specific form in order to authorize the release of information. Each health care facility should have an access policy. A letter addressed to the facility should suffice if it contains all of the elements of a valid authorization, but many facilities still require the use of a specific authorization form. HIPAA-compliant authorizations require the following core elements:

*Identification of the party being asked to release the information:* The owner of the actual documents (i.e., the facility or health care provider who has custody of the documents) is named.

*Patient name/identification:* The patient's name is the primary identifier. However, because many individuals have the same or similar names, additional identifiers such as date of birth or Social Security number should be documented. The medical record number or account number is also very useful, if known.

*Identification of the party to whom the information is to be released:* The person or class of persons to whom information is being released must be listed. This may be the name of a facility, a health care provider, or any other party. In other words, to whom does the patient want the information to be sent? It is also important to include the accurate address of this party.

*Specific information to be released:* The authorization must include description of the information to be used or disclosed that identifies the information in a specific and meaningful way.

*Description of the purpose of the use or disclosure:* Common purposes for disclosure are for treatment purposes, legal reasons, application for disability benefits, application for life insurance, or simply "at the request of the individual."

*Expiration date:* The authorization form must list an expiration date or expiration "event." For example, the patient may document an expiration event of "upon my death" or "upon the event that my favorite National Football League team [must be named] wins the Super Bowl."

*Signature of the patient or personal representative authorizing the disclosure:* If the personal representative of the patient signs the authorization, a description of such representative's authority to act for the individual must also be provided. For example, if a mother authorizes a disclosure on behalf of her minor child, she must sign and document the disclosure "as mother or parent." If a patient is deceased, the executor of the will provides such documentation as the patient's representative.

*Date:* This is the date on which the patient makes the consent and signs the authorization documenting his consent.

In addition to the core elements, there are some required statements:

*Patient's right to revoke the authorization:* The patient or authorized agent has the right to revoke the consent for release of information in writing at any time before the actual distribution of the information. This should be explicitly stated on the authorization form.

*Redisclosure statement:* The information used or disclosed may be subject to redisclosure by the recipient and may no longer be protected.

*Conditions of authorization:* Specifications as to whether the covered entity is permitted to condition treatment, payment, enrollment, or eligibility for benefits on the authorization.

---

## HIT-bit

### ASSISTING PATIENTS WITH AUTHORIZATION FORMS

When a patient visits the HIM department to obtain copies of his or her health record, the HIM professional must often help the patient complete the authorization form to ensure that it is properly filled out. Patients must always understand what they are signing.

---

**AUTHORIZATION VALIDITY CHECKLIST:**

_____ Discloser (facility) name listed (e.g., Hospital Medical Center)

_____ Requestor name listed (e.g., attorney John Doe)

_____ Specific description of information to be disclosed (e.g., mammogram 3/01/06)

_____ Is the disclosure purpose listed or does it state something to the effect "at the request of the individual"? (e.g., to take to new physician)

_____ Is there an expiration date or event that has not passed? (e.g., an actual date or an event like "upon completion of this request" or "upon my death")

_____ Is it signed by the patient or by a personal representative with his or her authority documented? (e.g., parent of a minor)

_____ Is it dated? (e.g., must include the date the patient signed it)

_____ Is there a statement of the individual's right to revoke the authorization?

_____ Is this authorization still valid (i.e., has not been revoked?) (Check for revocation.)

_____ All of the information in the authorization appears to be true. (If you know that any information in the authorization is false, it will not be valid.)

_____ Is the authorization written in plain language? (i.e., a non-lawyer can understand it)


DECISION: _____ VALID or _____ INVALID

Employee _____   Date _____

**Figure 12-7** A sample checklist to help ensure that an authorization is valid. Individual states may require additional elements for valid authorization.

## Defective Authorizations

An authorization is considered invalid if:
- Any of the core elements is missing
- The expiration date or event has passed
- It is filled out incorrectly
- It is known that it was revoked
- Any information in the authorization is known to be false
- The authorization is not in plain language (i.e., in simple language that a person with a sixth-grade education would be able to understand)
  Figure 12-7 provides a checklist to ensure authorization validity.

## Exceptions

Another aspect of release of information is **public priority exceptions**. These are permitted disclosures in which authorization is not required as long as state law allows these exceptions. For example, many states require reporting of conditions of public health interest. Some of these conditions include cancers, birth defects, and infectious diseases. In these cases, patient consent is not required to file reports with the appropriate governmental agency. Suspected child abuse is another instance in which reporting may occur without patient consent. Other examples are disclosures to coroners, law enforcement officials, and health licensing agencies and for organ transplant activities, for certain research, for prevention of a bioterrorism event, and for other specific government functions and workers' compensation activities.

**public priority exception** Permitted disclosure in which authorization is not required as long as state law allows the exception.

**disclosure** When patient health information is given to someone.

**workers' compensation** An employer's coverage of an employee's medical expenses due to a work-related injury or illness.

# Special Consents

Special consents require consideration of federal law, state law, and federal and state rules and regulations. In general, health records containing chemical dependency information, HIV and acquired immunodeficiency virus (AIDS) information, mental health information, and adoption information are often addressed in state laws and regulations. As previously mentioned, the regulations that give the patient the highest level of protection should be followed. Most health care facilities have designed their authorization forms to be compliant with HIPAA and any state laws or regulations, but some facilities have a separate authorization form for special consents. In general, the authorization must specifically list the special nature of the health information that is to be disclosed.

The *Code of Federal Regulations* (42 CFR Part 2), commonly referred to as the **Federal Drug and Alcohol Abuse Regulations**, outlines the requirements for disclosing chemical dependency information. A subpoena for disclosure of chemical dependency information is not good enough—a court order is required.

> **HIPAA** Health Insurance Portability and Accountability Act
>
> **Federal Drug and Alcohol Abuse Regulations** Regulations at the national level addressing requirements for disclosure of chemical and alcohol abuse patient information.
>
> **subpoena** A direction from an officer of the court.
>
> **court order** The direction of a judge who has made a decision that an order to produce information (on the record) is necessary.

## EXERCISE 12-5

### Release of Information

1. A patient comes to the HIM Department requesting a copy of the record for his recent appendectomy. Upon inquiry, the patient reveals that, in addition to wanting a record of the operation, he had an allergic reaction to the anesthesia and wants to keep a record of this event in order to prevent a similar problem in the future. What else should the patient be advised to request?

## PREPARING A RECORD FOR RELEASE

There are several steps to take to properly release health care information. Each facility should have formal written policies and procedures regarding these steps. The specific policies and procedures vary among facilities; however, the issues can be discussed in general. Care should be taken to train and continually remind personnel of the confidential nature of health information.

## Validation and Tracking

After a request for information is received, the request should be recorded either in a manual log or in a computer database. The purpose of recording the request is so that its status and disposition may be tracked. Many state regulations require that facilities fulfill such requests within a specific time frame. A correspondence-tracking log serves to document compliance and fulfill HIPAA's requirements regarding accounting of disclosures.

> **accounting of disclosures** The listing of the identities of those to which certain protected health information has been disclosed.

Every request should be fully read, and every accompanying authorization form should be analyzed to determine whether there is valid authorization. In addition, there should be **verification** that the patient indeed has consented. The signature of the patient should be validated in an appropriate manner. This may be as simple as comparing the signature on the authorization form with the signature on file in the health record. If such validation cannot be accomplished or is not clear, notarization of the signature or additional proof of identity may be required. It is also important to verify identity when a patient comes to the facility to obtain copies of records. Proof of identity should always be requested to verify that the person to whom records are disclosed is indeed the person who is authorized to receive them.

> **verification** Confirming accuracy.
>
> **consent** An agreement or permission to receive health care services.

Box 12-4 lists sample data elements contained in a typical correspondence-tracking log. Most logs today involve an electronic database.

## Retrieval

Retrieval of the patient's information is based on the specific information requested. It is very important to release only those portions of the record that are authorized for

From Andress AA: Saunders' manual of medical office management, Philadelphia, 1996, Saunders, p 150.

disclosure. Care should be taken to ensure that the information retrieved is complete. This verification may be complicated by the decentralization of paper-based records among facility clinics or by incomplete processing of the record. Incomplete records should not, as a general rule, be released unless the release is for treatment purposes and the facility is sending whatever is available. If an incomplete record is disclosed in response to a subpoena, the status of the record as incomplete should be clearly stated in the certification statement, affidavit, or cover sheet.

## Reproduction

Photocopies or printed reproductions are made of the specific information requested. Every effort should be made to ensure the quality of the reproductions. When photocopying, personnel should compare the reproduction with the original to ensure completeness and clarity.

## Certification

When a copy of a record is required as evidence in a trial, a certified or notarized copy is usually acceptable in court. However, sometimes the original record is subpoenaed, and the custodian of the medical record accompanies the record to court. The custodian may be required to testify on the facility's procedures regarding development and retention of the record. When appearance by the custodian is required, a witness subpoena is usually issued in addition to the subpoena duces tecum for production of the record.

A certified copy contains a certification cover sheet signed by the custodian of the medical records, which states that the copy is a true and complete reproduction of the original record that is on file at the facility. The facility's policies and procedures should include the process by which verification of completeness can be obtained. With a paper record, completeness can be verified by numbering all of the pages in the original record before it is copied. Every copy can then be verified as complete if they contain the same sequential numbering of the pages.

## Compensation

Most states permit facilities to charge a fee for providing copies of health records. Some states place a cap, or maximum, on the fees that may be charged. The fee covers the actual

**custodian** The person entrusted with the responsibility for the confidentiality, privacy, and security of medical records.

**retention** The procedures governing the storage of records, including duration, location, security, and access.

services performed: retrieval of the record (search fee), reproduction of the record, and delivery charges (postage). Therefore an important component of the release-of-information (ROI) process is the preparation of the invoice. Some facilities may require that requesters pay the fee in advance, particularly for large records. As a professional courtesy, health care providers do not generally charge other health care providers for copies of records. In many cases, insurance companies and other payers have established set amounts that they will pay for copies of records. These fees may differ from the fees charged by the facility to other parties. HIPAA does not allow facilities to charge a retrieval or search fee to patients. Generally, the rate should be based on the actual cost to the facility of providing copies to the patient.

**release of information (ROI)** The term used to describe the HIM department function that provides disclosure of patient health information.

**payer** The individual or organization that is primarily responsible for the reimbursement for a particular health care service. Usually refers to the insurance company or third party.

## Distribution

When a record is released, inclusion of a confidentiality notice is common practice. A typical notice might say, "This information is confidential and may not be used for other than the intended purpose and may not be re-released." This is to remind the recipient that the information belongs to the patient—not the recipient. Table 12-1 lists the general steps in release of information.

The individual to whom the record is being released may arrive in person to pick up the record. Policies and procedures should define how the patient or individual's identity should be verified, and the individual picking up the record should sign a receipt. Usually, the copies are mailed. Care must be taken to ensure that the address is correct and legible on the envelope so that the record is not misdirected. Records may also be sent electronically, by fax machine or e-mail. Extra care should be taken with electronic transmission of health information, as specifically addressed in the HIPAA Security Rule.

A cover sheet should accompany records sent by fax machine. The cover sheet should contain a confidentiality statement (Figure 12-8). Internet transmission of confidential information is becoming more common, particularly in the physician's office setting. Consideration should be given to the transmission security and whether the recipient is able

**TABLE 12-1**

**STEPS IN RELEASE OF INFORMATION**

| PROCEDURE | COMMENTS |
|---|---|
| 1. Log in request. | Log request into a computer tracking system or onto a paper form. |
| 2. Validate request. | Check signature; review the request for completeness. |
| | Obtain missing information if possible. |
| | Verify the validity of the subpoena or court order. |
| 3. Obtain record. | Retrieve the record from storage. |
| | Complete an incomplete record before releasing it. |
| 4. Copy record. | Photocopy or print from computer system. |
| | Copy only the required sections, as specified in the request. |
| 5. Prepare invoice. | Calculate charges, and prepare an invoice. |
| 6. Distribute copy. | Obtain signed receipt if requested information is picked up in person. |

This facsimile message and the document(s) accompanying this telefax transmission may contain confidential information which is legally privileged and intended only for the use of the addressee named above. If the reader is not the intended recipient or the employee of the intended recipient, you are hereby notified that any dissemination, copying, or distribution of this communication is strictly prohibited. If you received this communication in error, please notify us immediately by telefax or telephone and return the original documents to us via the U.S. Postal Service at the above address. Thank you for your help.

Figure 12-8 Sample confidentiality notice for faxed information. (From Andress AA: Saunders manual of medical office management, Philadelphia, 1996, Saunders, p 150.)

to handle the information confidentially. For example, many employers automatically monitor their employees' e-mails. Therefore sending medical information to a patient at his or her place of business may jeopardize confidentiality. The patient must be made aware of the issues before authorizing transmittal in this manner.

## ▪ EXERCISE 12-6

### ▪ Preparing a Record for Release

1. Your facility charges a $10 search fee plus $1.00 per page to copy records up to 100 pages. All pages in excess of 100 incur a charge of $.50 per page. Based on these rates, what is the fee for a 125-page record?

## INTERNAL REQUESTS FOR INFORMATION

**Go To** Review Chapter 11 for a detailed discussion on the use of health information within the facility.

**utilization review** The process of evaluating medical interventions against established criteria, on the basis of the patient's known or tentative diagnosis. Evaluation may take place before, during, or after the episode of care for different purposes.

**performance improvement (PI)** Also known as *quality improvement (QI)* or *continuous quality improvement (CQI)*. Refers to the process by which a facility reviews its services or products to improve quality.

**minimum necessary** A rule requiring health providers to disclose only the minimum amount of information necessary to accomplish a task.

**audit trail** A review of individual user access codes to determine who had access to patient health information and to ensure that the access was deemed necessary for patient care.

In everyday practice within a health care facility, there are numerous instances in which facility personnel routinely request health information. Some of these requests include utilization review, performance improvement, and a variety of ongoing clinical reviews (e.g., surgical case review and infection control). These requests should be documented in writing both for internal control purposes (chart tracking) and to ensure that the request is valid.

The routine release of information for patient care should be handled with some caution. Even within a facility, many attempts are made to obtain information inappropriately. The culprits range from overly curious friends and family members who inquire about a patient's condition to unethical health care professionals who spy on one another. In the case of a physician's request, authorization is easily determined by checking the record to ensure that the physician requesting the chart is listed as an attending or consulting physician for that particular case. HIM departmental policies and procedures should be clear and specific regarding the internal release of information and should also include the steps to be taken when the legitimacy of the request is in question. Staff members should be allowed access to health information only on a "need to know" basis. In other words, what is the minimum amount of information necessary for the staff members to do their jobs?

## SENSITIVE RECORDS

There are two major types of sensitive records: employee patients and legal files. Although there may be no statutory or regulatory requirement to handle these records differently from others, certain practical considerations apply. In the electronic environment, knowledge that an audit trail of access to the record will be monitored may serve as a deterrent to inappropriate access.

### Employee Patients

Maintaining the confidentiality of employee records is particularly difficult. In a small facility, a paper record can be maintained in a secure file. In a large facility, this arrangement may be impractical. Therefore facility policies and procedures should include specific language regarding the sensitivity of health information pertaining to fellow employees. The confidentiality statement shown in Figure 12-1 includes such language.

### Legal Files

**litigation** The term used to indicate that a matter must be settled by the court and the process of engaging in legal proceedings.

Special attention should be paid to records that have been requested for litigation involving the facility, health care personnel, or a physician. Every effort should be made to obtain control of those records immediately on receipt of the notification, and special care should be taken to safeguard these records in a special area inaccessible to all but authorized personnel. If possible, the records should be locked in a file used exclusively for that purpose.

Although photocopies of the records can be circulated for review and discussion, HIM personnel should safeguard the original records. Staff members may be tempted to alter or remove incriminating records when a health care practitioner is being sued. Safeguarding the records in the aforementioned manner removes that temptation and ensures the safety and availability of the records for legal proceedings.

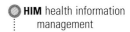 **HIM** health information management

## EXERCISE 12-7
### Internal Requests for Information

1. What special procedures, if any, should be in place to handle the records of employees who are patients in the facility?

## FEDERAL, CORPORATE, AND FACILITY COMPLIANCE

An increasingly important responsibility of the HIM professional is that of ensuring **compliance** with the many statutes, regulations, and other rules imposed on the facility and the professionals who work there. There are many functions that require oversight. Some of these are specific to patient care or patient complaints. Other compliance functions focus on monitoring data quality of ensuring the completeness and timeliness of records. The following sections discuss the most common areas of concern to HIM professionals.

**compliance** Meeting standards. Also the development, implementation, and enforcement of policies and procedures that ensure that standards are met.
**statute** A law that has been passed by the legislative branch of government.

### Licensure

As discussed in Chapter 1, individual states license facilities for operation within that state. A state's licensure requirements, which can be found in the state's administrative code, may contain very specific provisions for the content and retention of specific clinical documentation. These provisions may take the form of a listing of elements to be maintained in a health record. They may also be included in statements about a facility's medical staff. The provisions for health records may be as detailed as specifying which documents should be included or which types of data should be collected. Whatever provisions are listed for a specific type of facility, HIM personnel must be aware of these rules and must ensure that any activities under their span of control are in compliance with those rules.

**licensure** The mandatory government approval required for performing specified activities. In health care, the state approval required for providing health care services.

The first step in ensuring compliance with any rule is to review the rule and understand what it really means. Therefore every HIM professional should have access to a copy of the specific portions of the licensure regulations that apply to his or her activities. Although it is not necessary in terms of everyday practice for each person to have a copy of the document, it is certainly appropriate for such a document to be available to personnel in the facility.

In practice, each employee in the facility is responsible for a small portion of the compliance with the specific regulations. The responsibility for overall compliance with the particular regulations rests with the director of the particular department. In the case of the HIM department, the director typically is responsible for compliance. Regulations may also be identified in the medical staff bylaws, rules and regulations or Hospital Policy and Procedures.

One of the best ways to teach HIM employees how to comply with various regulations is to ensure that there are written policies and procedures in the department that address these particular issues consistent with organizational policies and procedures. Employees should be trained with these issues in mind. It is also important to cross-reference the policies and procedures to the specific regulations for compliance.

**Go To** Chapter 13 discusses the development of policies and procedures in the HIM department.

HIM professionals often become involved in researching and interpreting regulations and they assist in the development of policies and procedures to comply with those regulations. Frequently, HIM professionals aid in facility-wide compliance issues. This occurs because of the pervasive nature of the documentation that is handled after a patient's discharge. For example, if a regulation dictates that physician telephone orders be signed

**discharge** Discharge occurs when the patient leaves the care of the facility to go home, for transfer to another health care facility, or by death. Also refers to the status of a patient.

**accreditation** Voluntary compliance with a set of standards developed by an independent agent, who periodically performs audits to ensure compliance.

**continuity of care** The broad range of health care services required by a patient during an illness or for an entire lifetime. May also refer to the continuity of care provided by a health care organization. Also called *continuum of care.*

**The Joint Commission (TJC)** An organization that accredits and sets standards for acute care facilities, ambulatory care networks, long-term care facilities, and rehabilitation facilities, as well as certain specialty facilities, such as hospice and home care. Facilities maintaining TJC accreditation receive *deemed status* from the CMS.

**acute care facility** A health care facility in which patients have an average length of stay less than 30 days and that has an emergency department, operating suite, and clinical departments to handle a broad range of diagnoses and treatments.

**rehabilitation facility** A health care facility that delivers services to patients whose activities of daily living are impaired by their illness or condition. May be inpatient, outpatient, or both.

**long-term care (LTC) facility** A hospital that provides services to patients over an extended period; an average length of stay is in excess of 30 days. Facilities are characterized by the extent to which nursing care is provided.

**ambulatory care facility** An outpatient facility, such as an emergency department or physician's office, in which treatment is intended to occur within 1 calendar day.

**deemed status** The Medicare provision that an approved accreditation is sufficient to satisfy the compliance audit element of the Conditions of Participation.

within a certain time frame after being ordered, HIM personnel are frequently involved in the development of the procedures and controls to ensure the monitoring of that activity, because by analyzing the chart after the patient's discharge, they are in a position to note noncompliance with this regulation.

## Accreditation

State licensure of a facility is mandatory. Accreditation is optional. Remember that accreditation is the process by which independent organizations verify that a facility complies with standards of practice developed by that organization. There are accrediting bodies that deal with a specific type of health care facility, and there are accrediting bodies that deal with many different types of health care facilities across the continuity of care. **The Joint Commission (TJC),** known primarily for accrediting acute care facilities, also accredits other facilities such as rehabilitation, long-term care, and ambulatory care facilities. Because TJC is so important, it is used in this chapter to exemplify how accreditation works. The accreditation process is very similar, regardless of the accrediting body. Many health care payers mandate that an organization obtain accreditation in order to comply with their requirements for reimbursement. Currently, if a facility maintains TJC accreditation, it receives deemed status for its state and CMS survey requirements. Deemed status helped reduce the administrative costs of health care.

TJC publishes its standards annually in several formats, including a *Comprehensive Guide* that pertains to each level of health care the Commission accredits. The standards are updated annually to reflect changes in health care delivery, quality, organizational philosophy, evidence-based practices, and environment. To become accredited, a facility applies to the TJC, completes a detailed questionnaire, and undergoes an intensive site visit called a *survey.* TJC surveys facilities approximately every 3 years. Unannounced surveys or surveys focusing on previously identified problems may take place between formal surveys. Because TJC standards are modified frequently, reference to the most recent publications is essential to ensure compliance. See the TJC Web site for current publications and other information (http://www.jointcommission.org).

Ideally, a facility should be in continuous compliance with the standards; however, because the standards change annually, it may take facilities a little time each year to adjust their operations accordingly. Many facilities spend a great deal of time preparing for a survey, ensuring that documentation and various procedures are in compliance. Although it is important to discuss the preparation for a TJC survey, it should be stated that if a facility is in continuous compliance with TJC standards, continually updates its procedures to ensure compliance, and structures its reporting to document that compliance, very little preparation is needed before a TJC survey. Nevertheless, in reality, verifying TJC compliance is a time-consuming process, and facilities should scrutinize their compliance documentation and procedures on a periodic basis rather than a continuous basis.

The preparation for a routine TJC survey frequently begins with the appointment of a TJC steering committee or task force. It is very important that the HIM department be represented on the steering committee. In some cases, the director of the HIM department chairs or co-chairs that committee. Other members of the committee include a variety of department directors and managers. The director of nursing or his or her designee and a physician's representative are critical participants. There are a number of management-level staff members on the committee, and they divide the responsibilities for reviewing compliance among themselves.

Some of the activities of the TJC steering committee are to review current TJC standards and compare them with current policies and procedures, to ensure that the policies and procedures are updated, to conduct mock surveys, to prepare staff for the TJC visit, to review reports that will be required, and to assemble the large quantities of documentation required by the TJC surveyors. These activities are largely delegated to the appropriate department manager, but many employees become involved in preparing for the TJC survey. In corporate environments, a team from the home office usually conducts mock surveys in a facility before the actual TJC survey.

## Compliance

As a result of increasing pressure from the federal government, health care organizations have spent a great deal of time and effort in recent years demonstrating their commitment to data quality, particularly in terms of accurate billing. Some of this pressure comes from the DHHS's Office of the Inspector General (OIG), which has received increased funding for enforcing accurate billing through audits and penalties. In addition, the HIPAA legislation of 1996, the Balanced Budget Act of 1997, and the HITECH provisions in the ARRA legislation of 2009 increased the penalties for failure to comply with regulations. It is important to note that ARRA established tiered penalties and gives state attorneys general the power to take legal action against covered entities and business associates at the federal level. These officers can take this action if they find that their states' populations suffered because of a HIPAA violation.

A compliance program is a facility-wide system of policies, procedures, and guidelines that help to ensure ethical business practices. These policies, procedures, and guidelines should include, for example, ethics statements, strong leadership policy, commitment to compliance with regulations, and ways for employees to report unethical or noncompliant activities and behaviors. Part of a compliance effort is a coding compliance program. Such a program ensures accurate coding and billing through training, continuing education, quality assurance, and performance improvement activities. An excellent beginning reference source for learning about corporate compliance is the AHIMA practice brief "Seven Steps to Corporate Compliance: The HIM Role" (see Suggested Reading for bibliographic information).

## Professional Standards

Finally, there are professional standards with which health care professionals must comply. As mentioned in Chapter 1, each profession has a code of ethics and a set of standards that are imposed by the credentialing body or the licensing agency for that profession (or both). HIM professionals comply with the code of ethics of the AHIMA (see Box 1-2). In addition, AHIMA supports the profession by issuing a variety of publications designed to guide and promote excellence in professional practice. AHIMA regularly issues practice briefs, documenting best practices in areas of interest to HIM professionals.

### EXERCISE 12-8
#### Compliance

1. What is the purpose of the TJC Steering Committee?
2. What is compliance? Why is it important?

## SUGGESTED READING

Aiken TD: Legal and ethical issues in health occupations, Philadelphia, 2008, Saunders.
American Health Information Management Association (AHIMA): Practice Brief: Preemption of the HIPAA Privacy Rule. http://library.ahima.org/xpedio/groups/public/documents/ahima/bok1_048022.hcsp?dDocName=bok1_04802.2 Updated June 2010.
American Health Information Management Association: Notice of Privacy Practices (Updated). http://library.ahima.org/xpedio/groups/public/documents/ahima/bok1_048808.hcsp?dDocName=bok1_048808. Published February 2011a.
American Health Information Management Association: Patient Access and Amendment to Health Records (Updated). http://library.ahima.org/xpedio/groups/public/documents/ahima/bok1_048587.hcsp?dDocName=bok1_048587. Published January 2011b.
American Health Information Management Association: Practice Brief: Redisclosure of Patient Health Information. http://library.ahima.org/xpedio/groups/public/documents/ahima/bok1_042636.hcsp?dDocName=bok1_042636. Updated February 2009.
American Health Information Management Association: Practice brief: Facsimile transmission of health information. J AHIMA 72:64E–64F, 2001.

**CMS** Centers for Medicare and Medicaid Services

**billing** The process of submitting health insurance claims or rendering invoices.
**covered entity** Under HIPAA and HITECH provisions, any organization that collects and manages health information.
**business associate** Under HIPAA, a contracted vendor that uses confidential health information to perform a service on behalf of a covered entity.
**Health Insurance Portability and Accountability Act (HIPAA)** Public Law 104-191, federal legislation passed in 1996 that outlines the guidelines of managing patient information in terms of privacy, security, and confidentiality. The legislation also outlines penalties for noncompliance.

**DHHS** Department of Health and Human Services
**HITECH** Health Information Technology for Economic and Clinical Health (Act)
**ARRA** American Reinvestment and Recovery Act

**continuing education** Education required after a person has attained a position, credential, or degree, intended to keep the person knowledgeable in his or her profession.
**performance improvement** Also known as *quality improvement (QI)* or *continuous quality improvement (CQI).* Refers to the process by which a facility reviews its services or products to ensure quality.

**AHIMA** American Health Information Management Association

American Health Information Management Association: Regulations Governing Research. http://library.ahima.org/xpedio/groups/public/documents/ahima/bok1_048639.hcsp? dDocName=bok1_048639. Updated January 2011.

Department of Health and Human Services, Office of the National Coordinator for Health Information Technology: The Nationwide Privacy and Security Framework for Electronic Exchange of Individually Identifiable Health Information; Health IT Privacy and Security Toolkit. http://healthit.hhs.gov/portal/server.pt?open=512&mode=2&cached=true&objID=1173.

Haugen MB, Tegen A, Warner D: Fundamentals of the legal health record and designated record set, J AHIMA 82:44–49, 2011.

Hjort B: AHIMA Practice Brief: Release of Information Reimbursement Laws and Regulations. http://library.ahima.org/xpedio/idcplg?IdcService=GET_SEARCH_RESULTS&QueryText=dDocTitle+%3Ccontains%3E+%60Release+of+Information+Reimbursement+Laws+and+Regulations%60++%3CAND%3E++%28xPublishSite%3Csubstring%3E%60BoK%60%29&SearchProviders=master_on_ch1as13%2C&ftx=&AdvSearch=True&adhocquery=1&urlTemplate=%2Fxpedio%2Fgroups%2Fpublic%2Fdocuments%2Fweb_assets%2Fqueryresults.hcsp&ResultCount=25&SortField=xPubDate&SortOrder=Desc. Updated March 2004.

Hjort B: Practice Brief: Understanding the Minimum Necessary Standard (Updated). http://library.ahima.org/xpedio/groups/public/documents/ahima/bok1_018177.hcsp?dDocName=bok1_018177. Published March 2003.

Hughes G: Practice brief: Defining the designated record set, J AHIMA, 74:64A-664D, 2003.

United States Department of Health and Human Services: Summary of the Privacy Rule. http://www.hhs.gov/ocr/privacy/hipaa/understanding/summary/privacysummary.pdf. Revised March 2003.

Wiedemann LA: Practice Brief: HIPAA Privacy and Security Training. http://www.emron.com/pathways/downloads/ahima/Privacy_Security_Training.htm. Updated November 2010.

## CHAPTER ACTIVITIES

### CHAPTER SUMMARY

This chapter covered the legal and regulatory issues governing the development and retention of health information. Informed consent underlies patient admission, treatment, and release of information. Health information is confidential. Patient-physician privilege dictates confidentiality and release of records only with the consent of the patient. A valid consent for release of information comprises eight elements: identification of the party being asked to release the information, patient name/identification, identification of the party to whom the information is to be released, specific information to be released, description of the purpose of the use or disclosure, expiration date, signature of the patient or personal representative authorizing the disclosure, and date. However, in an emergency, records may be released without patient consent. Other important issues include compliance with regulatory, accrediting, and professional standards. Health care facilities should make every effort to ensure continuous compliance with the standards imposed by authoritative bodies.

### REVIEW QUESTIONS

1. What are the differences among privacy, confidentiality, and security?
2. Describe the ways in which HITECH has impacted regulations surrounding the privacy and security of health information.
3. Discuss the steps to release patient information.
4. List and describe the elements of a valid authorization for release of information.
5. Describe situations in which authorization is not necessary to release information.
6. Compare and contrast the procedures for preparing a record for release to the patient versus a certified copy for court.
7. Locate the licensure regulations for your state.
   a. What are the provisions for the content of a health record?
   b. What are the rules regarding the timeliness of completion of a record?
8. Locate any state laws regarding health information or medical records for your state.
   a. Are there retention statutes for medical records?
   b. Are there references to the costs of providing copies of medical records?
9. Describe the accreditation process.

## PROFESSIONAL PROFILE

### Customer Service Representative

My name is Zak, and I am a customer service representative with a company that performs release-of-information services for acute care facilities. The company and others like it are often referred to as copy services because our employees spend so much time making photocopies.

I am a registered health information technician. While I was in school, I was hired by the copy service to work as a copy representative. At the facility at which I was placed, health information management (HIM) department employees logged in the requests, validated the requests, and retrieved the records. Then I would copy the required sections, prepare an invoice, log the completion of the request, and send out the copies. Eventually, the facility turned over the entire function to me.

As a copy representative, I need to know the laws in my state governing the release of information as well as the hospital's policies and procedures. I need to know the contents of the record, how to retrieve it, and how to ensure that the record is complete. In addition, I had to learn the copy service's computer logging and invoicing system. Most important, I'm required to maintain a professional attitude at all times and employ good communication skills to ensure a cordial and professional relationship with my clients.

After I graduated from my HIT program, I was promoted to customer service representative. Now I am responsible for training new employees, scheduling and managing their assignments, solving problems that arise, and occasionally substituting for someone who is ill or on vacation. Sometimes, I accompany the marketing manager when she makes presentations to potential new clients. I like to travel to different hospitals and meet new people, and I enjoy the responsibilities, so I'm very happy in this new position.

## PATIENT CARE PERSPECTIVE

### Maria

After my experience with Mom and not having immediate access to medical records, I decided to make a file of all of our family's important health care records. I found a good Web site that let me enter key data and upload documentation. I wasn't sure what documentation was really important, so I called Diamonte and spoke with Zak. Zak helped me understand what documentation was important for continuing medical care, and he helped me fill out the consent forms that were needed to get it. He was also able to give me the documentation electronically! Now I'm all organized. I was really surprised to find out how much was missing from my own early records and my husband's. We should have started this process sooner, but we will have it all going forward.

## APPLICATION

### Is It Confidential?

You are the director of health information management (HIM) in a small community hospital. One day, an employee in the incomplete file area comes to you with a coat. One of the physicians left it in the dictation room, but the employee does not know to whom it belongs. You decide to look in the pockets of the coat to see whether any identification is present. You find in one of the pockets a prescription bottle of Antabuse (disulfiram), a medication given to alcoholics to help them stop drinking. The patient named on the bottle is a physician at your facility. What should you do with this information? What are the confidentiality issues? Should you have handled this situation differently?

# HIM DEPARTMENT MANAGEMENT

Melissa LaCour

## CHAPTER OUTLINE

HUMAN RESOURCES
ORGANIZATION CHARTS
  Facility Organization
  Delegation
  HIM Department Organization
HIM DEPARTMENT WORKFLOW
  Workload and Productivity
  Prioritization of Department
    Functions
EVALUATION OF DEPARTMENT
  OPERATIONS AND SERVICES
  Postdischarge Processing

Concurrent Processing
Electronic Record Processing
DEPARTMENT PLANNING
  Mission
  Vision
  Goals and Objectives
  Budget
  Planning for EHR Migration and
    Implementation
DEPARTMENT POLICIES AND
  PROCEDURES
HEALTH INFORMATION
  PERSONNEL

Job Descriptions
Job Analysis
Performance Standards
Evaluating Productivity
Employee Evaluations
Hiring HIM Personnel
DEPARTMENT EQUIPMENT AND
  SUPPLIES
  Supplies
  Monitoring Use of Department
    Resources
  Ergonomics

## VOCABULARY

capital budget
chain of command
delegation
ergonomics
full-time equivalent (FTE)
goals
job analysis

job description
matrix reporting
mission statement
objectives
operational budget
organization chart
outsourcing

performance improvement
  plan (PIP)
performance standards
policy
procedure
productivity
request for proposal (RFP)

span of control
stakeholder
system development life
  cycle (SDLC)
unity of command
vision
workflow analysis

## CHAPTER OBJECTIVES

*By the end of this chapter, the student should be able to:*

1. Explain the purpose of the organization chart.
2. Organize the appropriate workflow of health information management functions and services.
3. Develop plans, goals, and objectives for health information management employees.
4. Identify the stages in the systems development life cycle and considerations in the implementation of an electronic health record.
5. Develop department policy and procedures for health information management functions and services.
6. Perform job analysis.
7. Write job descriptions using the Americans with Disabilities Act requirements.
8. Develop health information management department policies for employee operations and conduct.
9. Establish standards for performance of employees in health information management functions and services.

10. Collect data to measure the productivity of a health information management employee and the productivity of the department.
11. Evaluate the effectiveness of operations and services in a health information management department.
12. Explain the steps associated with hiring health information management department employees.
13. Identify health information management functions that can be outsourced.
14. Monitor the use of department resources, including inventory, budget, and planning.
15. Identify technology, storage space, ergonomics, dictation/transcription area, and equipment and supply needs for health information management department functions and services.
16. Assess and design an ergonomically sound work environment for health information management personnel.

This chapter focuses on issues, tools, and techniques used to manage health information management (HIM) employees who perform HIM department functions. Previous chapters explained how to process, maintain, and secure health information. In these final two chapters, human resources, organization, planning, policy, procedures, equipment, and supplies are discussed in the context of their importance, relevance, or function in the HIM department.

**health information** Organized data that have been collected about a patient or a group of patients. Sometimes used synonymously with the term *health data*.

## HUMAN RESOURCES

Within an organization, the human resources (HR) department maintains personnel records; handles employee benefit issues; and advertises for, interviews, hires, disciplines, and terminates facility employees. HR works with the managers and supervisors in the health care facility when developing job descriptions and performance standards, conducting employee performance evaluations, handling employee conduct problems, and managing other technical aspects of employment. Supervisors, managers, and directors of an HIM department should consult the human resources department for advice and guidance as necessary on these matters when managing employees.

**HR** human resources

The phrase "human resources within the HIM department" refers to the employees, who are the source of effort and productivity required to accomplish health information functions. Along with physical resources such as buildings and technology, and capital resources that allow the operation to run, employees are resources that are essential to performing the work/job duties/tasks. Although many functions in a health care facility are electronic, humans are still needed to facilitate HIM functions to ensure timely, complete, and accurate health information. Furthermore, the appropriate management of HIM employees has an impact on the entire organization.

Managers are responsible for efficient and effective use of all the resources in an organization, including the people. They organize workflow, establish policy and procedures, hire, and monitor employee productivity and performance. In this chapter we discuss many of the tools HIM managers employ to coordinate these functions. Please note that HIM departments differ among health care facilities. The methods that work in one department may not work the same in another department.

Employees may be classified according to hours worked (full-time or part-time) or by position—such as management or staff. Those in management or supervisory positions have responsibility for other employees. Staff employees are responsible for daily tasks and functions, and they report to a supervisor or manager.

As shown in Table 13-1, employee classifications by hours worked are full-time, part-time, and temporary (also known as PRN [as needed], extra help, pool, or per diem). A **full-time** employee typically works 32 to 40 hours each week—up to 2080 hours per year—excluding overtime (or in some cases, 64 to 80 hours every 2 weeks), thereby earning full benefits as offered by the health care facility. Full-time status affects employees' benefits in terms of hours earned in paid time off (PTO), vacation, holiday benefits, and retirement options. For example, an employee who works 40 hours each week is considered a full-time

## HIT-bit

### FULL-TIME EQUIVALENT EMPLOYEES

If a full-time employee works 40 hours per week, then the staffing complement can be expressed not just by the number of employees, but also by how many full-time equivalents (FTEs) are used. The FTE calculation enables managers to better understand their utilization of human resources. FTEs are calculated as the total number of hours worked (allowed, or budgeted), divided by the number of standard full-time hours per week (in this case, 40). The resulting number, which may include a fractional employee, helps account for the part-time employees. For example: The HIM department is allowed 100 hours each work week for coding. How many FTEs equal 100 hours? The answer is 100 divided by 40 (1 FTE) equals 2.5 FTEs; 2.5 FTEs are allowed in the coding department each week. We discuss FTEs in more detail later in the chapter.

## TABLE 13-1

### EMPLOYEE CLASSIFICATIONS

| CLASSIFICATION | COMMON TERMS | DESCRIPTION |
|---|---|---|
| Full-time | FTE | Employee who works 32-40 hours each week, or 64-80 hours every 2 weeks, earning full benefits |
| Part-time | PT | Employee who typically work less than the minimum full-time hours; frequently less than 20 hours each week, occasionally earning benefits at half of the full-time rate |
| Temporary | Pool, PRN, per diem | Employee scheduled to work as necessary because of an increased workload |

**per diem** Each day, daily.

**full-time equivalent (FTE)** A unit of staffing that equals the regular 32 to 40 hour work week as defined by the organization.

**release of information (ROI)** HIM department function that provides disclosure of patient health information.

**coding** The assignment of alphanumerical values to a word, phrase, or other nonnumerical expression. In health care, coding is the assignment of numerical values to diagnosis and procedure descriptions.

**outsourcing** Refers to services that are provided by external organizations or individuals who are not employees of the facility for which the services are being provided.

employee, and he or she may earn 4 hours of vacation each week. Additionally, the organization might match retirement benefits for the full-time employee at a rate higher than for other classes of employees.

A part-time (PT) employee is one who typically works less than the standard, full-time hours (frequently less than 20 hours) per week, thereby earning benefits at half the weekly rate of a full-time employee, if at all. For example, a PT employee may earn 2 hours of vacation, sick leave, or paid time off for every 20 hours of work. Temporary or per diem employees rarely earn any type of employee benefit. Per diem employees are scheduled to work as needed in the facility when the amount of work exceeds what the regular employees can accomplish. These employees are valuable to the organization when there is an unexpected excess of work.

Staffing complements are often described by the number of **full-time equivalent** (FTE) employees. If the normal work week is 40 hours, an employee working 20 hours is one half of an FTE. Similarly, two part-time employees working 20 hours per week is equivalent to one employee working 40 hours per week. These two part time employees equal one FTE. All of the regularly scheduled hours for the week are added then divided by the full-time work week hours to arrive at the total number of FTEs for the department.

| | |
|---|---|
| Sue | 20 hours |
| James | 15 hours |
| Mary | 40 hours |
| Alison | 40 hours |
| Total hours | 115 hours |

Example:

In this example, the department staff are scheduled to work 115 hours per week. The full-time work week is 40 hours. Therefore the employee complement is 2.875 FTEs (115 divided by 40).

Some people who work in the HIM department are employed by an agency or company that "contractually" agrees to perform certain job functions for the HIM department or health care facility. These employees are paid by the agency or company, not the health care facility. A facility might choose to make this arrangement to acquire specialized help in a particular HIM function such as release of information (ROI), transcription, or coding. This type of contractual arrangement is also called **outsourcing**, whereby the work is performed by workers *other than those* employed by the facility. These categories are discussed in more detail later in the chapter, with regard to the HIM department structure.

## EXERCISE 13-1

### Human Resources

1. A(n) _____ works 32 to 40 hours each week excluding overtime, earning full benefits as offered by the health care facility.
2. An employee who works 16 to 20 hours each week, occasionally earning partial benefits, is:
   a. an FTE.
   b. a PRN.
   c. part time.
   d. an LPN.

3. A pool of employees used as needed when work load increases is:
   a. an FTE.
   b. part-time.
   c. a PRN.
   d. a coder.
4. The department within the health care organization responsible for employee management is the:
   a. HIM department.
   b. human resources department.
   c. materials management department.
   d. operations management department.
5. The HIM department is allowed 450 hours per week. This equals how many FTEs?
   a. 4.5
   b. 22.5
   c. 11.25
   d. 45

## ORGANIZATION CHARTS

One method used by health care facilities to describe the arrangement of departments and positions is the **organization chart**. The organization chart illustrates the relationships among departments, positions, and functions within the organization. The traditional structure of an organization chart resembles a pyramid, in which there are more departments and personnel at the bottom than at the top. An organization chart uses boxes and lines to represent departments and positions within the facility (Figure 13-1). Each box

**organization chart** An illustration used to describe the relationships among departments, positions, and functions within an organization.

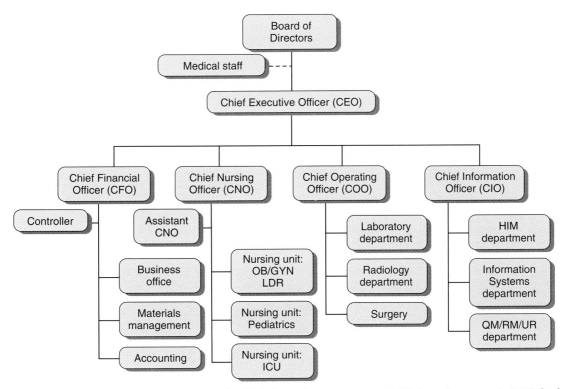

**Figure 13-1** Health care facility organization chart. HIM, health information management; ICU, intensive care unit; LDR, leader; OB/GYN, obstetrics/gynecology; QM, quality management; RM, risk management; UR, utilization review.

indicates a department or position. The higher the box is located within the chart, the higher the authority and responsibility of the position or department that it represents. Boxes on the same level indicate similar levels of authority or responsibility. Lines connecting the boxes indicate relationships. Solid lines indicate a direct relationship. Broken lines indicate an indirect (or shared) relationship.

The lines in the organization chart illustrate the subordination of positions in the chain of command. The **chain of command** refers to the order in which decisions are made within the facility. For decisions that require approval, the organization chart describes who must give that approval. Therefore the organization chart also represents the reporting structure; it indicates which individuals manage or have authority over another employee or department.

## Facility Organization

The traditional health care facility is composed of departments with specialized personnel or services; these are related to the health care professions discussed in Chapter 1. Figure 13-1 is a useful reference when you are considering the organization chart of a medium-sized acute care facility. The box at the top of the chart represents the ultimate authority and responsibility within the organization. This authority is usually called the *governing body, board of directors,* or *board of trustees.* Every health care facility has this type of authority at the top of the organization.

There are typically 8 to 25 members on the board, depending on the size of the facility. Members of the board include the chief executive officer (CEO), members of the medical staff, and members of the community. The board meets regularly to review the business of the health care facility, set direction, and monitor progress. The board has two distinct relationships, as shown in Figure 13-1. One is their delegation of authority to the CEO for the daily operations of the facility. The other is the relationship with the facility's medical staff.

The medical staff is organized as a membership group of physicians governed by the facility's medical staff bylaws, rules, and regulations. They admit patients to the health care facility and provide care during the patient stay. In addition, the medical staff has a responsibility to aid the administration in the longer-term planning of the health care facility. An example of medical staff structure is shown in Figure 13-2.

The CEO, under the governing board, is given the authority to oversee the daily management of the health care facility. The CEO must guide, motivate, and lead the organization, receiving direction of the governing board.

Below the CEO are several administrative positions. These positions have authority over specific departments within the organization. These administrators report to the CEO and are accountable for the operations of their departments. This level of the administration is also known as the chiefs, or the "C-Suite": chief operating officer (COO), chief nursing officer (CNO), chief financial officer (CFO), chief information officer (CIO); and assistant administrators, or vice presidents of finance, nursing, information, and quality.

The personnel responsible for managing specific departments report to the aforementioned administrators. The managers of the departments are known as directors, department heads, or managers. Below department directors are supervisors, and then staff

> **chain of command** The formal authority and decision-making structure within an organization.

> **acute care facility** A health care facility in which patients have an average length of stay less than 30 days and that has an emergency department, operating suite, and clinical departments to handle a broad range of diagnoses and treatments.

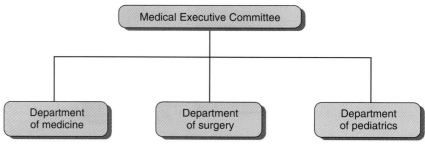

**Figure 13-2** Medical staff organization chart.

employees. The managers of each department have authority over the supervisors within their departments, and finally the staff employees within each department report to their respective supervisors.

### Span of Control

In an organization chart, the number of positions or employees shown below the box for an administrator, manager, or supervisor indicates the **span of control** for that position. The span of control is the number of employees or departments that report to one individual. The span of control for one supervisor must be appropriate so that management is efficient and effective. Too many varied responsibilities or employees under one supervisor can lead to ineffective management. A large facility may require more managers than a small facility because of the number of employees needed to accomplish tasks or functions.

**span of control** The number of employees who report to one supervisor, manager, or administrator.

---

### HIT-bit

#### MANAGEMENT STYLES

The previously discussed topics are affected by the HIM department director's management style. The three major categories of management are autocratic, democratic, and laissez-faire.

The *autocratic* manager controls everything. Employees function under strict control of this manager. All operations and decisions are overseen by this type of manager. Autocratic managers are sometimes called micromanagers, because they oversee even the smallest details of the department.

The *democratic* manager allows all employees to provide input in decision making or operations of the department. He or she seeks input and then typically makes decisions on the basis of this feedback.

The *laissez-faire* manager allows the employees to run the department and gets involved only when absolutely necessary. This is a true "hands-off" manager. Chances are that the laissez-faire manager will not pitch in when the work piles up.

---

### Unity of Command

It is equally important that any individual employee reports to only one manager. This concept is called **unity of command**. If one employee has two supervisors, this can cause a dilemma as to which manager's authority is higher or which manager's rules and requests take precedence. If both managers have deadlines, which one must be met first? Who decides? If the employee has only one manager, the employee knows that he or she is accountable to that manager according to the role and responsibility of the position.

**unity of command** Sole management of one employee by one manager.

In an increasingly challenging health care environment, it is not always possible or practical to maintain strict unity of command. Further, with performance improvement and other quality efforts crossing all aspects of a facility, the functional responsibility for a project may result in an employee, particularly a manager, reporting to multiple higher level individuals, either formally or informally. This type of cross-departmental chain of command is called **matrix reporting**. Matrix reporting is typically represented by broken or dotted lines on an organization chart, if the reporting line is permanent and inherent in the duties of the employee. Less formal matrix reporting that results from project work is not generally represented on the table of organization. The issues mentioned in the previous paragraph are inherent in matrix reporting. Clear communication, documentation of responsibilities, and measurable performance objectives are common ways to overcome these issues.

**matrix reporting** An employee reports to more than one manager.

## Delegation

**Delegation** describes what a manager does when he or she assigns responsibility to an employee to complete a project or task. The employee to whom the task is being delegated

**delegation** The transfer of a responsibility, task, or project from a manager to a lower level employee.

may need some authority to get the job done (e.g., signing forms, making changes in a process, and disciplining employees). Delegating empowers an employee with the responsibility and the necessary authority to accomplish the project or task. Delegation is not only a tool that managers use to accomplish multiple tasks; it is also an important motivator. It shows the employee that the manager trusts him or her to do a good job and allows the employee to take ownership of the project.

## HIM Department Organization

Figure 13-3 illustrates a table of organization within the HIM department. This is an organization chart for an HIM department with 30 employees. The box at the top of the chart represents the department director. The person in this position has the delegated authority from the administration of the facility to act as the custodian of health information. This position also has the responsibility and authority to manage the daily operations of the HIM department. Figure 13-3 shows a department with one director, one assistant director, three supervisors, and 32 staff employees. Keep in mind that job titles for positions within the HIM department vary among facilities.

---

### HIT-bit

**HEALTH INFORMATION MANAGEMENT DEPARTMENT IDENTITY**

The HIM department may also be called the *medical record department* or *health information services*. Names of HIM departments remain diverse across the country.

---

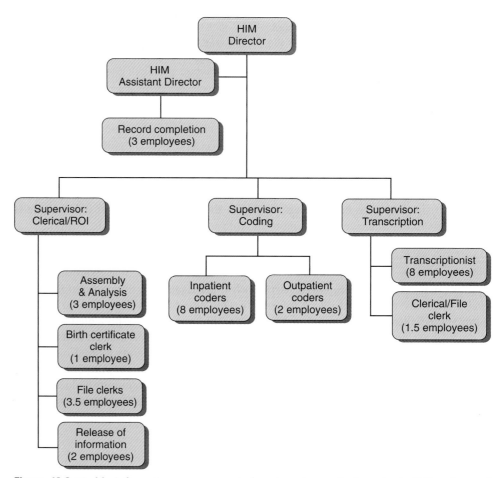

**Figure 13-3** Health information management department organization chart. ROI, release of information.

In addition, the organization chart in Figure 13-3 shows a department that is organized into three supervised sections of health information functions. Each supervisor is responsible for specific functions within the department. There is a supervisor for the assembly, analysis, release of information (ROI), and filing functions, also known as the *clerical, or ROI, supervisor*. Another supervisor, called the *coding supervisor*, oversees the coding and abstracting functions. The third supervisor, *the transcription supervisor,* is responsible for the transcription function.

Supervisors work at the staff level to ensure that the daily tasks in the HIM department are accomplished in a timely and accurate manner. Supervisors typically work in close proximity to or with the employees they supervise. They are on hand to handle in a timely manner issues, questions, and situations that arise. Responsibilities of the supervisor positions differ in each department, but they may include scheduling, hiring, training, disciplining, and terminating. The supervisor is responsible for ensuring that staff employees are performing their functions efficiently and consistently with the policies of the department.

**assembly** The reorganization of a paper record into a standard order.

**analysis** The review of a record to evaluate its completeness, accuracy, or compliance with predetermined standards or other criteria.

**ROI** release of information

---

## HIT-bit

### CHAIN OF COMMAND

*Chain of command* refers to the line of authority through which decisions are formally authorized. An employee should follow the chain of command for approval related to his or her job in the department, including discussion of disagreements with supervisors.

---

Within the HIM department, employees are further identified by the positions that they hold or job functions that they perform. HIM departments have clerical and technical staff positions (Table 13-2). The director of the HIM department or the human resources department determines the title for employee positions. Some titles are generic (e.g., HIM Tech I), whereas other titles describe the employee's responsibilities (e.g., inpatient coder, outpatient coder, scanning technician, ROI clerk, revenue cycle supervisor).

Clerical employees are responsible for the functions known as scanning (or assembly), indexing and data validity (analysis), and release of information (filing). Technical employees perform functions such as coding, abstracting, and transcription. (Table 13-2 describes possible job titles.) Such positions are sometimes referred to as HIM Tech II. These staff employees typically report to the first or lowest level of management, either the HIM supervisor or a team leader. The titles, roles, and responsibilities of positions

**inpatient** An individual who is admitted to a hospital with the intention of staying overnight.

**outpatient** A patient whose health care services are intended to be delivered within 1 calendar day or, in some cases, a 24-hour period.

**revenue cycle** The groups of processes that identify, record, and report the financial transactions that result from the facility's clinical relationship with a patient.

**indexing** The process of sorting a record by the different report types, making the viewing of the record uniform.

**data validity** The quality that data reflect the known or acceptable range of values for the specific data.

---

## TABLE 13-2

### STAFF POSITIONS IN THE HEALTH INFORMATION MANAGEMENT DEPARTMENT

| POSITION | RESPONSIBILITY/FUNCTION | HOURS | STATUS |
|---|---|---|---|
| HIM Director | Daily management of the HIM department | Monday through Friday, 8:00 AM to 4:30 PM | Full-time |
| Supervisor | Clerical/ROI/filing | Monday through Friday, 7:00 AM to 3:30 PM | Full-time |
| Scanning Clerk | Assembly and analysis of all patient records | Sunday through Thursday, 6:30 AM to 3 PM | Full-time |
| Birth Certificate Clerk | Birth certificates Saturday assembly/analysis | Tuesday through Saturday, 8:00 AM to 4:30 PM | Full-time |
| HIM Tech I | File clerk | Monday through Friday, 5:00 PM to 9:00 PM | Part-time |
| Inpatient Coder | Inpatient coding | Monday through Friday, 8:30 AM to 5:00 PM | Full-time |
| Outpatient Coder | Outpatient coding | Monday through Thursday, 4:00 PM to 9:00 PM | Part-time |
| ROI Clerk | Release of information | Monday through Friday, 8:30 AM to 5:00 PM | Full-time |
| Revenue Cycle Manager | Daily management of revenue cycle activities, including quality of claims-related data | Monday through Friday, 7:30 AM to 4:00 PM | Full-time |
| Transcriptionist | General transcription and STAT requests | Saturday through Sunday, 8:00 AM to 4:30 PM | Part-time |

HIM, health information management; ROI, release of information; STAT, immediate.

**admission** The act of accepting a patient into care in a health care facility, including any nonambulatory care facility. Admission requires a physician's order.

within the HIM department vary. Smaller facilities with few patient admissions have fewer positions as well as fewer levels of management. However, larger health care facilities have several employees performing one function, and they require more supervisors and levels of management to oversee daily functions.

## HIT-bit

### EXEMPT OR NONEXEMPT

The Fair Labor Standards Act (FSLA) of 1938 addressed many workers' rights issues of the time. In addition to the implementation of strict rules surrounding child labor, the FSLA set a national minimum wage, and it guaranteed overtime pay for some jobs. Although the provisions of the FSLA continue to cover most industries in the United States, some jobs are "exempt" from the rules regarding overtime. In health care, *exempt* employees are salaried—most are not required to punch a time clock— and usually have a supervisory role. There are some exceptions, depending on record-keeping practices. *Nonexempt* employees are paid according to the number of hours worked, and under the FSLA must be paid overtime, usually for work beyond 40 hours in any given week, although some states set stricter guidelines.

U.S. Department of Labor, 2012. http://www.dol.gov/elaws/esa/flsa/screen75.asp

## EXERCISE 13-2
### Organization Charts

1. The _____ is an illustration used to describe the relationships among departments, positions, and functions within an organization.
2. As the new supervisor over the file area, release of information, and assembly and analysis, Sandra feels overwhelmed by the number of projects requiring her attention. One way that Sandra may relieve the pressure from these projects is to _____ some of the projects to her employees.
3. Judy, the physician record clerk in the HIM department, is responsible to Jovan, the supervisor, and Michelle, the director. This situation violates the _____ principle.
4. Janet is a supervisor responsible for eight coding employees; this statement represents Janet's _____.
5. The governing body:
   a. has the authority to grant privileges to members of the medical staff.
   b. is responsible for quality services provided by the facility.
   c. Both A and B are correct.
   d. None of the above is correct.

**abstracting** The recap of selected fields from a health record to create an informative summary. Also refers to the activity of identifying such fields and entering them into a computer system.

**workflow** The process of work flowing through a set of procedures to complete the health record.

**workflow analysis** A careful examination of how work is performed in order to identify inefficiencies and make changes.

**electronic health record (EHR)** A secure real-time, point-of-care, patient centric information resource for clinicians allowing access to patient information when and where needed and incorporating evidence-based decision support.

## HIM DEPARTMENT WORKFLOW

The collection, organization, coding, abstracting, analysis, storage, and retrieval of patient health information are organized into a workflow within each health care organization to best suit that facility. Workflow is the order in which tasks are organized to progress from one function to the next. Efficient workflow allows department employees to accomplish their functions in a timely, accurate, and complete manner. Although managers should continually look for ways to remove obstacles and streamline the workflow in their departments, **workflow analysis**, or a careful look at how work is performed, is especially crucial when a facility is implementing new software, or in the process of migrating to an electronic health record (EHR).

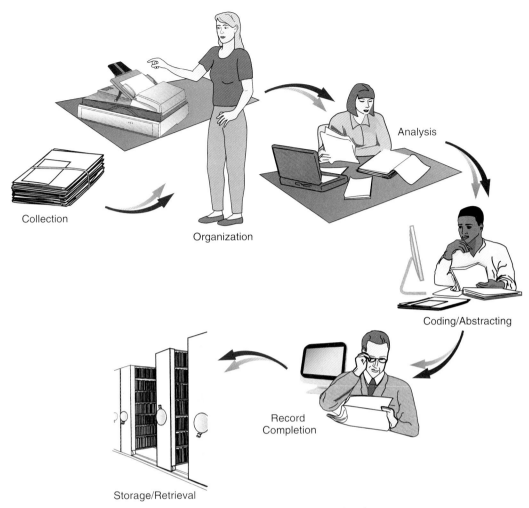

**Figure 13-4** Retrospective processing of health information.

Because every HIM department is different, this section covers general workflow concepts such as the management and organization of HIM functions with only a few variations. Variations in the workflow among different facilities are necessary to accommodate the type, size, and structure of each health care facility.

First let's review HIM functions and responsibilities as they are commonly conceived in health care facilities that use paper-based records. As shown in Figure 13-4, health records undergo several distinct processes which enable the current and future use of the data they contain:

*Collection*—the retrieval of a health record from the patient care unit for every patient treated by the facility

*Organization*—the assembly of the record into a format usable by others; this might mean scanning or attaching the record to a file folder labeled appropriately for identification and storage

*Analysis*—the review of quantitative (and sometimes also the qualitative) health information to ensure timely, accurate, and complete records

*Coding*—the assignment of alphanumerical or numerical codes to patient diagnoses and procedures for reimbursement and data retrieval

*Abstracting*–the method by which the information in the health record is reviewed and key data elements identified and entered in to a database

*Record completion*—the processing of an incomplete record as more health data are entered from appropriate health care personnel

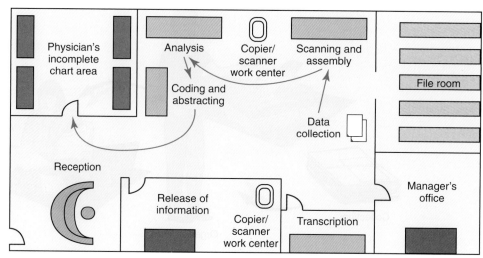

Figure 13-5 The layout and workflow of a typical health information management department.

*Storage*—the filing methods used to maintain records for future use

*Retrieval*—the function that locates a record for future use following patient care

*Transcription*—the method by which the physician's dictation is turned into a medical report for placement in the patient's record

Figure 13-5 shows a typical HIM department layout and the locations where these actions might occur for the most efficient workflow.

These HIM functions occur sequentially and are typically grouped into sections under a supervisor for efficient management (see Figure 13-3). The need for supervisors within a department, as discussed previously, is determined by the number of employees in the HIM department and their varied functions. Typically, supervisors oversee 6 to 12 employees, depending on the functions performed by the group and the employees' need for direct supervision. If there are 12 transcriptionists, only one supervisor may be necessary. However, if the department is relatively small and there are only 12 employees total, 6 of whom are clerical workers, 3 of whom are coders, and 3 of whom are transcriptionists, the department may have 3 supervisors, 1 each for the clerical, coding, and transcription sections. In this situation the supervisor is likely an employee who performs the job functions well and actually leads the others to ensure the work is performed. Other areas where it can be important to have a supervisor is over revenue cycle (all processes that help generate revenue from the time of discharge), and another may be over release of information with responsibility for patient interaction, audits, and HIPAA.

## Workload and Productivity

Each department must have a method for completing its workload. The amount of work in the HIM department is determined by the number of discharges, by the type (e.g., outpatient, inpatient, rehab), and length of stay (LOS). The number of patients discharged each day will be equal to the number of records that must be processed. The patient type (e.g., inpatient, outpatient, rehab, psych) determines the extent of the processing. For instance, ambulatory/outpatient records are very brief and are relatively easy/quick to process. Ambulatory surgery records require less time to review than inpatient stays. Likewise, the LOSs for patients who have been discharged affect the length of time that it will take to process (and code) the patients' charts. If a patient has an LOS in the facility of 2 days, the record is relatively thin (e.g., approximately 1 inch). However, if the patient remains in the facility for 21 days, the record is relatively thick (approximately 2 to 3 inches) and may require two folders to contain the papers for that one stay. If your facility has many discharges with long LOSs, then the assembly process will take longer than in a facility that has few discharges with short LOSs.

Supervisors may use time studies to determine the appropriate number of employees for the workload. A time study can be accomplished by monitoring the employee(s) performing the function and the time that it takes to complete each task. This helps the supervisor identify how much work can be done by one employee in a specific period. It also determines the percentage of accuracy with which the work should be completed. If the supervisor is actually present while the employee performs the job, the employee may become nervous or irritated. Likewise, a supervisor does not want to waste valuable time watching employees work. Other methods exist to capture this information without physically watching employees. Employees can fill out forms to indicate their performance, productivity, and time (Figure 13-6). In an electronic system or with document conversion, data may be available from the system through reporting.

The standards set for the department must comply with organizational, professional, licensing, and regulatory requirements. These standards determine when many of the functions must be performed (e.g., scanning/assembly and analysis within 24 hours of discharge and coding within 48 hours of discharge; Table 13-3). Some internal standards may lead

| Coder: _____ | | | | | Month/year: _____ | | | | | | | | | | | | | | | |
|---|---|---|---|---|---|---|---|---|---|---|---|---|---|---|---|---|---|---|---|
| | M | Tu | W | Th | F | M | Tu | W | Th | F | M | Tu | W | Th | F | M | Tu | W | Th | F |
| Date | | | | | | | | | | | | | | | | | | | | |
| Inpatient | | | | | | | | | | | | | | | | | | | | |
|   Medicare | | | | | | | | | | | | | | | | | | | | |
|   Non-Medicare | | | | | | | | | | | | | | | | | | | | |
| Outpatient | | | | | | | | | | | | | | | | | | | | |
|   Observation/surgeries | | | | | | | | | | | | | | | | | | | | |
|   Diagnostics | | | | | | | | | | | | | | | | | | | | |
|   Emergency department | | | | | | | | | | | | | | | | | | | | |
| | | | | | | | | | | | | | | | | | | | | |
| Hours worked | | | | | | | | | | | | | | | | | | | | |
| Physician contacts | | | | | | | | | | | | | | | | | | | | |
| Other (please comment below) | | | | | | | | | | | | | | | | | | | | |
| Comments: | | | | | | | | | | | | | | | | | | | | |

Figure 13-6  Coding productivity sheet.

## TABLE 13-3

### TYPICAL HIM DEPARTMENT STANDARDS*

| DEPARTMENT FUNCTION | STANDARD |
|---|---|
| Assembly and analysis Scanning | Completed within 24 hours of patient discharge |
| Coding and abstracting | Completed within 48-72 hours of patient discharge |
| Record completion | Completed within 30 days of discharge |
| Filing | Completed daily |
| Release of information | Completed within 48-72 hours of receipt of an appropriate authorization or request for information |
| Transcription: | |
|   History and physical | Transcribed within 4 hours of dictation |
|   Consults | Transcribed within 12 hours of dictation |
|   Operative reports | Transcribed within 6 hours of dictation |
|   Discharge summary | Transcribed within 24 hours of dictation |

*Note: These standards are for example only; standards in HIM departments may vary.

the way for new processes, such as concurrent analysis or coding, to successfully accomplish department functions within the set time frame.

The standards, along with the amount and type of work, dictate the operating hours of the HIM department and the scheduling of the employee(s) work hours. Some departments in large health care facilities are open 24 hours a day, 7 days a week. Other departments have limited hours (Monday through Friday 7 AM to 9 PM and part-time on weekends) and use cross-trained staff (i.e., nursing) to cover emergency issues when the department is closed (see Table 13-2).

Workload is also affected by the amount of computerization in the HIM department. In some instances, technology reduces the complexity of a function, making it easier to complete HIM processes in a timely manner, and at other times it increases the steps in the process to complete a function. For example, in a hybrid record, the time needed to process a record for scanning and indexing can add complexity to the process formerly called assembly and analysis.

## Prioritization of Department Functions

Prioritization of health information functions can occur once the department has established its goals and objectives. Earlier in the chapter, Table 13-3 provided a list of potential HIM department standards. Standards for department functions are necessary to keep the processes flowing. For example, in this textbook HIM functions are discussed in the following order: assembly, analysis, or postdischarge processing (Chapter 5), coding (Chapter 6), and filing (Chapter 9). However, coding may actually be a function that should occur very early in the workflow. The department may have a goal to reduce accounts receivable (AR) days, a measure of the average length of time it takes to collect on outstanding accounts, which may be lessened by prioritized coding in the workflow.

Typically, though, scanning and analysis are the first tasks performed to organize the record for the other HIM processes like coding, abstracting, and record review. The HIM director must also make sure that the records are analyzed for deficiencies quickly to meet The Joint Commission (TJC) or state standards for record completion—whichever is the most stringent. TJC standards require a complete record within 30 days of discharge, although some states preempt this standard, requiring a completed record within 14 days of discharge. The longer it takes for HIM staff to analyze a record, the less time is available to get the record completed by a physician.

The manager also sets standards for functions such as ROI and transcription. Timely completion of requests for ROI can affect continuity of patient care and possibly reimbursement, if the request is related to payment. The transcription team processes the dictated patient health information into a report that is used in communication and decision making during patient care. Timely completion of transcription affects patient care.

Department standards set the framework for efficient and effective management of health information. The standards direct the employees within the department workflow to accomplish their tasks in a timely manner. Sometimes, the task affects patient care directly; at other times, the task is part of department workflow and could impact the revenue cycle or customer service. Standards can then be used to evaluate the function of the HIM department.

## EVALUATION OF DEPARTMENT OPERATIONS AND SERVICES

It is important that supervisors and managers continually evaluate their departments according to department goals, objectives, and standards. If the standard is to assemble and analyze records within 24 hours, then the HIM manager must ensure that his or her employees are doing that. Evaluation of goals and objectives takes place annually, but employee-specific productivity should be evaluated at least monthly to ensure quality in the HIM department.

---

**hybrid record** A record in which both electronic and paper media are used.

**postdischarge processing** The procedures designed to prepare a health record for retention.

**analysis** The review of a record to evaluate its completeness, accuracy, or compliance with predetermined standards or other criteria.

**abstracting** The recap of selected fields from a health record to create an informative summary. Also refers to the activity of identifying such fields and entering them into a computer system.

**deficiencies** Required elements that are missing from a record.

**The Joint Commission (TJC)** An organization that accredits and sets standards for acute care facilities, ambulatory care networks, long-term care facilities, and rehabilitation facilities, as well as certain specialty facilities, such as hospice and home care. Facilities maintaining TJC accreditation receive *deemed status* from the CMS.

**preemption** The legal principle supporting the HIPAA stipulation that when the privacy regulations conflict with state law, the regulation or law that gives the patient more rights or is more restrictive should prevail.

**reimbursement** The amount of money that the health care facility receives from the party responsible for paying the bill.

**workflow** The process of work flowing through a set of procedures to complete the health record.

**revenue cycle** The groups of processes that identify, record, and report the financial transactions that result from the facility's clinical relationship with a patient.

**ROI** release of information

**Coding Productivity Report**
**02/20/2012**

| Coder | IP Total | IP Mcare | IP Non-Mcare | OP Total | ER | OP Refer | OBS | SDS |
|-------|----------|----------|--------------|----------|-----|----------|-----|-----|
| JBG | 22 | 20 | 2 | 40 | 0 | 40 | 0 | 0 |
| CRB | 15 | 15 | 0 | 55 | 48 | 0 | 7 | 0 |
| TLM | 30 | 25 | 5 | 12 | 0 | 0 | 0 | 12 |
| SNK | 32 | 20 | 12 | 5 | 0 | 0 | 0 | 5 |

**Figure 13-7** Productivity report of coders in a health information management department.

HIM managers and supervisors continually monitor the effectiveness and efficiency of the department through employee productivity reports (Figure 13-7) and through quality assurance monitoring. These measures alert the supervisors to any problems. Significant problems can then be addressed through employee training, performance improvement, or quality improvement efforts.

## Postdischarge Processing

Workflow in the HIM department that performs retrospective or postdischarge processing begins when the patient is discharged from the facility. The postdischarge process often follows the traditional processing (see Chapter 5) of paper health records. In this process the records are assembled or scanned, analyzed, coded, abstracted, completed, and filed (see Figure 13-4).

But workflow depends on the priorities set within the department. Specifically, the productivity standards for a function may require that one function be performed before another. For instance, if the department is motivated to code the health record within 24 hours of the patient's discharge, the coding function may need to take place before the analysis, and coding may be separated from the abstract function to promote coders' productivity. This workflow would be different from what was discussed in Chapter 5, because the health care facility has set the standard for coding in a shorter time frame. This is often the case when the facility is trying to reduce its AR days, the length of time it takes to send insurance claims ("bill") and receive payment (reimbursement) for health care.

## Concurrent Processing

In concurrent health information processing, the assembly, analysis, coding, and abstracting of the health record occur while the patient is in the facility. The analysis, such as the review for signatures, forms, and content of the documentation in the health record, takes place on the patient care unit. Concurrent analysis of health information is designed to have an impact on the quality of patient care by promoting timely, accurate, and complete documentation of patient health information.

Which functions occur first during concurrent analysis: coding, abstracting, assembly, or analysis? Priority is ultimately determined by the goals and objectives of the HIM department. The performance of concurrent analysis can include several scenarios. One situation may involve physically relocating employees to the patient care units. Another scenario may involve sending HIM employees to the patient care units to perform the analysis and then having them report back to the department for follow-up or further processing. For instance, an HIM clerk can go to a patient care unit to review the chart of

**performance improvement (PI)** Also known as *quality improvement (QI)* or *continuous quality improvement (CQI)*. Refers to the process by which a facility reviews its services or products to ensure quality.

**postdischarge processing** The procedures designed to prepare a health record for retention.

**AR** accounts receivable

**claim** The application to an insurance company for reimbursement of services rendered.

**concurrent analysis** Any type of record analysis performed during the patient's stay (i.e., after admission but before discharge).

## TABLE 13-4

### TYPICAL CONCURRENT PROCESSING STANDARDS*

| FUNCTION | EXAMPLE OF CONCURRENT PROCESSING STANDARD |
|---|---|
| Analysis | Initial analysis for patient signatures, forms, history and physical, and physical signatures completed within the first 24 hours of the patient's stay; routine (daily) analysis performed until the patient's discharge |
| Coding and abstracting | Initial coding performed during the first 24-48 hours of the patient's stay; updated periodically during the patient's stay, as the patient's condition warrants; final coding completed after discharge |
| Transcription | |
|   History and physical | Transcribed within 12 hours of dictation |
|   Consults | Transcribed within 12 hours of dictation |
|   Operative reports | Transcribed within 6 hours of dictation |
|   Discharge summary | Transcribed within 24 hours of dictation |

*Note: These standards are for example only; standards may vary depending on process.

**Go To** Review Chapter 5 for examples of detective controls.

**history and physical (H&P)** Health record documentation comprising the patient's history and physical examination; a formal, dictated copy must be included in the patient's health care record within 24 hours of admission for inpatient facilities.

**physician's orders** The physician's directions regarding the patient's care. Also refers to the data collection device on which these elements are captured.

**H&P** history and physical

**accreditation** Voluntary compliance with a set of standards developed by an independent agent, who periodically performs audits to ensure compliance.

**Go To** The quantitative analysis process is detailed in Chapter 11.

each patient who was admitted the previous day for the history and physical (H&P), physician's order signatures, and so on. This process of concurrent analysis is a detective control that provides an opportunity to take corrective action to achieve compliance with standards.

Regardless of the method, productivity standards must be designed to ensure timely processing. Table 13-4 provides an example of the productivity standards for concurrent processing in an HIM department.

## Electronic Record Processing

As described in Chapter 5, processing of health information in the hybrid record and electronic health record (EHR) environment changes the HIM workflow previously mentioned. The EHR is populated from intelligent software capable of recognizing patient record information and identifying any problems. A system that recognizes the requirements of a timely, accurate, and complete health record shifts from the need for an employee to perform assembly of the clinical documentation and to requirement for an audit. Here the audit process involves review of information that is inconsistent or incomplete. The EHR system changes the quantitative analysis process, assuming that the computer/software program recognizes pertinent information and automatically flags what is incomplete or missing. For example, the software can identify that the H&P is complete but missing a signature. The audit of patient health information in the EHR requires the technical skills of the registered health information technician (RHIT). Data integrity, record completion standards, system design and analysis are also part of a process that requires the knowledge of accreditation requirements, coding guidelines, and the clinical aspects of patient care. These functions resemble those of an auditor or database manager.

### EXERCISE 13-3

#### Health Information Management Department Workflow

1. List the HIM functions in postdischarge processing.
2. The amount of work in the HIM department is determined by:
   a. the CEO.
   b. the department director.
   c. admissions.
   d. the number of discharges, patient type, and length of stay.
3. Processing of the health care record after patient discharge is called:
   a. postdischarge processing.
   b. concurrent processing.
   c. HIM processing.
   d. analysis.

4. Processing of the health care record during patient care is called:
   a. retrospective processing.
   b. concurrent processing.
   c. HIM processing.
   d. analysis.
5. One method of monitoring the amount of work an employee performs is:
   a. reviewing the organization chart.
   b. reviewing the productivity report.
   c. monitoring payroll.
   d. limiting employee breaks.

## DEPARTMENT PLANNING

Planning is used by organizations to prepare for the future: expansion of the facility, providing new services that require knowledge of regulations and guidelines, and even conversion to an EHR. Some situations require more planning than others, and some plans are more formal and elaborate than others.

The plan itself is a guide that describes the manner in which events are expected to take place in the department. For example, the workflow in a department, discussed previously, is the result of a plan. Before employees begin performing the functions of assembly, analysis, and coding, HIM managers must plan to ensure optimal productivity.

The HIM department may also plan for changes or improvements. Managers can plan to implement a new procedure—for example, concurrent coding, purging of records, or scanning of paper files into digital images. Planning involves analyzing the current situation, determining the goal, and strategizing to accomplish goals.

**productivity** The amount of work produced by an employee in a given time frame.

### Mission

A **mission statement** is a declaration of the organization's purpose. Traditionally, the organization's mission statement shows careful thought for those it serves. A mission statement is very important to an organization because it provides a common purpose, which helps the organization unify, serving its community as a team with a specific direction. An example is the mission statement for Diamonte Hospital (our hypothetical acute care facility): "Diamonte Hospital provides high-quality health care through dedication and commitment to excellence." The mission statement is important for the development of a *culture*. If the employees demonstrate the mission in their actions, it impacts how the organization functions.

**mission statement** The strategic purpose of the organization documented in a formal statement.

HIM departments may also have a mission. For example, the HIM department of Diamonte Hospital exists to provide efficient, high-quality health information to all customers to promote high-quality health care in the organization. The department mission should coincide with the mission for the entire facility. The following is the mission statement for the HIM Department of Diamonte Hospital: "The Health Information Management Department of Diamonte Hospital exists to provide timely, complete, accurate, confidential, and secure health information to all users." As with the mission statement for the organization, when the HIM employee actions reflect the HIM mission statement, their purpose is evident to the customers.

### Vision

Another common element to be considered when planning in an organization or department is a vision. A **vision** statement clearly states the organization's expected future. Although the mission is to provide high-quality patient care and to exceed customers' expectations, the vision may state the desire to become the leading health care provider in the community. By definition, *vision* conveys an intelligent foresight. A vision for the

**vision** The goal of the organization, above and beyond the mission.

**electronic health record (EHR)** A secure real-time, point-of-care, patient centric information resource for clinicians allowing access to patient information when and where needed and incorporating evidence-based decision support.

**goals** Desired achievements.

**objectives** Directions for achieving a goal.

**capital budget** Money set aside for larger purchases, usually over a certain dollar amount, whose use will span multiple fiscal years.

**operational budget** Costs related to the operation of the health information department, such as utilities and supplies.

HIM department might be to implement an EHR in order to ensure quality health care services; this would be in line with the vision of the organization, because an EHR supports the quality patient care needed to become a leading health care provider.

## Goals and Objectives

Managing the daily operations in an HIM department can be a very demanding job. HIM departments annually set *goals* to accomplish new or improved functions. **Goals** are statements that provide the department with direction or focus. Goals state that the department will strive to achieve something new. Goals can reflect different time frames; they can be annual, short-term, or long-term. Examples of goals for an HIM department are listed in Table 13-5.

To reach a goal, the department sets *objectives* to direct how the goal will be achieved. **Objectives** specify what must be accomplished. The expectation is that when the action for each objective is implemented, the goal is attained. In this text, each chapter has learning objectives. The material in each chapter is presented so that the reader is able to perform the objectives. Table 13-5 provides some examples of HIM department objectives.

The goals and objectives of the HIM department are typically more concrete than its mission and vision statements. The department's goals and objectives should complement the organization's mission and vision. In other words, if the organization is committed to quality, then the HIM goals and objectives should address and support quality. The purpose of the goals and objectives is to keep the department focused and to provide a guide for improvement.

## Budget

In addition to managing an efficient and effective HIM department, the HIM director (and supervisors) is responsible for the HIM budget. There are several different types of budget, but for the purposes of this discussion, only *capital* and *operational budgets* are pertinent. The **capital budget** is money set aside to make purchases that are over a certain dollar limit. For example, any purchase costing more than $1500 might need to be part of the capital budget. The specific dollar amount limit is set by the administration. EHR implementation is an example of a capital budget item. Typically, capital equipment, like furniture and computers, is depreciable on the basis of certain tax systems.

The **operational budget** includes those expenses necessary to run the department. Supply costs, maintenance contract expenses, and utilities are some common expenditures

**TABLE 13-5**

**HIM DEPARTMENT GOALS AND OBJECTIVES***

| GOALS | OBJECTIVES |
|---|---|
| 1. Maintain continuous compliance with TJC accreditation standards for timely record completion. | 1a. The monthly number of delinquent health records will be less than 50% of the average monthly discharge (AMD). |
| | 1b. The number of delinquent history and physical records will not exceed 1%. |
| | 1c. The number of delinquent operative reports will not exceed 1%. |
| 2. Transcription services will facilitate compliance with TJC requirement for timeliness of documentation regarding history and physical records, discharge summary records, consults, and operative reports. | 2a. History and physical records will be transcribed within 6 hours of dictation. |
| | 2b. Consultation reports will be transcribed within 12 hours of dictation. |
| | 2c. Operative reports will be transcribed within 12 hours of dictation. |
| | 2d. Discharge summaries will be transcribed within 24 hours of dictation. |

*These goals are for example only; they are not all-inclusive.

of the HIM department's capital budget. The budget is calculated for a 12-month period, or 1 year. This year, also known as the fiscal year (FY), is not always identical to a January-through-December calendar year, and the fiscal year period is determined by the facility. For example, a fiscal year may run July 1 through June 30, or October 1 through September 30.

Typically, each hospital department in the organization is responsible for developing and presenting its budget to the financial administrators for approval. The capital budget is approved separate from the operational budget. Fortunately, when planning for the next year, the department managers are able to use the operational budget from the previous and current years. This information allows the manager to make sound decisions regarding the proposed budget, which is important because the manager will be held accountable for staying within the budget that is approved for his or her department. The budget contains an estimate for revenue each month and allows the department a set amount of money for each expense (e.g., supplies, employee salaries, contracts). The HIM department is not typically a revenue-generating department. Seeming exceptions, such as the charges a department that collects for copying and ROI, are nominal, as mandated by HIPAA, and should cover only the costs of copying and postage. However, some HIM departments may offer transcription or coding services to area physicians for a fee.

Each month, the director must compare the actual expenses and revenue with the budgeted expenses and revenue. Figure 13-8 displays limited budget items for the HIM department during the month of July. An actual budget report would include many more line items or expenses. The "Budget" column displays the amount allocated for the corresponding expense. The "Actual" column displays the amount of money spent during the month of July. Notice that this information, budget and actual, is also displayed for year to date (YTD) expenses. The YTD information allows the manager to determine whether the budget is being met for the year. This is helpful because sometimes one month's expenses will be more or less than the actual budget, and knowing the YTD expenses helps the manager determine whether they will meet the budget for the entire year. The last column displays the difference, or the actual amount that the department is over or under budget.

**FY** fiscal year

**release of information (ROI)** HIM department function that provides disclosure of patient health information.

**HIPAA** Health Insurance Portability and Accountability Act

**YTD** year-to-date

| HIM Department Budget – July (month 7 of Fiscal Year) | | | | | |
|---|---|---|---|---|---|
| | Budget | YTD-Budget | Actual | YTD-Actual | Difference |
| Revenue: | | | | | |
| Expenses: | | | | | |
| Salaries | $12,000 | $84,000 | $11,458 | $82,880 | ($1120) or 1.3% |
| Supplies | $250 | $1750 | $308 | $1800 | $50 or −2.9% |
| Maintenance contract | | | | | |
| Copy machine | $500 | $3500 | $500 | $3500 | 0% |

Figure 13-8 HIM (health information management) department budget for July (month 7 of the fiscal year). YTD, year to date.

## EXERCISE 13-4

### Department Planning

1. For the 2013 to 2014 fiscal year, the manager has set a _____ to implement a document imaging system.
2. To reach a desired goal, the department must establish _____, directions for achieving a goal.
3. The purpose of the organization documented in a formal statement is known as the _____.
4. Above and beyond the mission statement, _____ sets a direction for the organization for the future.

5. The HIM director established the following: "The HIM department delinquency percentage will not exceed 50% of average monthly discharges by July 1." This is an example of a(n):
   a. plan.
   b. goal.
   c. objective.
   d. mission.
6. In addition, the director stated that the suspension procedure will be performed weekly (as approved in the bylaws). This is an example of a(n):
   a. plan.
   b. goal.
   c. objective.
   d. mission.
7. The HIM department is allowed $300 per month for supplies. At the end of the third quarter, the department has spent $3000 on supplies. This means that the HIM department is:
   a. under budget YTD by $300.
   b. over budget YTD by $300.
   c. exactly as it should be on budget for supplies.
   d. over budget $250.
8. Diamonte Hospital's fiscal year runs July 1 through June 30. Which of the following months are in the third quarter?
   a. January, February, March
   b. April, May, June
   c. July, August, September
   d. October, November, December
9. The employees who should be involved in the selection process of an EHR because they will use and maintain the system are called _____.

**meaningful use** A set of measures to gauge the level of health information technology used by a provider, and required, in certain stages, in order to receive financial incentives from the CMS.

**system development life cycle (SDLC)** The process of planning, designing, implementation, and evaluation used in updating and improving, or implementing a new health information system.

**stakeholder** Regarding EHR implementation and selection, an individual or department with an interest in the process, either in the implementation or the outcome.

## Planning for EHR Migration and Implementation

Federal meaningful use mandates, driven by the need for improved patient care and the long-term reduction in health care costs, have meant that facilities across the United States are planning their migration to an EHR. Today's HIM department managers are working within the mission, vision, and budget of their organizations to implement a fully functional electronic health record.

There are many things that must be considered in order to successfully implement an EHR in a health care facility. Health care organizations and HIM professionals can use the **system development life cycle (SDLC)** for the large-scale design and implementation of information systems. Box 13-1 shows the phases of the system development life cycle.

### Selection

Selection of an EHR product is a major project for the health care organization. It requires involvement from those employees that will use and maintain the system. These employees are often called **stakeholders**. Corporate facilities often choose one product to use in *all* of their facilities; while in independent health care facilities, the product may be chosen/

| BOX 13-1 | PHASES OF INFORMATION SYSTEM DEVELOPMENT LIFE CYCLE |
|---|---|

1. Selection
2. Design
3. Implementation
4. Evaluation
5. Support

dictated by the CEO, governing board, or partner organizations. Health care facilities start by identifying their needs or system requirements. The needs are incorporated into a "list" that will serve as the *rubric* or method for evaluating each proposed EHR product.

With the list of system requirements, a facility can formulate a **request for proposal (RFP)**. The RFP is used to explain to EHR vendors what the health care organization intends to accomplish and requires of an EHR product. EHR vendors who are interested in doing business with the health care organization will review the RFP and submit a proposal explaining how their product can fulfill the needs of the health care facility/organization.

> **request for proposal (RFP)** A document composed from provider's list of system requirements used to explain to EHR vendors what the health care organization intends to accomplish and requires of an EHR product.

---

## HIT-bit

### REQUEST FOR PROPOSAL PROCESS

The RFP is a document created by the health care facility to explain its expectation for a particular service or product to potential vendors —for example, EHR software or an outsource service contract. The RFP describes the health care facility and also explains what the facility requires in the software product it wishes to purchase. A vendor who is interested in being chosen to provide the system or service for the health care organization reviews the RFP and submits a proposal explaining how his/her product/company can fulfill the needs listed in the RFP.

---

Once proposals are received, then a committee of stakeholders reviews the proposals to determine the vendor that best meets their needs, keeping in mind costs and the vendor's ability to provide support. Once a vendor is chosen, the stakeholders can move to the next SDLC phase: design.

> **SDLC** system development life cycle

### Design

During the design process, the stakeholders work to ensure that the product performs to meet the needs of the health care organization (as they requested in the RFP). The EHR vendor will help the organization establish a time line for the implementation. Some vendors have products that are easy to implement but allow very little flexibility in custom design. Other vendors allow the organization options to customize the product so that it meets their specific needs. Generally speaking, without compromising quality a facility will work within time and budget constraints to ensure that the new technology matches their current or anticipated workflow needs.

> **workflow** The process of work flowing through a set of procedures to complete the health record.

In addition, this is the point at which the facility will ensure that the product can work with other information systems or software products being used in the facility. This is often called *integration*, making sure that the data from one system can be integrated into another system for optimal use. Integration can require additional cost and time to make sure all of the data are shared accurately in a way that functions correctly.

### Implementation

As the organization transitions from the Design to the Implementation phase, there is a period when the stakeholders and the vendor create a "test" environment so that they can determine whether the product works as it was designed. Once testing is complete, the facility is ready to implement the system in the "live" environment. There are several ways to accomplish this. One way is to implement in pilot stages, by which it is used only partially in small areas until the stakeholders are sure that the product functions correctly. Another method is to run the new system parallel (at the same time) with the old system, and still another way is to switch over, to simply stop using the old system on a particular date and start using the new system. There are pros and cons to each system, so the implementation method should suit the size and capability of the new system and the method for implementation is chosen by the stakeholders or implementation team.

**computerized physician order entry (CPOE)** A health information system in which physicians enter orders electronically. Includes decision support and alerts.

**stakeholder** Regarding EHR implementation and selection, an individual or department with an interest in the process, either in the implementation or the outcome.

**document imaging** Scanning or faxing of printed papers into a computer system or optical disk system. See also Computer output to laser disk.

A pilot phase implementation could work well when a system like computerized physician order entry (CPOE) is being implemented. The implementation could begin on a particular patient care unit in the health care facility. Prior to implementation, the training would be focused and specific to the needs of the group of physicians and nurses who work on the unit. The implementation date would be chosen, and the progress of the implementation would be localized to one unit and group of stakeholders. Then, as the comfort level and function of the new system become stable, a new unit would be chosen for the next phase of implementation to include training, and so on.

When systems are implemented in a parallel situation, the health care facility chooses to keep the old system operational while training and beginning to use the new system. This may happen when a health care facility begins to scan health care records into a document imaging system. This method requires double processing of health care records. Training would begin with the HIM scanning technicians learning the new process to prepare records for scanning into the document imaging system. The double processing would occur once the paper pages of the record were scanned, the HIM technicians would still assemble the record in the paper method (organizing them and attaching them to a file folder labeled accordingly) for maintenance and record completion. The parallel systems would continue for a time to allow comfort with the new system and to ensure that the new system facilitated the accurate storage, retrieval, and record completion requirements of the HIM department. At some point the old method of assembly and paper record identification and storage would stop, and the document imaging system would be the primary method of record processing.

The switch-over implementation method is simple in explanation: The health care facility simply "stops" using the old method and from that date forward only uses the "new" system. It is best to prepare for this method of implementation by performing a significant amount of testing prior to the "go live" date. The employees who will use the new system need to be trained and comfortable with the new system. It is also a good idea to have a number of support tools available to employees when they begin using the system; for instance, a team of super-users well trained and able to monitor the implementation from all areas, help desk contact numbers and/or specific employees in their unit to report problems and ask questions, and easily accessible training modules/policy (online knowledge base) to access online if they forget a procedure.

Regardless of the method used for implementation, it is important to manage this stage closely and to prepare/plan ahead of time for the transition period. Implementation is exciting and daunting. Proper planning is required. Training is essential. Support tools and problem-reporting methods provide mechanisms to keep the implementation on track.

### Evaluation

Once the system is implemented in the real work environment, it is evaluated to ensure that it is working the way it was designed. This is different from testing because the system is being evaluated in the real or live situation it is serving. The evaluation process can include feedback from users, surveys of satisfaction, and monitoring of reported problems where the system does not perform correctly. These indicators help pinpoint places where modifications can be made in the system to ensure that it functions as intended.

### Support

As with any information system there must be a way for users to report problems associated with the function or access to the system. The support is typically called a "help desk" or technical support hotline. In some organizations there may be one phone number to report these problems, although more advanced systems also have an e-mail, live chat feature, or online knowledge base so that users have access to technical support 24 hours a day, 7 days a week. Reporting a problem with the system usually results in a ticket, or record of the reported problem, so that the problem can be tracked through the process until it is resolved. This allows technical support to keep a record of frequent problems, have answers ready when a similar problem arises, and work on ways to correct the problem permanently, improving overall efficiency.

## EXERCISE 13-5

### Planning for EHR Implementation

1. List three important items that must be considered in the selection of an EHR.
2. What is the purpose of an RFP?
3. Explain why (or a situation in which) a pilot, phased implementation would be the preferred method.
4. Running two systems simultaneously is called _____ implementation.
5. Identify three methods used to evaluate an EHR.
6. Explain why it is important for the health care organization to have a method for reporting technical problems.

## DEPARTMENT POLICIES AND PROCEDURES

The policies and procedures of a health care facility are documented so that the employees, customers, accreditation agencies, licensing bodies, regulatory agencies, and legal authorities can identify the philosophy and methods under which the facility operates. A **policy** is a statement, in broad terms, of what the facility does on a routine basis. For example, a policy might require that a health record be maintained for every patient treated in this facility. The **procedure** is the process of how the policy is carried out. For example, a procedure might require that an assembly clerk retrieve all discharge records from the nursing units immediately following the patients' discharge. Policies and procedures provide details about the following:

- How, when, and why things are done
- Who performs which tasks, jobs, and functions
- Who is responsible for an activity, an authorization, and so forth
- Quality controls and audits
- Historical, routine, and emergency situations

Figure 13-9 shows an example of the previously mentioned policy—that is, a health record is maintained for every patient treated in this facility.

The entire health care organization has policies and procedures that affect everyone in the facility. Each department in the health care facility should have specific policies and procedures that outline their processes, responsibilities, and services. All employees of the facility must have access to the *policy and procedures manual*, or *PPM*. Today PPMs are often stored electronically so that all employees have easy access from any computer. The HIM department manual contains policies and procedures that relate specifically to health information. Figure 13-10 contains a list of contents for an HIM department policy and procedures manual.

> **accreditation** Voluntary compliance with a set of standards developed by an independent agent, who periodically performs audits to ensure compliance.
>
> **policy** A statement of something that is done or expected in an organization.
>
> **procedure** A process that describes how to comply with a policy. Also, a medical or surgical treatment. Also refers to the processing steps in an administrative function.

> **PPM** policy and procedures manual

### HIT-bit

#### POLICIES AND PROCEDURES ON AN INTRANET

Special consideration for a facility's policies in the digital environment includes securing access to prevent unauthorized people from making changes to policies. It is also important to have a paper copy of the policy statements in case the computer is inaccessible.

For example, a policy in the HIM department for coding and abstracting of health care records might read as follows: "The HIM department will maintain accurate diagnosis and procedure indices. The HIM department will maintain appropriate indices by accurately coding all diagnoses and procedures found in the patient's medical records." The procedure then details how coders should go through these records and identify the primary diagnoses and primary procedures and how they should assign the codes. It should also stipulate or explain how the information is entered into a computer system (e.g., how data are collected for compilation of a patient abstract).

> **index** A system that places specific data items within a frame of reference, creating collections of patient data (or a database) specific to a diagnosis, procedure, or physician.
>
> **abstract** A summary of the patient record.

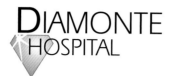

**DIAMONTE HOSPITAL**

Diamonte, Arizona 89104 • TEL. 602-484-9991

**Health Information Management Department**
Policy No. 3.01
Health Record Creation and Definition, Unit Medical Record
   Number Assignment

| **Effective:** 01/15/2011 | **Reviewed:** 01/2012, 01/2013 |

**Approved:**

**Policy:**

The Health Information Management Department will maintain a health record for all patients receiving treatment at Diamonte Hospital. The record will be kept in accordance with state, federal, accreditation, and professional guidelines. Each patient record will be identified using a unit numbering system.

**Procedure:**

1. Upon registration at Diamonte Hospital for any service, the patient will be assigned a medical record number and a health record will be initiated.

2. During the patient visit, health information shall be documented in a timely manner on approved facility forms.

3. Following discharge, all patient records will be collected by the Health Information Management Department.

4. The Health Information Management clerk will use the daily ADT (Admission-Discharge-Transfer) reports to verify collection of *all* health records.

5. Records not retrieved the day following discharge will be reported to the Health Information Supervisor immediately, for appropriate action.

*Example Policy Only*

Figure 13-9 Policy and procedure for maintenance of health records for all patients receiving care in a facility.

The HIM department director is responsible for ensuring that the departmental policies and procedures are current. This is accomplished by making sure that policies exist for all necessary functions, responsibilities, and services under his or her control. All policies and procedures should be reviewed annually and as significant changes occur in procedures, regulations, or legislation. Review is as simple as reading through each policy and procedure to verify that the contents are accurate, then initialing and dating the review for authentication.

# EXERCISE 13-6

## Department Policies and Procedures

1. The following is _____ of Diamonte Hospital, an equal opportunity employer: "All new hires will be drug tested."
2. A process that describes how to comply with a policy is a _____.
3. To maintain a high-quality HIM department, the supervisors and managers should:
   a. monitor employee dress code.
   b. continually evaluate the functions of the HIM department on the basis of the goals and standards set.
   c. convert to concurrent processing.
   d. never promote from within.

4. Policy and procedures should be:
   a. reviewed annually.
   b. updated as necessary in accordance with changes in policy or procedure.
   c. maintained in an area or manner accessible to all employees.
   d. all of the above.
5. The HIM department is the only department in the organization that has a policy and procedures manual.
   True
   False
6. Policy and procedures should be updated:
   a. annually and as needed due to change.
   b. only as needed due to change.
   c. by the CEO.
   d. by the nursing administrator.

## HEALTH INFORMATION PERSONNEL

With the workflow organized, it is time to consider the way in which job functions are organized into job descriptions with performance standards that communicate the manager's expectation of the employee. Hiring practices and priorities are also discussed. Certain jobs in the HIM departments are staffed by credentialed employees. For example, the director of the HIM department must hold a current RHIT or Registered Health Information Administrator (RHIA) credential. Coding positions may require the Certified Coding Specialist (CCS), Certified Coding Specialist–Physician (CCS-P), or Certified Coding Associate (CCA). At the very core HIM credentialed employees must adhere to the American Health Information Management Association (AHIMA) code of ethics in handling HIM procedures and health information. Hiring credentialed employees is one way to ensure that the fundamental tenants of HIM were a part of the employees training. It is important to note that the topics discussed may vary by state, region, and employee associations. Department managers should be very careful to understand the labor rules and regulations associated with the employees in their department. When in doubt, one should consult the facility's human resource department.

**workflow** The process of work flowing through a set of procedures to complete the health record.

**performance standards** Set guidelines explaining how much work an employee must complete.

**RHIT** Registered Health Information Technician

## Job Descriptions

The **job description** is a list of the employee's responsibilities. Each position in the department should have a job description. The job description communicates the expectations of the job to the employee. If an old job description needs to be updated, it is appropriate to give the employee a copy of the job description for review. Allow the employee to review the job description and ask him or her to identify how the job has changed. This involvement gives the employee an opportunity to clearly communicate to the manager/supervisor how the job is currently being performed. Job descriptions should be reviewed annually by managers and employees. Employees sign the job description to acknowledge their awareness of their responsibilities and job function.

**job description** A list of the employee's responsibilities.

### Writing a Job Description

A job description contains several key elements that describe the job specifically. The job description has a heading that briefly describes the position. The heading should include the facility in which the position is located, the title of the position, the supervisor for the position, and the effective date of the job description (Figure 13-11). The remainder of the job description includes information regarding hours worked, the purpose of the job, its responsibilities and skills required. It also includes a description of the physical demands of the environment in which the work is performed, and the basic physical requirements of the position. It is important to list only physical requirements that are essential to the performance of the job, in accordance with the stipulations of the Americans with

| Diamonte Health Information Management Department Policy and Procedure Manual | |
|---|---|
| **Table of Contents** | |
| **Section 1** | **Introduction** |
| 1.01 | Purpose |
| 1.02 | Responsibility for policy development, update, and approval |
| 1.03 | Distribution and access of policies |
| 1.04 | Diamonte mission statement |
| 1.05 | Diamonte organization chart |
| 1.06 | Health information management department mission statement and organization chart |
| **Section 2** | **General Department Policies** |
| 2.01 | Centralized health information management department |
| 2.02 | Scope of service |
| 2.03 | Hours of operation |
| 2.04 | Confidentiality, privacy, and data security considerations |
| 2.05 | Confidentiality statement |
| 2.06 | Department orientation |
| 2.07 | Training and education of department employees |
| 2.08 | Employee competency |
| 2.09 | General policies of the health information management department |
| 2.10 | Health information management department organization chart |
| **Section 3** | **The Health Record** |
| 3.01 | Creation and definition, unit medical record number assignment |
| 3.02 | Ownership of the health record |
| 3.03 | Guidelines for entries into the health record |
| 3.04 | Abbreviations list |
| 3.05 | Fax copies in the health record |
| 3.06 | Completion of discharge summaries |
| **Section 4** | **Assembly and Analysis** |
| 4.01 | Health record assembly and chart order |
| 4.02 | Retrospective record analysis |
| **Section 5** | **Storage, Access, and Security** |
| 5.01 | Health record storage system |
| 5.02 | Security of health information |
| 5.03 | Confidentiality and security of computerized information |
| 5.04 | Retention schedule for health records and related documents |
| 5.05 | Procedure to access health records |
| 5.06 | Health record locations |
| 5.07 | Removal of health records from the health information management department |
| 5.08 | Destruction of records |
| **Section 6** | **Record Completion** |
| 6.01 | Incomplete chart/record completion process |
| 6.02 | Notification of incomplete health records for physicians |
| 6.03 | Suspension process |
| **Section 7** | **Release of Information** |
| 7.01 | General policies for release of information |
| 7.02 | Consent for release of information |
| 7.03 | Notice of recipient of information, disclosure laws |
| 7.04 | Patient's right to health information, copies of health records |
| 7.05 | Copy and retrieval fees |
| **Section 8** | **Quality of Health Information** |
| 8.01 | Monitoring and evaluation of quality in the health information management department |
| 8.02 | Record review process/clinical pertinence |
| 8.03 | Compliance with regulations and standards |
| **Use of Contract Services or Agencies–Business Associate Agreements** | |
| **Job Descriptions** | |
| **Safety in the Health Information Management Department** | |
| Materials Safety Data Sheets (MSDS) | |

**Figure 13-10** Table of contents of a health information management department policy and procedures manual.

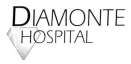

**Health Information Management Department**
**Position Title:** Birth Certificate Clerk

| **Position #:** 070530 | **Grade:** G2 |
| **Reports to:** HIM Manager | **Effective:** 01/15/2013 |

Position Description: Under the general supervision of the HIM Manager, the Birth Certificate Clerk completes a birth certificate, and supporting forms as necessary, for each baby born at Diamonte Hospital. The birth certificates are electronically submitted to the Office of Vital Records, and original certificates with signatures are mailed to the Office of Vital Records in a timely manner. The clerk must maintain a current knowledge of the rules regarding birth certificates. The Birth Certificate Clerk is a member of the Health Information Management department team and maintains knowledge of various other functions in the department to assist as necessary.

**Position Qualifications:**

*Education:* High school diploma

*Licensure/Certification/Registration:* None necessary

*Experience:* Excellent communication skills. Ability to type 30 WPM. Previous clerical experience preferred. Ability to function in busy office environment with multiple shifting and evolving priorities.

**Responsibilities:**

1. Monitors Labor and Delivery log and Admission reports to identify all patients requiring a birth certificate.

2. Collects birth certificate information from parent(s) and completes birth certificate accurately. Parent(s) review birth certificate to verify accuracy and sign in appropriate areas.

3. Maintains current knowledge of all birth certificate rules, regulations, and issues. Reviews and implements state laws governing completion of birth certificates.

4. Ensures completion of other forms relating to the birth as necessary (e.g., paternity, social security verification).

5. Maintains current and accurate birth certificate log.

6. Contacts any parents who have left the hospital prior to completion of the birth certificate. Processes new, delayed, or corrected birth certificates.

7. Obtains physician's signature on the birth certificate within 1 week of completion.

8. Submits electronic birth certificates immediately following completion, mailing completed original certificate within 15 days of completion.

9. Maintains electronic birth certificate software in working condition; performs backups regularly.

10. Follows established policies and procedures regarding confidentiality and security of health information, infection control, safety and security management, and emergency preparedness.

Figure 13-11 Job description for a health information management (HIM) department position. WPM, words per minute.

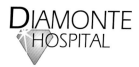

**JOB DESCRIPTION, continued**

**Health Information Management Department**
**Position Title:** Birth Certificate Clerk

| **Position #:** 070530 | **Grade:** G2 |
| **Reports to:** HIM Manager | **Effective:** 01/15/2013 |

11. Displays a positive and courteous manner toward patients, visitors, customers, and co-workers.

12. Follows all policies and procedures of the facility and HIM department.

13. Completes annual employee in-service and required department training.

**Physical Requirements:**

*Mental and emotional requirements:*  Employee must be able to manage stress appropriately, work independently, handle multiple priorities.

*Working conditions:*  Employee spends approximately 90% of time inside the health care facility. The work area has adequate lighting, good ventilation, comfortable temperature.  Employee work station provided with appropriate access to rest rooms and lunch and break areas.

*Physical demands:*  Employee is responsible for light work—lifting maximum of 20 lb, with frequent lifting or carrying of objects weighing up to 10 lb.  Work positions include sitting 50%, standing 20%, walking 20%, lifting/carrying 10%.

**Example only**

Figure 13-11, cont'd

Disabilities Act (ADA) requirements. The job description also contains any numbers, grades, and classification (exempt or nonexempt) used by the human resources department or the organization to describe that position.

## Job Analysis

**job analysis** Review of a function to determine all of the tasks or components that make up an employee's job.

It is important to have the right employee performing the appropriate function at the right time in order to effectively manage the HIM department. **Job analysis** is the review of a specific function to determine all of the tasks or components from the job. When a job analysis is performed, the job tasks are reviewed to ensure that the process works efficiently.

**HIT-bit**

**FROM JOB ANALYSIS TO JOB DESCRIPTION**

If you have involved the employee in a job analysis, the employee should review the job's functions and responsibilities when the job description is complete.

Job analysis can be performed by a supervisor or manager working with the employee; together, they review and perform the employee's job function. As the supervisor works with the employee, he or she is able to determine the procedures performed by the employee. The supervisor must document the procedures as performed by the employee so that they can be reviewed in total. Following this observation, which can take a few hours or even

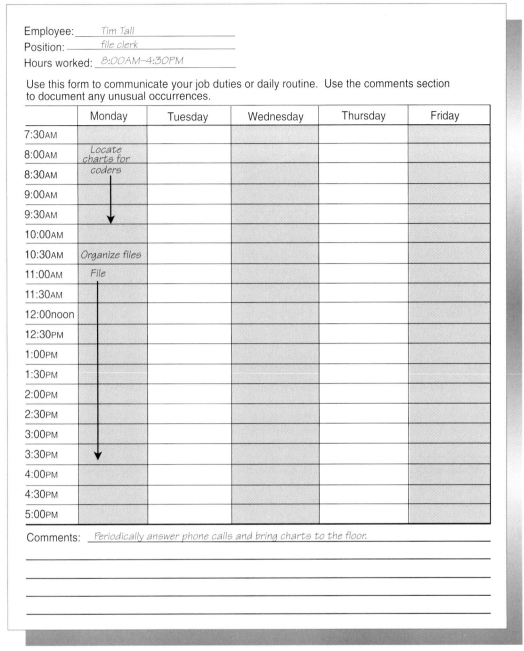

Employee: _____Tim Tall_____
Position: _____file clerk_____
Hours worked: _8:00AM–4:30PM_

Use this form to communicate your job duties or daily routine.  Use the comments section to document any unusual occurrences.

|  | Monday | Tuesday | Wednesday | Thursday | Friday |
|---|---|---|---|---|---|
| 7:30AM |  |  |  |  |  |
| 8:00AM | Locate charts for coders |  |  |  |  |
| 8:30AM |  |  |  |  |  |
| 9:00AM |  |  |  |  |  |
| 9:30AM |  |  |  |  |  |
| 10:00AM |  |  |  |  |  |
| 10:30AM | Organize files |  |  |  |  |
| 11:00AM | File |  |  |  |  |
| 11:30AM |  |  |  |  |  |
| 12:00noon |  |  |  |  |  |
| 12:30PM |  |  |  |  |  |
| 1:00PM |  |  |  |  |  |
| 1:30PM |  |  |  |  |  |
| 2:00PM |  |  |  |  |  |
| 2:30PM |  |  |  |  |  |
| 3:00PM |  |  |  |  |  |
| 3:30PM |  |  |  |  |  |
| 4:00PM |  |  |  |  |  |
| 4:30PM |  |  |  |  |  |
| 5:00PM |  |  |  |  |  |

Comments: _Periodically answer phone calls and bring charts to the floor._

**Figure 13-12** Job analysis tool.

an entire day, the evaluator or supervisor has actual information with which to develop a job description and performance standards.

Another effective way to perform a job analysis is by asking the employee to explain how he or she performs the job. This method employs a data collection device used by the employee to analyze his or her job. The form shown in Figure 13-12 is an example of this sort of tool. The employee uses this form to communicate to the manager in detail what the job involves on a daily basis, using his or her own words.

## Performance Standards

Managers can use the information they gathered in job analysis to set **performance standards**. Performance standards determine how much work should be accomplished within a specific time frame. Additionally, performance standards let the employee know that

**performance standards** Set guidelines explaining how much work an employee must complete.

**TABLE 13-6**

**PERFORMANCE STANDARDS***

| EMPLOYEE/POSITION | STANDARD | PERFORMANCE RATING SCALE |
|---|---|---|
| Coder | All health records will be coded within 48-72 hours of patient discharge. | Exceeds expectations: 36 or more records coded daily<br>Meets expectations: 28-35 records coded daily<br>Does not meet expectations: Fewer than 28 records coded daily<br>*Supervisor uses daily productivity reports to average the coder's performance.* |
| Coder | Health records will be assigned appropriate and accurate codes according to applicable coding guidelines. | Exceeds expectations: 96%-100% of records reviewed coded appropriately and accurately<br>Meets expectations: 90%-95% of records reviewed coded appropriately and accurately<br>Does not meet expectations: Less than 90% of records reviewed coded appropriately and accurately<br>*Supervisor will review a representative sample of the coder's work to ensure appropriateness and accuracy of coding.* |
| Assembly/ analysis clerk | All patient health records will be assembled and analyzed within 24 hours of patient discharge. | Exceeds expectations: 95%-100% of all records assembled and analyzed within 24 hours of patient discharge<br>Meets expectations: 85%-95% or all records assembled and analyzed within 24 hours of patient discharge<br>Does not meet expectations: Less than 85% of all records assembled and analyzed within 24 hours of patient discharge<br>*Supervisor will routinely assess and document the clerks' productivity to determine score.* |
| File clerk | Accurate filing of all patient health records will be completed daily. | Exceeds expectations: 100% of all health records filed accurately on a daily basis<br>Meets expectations: 96%-99% of all health records filed accurately on a daily basis<br>Does not meet expectations: Less than 96% of all health records filed accurately on a daily basis<br>*Supervisor will perform routine checks of filing area to determine accuracy; results will be documented to determine file clerk's score.* |

*Note: These standards vary in each facility.

quality (percentage of accuracy) is required for this position. It is not only important for the employee to complete the job; the work must also be done correctly. Supervisors can use these standards to evaluate employee performance.

Performance standards are drawn from the job description and job analysis. Table 13-6 provides example of performance standards for various job descriptions in the HIM Department birth certificate clerk. These performance standards establish a time frame in which the employee's work is to be completed and include a scale that explains how each score is achieved. The birth certificate clerk is responsible for completing a birth certificate for all newborn admissions according to the facility's policy and state law. Performance standards for this requirement might be stated as follows: "A birth certificate is completed on all newborn admissions according to facility policy and state law prior to the newborn's discharge. If at any time a birth certificate is not completed before the newborn is discharged, the employee has not met the standard, thereby affecting the employee's performance rating."

Employee performance affects the productivity of the entire department. Therefore the standards are developed specifically for each position to ensure that each employee's performance promotes effective and efficient progress in the HIM department.

## Evaluating Productivity

**productivity** The amount of work produced by an employee in a given time frame.

There are several ways to collect information on the employee's performance and **productivity**: manually, by observation, or by using computerized reports from computer applications. The goal is to have an objective tool that reflects the amount of work performed by the employee. Later, the accuracy and quality of the employee's work can be assessed by sample review of his or her work.

### Manual Productivity Reports

Manual productivity reports can be designed to obtain information about the employee's performance. Figure 13-6 gives a sample form for collection of data on the productivity of a coding employee.

This form contains information to identify the employee, the time frame in which the information is collected, and specifics about the employee's job. Because the employee in our example is responsible for inpatient coding, the form shown in Figure 13-6 collects information about the number of records coded each day. In addition, the form collects information about activities related to the employee's job, including conversations with physicians, problems with chart documentation, and other activities as they occur.

This form can be developed by reviewing the job description and creating categories for each responsibility. The employee uses the form to collect statistics regarding his or her job performance. The completed form is turned in to the supervisor. The supervisor is then able to review the employee's productivity against the job's performance standards. This information, collected on a regular basis, provides a picture of the employee's job performance for the entire review period, discussed later in the chapter. Routine collection of this information over time provides a larger picture of the employee's performance so that the evaluation is not skewed in one direction toward his or her performance over a limited time period.

### Computerized Productivity Reports

Some of the functions in the HIM department are performed in a computer system that produces a productivity report. The report is maintained by the computer system as the employee logs on to the system and completes job tasks. Some electronic reports not only tell the supervisor how much work is performed but also indicate the time frame in which the work was done. With regard to our coding example, coders are often expected to code a specific number of records within an hourly time frame (i.e., six to eight charts per hour). The software system used by the coders keeps track of productivity without additional effort from the coder. Figure 13-7 illustrates this type of productivity report.

## Employee Evaluations

Employee evaluations allow management to provide feedback to the employee on the basis of the employee's job performance. Feedback is an important aspect of a manager's communication with employees. The evaluation entails one-on-one communication from the manager about an employee's job performance. Performance standards, measures of productivity, and the job description are used as a rubric to perform the employee rating. This rating of the employee's performance is called an *evaluation*. Evaluations should be performed at the end of the probationary period and annually thereafter for each employee. Sometimes, the employee's annual evaluation is tied to a merit pay increase. The result of an evaluation can determine whether an employee receives a 1%, 2%, or 5% increase in pay, and occasionally it affects an employee's promotion. Figure 13-13 illustrates a sample evaluation form.

## HIT-bit

### EMPLOYEE EVALUATION

The employee evaluation is not the first communication that the employee receives regarding his or her job performance. Each employee is given performance expectations and performance standards when he or she receives a copy of the job description. Routine communication between the employee and the supervisor should indicate whether the employee's performance is acceptable. The employee evaluation should not be the first occasion on which an employee learns that he or she is not meeting expectations. The manager or supervisor should regularly communicate with the employees, especially when their performance is unacceptable. Poor communication by the management can negatively affect functions in the HIM department.

## FY 2013 Employee Evaluation – Criteria-Based Appraisal

**Employee Name:** Erin Rene Ory       **Position:** Emergency Department Coder

**Supervisor:** Tami JoAnne Davi       **Date:** March 23, 2013

Ratings scale to assess performance: **Exceeds (E=3 points)** – consistently performs at a level over and above standards; **Satisfies (S=2 points)** – consistently performs at the level defined by the standards; **Opportunity (O=1 point)** – generally meets more standards in the function, but needs improvement; **Unsatisfactory (U=0 points)** – Consistently performs at a level below the standards.

| Job Functions | % Weight | Rating | Score=: Weight × Rating |
|---|---|---|---|
| 1. **Job Function: Codes patient medical record information for diagnosis and procedures.**<br>• Assigns ICD-10-CM codes accurately in accordance with coding guidelines, CMS regulations, and hospital policies.<br>• Assigns CPT-4 codes accurately in accordance with coding guidelines, CMS regulations, and hospital policies.<br>• Assigns ED charges, as needed, in accordance with coding guidelines, CMS regulations, and hospital policies. | 40% | ☐ E (3)<br>☐ S (2)<br>☐ O (1)<br>☐ U (0) | 1.20 |
| 2. **Job Function: Maintains acceptable coding productivity for outpatient claims.**<br>• Codes, charges, and abstracts an average of at least 110 ED charts per day.<br>• Maintains a minimum 99% accuracy rate as determined by independent audit. | 30% | ☐ E (3)<br>☐ S (2)<br>☐ O (1)<br>☐ U (0) | 0.90 |
| 3. **Job Function: Employs full use of encoding software and abstracting system.**<br>• Uses the encoder to ensure proper coding and sequencing.<br>• Accurately abstracts all information in the abstracting system to reflect correct UB-04 data.<br>• Correctly refers to the computer system when necessary for lab results, transcription, and older claims information. | 15% | ☐ E (3)<br>☐ S (2)<br>☐ O (1)<br>☐ U (0) | 0.45 |
| 4. **Job Function: Performs other financial and compliance duties as necessary.**<br>• Assists patient financial services personnel with any claims issues to ensure that proper billing is facilitated.<br>• Works with the registration department to ensure data integrity on patient information.<br>• Complies with the standards set by department policy, CMS, and other regulatory agencies. | 5% | ☐ E (3)<br>☐ S (2)<br>☐ O (1)<br>☐ U (0) | 0.05 |
| 5. **Job Function: Continuing Education**<br>• Maintains credentials through ongoing education.<br>• If uncredentialed, seeks to obtain a coding credential, as appropriate.<br>• Attends mandatory educational sessions for coding information. | 10% | ☐ E (3)<br>☐ S (2)<br>☐ O (1)<br>☐ U (0) | 0.20 |
| | | **TOTAL** | **2.8**<br>Performance above standard |

**Figure 13-13** Sample evaluation form. CMS, Centers for Medicare and medicaid Services; CPT, Current Procedural Technology; ED, emergency department; ICD-10-CM, International Classification of Diseases, 10th Revision—Clinical Modification; UB-04, Uniform Bill.

Routine feedback to employees about their job performance improves effectiveness if there is a problem and makes the employee performance evaluation go more smoothly because the necessary information has been gathered over the entire evaluation period (i.e., over the course of an entire year). If the manager does not gather information over the course of the entire evaluation period and waits instead until the evaluation is due to complete it, the manager may be able to recall only the most recent incidents. If these are not favorable, the manager may not consider the employee's positive performance during the entire evaluation period. In other words, employees should receive regular feedback, both positive and negative, from the supervisor. These conversations should be documented for future reference. Because employees have job descriptions and understand the productivity expectations, evaluations should not be a surprise to them.

The employee evaluation should be performed in person by the employee's direct supervisor. If at all possible, the employee should sit down with his or her manager to discuss the evaluation; this is an excellent opportunity for feedback and communication. The employee evaluation is the formal summary of the employee's performance (as required in the performance standards) for the evaluation period. It is documented and maintained in the human resources department, and a copy is kept in the employee's file maintained by the HIM manager.

What occurs if the evaluation is not favorable? Is the employee immediately terminated for poor performance? Typically, an employee who has successfully completed a probationary period and later performs poorly is put on a **performance improvement plan (PIP)**. The PIP informs the employee of the poor performance and describes the consequences of not performing according to the acceptable standards. The standard disciplinary process requires counseling, a verbal warning, and then suspension. This can vary, depending on specific human resource guidelines at the organizational level or being based on union contracts. Regardless of the process, regular communication that includes both positive and negative feedback fosters an environment in which the results of an evaluation should not be a surprise to an employee.

> **performance improvement plan (PIP)** A plan to explain the required responsibilities and competencies expected of an employee's job performance.

---

**HIT-bit**

**PIP**

The acronym PIP stands for various things. For example, the CMS has a program called PIP, which stands for "periodic interim payments." PIP might also stand for "preferred Internet provider" or "performance improvement program." When using an abbreviation or acronym, be sure that you understand the meaning in the context in which it is being used.

---

## Hiring HIM Personnel

Hiring the right employee is a very important task performed by the managers and supervisors in a department. When a person is hired to perform a job, an agreement is made between the organization and the employee. The agreement is that the employee will perform the job required for compensation. Sometimes, finding the right person for the job is quite challenging. One strategy for filling positions is to hire from within—identifying an employee of the organization that may be a good fit for a new position, or even a promotion. This option promotes a positive environment in which employees can realize the benefits of their good performance, productivity, and work ethic.

### Advertisement

To locate potential candidates for a job, the organization must let others know that the position is open. An open position can be publicized in a number of ways, such as by placement of an advertisement on the organization's employment Web site, on popular recruiting Web sites, and in local newspapers, professional journals, and community and association newsletters.

The right advertisement should include all of the qualifications that a candidate should possess. The advertisement must specify how much education is required (e.g., college degree, high school degree, or equivalent) along with specific training or credentials (e.g., training in anatomy and physiology, medical terminology, or transcription). The advertisement should also specify (1) the amount of prior experience that a candidate should have, (2) whether the experience needed is specific to a job function or generally related to the HIM field, and (3) the means by which candidates should apply for the position (e.g., by sending a résumé by fax or e-mail or applying in person to the human resources department) (Figure 13-14). Other information about the position that may be included in the advertisement pertains to employment status: full-time or part-time, the hours worked per week, responsibilities, benefits, and pay scale. Interested candidates should follow the instructions in the advertisement to apply for the position.

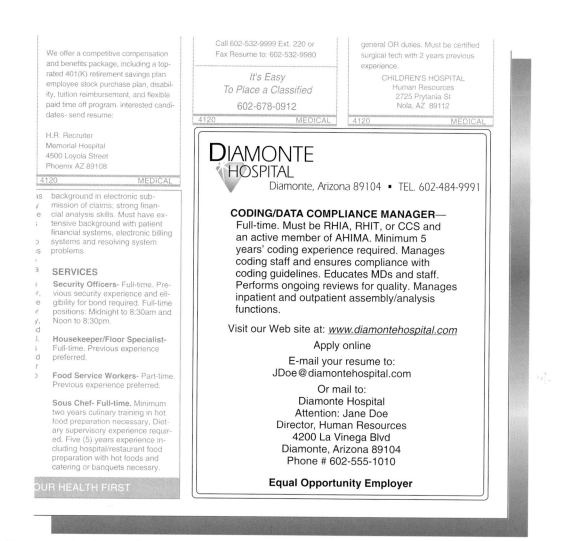

**Figure 13-14** Newspaper advertisement for health information management (HIM) personnel. AHIMA, American Health Information Management Association; CCS, Certified Coding Specialist; MDs, medical doctors; RHIA, Registered Health Information Administrator; RHIT, Registered Health Information Technician.

### ADVERTISING AND HIM ASSOCIATIONS

Many HIM positions are advertised by word of mouth. Participation in local HIM associations can put you in touch with large numbers of professionals who are potential candidates for open positions in the department. This activity is often called "networking"—getting to know other HIM professionals and sharing information, knowledge, and strategies as appropriate.

## Application

Typically, candidates must complete an application for employment to be considered for a position. Today most applications are completed on a Web site and submitted to the hiring authority electronically. All applicants must provide accurate and complete information on the application (Figure 13-15).

### CORRESPONDENCE TO APPLICANTS

Those job applicants who are screened but not interviewed, at a minimum, should receive some correspondence letting them know how their applications will be handled. The correspondence may thank candidates for the application before explaining that their qualifications did not match those of the position; in addition, it can inform them that their applications will be kept on file for a specific period in case any future openings occur.

The manager uses the applications to determine which candidates meet the minimum qualifications of the job to receive an interview. Qualifications include the type of education, training, and experience required to perform the job duties. An applicant should expect that inconsistent, vague, or incomplete information on any part of the application may require further explanation during the interview. Therefore, when reviewing applications, the hiring authority looks to see that each question on the application is answered. The candidate should not leave any spaces blank, even if he or she believes that the information is covered on the résumé and attached to the application. Inconsistencies on an application are a "red flag" to the manager that the candidate is not honest. References should be current and appropriate, because employers will check the references before making a final hiring decision.

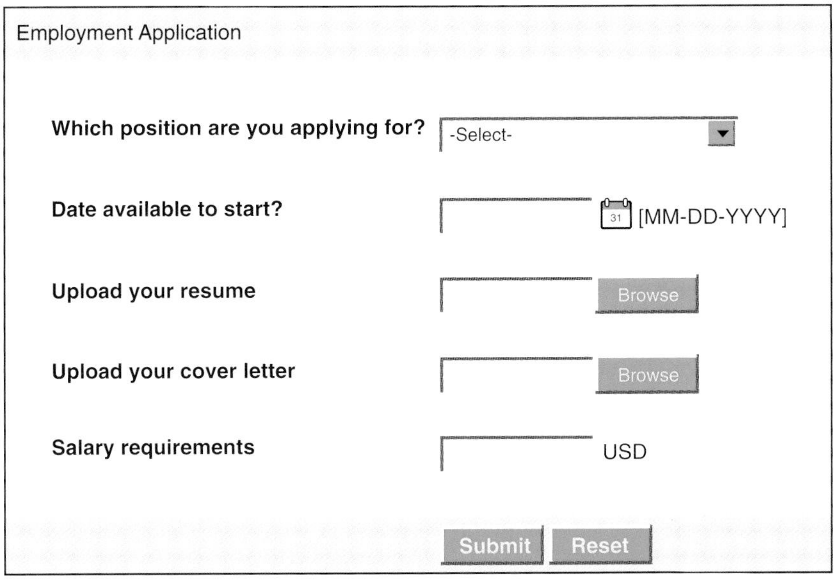

Figure 13-15 Sample of online submission of resume and cover letter.

**HIT-bit**

**SUBMITTING ELECTRONIC APPLICATIONS**

Electronic applications must be completed carefully. Be sure to complete each portion or field in the application accurately. Read all of the instructions carefully before finishing the application and "hitting" the submit button!

Electronic applications typically offer the opportunity to attach a copy of your résumé, letters of reference, and other transcripts, certificates, or supporting documents. It is a best practice to convert documents into a pdf file so that they can be opened by the hiring personnel for review—that way they can read the documents regardless of the software suite they use.

### Interviewing

The interview is typically a face-to-face meeting between the applicant and the organization's representative. Each organization has a specific process for performing an interview. Sometimes, the applicant is interviewed over the phone or with the human resources department before meeting with the HIM department manager. Other organizations perform a group interview, in which the applicant meets with several different members of the organization at the same time. For the applicant, the interview is an opportunity to learn about the organization and the responsibilities of the position. For the organization, the interview is a way to assess the candidate's qualifications for the position. Interviews may be very formal and structured, informal, or somewhere in between. The interviewer should plan ahead, determine an appropriate location, decide on the style, and write down the questions he or she wants to ask.

All interviews begin with a greeting between the candidate and the interviewer. Experienced interviewers can tell a lot about a candidate within these first few moments. Therefore the interviewer must be prepared and must pay close attention to the responses given by the interviewee.

During the interview in the HIM department, the manager describes the position to the candidate, explaining expectations, requirements, environment, and philosophy of the organization or management style. The manager also asks questions to obtain further information about the candidate's qualifications. This exchange gives the candidate and the manager more information with which to develop an opinion about the candidate's suitability for the position. The interview is the opportunity to find out whether the candidate is appropriate for the job and a good fit for the department. Box 13-2 provides a list of the questions often asked during an interview. The same questions are used for each person interviewed for the position.

In the United States, a series of federal laws enacted since the 1960s govern job discrimination (Table 13-7). Known collectively as Equal Employment Opportunity (EEO) laws,

---

**BOX 13-2   INTERVIEW QUESTIONS**

- Tell me a little bit about yourself.
- Describe your last job. What did you like or dislike about the job?
- What expectations do you have for your supervisor?
- Describe your relationship with your former supervisor.
- Explain a stressful situation and how you handled it.
- What is the one word that best describes you? Which of your strengths best suit you for this job?
- Which of your weaknesses may cause a problem for you in this job?
- Do you have any future education goals?
- Where do you see yourself in 5 or 10 years?
- Are you available to work weekends, evenings, or some holidays?

**TABLE 13-7**

**EMPLOYMENT LAWS**

| LAW | AREA OF CONCERN |
|---|---|
| Age Discrimination in Employment Act (1967) | Protects employees between the ages of 40 and 70 years |
| Americans with Disabilities Act (ADA) (1990) | Outlaws discrimination against disabled people and ensures reasonable accommodation for them in the workplace |
| Title VII of the Civil Rights Act (1964) | Prohibits discrimination on the basis of race, color, religion, sex, or national origin and ensures equal employment opportunity |
| The Pregnancy Discrimination Act (1978) | Amended to Title VII, this law makes it illegal to discriminate against a woman because of pregnancy, childbirth, or related medical complications |
| Fair Labor Standards Act (1938) | Sets minimum wage, overtime pay, equal pay, child labor, and record-keeping requirements for employers (Equal Pay Amendment [1963] forbids sex discrimination in pay practices) |
| Family Medical Leave Act (1993) | Grants unpaid leave and provides job security to employees who must take time off for medical reasons for themselves or family members |
| Genetic Information Nondiscrimination Act (GINA) (2008) | Makes it illegal to discriminate against employees or applicants on the basis of genetic information, including genetic tests of an individual or his/her family, as well as any disease, disorder, or condition |

Modified from U.S. Equal Employment Opportunity Commission: Laws Enforced by EEOC. www.eeoc.gov/laws/statutes/index.cfm. Accessed November 15, 2012.

they prohibit employment discrimination based on age, gender, race, color, religious beliefs, nation of origin, disabilities, genetics, and plans to marry or have children. Interviewers must consider carefully whether their inquiry is relevant to the applicant's capacity to perform the job. Table 13-8 lists some examples of questions that may be discriminatory. Fair employment practices are discussed in more detail later.

## HIT-bit

**THE HANDSHAKE**

The handshake is often part of an introduction. The manner in which you participate in the handshake will make an impression on the other party. A good handshake is assertive and has a firm grip. Try out your handshake on a classmate.

### Assessment

Although the questions asked in an interview are necessary and inform a manager about a candidate's ability and knowledge, it is often necessary to test the candidate's skills. The interviewer must determine whether the candidate is competent to perform the job. For example, if the manager wants to hire a skilled coder, he or she should give an assessment to each candidate that resembles actual coding work to determine whether the candidate is capable of performing the work required for this job. Health care workers are also required to pass a criminal background check and drug tests before being formally offered a position with the organization.

There are at least two different types of applicant assessments—one for skills and the other for aptitude. A skills assessment is designed to identify the applicant's ability to perform the job. The aptitude assessment evaluates the applicant's inclination, intelligence, or appropriateness for a position and the likelihood of his or her fitting into a particular

**TABLE 13-8**

**INTERVIEW GUIDELINES***

| CATEGORY | MAY ASK | MAY BE DISCRIMINATORY BY ASKING |
|---|---|---|
| Gender and family | Whether applicant has relatives who work for the health care facility | Gender of applicant<br>Number of children/childcare arrangements<br>Marital status/living situation<br>Spouse's name or occupation<br>Plans to have children<br>Any question that could determine gender or family status |
| Race | – | Applicant's race or color of skin, hair, or eyes<br>Request for a photo before hire |
| National origin or ancestry | Whether applicant can be legally employed in the U.S.<br>Ability to speak/write English (if job related)<br>Other languages spoken (if job-related) | Nationality/ethnicity of name<br>Birthplace, or birthplace of applicant's parents<br>Nationality<br>Nationality of spouse<br>Country of citizenship<br>Applicant's native language/English proficiency<br>Maiden name |
| Religion | – | Religious affiliation/church or services the applicant attends<br>Religious holidays observed |
| Age | Whether applicant is over age 18<br>Whether applicant is over age 21 if job-related | Date of birth<br>Date of graduation<br>Age<br>Length of time until applicant plans to retire |
| Disability | Whether applicant can perform the essential job-related functions[†] | Any question about an applicant's mental or physical disability, including its nature or severity<br>Whether applicant has ever filed a workers' compensation claim<br>Current, recent, or past diseases, treatments, or surgeries |
| Other | Academic, vocational, or professional schooling<br>Training received in the military<br>Membership in any trade or professional association<br>Job references | Number and kinds of arrests<br>Height or weight<br>Veteran status, discharge status, branch of service |

*The goal of the interview is to determine the applicant's qualifications for the position. Interviewers must avoid any inquiry that may be discriminatory. This table lists common examples, but it is not comprehensive. Consult the organization's human resources department for guidance on the interview process.
[†]The physical requirements essential to the performance of the position are included in the job description. The ADA requires employers to make reasonable accommodations to qualified individuals with disabilities, unless those accommodations cause undue hardship to the employer. Refer to http://www.eeoc.gov/policy/docs/accommodation.html#reasonable for more information.

organization or position. The assessment is typically a test given during the interview. Some tests are lengthy. Skills assessments should include activities that the applicant would encounter on the job; for instance, if the position is for outpatient coding, have the applicant code some of the emergency room or outpatient records. It is not fair practice to assess an applicant with a test that is different from the actual work that he or she will be expected to perform. HIM managers should always test the coding skills of an applicant for a coding position and test the keyboarding/typing and terminology skills for a transcription position. There are different screening practices for clerical positions, such as testing filing skills for a file clerk.

### Outsourcing

It is increasingly common for HIM departments to outsource functions performed within the HIM department. To outsource means to hire a vendor or consultant from outside of

**outsourcing** Services that are provided by external organizations or individuals who are not employees of the facility for which the services are being provided.

the facility to perform the HIM function; another term for this practice may be to contract out the function. For example, many facilities use contract coders when they have a backlog or need temporary help during an employee's vacation or sick leave. However, some facilities permanently outsource these functions—meaning that a facility signs a contract for a period with a company who will perform the function and bill the facility for the services. Another HIM function that is commonly outsourced is ROI. HIM departments use a contract service to perform this very important and specialized function on a full-time basis for a specific contract period. The advantage for the facility is the shift of employee management responsibility to the company/consultant. The facility must be careful to hire a reputable company/consultant and to monitor the outsourced work just as they would that of an onsite employee. Even though a contract exists, the facility remains responsible for the overall quality and integrity of the HIM department.

**ROI** release of information

### Fair Employment Practices

It is extremely important that HIM managers and supervisors comply with appropriate and legal hiring practices. Over many years the United States has passed a number of laws pertaining to age, gender, race, religion, and disability that affect hiring practices, outlined in Table 13-7. The U. S. Equal Opportunity Commission (EEOC) is the federal agency charged with enforcing these laws, which apply not only to discrimination in hiring and firing, but also regarding fair compensation and harassment (EEOC, 2012a).

Employers must be certain that their hiring practices do not discriminate among candidates. Additionally, employers must be sure that all employees are managed in an appropriate, law-abiding manner. The Americans with Disabilities Act (ADA), passed into law in 1990, makes it illegal for any employer to discriminate against a person qualified to perform a job on the basis of his or her disability. Under this legislation, as long as a disabled individual has the necessary background, experience, and skill set and is able to perform the "tasks that are essential to the job, with or without reasonable accommodation," he or she may not be discriminated against in any employment practice (EEOC, 2012b). For this reason HIM managers must be sure to consider this law when writing job descriptions and must include the necessary physical requirements of the job.

Employers are allowed to hold their employees to certain standards; for example, the law allows health care employers to perform a drug screen before making a job offer. An employee working under the influence of certain substances does not have the ability to provide high-quality health care and would expose the employer to liability. Department standards, however, must not contradict the law at any level—local, state, or federal.

### EXERCISE 13-7

#### Personnel

1. A formal list of the employee's responsibilities associated with their job is called a _____.
2. _____ are set guidelines explaining how much work an employee must complete.
3. A _____ involves the review of a function to determine all of the tasks or components that make up an employee's job.
4. Performance standards measure:
   a. quantity.
   b. quality.
   c. both a and b.
   d. the number of employees.
5. The job description must contain information about the work environment and the necessary skills and abilities that the employee must have to complete the job. These statements are known as the:
   a. salary information.
   b. OSHA requirements.
   c. ADA information.
   d. performance standards.
6. The _____ is an opportunity for management to provide feedback to the employee on the basis of the employee's performance.

7. Explain the best method of delivering an employee evaluation.
8. Identify some HIM functions that may be outsourced.
9. Which of the following Fair Employment Laws prohibit discrimination based on race, color, religion, or sex?
   a. Fair Labor Standards Act
   b. Civil Rights Act
   c. Americans with Disabilities Act
   d. Age Discrimination in Employment Act
10. Which of the following Fair Employment Laws sets minimum wage, overtime pay, and equal pay?
    a. Fair Labor Standards Act
    b. Civil Rights Act
    c. Americans with Disabilities Act
    d. Age Discrimination in Employment Act
11. Which of the following Fair Employment Laws prohibits discrimination of handicapped people and ensures reasonable accommodation for them in the workplace?
    a. Fair Labor Standards Act
    b. Civil Rights Act
    c. Americans with Disabilities Act
    d. Age Discrimination in Employment Act

## DEPARTMENT EQUIPMENT AND SUPPLIES

The equipment most often recognized in an HIM department includes employee workstations' computers, scanners, printers, filing mechanisms, copiers, fax machines, and telephones. Old, faulty equipment can have a negative impact on the productivity of an employee, which ultimately affects the entire department. Once an employee has notified the manager of an equipment problem, the manager should begin the maintenance process in a timely manner.

Reference material is another necessary tool for any department providing coding and transcription services. Reference material is used to look up information for clarification or knowledge; *Dorland's Medical Dictionary* and the *Physicians' Desk Reference*, for looking up drugs, are a few common ones. The references can be viewed electronically and accessible to all appropriate employees. Reference materials should be updated routinely to ensure access to current information. Table 13-9 provides a list of suggested reference

**TABLE 13-9**

**SUGGESTED REFERENCE MATERIALS FOR THE HIM DEPARTMENT**

| REFERENCE | UPDATES | WHO NEEDS THIS REFERENCE MATERIAL? |
|---|---|---|
| *Physician's Desk Reference* (PDR) | Published annually | One copy each for transcription and coding functions |
| Medical dictionary | Updated occasionally | One copy each for transcription and coding functions |
| Human disease reference | — | Coding function |
| Specialized word books (e.g., surgical word book, drug book, abbreviation book) | — | Transcription function |
| International Classification of Diseases, Tenth Revision—Clinical Modification (ICD-10-CM) coding book | Updated annually October 1 | Coding function must have current codes as of October 1 each year |
| *Coding Clinic for ICD-10-CM* | Quarterly newsletter published by AHA | Coding function: provides knowledge and advice on implementation of ICD-10-CM coding guidelines |
| Healthcare Common Procedure Coding System (HCPCS) | Updated annually by CMS | Coding function and the person responsible for the maintenance of the facility |
| Current Procedural Terminology (CPT) | Updated annually | Coding function: necessary for outpatient services and physician's office to have current codes |
| *CPT Assistant* | Monthly newsletter published by AHA | Coding function: provides examples, explanation, and scenarios for implementation of CPT coding |

materials for these areas. Other tools and equipment (e.g., pens, paper, toner, file folders, envelopes, and labels) need to be appropriately maintained and on hand so that employees can effectively perform their jobs. This includes necessary equipment and supplies for contract employees and those employees who work for the facility from their homes.

## Supplies

The manager should ensure that the supply of each stocked item is adequate. A lack of supplies can limit productivity. Running out of copy paper delays printing paper copies of records, reports (delaying patient care), or insurance requests for timely payment. Orders for additional supplies should be placed in a timely manner to prevent delay, and the manager must stay within the budget for supplies.

### Filing

A significant number of supplies are associated with filing, such as folders, color-coded labels, and year-band labels. File folders are typically ordered annually; therefore the manager must consider how many folders will be used every year before purchasing the items. The manager must remember to account for each type of patient that will require a folder—inpatient, outpatient, patients in for observation, and newborns. Of course, the number of folders needed depends on the filing system used, whether serial, unit, or serial-unit. In the unit numbering system, the patient uses the same number for all visits; therefore one folder could conceivably store data for more than one discharge. However, for serial and serial-unit numbering systems, each patient needs a new folder. To simplify matters, one can assume that each discharge requires a new folder. The number of discharges for the year should almost equal the number of folders used; the manager should order enough extra folders to allow for errors, mistakes, repair of torn folders, and other unforeseen events. Also, he or she should be sure to order sufficient quantities of year-band labels and number labels (see Chapter 9).

### Copy Machines, Scanners, and Printers

HIM departments rely on copy machines and printers for many different tasks. Today copy machines can make a paper copy, or scan a document into a digital file, such as a portable document format (pdf) file, and e-mail. HIM personnel use these machines to make traditional paper copies of information, release information to third parties, transfer patient information to a new facility or health care provider, and provide reports as requested by other departments. Scanners are necessary in departments that use document imaging, as discussed in Chapter 9. Copy machines require an adequate supply of paper and toner. Additionally, the department should have a maintenance agreement for each machine so that it can be serviced routinely. Printers also require paper, as well as ink, which comes in the form of cartridges. Managers must keep a sufficient supply of cartridges on hand so that the department is able to operate efficiently. A good way to stock this supply is always to have one extra ink or toner cartridge for every two printers so that a replacement is always available.

**Go To** Chapter 9 details document imaging as a health record storage method.

**document imaging** Scanning or faxing printed papers into a computer system or optical disk system. See also *computer output to laser disk (COLD)*.

### HIT-bit

#### MAINTENANCE CONTRACTS

Equipment such as computers, copiers, and transcription and dictation devices is typically purchased with a maintenance contract option. It is important for managers to update these items and budget for them annually. The maintenance contract provides for repair, assistance, and sometimes replacement of certain equipment. The contract option can usually be purchased at minimal cost for maintenance coverage from Monday through Friday, 9 AM to 5 PM, or for the first 90 days. For a higher fee, the contract may cover the equipment 24 hours per day, 7 days per week, including holidays.

**master patient index (MPI)** A system containing a list of patients who have received care at the health care facility and their encounter information, often used to correlate the patient with the file identification.

**chart locator system** A system for locating records within a facility.

**grouper** The software used to derive the diagnosis related group from the ICD-10-CM diagnoses and procedures.

**reimbursement** The amount of money that the health care facility receives from the party responsible for paying the bill.

**ROI** release of information

### Transcription and Dictation Equipment

Transcription and dictation equipment is important in the communication of patient health information. The dictation equipment is used by the health care professional to record the patient's health information. The transcription equipment is the machine used by the transcriptionist to listen to and type the dictated reports (which may be the computer in newer digital systems), the foot pedal, and the headset. Transcriptionists use the dictation system to retrieve the recorded voice. They then listen to the voice to type the report. This equipment should have a maintenance agreement, preferably one that ensures 24-hour, 7-day-per-week coverage.

### Software and Hardware

Many of the operations in the HIM department require the use of computer software. Typical software in a HIM department includes the master patient index (MPI), chart locator system, ROI tracking software, electronic birth certificate software, and encoders and groupers for coding. This software is critical to the operation of the department. For example, annual updates to coding software are essential to the reimbursement and proper classification of health information. Software that is not updated in these areas will cause bills to be rejected, delaying payment to the facility. Therefore each software system should be maintained in an appropriate environment, on computer equipment sufficient to support the applications, with adequate maintenance contracts for upgrades and support.

---

**HIT-bit**

**UPGRADE**

An *upgrade*, in software terminology, refers to a new version of software that is improved in some way.

---

### Miscellaneous Supplies

The manager must remember to coordinate appropriate ordering practices for even routine supplies, such as pencils, pens, paper, and flags for analysis. An inadequate supply of these critical tools may cause unnecessary delays in the processing of health information.

## Monitoring Use of Department Resources

HIM department managers must carefully monitor the equipment and supplies so that workflow is not affected. Poor equipment management—whether in buying new equipment, maintaining existing equipment, or converting from one system to another—can negatively affect productivity in the department. It is important to maintain adequate supplies for the employee workforce (onsite, contracted, and at home); important supplies include files, labels, printer or copier paper, and toner or ink cartridges. Minor oversights in department equipment and supplies can cause the workflow to backlog, which negatively affects employee performance and sometimes even department budgets.

## Ergonomics

**ergonomics** Alignment of the work environment to accommodate the employee's job function.

**Ergonomics** is the science of suiting the work environment to the worker. The work environment should be comfortable, allowing the employee to perform the job as necessary, free from injury or harm. Ergonomics is sometimes thought of as proper body positioning of the employee at his or her desk (Figure 13-16). However, the desk and chair are not the

# ANATOMY OF AN ERGONOMIC WORK STATION

## WORKPLACE ENVIRONMENT
- Most important consideration is working comfortably and efficiently
- Sufficient desk area for keyboard, monitor, mouse, document holder, telephone, etc.
- Organize the area so that it reflects the way you use equipment
- Things you use most often should be within easiest reach
- Vary your tasks
- Take frequent breaks
- If area is shared, be sure all who use it can adjust everything to their needs
- Document holders same height and distance from monitor
- Adequate leg room
- Unobscured line of sight

## Avoid:

### Awkward posture
Can include reaching behind, twisting, working overhead, kneeling, bending, and squatting. Deviation from ideal working posture can lead to fatigue, muscle tension, and headaches.
**Correct working posture** – arms at sides, elbows bent approximately 90 degrees, forearms parallel to floor, wrists straight.

### Repetitiveness
Judgment is based on frequency, speed, number of muscle groups used, and required force. Not all people react to the same conditions, so carefully monitor your personal physical response to repetitiveness.

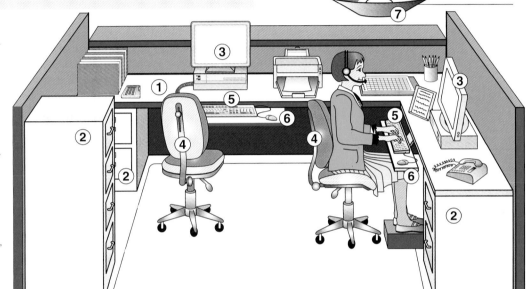

## (1) WORK SURFACE
- Proper height and angle
- Neutral postures
- Adjustable
- Standing—prevent slipping, adequate traction
- Sit/stand tools
- Antifatigue floor mats
- Darker, matte finishes are best

## (2) STORAGE AREAS
- Good body positions
- Reduce muscular forces
- Avoid excessive reach
- Heavy items between knee and shoulder height
- Frequently used storage closest to worker

## (3) VIDEO DISPLAY TERMINAL (VDT) [MONITOR]
- Position to minimize glare and reflections
- Top of screen is slightly below eye level
- Tilted slightly backward (less than 15 degrees)
- Distance from display 18–30 inches
- Perpendicular to windows
- Keep your head upright
- Set contrast and brightness
- Clean the screen (and your glasses)
- Antiglare filters
- Adjustable monitor arm

## (4) CHAIRS
- Comfortable (padded seats that swivel)
- Back and seat are adjustable while seated
- Provide good back support (can add additional cushion if necessary)
- Adjustable arm support
- Back straight
- Knees slightly higher than chair bottom
- Thighs horizontal
- Feet flat on the floor (use a footrest if necessary)
- Change positions occasionally

## (5) KEYBOARD
- Back should be lower than front
- Rounded edges
- Wrist rests (sharp edges, neutral position) same height as front of keyboard
- Type properly: don't force your fingers to stretch to incorrect keystrokes

## (6) MOUSE
- Keep it on the same level as the keyboard or slightly above
- Keep wrist straight
- Do not stretch your arm; keep mouse within immediate reach
- Use the whole arm to move the mouse ... not just the forearm

## (7) LIGHTING
- Less illumination for computer work
- Indirect lighting is best

**Figure 13-16** Ergonomic environment of a health information management department. (Redrawn from Gaylor LJ: The administrative dental assistant, ed 3, Philadelphia, 2011, Saunders, pp 198-199.)

only office equipment that can be adjusted to keep employees free from injury or harm. Other ergonomic issues involve lighting, appropriate climate, and the frequency and duration of rest breaks. Because many HIM functions are performed at a computer terminal or desk, appropriate coordination of employees with their workstations is required. Significant time spent in a harmful work environment can compromise employees' health, costing the facility valuable assets when workers' compensation claims are filed.

---

### HIT-bit

#### WORKERS' COMPENSATION

Workers' compensation is the benefit that pays an employee for time away from the workplace because of a work-related injury.

---

Areas in the HIM department that require significant ergonomic consideration are the transcription stations, coding workstations, and all computer terminals. The height of the chair in relation to the desk or workstation must be adjusted correctly to fit each employee, and the general office space should be configured to promote efficient workflow. The lighting, air conditioning, and heating should also be appropriate. The environment must provide safe and appropriate working conditions. For example, if the employee spends a significant amount of time reading, the lighting should be adjusted accordingly. If the employee spends most of the day facing a computer screen, dim or indirect lighting may better protect the employee's eyesight.

### EXERCISE 13-8

#### Department Equipment and Supplies

1. Which type of filing system requires more file folders: unit numbering or serial numbering?
2. It is the responsibility of the employer to provide a safe work environment for the employee to perform his or her job function. One way that this can be accomplished is through design of a(n) _____ work space.
3. It is the responsibility of the employer to provide a safe work environment for the employee to perform his or her job function. One way that this can be accomplished is through design of a(n) _____ work space.

## WORKS CITED

United States Department of Labor, Office of the Assistant Secretary for Policy: elaws—Fair Labor Standards Act Advisor. http://www.dol.gov/elaws/esa/flsa/screen75.asp. Accessed February 22, 2012.

United States Equal Opportunity Commission (EEOC): About EEOC. http://www.eeoc.gov/eeoc/. Accessed February 22, 2012a.

United States Equal Opportunity Commission: The ADA: Your Responsibilities as an Employer. http://www.eeoc.gov/facts/ada17.html. Accessed 22 February 22, 2012b.

## SUGGESTED READING

Burns L, Bradley E, Weiner B: Shortell and Kaluzny's Healthcare management: organization design and behavior, ed 6, Albany, NY, 2011, Delmar Cengage Learning.

## CHAPTER ACTIVITIES

### CHAPTER SUMMARY

The management of health information includes the management of the people performing HIM functions. Appropriate organization and management of the department's human resources significantly affects the quality of health information. A great place to begin effective management is in the clear communication of the employee's responsibilities in the job description and the performance standards for the position.

HIM supervisors and managers are responsible for the daily operations of the HIM department as well as future planning in keeping with the facility's mission and vision. Establishing mechanisms to monitor the quality and productivity of HIM functions keep the daily operations on track. To guide the department into the future, HIM managers must plan, set goals and objectives, and navigate the transition to the EHR. The system development life cycle—selection, design, implementation, evaluation, and support—of the EHR, transition to ICD-10, or any major changes in software products will certainly capitalize the time and attention of HIM managers. Therefore knowledge of health information, combined with management skills, sets the stage for continuous efficient and effective management of HIM departments.

## REVIEW QUESTIONS

1. How can the human resource department assist the HIM department managers/ supervisors?
2. Explain the purpose of an organization chart.
3. Explain the difference between unity of command and span of control.
4. Identify some of the considerations that will affect the priority for workflow in the HIM department.
5. Explain one method of determining productivity standards for HIM functions.
6. List the HIM functions in a paper processing department and compare them with the functions required for processing in an EHR environment.
7. List three circumstances that will require planning in the HIM department.
8. List and briefly explain the steps in the system development life cycle.
9. Explain the importance of a job description.
10. What is the purpose of performance standards?
11. List and describe some of the equipment and supplies necessary in the HIM department.
12. Identify some of the issues that must be considered in the design of an ergonomic workstation.
13. Explain the importance of having maintenance agreements or service contracts on HIM department equipment.

## PROFESSIONAL PROFILE

### Health Information Management Director

My name is Beth Catherine, and I am the director of the health information management department at Diamonte.

My responsibilities include overseeing the operations of the department and planning and organizing the direction of health information operations. I attend several meetings each week. I am a member of the quality management committee and the risk management committee. I am also the coordinator for the health information management committee. As coordinator, I work closely with the chairman of the committee, a member of the medical staff, to organize the meetings, coordinate record reviews, and compile minutes of the meetings.

I also attend a monthly meeting with all the department directors, at which we share important information about our department operations, perform facility-wide strategic planning, and receive communication from administration.

Once a month, I hold a department meeting for all HIM employees. During the meeting, we discuss department business and quality, and employees receive updates about various things that are occurring throughout the facility.

My education began at a community college where I earned an associate degree in Health Information Technology. The program was accredited by CAHIIM so I was able to sit for the RHIT exam, which I passed successfully on my first attempt. My current employer quickly realized I was a likely candidate to replace our long-time

### ⊙ CAREER TIP

Depending on state licensure regulations and the regional marketplace, the requirements for an HIM department director vary. In general, a minimum of a bachelor's degree is necessary and a master's degree is preferred. HIM professionals with an associate degree may want to expand their skill set to obtain a bachelor's degree in business administration or computer science. HIM professionals with a bachelor's degree may choose a master's degree in business administration, public administration, health administration, information systems, or health informatics, for example. It is important to obtain experience in an HIM department. Networking with HIM professionals at professional association meetings is helpful in obtaining an understanding of the marketplace and identifying opportunities early.

director, who was ready for retirement. I returned to school online to receive my bachelor's degree in Health Information Management. After I obtained my degree, things moved faster than I expected; our HIM director retired and I was promoted to Director while working with a consultant for an interim period to make sure I was comfortable handling the department.

I really enjoy my job. Every day is a new challenge—sometimes from administration, physicians, or employees; at other times, accreditation or federal government requirements present a challenge. Working as a team, we always manage to reach our goals.

## PATIENT CARE PERSPECTIVE

### Dr. Lewis's Other Partner, Dr. Simowitz

I am a consultant with privileges at four different hospitals. Between office hours and visiting inpatients for consultations, I have very little time left in the day to make my way to the HIM department to complete my records. It seemed to me that I was constantly in imminent danger of being suspended and was receiving warning notices almost daily. I complained to Beth that I signed my dictations electronically on a regular basis, so why was I having problems? She explained that I wasn't always signing my progress notes and I gave too many telephone orders, which also had to be signed. I agreed to be more careful in the future with the progress notes but the telephone orders are problematic. Since I often don't see those patients a second time, I don't notice that the orders aren't signed. Beth worked with me to identify a day and time when I would regularly be in the hospital and her staff would bring outstanding records to me on the nursing unit so that I could finish them in a timely manner. I'm not the only physician with this problem, so Beth is meeting with nursing leadership to develop and implement a process for helping physicians complete their charts while their patients are still in the hospital.

## APPLICATION

### Hiring a Coder

You recently lost a coder at your facility. The department director has asked that you, the coding supervisor, create an advertisement for the local newspaper and participate in the interview for this vacant position. Using your knowledge of hiring practices, create an advertisement for this new position.

Before the interview, document at least three questions that you would like to ask the applicant. Be sure to check the list of appropriate interview questions (see Box 13-2).

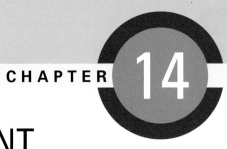

CHAPTER 14

# TRAINING AND DEVELOPMENT

Melissa LaCour

## CHAPTER OUTLINE

## VOCABULARY

agenda
continuing education (CE)
credentials

cross-training
inservice

memorandum (memo)
minutes

orientation
training

## CHAPTER OBJECTIVES

*By the end of this chapter, the students should be able to:*

1. Orient a new employee to the department and his or her job function.
2. Train an employee on a new job procedure.
3. Assess the training needs for the HIM department.
4. Prepare a development plan for HIM staff.
5. Identify inservice topics for HIM department personnel.
6. Create a presentation on an inservice topic.

7. Identify continuing education needs for HIM employees.
8. Document minutes from an inservice, a continuing education session, or a department meeting.
9. Organize an agenda for HIM department meetings.
10. Identify key aspects of effective communication.
11. Identify key qualities of effective leadership.

A well-managed health information management (HIM) department spends considerable time on the training and development of its employees. Training involves orientation, education, and practical application for a specific HIM job position. *Development* is the ongoing improvement of staff professionally. The HIM director is responsible for the hiring, training, development, and retention of employees who perform all department functions. Training is essential to the HIM department; well-trained employees provide high-quality service. Training is necessary at many times: at the beginning of employment, as procedures and policies change and processes are improved, and as technology and equipment are improved. Development is equally important because it improves the quality of service. A department that develops its employees is making an investment in the quality of its future service.

The previous chapter discusses setting standards for job responsibilities, hiring the right candidate, and monitoring performance. In this chapter, we emphasize training and developing employees to be assets in the HIM department.

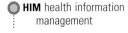
**HIM** health information management

**459**

## ORIENTATION

**orientation** Training to familiarize a new employee with the job.

When he or she begins a job at a health care facility, it is very important for an employee to learn about the environment and the new job, so an orientation is essential for employee success. The purpose of **orientation** is to make the employee familiar with the surroundings. Some facilities hold organization-wide orientations weekly, which are followed by second orientations specific to an employee's job within the department, led by his or her direct supervisor. The organization-wide orientation is general and introduces the employee to the organization, its corporate structure, along with regulations, policies, and procedures that are required of all employees.

### Organization-Wide Orientation

**mission statement** The strategic purpose of the organization documented in a formal statement.

**vision** The goal of the organization, above and beyond the mission.

**Health Insurance Portability and Accountability Act (HIPAA)** Public Law 104-191, federal legislation passed in 1996 that outlines the guidelines of managing patient information in terms of privacy, security, and confidentiality. The legislation also outlines penalties for noncompliance.

Typically, before new employees report to their departments, they attend an organization-wide orientation in which they learn about the organization, mission, vision, or values and have an opportunity to ask questions regarding employment. In most cases, an organization orientation includes the organization chart for the entire facility and the following topics:
- Personnel considerations
- Customer service expectations
- Quality
- Building safety and security
- Infection control
- Body mechanics
- Confidentiality/HIPAA
- Information systems
- Tour of the facility

Other topics may include incident reporting, compliance, and the phone and e-mail systems. This orientation should take place before employees begin their job activities; however, because these orientations are sometimes offered only once a month, employees may actually begin work before their organization orientation. It is important that all employees receive orientation, including those employees who work from home.

**compliance** Meeting standards. Also the development, implementation, and enforcement of policies and procedures that ensure that standards are met.

#### Personnel Considerations

Some of the first materials that employees receive during the orientation explain the benefits to which they are entitled as employees of the organization. During this part of the orientation, employees complete necessary forms for income tax purposes and learn about enrollment in other special savings plans, insurance, or retirement accounts. Because compensation for the job is important, orientation is an opportunity to ask about pay periods, proper completion of payroll forms, and use of the time clock. Employees are also informed of health care facility policies and procedures that affect their employment, and they must receive a copy of the employee handbook. Information in the employee handbook includes facility dress code, attendance policy, hours earned for vacation and sick leave (paid time off, or PTO), grievance procedures, and holidays.

**PTO** paid time off

#### Customer Service

During the initial orientation, the new employee learns about the organization's expectations in relation to all customers. Customer service is an important part of health care, and many facilities use this orientation as an opportunity to inspire a positive customer focus in all employees. Employees are encouraged to:
1. Identify all of their customers by name.
2. Greet each customer with a smile.
3. Provide assistance or find someone who can assist the customer.
4. Follow up on a customer's request.

Employees may have an opportunity to participate in a role-playing exercise in which they learn how to deal with a disgruntled customer.

## Quality

As discussed in Chapter 11, quality is critical to all aspects of health care. Because of its importance, employees are informed about the expectations and methods that the organization uses to ensure quality. The orientation should introduce the employee to the performance improvement (PI) method used by the organization. New employees learn that everyone in the facility is responsible for quality. As appropriate, employees are encouraged to identify and report opportunities to improve quality.

## Building Safety and Security

The health care environment should be safe for patients, visitors, and employees. Safety issues are covered in the organization orientation to make the employee aware of the policy and procedures for maintaining a secure environment and for handling situations in the event of an emergency (i.e., the disaster plan). Two commonly discussed topics are fire safety and response to "code" emergencies. A common fire response uses the acronym RACE—rescue, alarm, confine, and extinguish. Every employee learns to rescue patients, employees, or visitors from the area of the fire. He or she should go to the closest fire alarm and inform the operator of his or her name and the location and status of the fire. Then the employee should confine the fire by closing all doors in the area. If possible, he or she should extinguish the fire with a fire extinguisher or other appropriate device.

> **performance improvement (PI)** Also known as *quality improvement (QI)* or *continuous quality improvement (CQI)*. Refers to the process by which a facility reviews its services or products to ensure quality.
>
> **Go To** Review the HIM department's role in monitoring and improving quality in Chapter 11.
>
> **RACE** rescue, alarm, confine, extinguish

### HIT-bit

#### CUSTOMER SATISFACTION SURVEY

Many organizations use a customer satisfaction survey to measure their service to customers. The results are used to improve the quality of customer service, and when the survey results are overwhelmingly favorable, the organization can use them in marketing efforts.

During a visit to a health care facility, you may have heard the operator announce a "code" over the intercom system. Common codes are "code blue" for cardiac arrest and "code red" for fire. These codes alert the employees to an emergency that is occurring in the facility (Table 14-1). These codes may also be announced as fictitious physician names (e.g., Dr. Red instead of "code red," or Dr. Strong for "security"). All employees must recognize the codes in the facility and know their roles in the response to the emergency.

## Infection Control

By nature of the job environment, health care workers may be exposed to a number of infectious agents. For this reason, several significant issues are covered under the topic of infection control, including hepatitis, acquired immunodeficiency syndrome, and universal

### TABLE 14-1

#### SAMPLE EMERGENCY CODES

| CODE | EMERGENCY |
|---|---|
| Dr. Strong | Security requested in a specific area of the facility |
| Black | Bomb threat |
| Red | Fire |
| Orange | Radiation disaster |
| Pink | Infant abduction |
| Blue | Cardiac arrest |
| Yellow | External disaster |

precautions for blood and body fluids. During this part of the orientation, new employees learn how to protect themselves and others from infection; the discussion provides information about how these infections are spread and then shares procedures that help protect employees.

In a discussion about universal precautions for blood and body fluids, employees are informed that one of the best and easiest methods to prevent the spread of infection is by washing their hands. Employees are encouraged always to wash their hands before and after having contact with a patient, eating, and using the restroom. Universal precautions also include wearing masks and gloves when interacting with potentially infectious material and properly discarding needles and other contaminated objects.

Because some blood-borne organisms can survive for days outside the body, health care workers are advised to exercise caution when handling items contaminated with body fluids. For example, a paper record contaminated with blood should be filed in a sealed plastic sheet protector.

---

### HIT-bit

#### WHO IS A CUSTOMER?

By definition, a *customer* is one who receives goods or services from another. Each person who interacts with the HIM department, whether that person receives materials or services, is a customer. Therefore fellow employees in another department in the hospital can be customers, as well as physicians, patients, and third party payers.

---

### Body Mechanics

All employees should maintain proper body mechanics, particularly while sitting at the work station and when lifting, pushing, pulling, or transporting patients or equipment. Employees can be injured if they use poor body mechanics, and injuries are very costly to the entire organization; injuries could lead to missed work, workers' compensation claims, and reduced productivity. The orientation may include demonstration of proper body mechanics for employees to use in their job duties.

### Confidentiality

Confidentiality has always been an important part of the new health care employee orientation. HIPAA legislation increased the need for organizations to ensure that all employees and contractors receive training regarding the confidentiality and security of health information. Typically, this topic is presented by an HIM professional. All employees must recognize the sensitivity of confidential information in a health care facility and the proper manner in which it should be handled. The confidentiality policy is reviewed, and all employees are asked to sign a confidentiality statement, as discussed in Chapter 12 (see Figure 12-1). Additionally, all employees must be made aware of any applicable federal and state laws and organization policies regarding patient confidentiality and security. Security matters can include review of the information technology policy on password security and access to the organization's electronic health information. All employees will be asked to review the guidelines for security and to sign statements acknowledging their understanding and compliance.

### Information Systems

Many facilities require a training session before a new employee is given access to its computer systems, and The Joint Commission (TJC) requires that new employees complete this training within 7 days. During orientation new employees receive their login or user names, even though access will be limited until training on the various computer systems is complete. They also are given information on rules for setting passwords and the frequency that passwords must be changed, and learn about the use policies surrounding the facility's information systems. This information, along with training on the use of software applications, may be presented by an information technology (IT) professional, although the use of computer-based learning modules for this procedure is common.

---

**Go To** Review the discussion on ergonomics in Chapter 13.

**confidentiality** Discretion regarding the disclosure of information.

**health information** Organized data that have been collected about a patient or a group of patients. Sometimes used synonymously with *health data.*

**TJC** The Joint Commission

# Health Information Management Department Orientation

After the organization-wide orientation, employees report to their supervisors in their assigned departments for orientations specific to their jobs. Each employee is given an opportunity to become acclimated to the work environment, meet the employees who are part of the work group or team, and learn what is expected by management.

During this orientation, a new employee in the HIM department is given a copy of the job description, performance standards, rules, and policies and procedures of the department. The employee becomes familiar with the physical layout of the HIM department, including the evacuation route in case of fire and other related departments within the organization.

One way to orient new employees is to have them sit with coworkers in each section of the department to allow them to familiarize themselves with everyone's tasks. This experience helps new employees understand the impact of their roles in the department.

Although the organization-wide orientation covers payroll issues (as discussed earlier), there may be more specific schedule policies within the department. HIM employees should know the hours (shift) that they are expected to work. HIM employees also need to understand which holidays they may be required to work and how to request time off.

Another topic discussed in the organization-wide orientation is security of health information. HIM employees are given a password with access to appropriate systems that they will use to perform their job duties. In the HIM department orientation the employee is reminded of the rules associated with the password—for instance, employees cannot share passwords with others, and when they leave a computer station they should log out to prevent unauthorized access by someone who might try to access that computer after they walk away. Once their passwords are assigned, employees can begin training on the computer systems associated with their jobs.

An excellent way to keep track of everything that must be covered with a new employee is to complete an orientation checklist (Figure 14-1). The employee should initial and date each item as it is completed. This form is kept in the employee's file folder for future reference, as verification of the orientation.

> **job description** A list of the employee's responsibilities.
> **performance standards** Set guidelines explaining how much work an employee must complete.

## HIT-bit

### ORIENTATION PRESENTATIONS

Each topic in the organization-wide orientation is typically presented by the employee within the organization who is the authority on that issue. For example, the safety topic is presented by the facility's security officer; body mechanics is presented by a physical therapist; infection control is presented by the infection control nurse; and confidentiality is presented by an HIM professional.

## Clinical Staff Orientation

HIM department employees are not the only members of the organization who require an orientation about the department. Clinical staff, physicians, and members of other departments should be familiar with the functions and services of the HIM department. A general orientation explaining HIM department operations will help these members when they interact with the department. HIM customers need to know the requirements for requesting information or records and the procedures for completing or reviewing records.

## HIT-bit

### ORIENTATION TO NEW JOB DUTIES

Employees who change positions within an HIM department should undergo a formal orientation to their new duties and responsibilities.

## DIAMONTE HOSPITAL

Diamonte, Arizona 89104 • TEL. 602-484-9991

### *EMPLOYEE ORIENTATION CHECKLIST*

Employee: _____ Date: _____

Position: _____ Supervisor: _____

The following items have been reviewed with the employee.
(The employee and supervisor should initial and date items as they are reviewed.)

| | Employee | Supervisor | Date |
|---|---|---|---|
| Employee identification card policy | | | |
| Explanation of payroll procedures, including time clock location | | | |
| Absence and tardiness policy | | | |
| Employee job description | | | |
| Employee performance standards | | | |
| Introduction to department employees and physical layout | | | |
| Review of department functions | | | |
| Review of functions involving related departments | | | |
| Departmental Policy and Procedure manual | | | |
| Review of specific job-related policies and procedures | | | |
| Dress code | | | |
| Performance improvement activities | | | |
| Security and confidentiality policies | | | |
| Review and sign confidentiality statement | | | |
| Safety policy, disaster plan, and safety manual | | | |
| Review of break schedule | | | |
| Location of restrooms and area to secure belongings | | | |
| Password assigned and related policies covered | | | |

Employee signature: _____ Date: _____

Supervisor: _____ Date: _____

*Example only. This list is not all-inclusive.*

**Figure 14-1** Employee orientation checklist.

---

## HIT-bit

### PROBATION PERIOD

The first 90 days of employment for a new employee are often called the probation period. During the probation period, employees are allowed ample time to learn their new tasks and responsibilities. At the end of this time, employees who are performing at an acceptable level are considered permanent.

If at any time during this probation period the employer feels that an employee is not performing as expected, the employee can be released from the job.

---

Physicians require orientation to the HIM department because they will visit the department to complete their health records and perform research. Physician orientation can be by personal appointment or in the form of a letter (Figure 14-2) introducing or explaining HIM department functions.

Department managers must understand the proper way to request records from the HIM department. Managers often request records for a study or project in which they are

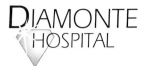

**D**IAMONTE **H**OSPITAL          Diamonte, Arizona 89104 • TEL. 602-484-9991

November 30, 2012

Eileen Dombrowski, MD
1101 Medical Center Blvd.
Diamonte, Arizona 89104

Dear Dr. Dombrowski,

On behalf of the Health Information Management department, welcome to Diamonte Hospital.
I would like to introduce you to the HIM department staff and the services provided.

**Release of Information**
To obtain copies of health information for a patient under your care, please contact Shelly Pontiac,
565-1411. She will be happy to provide the appropriate forms and process your request.

**Coding**
Our coding department is supervised by Joanne Davis, CCS.  If you have any questions regarding
coding, please feel free to contact her.

**Request for an old chart for patient care**
The unit coordinator will typically request previous records for patients under your care by contacting
the Health Information Management department at 565-1400.  If you encounter difficulty retrieving a
previous patient record, please feel free to contact John Brown, Supervisor.

**Medical record completion**
In keeping with our policy for timely completion of health records, we will e-mail weekly reminders to
your office to notify you of any incomplete records. If you plan to come by our office to complete your
records, please call in advance, 565-1455.  We will be happy to pull your records and leave them in
the physicians' lounge for 48 hours.

I look forward to working with you.  If you need any further assistance, I can be reached at 565-1416.

Sincerely,

Michelle Parks, RHIA
Director, Health Information Management

**Figure 14-2** Orientation letter to physicians.

involved or to obtain information for a meeting. They need to know how much notice the
department needs to complete the request. Does the request need to be specific? Does the
person requesting the information need to include the patient's name, medical record
number (MR#), and discharge dates on the request form? Covering these policies in an
orientation eliminates a great deal of confusion and stress in the future.

> ● **medical record number (MR#)** A
> unique number assigned to each
> patient in a health care system;
> this code will be used for the
> rest of the patient's encounters
> with that specific health system.

**HIT-bit** ·······································································

**PHYSICIAN ORIENTATION**

Physician orientation is an excellent opportunity to cover information relevant to
completion of records, specifically the suspension policy. The suspension policy is
typically found in the medical staff bylaws. But even if the orientation is no more than
a simple letter of correspondence, it tells the physician how to avoid negative correspondence and unfortunate consequences as a result of delinquent records. Whatever format, the physician orientation should let the physician know whom to contact
to gain access to incomplete records and how the HIM department can assist the
physician in record completion.

## EXERCISE 14-1

### Orientation

1. To become familiar with a new job and surroundings, the employee must attend which of the following?
   a. Training
   b. Orientation
   c. Inservice
   d. Department meeting
2. Which of the following organization-wide orientation topics should be presented by a HIM employee?
   a. Safety
   b. Infection control
   c. Personnel issues
   d. HIPAA, Confidentiality, and Security
3. The "R" in the common safety acronym *RACE*, which is used to describe the employee's expected response to a fire, stands for which of the following words?
   a. Red
   b. Run
   c. Rescue
   d. Reassure
4. What topics are important to cover in an HIM department physician orientation?

## TRAINING AND DEVELOPMENT

**training** Education in, instruction in, or demonstration of how to perform a job.

**inservice** Training provided to employees of an organization for continued or reinforced education.

**release of information (ROI)** The term used to describe the HIM department function that provides disclosure of patient health information.

**performance standards** Set guidelines explaining how much work an employee must complete.

**Training** is an important part of all jobs. Employees obviously need training when they begin a job, but they need it just as much when processes, procedures, and equipment are changed. Training is the education of employees in new techniques and processes within the organization. It is provided to employees in the health care facility through inservice training sessions, seminars, workshops, and continuing education, to ensure the quality of service.

*Development* is a term that can be used to describe training, but more specifically it indicates an investment by the organization—in an employee—with the expectation that the development will indeed pay off somehow in the future performance of the employee. For instance, an employee is hired to perform release of information (ROI). Over time and with experience, the managers recognize that this employee could be developed for a supervisor position. Development is an investment in the employee, enhancing skills and increasing his or her ability to perform necessary job duties.

### Planning a Training Session

#### Assessment of Education Needs

Training sessions should be planned with specific goals in mind, because they are essential to successful staff development. The first step in planning a training session involves an assessment of current staff training needs. The assessment helps the HIM director identify which areas need focus. Training topics can be identified through the following means:
- A management observation from performance standard reviews
- Employee surveys
- Updated or new equipment
- Legal or regulatory changes

In Chapter 13 we discuss performance standards. Performance standards tell employees the amount and the quality of work they are expected to accomplish. When performing employee evaluations, the manager may determine that additional training is needed in a particular area because of an employee's low performance.

Occasionally, employees may be asked to identify areas in which they would like to acquire more expertise. This is an opportunity for development. A survey can identify areas of interest to the employees, and training sessions can be developed accordingly. Surveys may also identify ideal areas for **cross-training**, which teaches employees how to perform job functions in the department that are not part of their job descriptions. Cross-training is a way to prepare a department to handle increased workloads and vacant positions when employees are on a break, are out sick, are on vacation, or leave their positions. It can also provide job enrichment for some employees.

**cross-training** Training of employees for additional jobs or functions within the department so that they can help with those jobs when necessary.

## Audience

An important part of planning a training session is learning about the audience. The presenters do not have to know each person individually, but they should know the participants' backgrounds. These backgrounds, with regard to education and work-related experience, tell the presenters how to begin the training. When the topic is new to the audience, the presenters begin with an elementary overview of the topic. If participants are knowledgeable about the topic and have practical experience, the training session can be more advanced. Additionally, knowing the backgrounds of participants affects the organization of the presentation—that is, the vocabulary and knowledge pertinent to the audience. In other words, significantly different vocabulary words and examples are used to train physicians and college students.

## Format

There are many different learning styles, and it follows that training should provide information in a variety of formats. Training formats can be passive, active, or collaborative. Traditional lectures are passive; the trainer does all the talking, and the trainees just listen to learn. Active training requires that the employees/trainees participate in some activity to achieve the learning outcome, and collaborative learning puts trainees in groups to work together to learn. The best training incorporates all of these formats to ensure that employees learn what is intended by the training.

The format of a training session explains how the information or topic will be presented. For example, will the training take place as a lecture, or will it be hands-on? Will the presentation include a video or demonstration? Will there be an instructor or a self-guided manual? The format is determined by the topic of the presentation and the audience. It is very important to explain the purpose of the training to the attendees. The explanation will allow them to examine how this new skill or information will be required in the performance of their jobs. If the topic involves procedures and use of equipment, a demonstration that includes hands-on participation by each attendee will enhance their understanding. Another common training session involves explaining annual coding updates. This type of training should involve explanation, examples, and case studies so that the coders can practice applying the new coding guidelines.

**coding** The assignment of alphanumerical values to a word, phrase, or other nonnumerical expression. In health care, coding is the assignment of numerical values to diagnosis and procedure descriptions.

The format of the presentation also determines whether the presenter needs audiovisual equipment. If the training session involves a video, access to that video must be available in the training room. Other audiovisual equipment includes overhead projectors, slide projectors, computer equipment with speakers and video capability, and microphones.

## Environment

The location of the training session is another element that can be determined by the topic of the presentation and the audience. Training sessions can be held in classrooms or auditoriums, via video conference or the Internet, or in the HIM department. If the training requires demonstration of equipment, the training should happen near the equipment or a demonstration model should be available in the classroom. The location of the training session is also affected by the number of participants. The larger the audience, the more space is required. Sometimes multiple sessions can be held to accommodate a large number of participants. However, if the number of participants is small, the training session may be held in the HIM department. If audience members are expected to take notes, chairs at tables or desks should be considered. If a computer terminal is used for the training, make sure there is adequate seating for one person per computer.

*Technology Training*

With all of the technological advances that occur in today's health care environment, equipment and computer software are continuously being updated and replaced. These changes certainly require training. Imagine the scenario in which a new time clock system for payroll is implemented. Leaders in the organization must create a presentation to explain the new time clock system and provide a method for employees to practice using the new system to clock in and out of work.

---

### HIT-bit ····································································

#### ONLINE TRAINING

Because of the increased performance expectations in health care organizations, many employers are looking for efficient and effective methods to train their employees. One method being used is online training. Training that can occur *asynchronously*— whenever any employee is available or able to fit it into the work schedule—is one advantage of online methods. *Synchronous* learning happens when the learner and the instructor are together, whether in person or online. Asynchronous learning can occur as a result of recorded materials or presentations (e.g., Microsoft's PowerPoint).

---

**computerized physician order entry (CPOE)** A health information system in which physicians enter orders electronically.

Now imagine the case of a more involved training scenario—implementation of a new computerized physician order entry (CPOE) system. Leaders in the organization need to prepare training for many different users: nurses, physicians, pharmacists, and HIM employees. For a training scenario like this, the vendor (product seller) is often very helpful in providing a test environment for practice, tutorials for Web training, and onsite workshops to "train the trainers" in the organization. This training requires coordination of efforts between the health care organization and the vendor. A communication from the leadership to the employees and medical staff is needed to explain the purpose and usefulness of the CPOE. Sometimes, a Web page on the health care organization's intranet can be created to provide additional video tutorials, information about the product, a training calendar, and contact information for technical support. At each step of the implementation process, the project leader should communicate with the organization to keep everyone informed about the progress.

## Calendar of Education

**confidentiality** Discretion regarding the disclosure of information.

How often should employees be trained? At a minimum, all employees in the facility should receive annual training in customer service, quality, safety, infection control, confidentiality and security, and body mechanics. Additional training sessions can be organized according to an employee's job function or as the need arises.

**credentials** An individual's specific professional qualifications. Also refers to the acronym or abbreviation representing a degree or certification that a professionally qualified person is entitled to list after his or her name.

**inpatient** An individual who is admitted to a hospital with the intention of staying overnight.

**outpatient** A patient whose health care services are intended to be delivered within 1 calendar day or, in some cases, a 24-hour period.

**ROI** release of information

In addition to credential continuing education requirements, several HIM positions (regardless of employee **credentials**) require routine training, particularly in the areas of coding and ROI (Table 14-2). Coding employees should participate in quarterly training sessions. Inpatient coding changes occur twice a year, in April and October; these changes affect all of the employees responsible for inpatient coding. A training session should be organized to inform these employees of any upcoming coding changes that will affect their jobs. Outpatient coding changes occur in January. A training session should be organized accordingly to cover these changes. Additionally, other regulations, such as the implementation of prospective payment systems, occur at various times during the year and require further training sessions. Employees who handle release of information requests should receive annual training, and additional sessions should be organized when there are changes in federal or state laws that affect the release of health information.

It is very important that a record be kept of employee attendance at training sessions. The record of an employee's attendance supports the communication of a new policy, procedure, or method required as a part of his or her job.

## TABLE 14-2

### AREAS OF ROUTINE TRAINING

| EMPLOYEE | CHANGES | TIME FRAME |
|---|---|---|
| Inpatient coder | Annual coding changes | April and October |
| Outpatient coder | Annual coding changes | January |
| Release-of-information clerk | Regulatory (federal and state law) changes | As needed; review sources daily |
| Revenue cycle manager | Regulatory (federal and state law) changes | As needed; review sources daily |
| All employees | The Joint Commission, Health Insurance Portability and Accountability Act, and U.S. Occupational Safety and Health Administration requirements | Annually |

A sign-in sheet should be used to document employee attendance. The heading at the top of the sign-in sheet should include the date topic is covered and the objectives that apply. This sign-in sheet can be kept in a binder to record employee education, or the information can be transferred to each employee's file. In addition, the information can be transferred to a computer system to track employee education.

Training is an ongoing process. Often it is important to involve other departments so that employees learn the necessary information from the appropriate source. Some topics can be coordinated with members of other departments, such as quality management, nursing, infection control, and business. All of the employees who are affected by the new information, including employees who work at home, should participate in the training for it.

## EXERCISE 14-2

### Training

1. Which of the following is the first step in planning a training, inservice, or continuing education program?
   a. Assessment of education needs
   b. Audience
   c. Area
   d. Inventory of skills
2. Continuing education is critical for coding employees. Which of the following dates is/are critical in the education of inpatient coders?
   a. January 1
   b. October 1 and April 1
   c. January 1, April 1, and October 1
   d. July 1
3. A general term for education, instruction, or demonstration of how to perform a job is _____.
4. The specific time, also known as a grace period, given to a new employee to learn the job and reach the performance standards associated with that job is known as the _____.

## Inservice Education

**Inservice** education is training for an organization's employees. A training session can be called inservice when it provides continuing or reinforced education for current employees. An inservice session can be part of a monthly department meeting, or it can be held separately to cover a new topic (e.g., use of new equipment). Inservice sessions reinforce and develop new skills and can also be used as methods of cross-training staff. Box 14-1

**inservice** Training provided to employees of an organization for continued or reinforced education.

**TJC Mandatory Annual Inservices**

| Topic | Date of attendance MM/DD/YYYY | Employee Initials | Witness Initials |
|---|---|---|---|
| HIPAA | | | |
| Fire and electrical safety in a health care facility (could be 2 separate) | | | |
| Cultural diversity and sensitivity | | | |
| Universal precautions | | | |
| Hazardous materials | | | |
| Infection control | | | |
| Blood-borne pathogens, hepatitis, AIDS | | | |
| Age-appropriate care | | | |
| Patient lifting, moving, restraints | | | |
| Yearly national safety goals | | | |
| N95 Respirator fitting and training | | | |

Signature of employee          Signature of witness

Original to Human Resource employee file
Copy for employee and HIM Department file

**Figure 14-3** Form showing employee attendance at The Joint Commission's mandatory annual inservice training sessions.

---

**BOX 14-1 EXAMPLES OF INSERVICE TOPICS**

- How to use a new scanner, copier, or printer
- How to respond to a fire emergency code, including the use of a fire extinguisher
- How to handle a walk-in request for copies of a health record
- How to use a clinical pathway
- Explanation of a new prospective payment system and how it will affect the organization

---

provides a list of inservice sessions for HIM employees. All of the elements of a training session apply to the development of an employee inservice session. Some accreditation agencies, such as TJC, mandate specific annual employee inservice sessions for compliance (Figure 14-3).

## Educating the Public

Health care professionals are often called on to educate the public about changes in laws relating to health care or health information as well as health-related topics, such as cancer awareness, diabetes, and infectious diseases. Therefore each of the topics associated with planning a training session for employees can be modified for use in planning a training session for the public.

**TABLE 14-3**

**CONTINUING EDUCATION IN CORE CONTENT AREAS FOR THE REGISTERED HEALTH INFORMATION TECHNICIAN (RHIT)**

| CORE CONTENT AREA | DESCRIPTION | CONTINUING EDUCATION EXAMPLE |
|---|---|---|
| Technology | Applications of existing and emerging technologies for collection of clinical data, the transformation of clinical data to useful health information, and the communication and protection of information | Attend a presentation explaining the process of converting paper records to a virtual file room |
| Management development | Application of organizational management theory and practices as well as human resource management techniques to improve departmental adaptability, innovation service quality, and operational efficiency | Attend inservice training to learn how to use a new employee evaluation system |
| Clinical data management | Application of data analysis techniques to clinical databases to evaluate practice patterns, assess clinical outcomes, and ensure cost-effectiveness of health care services | Attend a meeting of the community health information network to learn how to submit information and interpret results |
| Performance improvement | Study of fundamental organizational changes and how they are functionally organized or how they deliver patient care, with special focus on the requisite changes made in health information systems and services | Attend a meeting to learn how to facilitate quality improvement in your organization |
| External forces | Knowledge of strategies that organizational and HIM professionals in particular have used to effectively address emerging legislative, regulatory, or other external party action that has the potential to significantly affect the collection and use of health data | Attend a seminar explaining implementation of HIPAA requirements |
| Clinical foundations | Understanding of human anatomy and physiology, the nature of disease processes in humans, and the methods of diagnosis and treatment of acute and chronic medical conditions and diseases | Attend a conference on breast cancer |
| Privacy and security | Understanding and application of current health care regulations that promote protection and the electronic transmission of health information; to act as the patient's advocate and teach them about their rights with regard to protected health information | Attend a meeting on the implementation of the provider identification number (PIN) for your organization |

HIM, health information management; HIPAA, Health Insurance Portability and Accountability Act.
Adapted from Commission on Certification for Health Informatics and Information Management (CCHIIM): Recertification Guide: Maintenance of Certification. Revised Spring 2012. http://www.ahima.org/downloads/pdfs/certification/Recertification_Guide.pdf.

## Continuing Education

Education does not stop simply because a person has completed a degree or program or obtained employment. Professionals understand that education will continue over the course of their careers. All HIM professionals should recognize that their credentials are accompanied by a commitment to lifelong learning. In all health care fields, regulations change, technology advances, and processes improve. Because of such changes, you must continue your education as it relates to your job, your career, and your special interests.

Keeping a record of professional **continuing education (CE)** hours is very important. Because CE periods vary with each association, it is difficult to remember all of the hours earned unless you maintain personal attendance records. The easiest method for keeping track of CE hours is to designate a file folder for material from the meetings you attended, journal article questionnaires you submitted, and Web site tutorials you completed. Using a summary form in the file folder provides a quick reference for how many hours have been completed (Figure 14-4). This file folder and tracking form are also helpful in the event of an audit of CE hours. Using this file folder and tracking form makes it easier to fill out the CE form when a report of your continuing education hours is due. Additionally, some organizations, such as American Health Information Management Association (AHIMA), allow their members to track and maintain a record of their CE hours online (Figure 14-5). HIM department managers should also maintain record of all employees' CE activities in their employee files.

**credentials** An individual's specific professional qualifications. Also refers to the acronym or abbreviation representing a degree or certification that a professionally qualified person is entitled to list after his or her name.

**continuing education (CE)** Education required after a person has attained a position, credential, or degree, intended to keep the person knowledgeable in his or her profession.

**AHIMA** American Health Information Management Association

Continuing education for: _____

No. of hours needed: _____

Cycle ends: _____

| Date | Topic/Title | Location | Core Content Area | No. of Hours |
|------|-------------|----------|-------------------|--------------|
|  |  |  |  |  |
|  |  |  |  |  |
|  |  |  |  |  |
|  |  |  |  |  |
|  |  |  |  |  |
|  |  |  |  |  |
|  |  |  |  |  |
|  |  |  |  |  |
|  |  |  |  |  |
|  |  |  |  |  |
|  |  |  |  |  |
|  |  |  |  |  |
|  |  |  |  |  |
|  |  |  |  |  |
|  |  |  |  |  |

**Figure 14-4** Continuing education tracking form.

AHIMA

**Alert Messages**
No Messages

| | Type | Program Title \| Activity | Sponsors | Completed Date | CEUs | Domain | Documents |
|---|------|-------------------------|----------|----------------|------|--------|-----------|
| Edit \| Delete | Webinar | Health Care Reform | Other | 12/15/2011 | 1 | Management Development | |
| Edit | In Person Meeting | 2011 Annual Convention | AHIMA | 10/31/2011 | 3 | Clinical Data Management | |
| Edit \| Delete | Author | Review Principles of Finance | AHIMA | 06/30/2011 | 6 | Management Development | |
| Edit \| Delete | Speaker | NJHIMA Annual - ICD10 prep | Other | 06/16/2011 | 4 | Performance Improvement | |
| Edit \| Delete | In Person Meeting | HFMANJ Compliance/Audit Educational meeting | Other | 03/08/2011 | 6 | Management Development | |
| Edit \| Delete | In Person Meeting | HFMA Dode Institute | Other | 02/24/2011 | 5 | Performance Improvement | |
| Edit \| Delete | Webinar | Payment Audits in Hospitals, Part II | Other | 02/10/2011 | 1 | Clinical Data Management | |
| Edit \| Delete | Webinar | Payment Audits in Hospitals, Part I | Other | 01/26/2011 | 1 | Clinical Data Management | |
| Edit \| Delete | Webinar | Cardiovascular and Endovascular CPT Code Update | Other | 01/20/2011 | 1 | Clinical Data Management | |
| Edit \| Delete | Webinar | Cloud Computing | Other | 01/04/2011 | 1 | Technology | |
| Edit \| Delete | Webinar | Excel - Pivot Tables | Other | 12/27/2010 | 1 | Clinical Data Management | |
| Edit \| Delete | Webinar | CPT Coding Updates | Other | 11/23/2010 | 1 | Clinical Data Management | |
| Edit \| Delete | Webinar | CPT Coding Updates | Other | 11/22/2010 | 1 | Clinical Data Management | |
| Edit \| Delete | In Person Meeting | ICD-10 Overview | Other | 07/15/2010 | 6 | Clinical Data Management | |
| Edit \| Delete | In Person Meeting | HFMANJ Compliance/Audit Educational meeting | Other | 03/09/2010 | 6 | Management Development | |

**Figure 14-5** Using an online tracker to log continuing education units (CEUs). (Adapted and Reprinted with permission from the American Health Information Management Association. Copyright © 2012 by the American Health Information Management Association. All rights reserved. No part of this may be reproduced, reprinted, stored in a retrieval system, or transmitted, in any form or by any means, electronic, photocopying, recording, or otherwise, without the prior written permission of the association.)

AHIMA includes a continuing education requirement as a part of the certification/ registration process. To maintain your credential, you must earn continuing education credits pertinent to the HIM profession. The requirement for the Registered Health Information Technician (RHIT) and Registered Health Information Administrator (RHIA) states that the professional must earn 80% of the required hours in a core content area (see Table 14-3). AHIMA has designated the following areas as core content for the HIM profession: technology, management development, clinical data management, performance improvement, external forces, clinical foundations, and privacy and security.

The RHIA must earn 30 continuing education hours every 2 years with at least 24 (80% of the 30) hours in any one or multiple core content areas. These are sometimes referred to as continuing education units, or CEUs. The cycle runs January through December of the following year. The RHIT must maintain 20 continuing education hours every 2 years, and at least 16 of the 20 hours in one or multiple core content areas.

Because certification rules can change, always refer to the AHIMA Web site for the current requirements.

CEUs can be earned in a variety of ways. Most professionals earn their CEUs by attending local, state, or national HIM association meetings. Some may earn the hours by attending meetings within their facility. Yet another method for earning CEUs is by reading and responding to the education quizzes found in the *Journal of the American Health Information Management Association* or on the AHIMA Web site.

Additional AHIMA certifications also require a commitment to lifelong learning. The Certified Coding Specialist (CCS) and Certified Coding Specialist—Physician-based (CCS-P) credentials require an annual self-assessment (worth 5 CEUs), including health record coding scenarios. Depending on the number and nature of coding changes for that year, the number of multiple-choice questions may be as few as 10 or as many as 30.

Professionals who earn and maintain more than one credential will need to earn 10 additional continuing education hours for each credential but no more than 60 hours per cycle. For example, if Jane has the credentials RHIT and CCS-P, she will need to earn 30 CE credits, 20 for the RHIT and 10 for the CCS-P, in addition to the annual assessment. Table 14-4 lists the CEU requirements for various credentials.

> **RHIA** Registered Health Information Administrator
> **RHIT** Registered Health Information Technician

> **CEU** continuing education unit

## TABLE 14-4

### CREDENTIALS AND THEIR CONTINUING EDUCATION UNIT (CEU) REQUIREMENTS

| CREDENTIAL | | CEU REQUIREMENTS |
|---|---|---|
| RHIT | Registered Health Information Technician | 20 CEUs |
| RHIA | Registered Health Information Administrator | 30 CEUs |
| CCA | Certified Coding Associate | 20 CEUs, including two mandatory annual coding self-reviews (self-assessments)* |
| CCS | Certified Coding Specialist | 20 CEUs, including two mandatory annual coding self-reviews (self-assessments)* |
| CCS-P | Certified Coding Specialist—Physician-based | 20 CEUs, including two mandatory annual coding self-reviews (self-assessments)* |
| CHDA | Certified Health Data Analyst | 30 CEUs |
| CHPS | Certified in Healthcare Privacy and Security | 30 CEUs |
| CDIP | Clinical Documentation Improvement Practitioner | 30 CEUs |

*Each mandatory annual coding self-review is worth five (5) CEUs toward the total CEU requirement of a coding credential.
(Modified from Commission on Certification for Health Informatics and Information Management (CCHIIM): Recertification Guide: Maintenance of Certification. Revised Spring 2012. http://www.ahima.org/downloads/ pdfs/certification/Recertification_Guide.pdf. Adapted and Reprinted with permission from the American Health Information Management Association. Copyright © 2012 by the American Health Information Management Association. All rights reserved. No part of this may be reproduced, reprinted, stored in a retrieval system, or transmitted, in any form or by any means, electronic, photocopying, recording, or otherwise, without the prior written permission of the association.)

## EXERCISE 14-3

### Inservice Education

1. _____ indicate(s) a person's specific professional qualifications.
2. To maintain the RHIT credential, the professional must maintain:
   a. 20 hours of continuing education each year.
   b. 30 hours of continuing education each year.
   c. 20 hours of continuing education during a 2-year cycle.
   d. 30 hours of continuing education during a 2-year cycle.
3. A name for the training provided to employees of an organization is _____.
4. _____ may be required after attaining a position, credential, or degree; this is intended to keep those persons knowledgeable in core content areas.

## COMMUNICATION

Employees in the HIM department communicate daily using written, verbal, physical, and electronic methods. The HIM department also communicates with other departments in and outside the facility—clinicians and physicians, other health care facilities, insurance companies, attorneys, and patients. Communication should always be clear and appropriate regardless of the parties involved (Figure 14-6).

Communication requires two parties and the conveying of a message. First, the message must be transmitted by one party to another party. The message can be written, verbal, or electronic or can be expressed by body language. The first party—called the sender—initiates the message. The second party—the receiver—is the recipient of the message. With this understanding, consider typical communication within the HIM department. The following sections discuss communication among the following:
- Employees within the HIM department
- HIM department personnel and physicians
- HIM department personnel and other departments
- HIM department personnel and outside agencies or parties

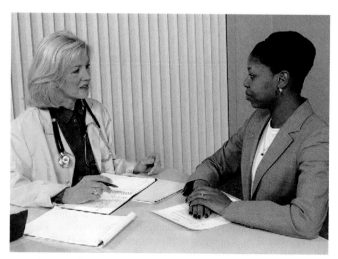

**Figure 14-6** Communication. (From Adams AP, Proctor DB: Kinn's the medical assistant, ed 10, St Louis, 2007, Elsevier Saunders.)

## Employee-to-Employee Communication

Communication occurs among employees within the HIM department and throughout the organization. Communication may be verbal, written, or electronic and may involve job-related or personal subjects. Positive, appropriate communication among employees enhances productivity.

Most important, communication about or to patients should be kept confidential. Patient health information should be communicated in an appropriate method to employees on a need-to-know basis in accordance with HIPAA regulations and health care facility policy.

Communication between employees and their immediate supervisors is very important. Employees need to know how their performance is perceived by management. They also need to be informed of changes in their work, processes, and functions that affect their daily operations.

## Health Information Management Department and Physicians

The HIM department communicates routinely with physicians regarding record completion, release of information (ROI), continuity of care, and documentation of health information for case management or reimbursement. Communication with a physician should be respectful. Consider the physician's time, and make your communication appropriate. To communicate record completion requirements, HIM employees use e-mail and official mail, and for questions on health record documentation, they post notes on electronic health records (EHRs) or attach paper memos to health record files, if appropriate. The message/communication must be meaningful, brief if possible, and most important, clear.

## Health Information Management Department and Outside Agencies or Parties

HIM departments often communicate with agents external to the organization. For example, the HIM department ROI employees receive requests from attorneys and third party payers (insurance companies) for copies of health records. As discussed in Chapter 12, information should be released only according to applicable policy or state or federal law. As a part of the release process, the HIM/ROI employee may need to discuss with the requestor the circumstances, charges, or additional forms necessary to comply with the request. Communication should be clear, preferably in writing, and should provide information so that the recipient can reply as necessary. Many departments create form letters to handle this type of communication in a standard, law-abiding, and professional manner.

## Written Communication

Written communication provides documentation of the message intended for the recipient. Therefore written communication serves two purposes: it conveys a message and records it. A common form of written communication in a health care facility is the memorandum, better known as the *memo* (see later). Memos can be written on paper and delivered individually to each employee or communicated in electronic form via e-mail.

### Electronic Communication

It is extremely common for health care facilities to use e-mail for communication and notification. This method of communication allows the same message to be sent to all employees instantly. E-mail systems provide a record of a communication sent as well as indication, using a read receipt function, that the receiving party has opened the e-mail.

---

**Health Insurance Portability and Accountability Act (HIPAA)** Public Law 104-191, federal legislation passed in 1996 that outlines the guidelines of managing patient information in terms of privacy, security, and confidentiality. The legislation also outlines penalties for noncompliance.

**continuity of care** The broad range of health care services required by a patient during an illness or for an entire lifetime. May also refer to the continuity of care provided by a health care organization. Also called *continuum of care*.

**case management** The coordination of the patient's care and services, including reimbursement considerations.

**reimbursement** The amount of money that the health care facility receives from the party responsible for paying the bill.

**third party payer** An entity that pays a provider for part or all of a patient's health care services; often the patient's insurance company.

> ## HIT-bit
>
> ### E-MAIL ETIQUETTE
>
> Do not type an e-mail message using all capital letters. In the e-mail context, all-capital letters are considered the equivalent of shouting. Use all-capital letters sparingly, only to emphasize a word.
>
> Avoid long messages. Keep the message brief and to the point.
>
> If someone sends you an e-mail message that requires a response, be careful to reply to the sender as appropriate. Include the previous message so that the person knows why you are communicating a specific message.
>
> In a business e-mail, end your message with your name, title, and business address, including phone numbers as appropriate. You want the person to be able to contact you appropriately.
>
> E-mail is not private. Be careful what you send via e-mail. Messages can be read by others or misdirected. Send only what you feel comfortable expressing to the whole world.
>
> Use punctuation appropriately.
>
> E-mail is faster than conventional mail. However, the quicker arrival of e-mail does not mean that the intended recipient will actually read the message any faster.

With the use of e-mail, messages can be conveniently tracked for receipt, returned, forwarded, or saved. When sending an e-mail, it is easy to send a copy to others (cc: carbon copy) in receipt of the message so that they have the information. Additionally, copies of e-mails can be sent to others in such a way that the intended original recipient does not know that others are included or copied in the message (bcc: blind carbon copy).

Because e-mail is a form of written communication, appropriate grammar, punctuation, and etiquette must be used in creating it. Additionally, e-mail is not a private method of sending communication; therefore health care facilities must use encryption to enhance security of this communication and employees must comply with HIPAA guidelines for release of information by e-mail.

### Memos

**memorandum (memo)** A communication tool used to inform members of an organization.

A **memorandum (memo)** is typed communication for informational purposes. A memo is used to provide clear, concise information about a new procedure, process, or policy to all those affected by it (Figure 14-7). The memo is more formal than verbal communication. Memos can be addressed to a group or an individual but are not as formal as a letter addressed specifically to an employee.

Memos can also serve as proof of communication to an employee. When a memo is shared with employees in a department, it may be posted in a highly visible and frequented place (e.g., near the time clock or in the break room). At other times, memos are copied for each employee and handed to the employee personally by another staff member. Regardless of the means, the manager wants to be sure that the message is communicated. One easy method for attaining confirmation of the employee's receipt of the memo is to have the employee initial a master copy of the memo. This system allows management to record employees' receipt of the memo.

## EXERCISE 14-4

### Communication

1. A written/typed communication tool used to communicate or provide information to members of an organization is a _____.
2. A popular form of electronic communication is a(n):
   a. memo.
   b. e-mail.
   c. fax machine.
   d. telephone.

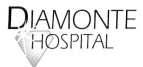

**MEMO**

TO: Health Information Management Employees

FROM: Michelle Parks, RHIA
    Director, Health Information Management

DATE: May 8, 2012

RE: Monthly Department Meeting

A Health Information Management department meeting will be held Wednesday, May 31, in the hospital auditorium at 2:00 PM.

We will have a brief presentation by the Human Resources department followed by the regular monthly agenda. Please make necessary arrangements to attend this meeting.

Thank you.

**Figure 14-7** A memo.

## DEPARTMENT MEETINGS

HIM department meetings are another method of face-to-face communication. Department meetings should be held monthly or more often as the need arises. A good way to schedule the meetings is to set aside one day each month for the meeting. This routine helps employees and managers know when to expect the next department meeting so that scheduling conflicts do not arise. The department meeting is an opportunity for HIM employees to come together to discuss, learn, communicate, and share information. The department meeting is an ideal forum for reviewing policies and procedures to ensure that everyone understands the appropriate course of action. HIM department meetings are an excellent opportunity for holding annual inservice training, discussing productivity goals, planning for major workflow changes, and providing development opportunities.

In a small department, a single meeting may suffice to communicate necessary information to all employees. However, in a large department, more than one meeting is necessary during different shifts so that all employees can attend.

**inservice** Training provided to employees of an organization for continued or reinforced education.
**productivity** The amount of work produced by an employee in a given time frame.
**workflow** The process of work flowing through a set of procedures to complete the health record.

> **HIT-bit**······················································································································
>
> ### ROBERT'S RULES OF ORDER
>
> To conduct an orderly meeting, many managers have adopted some form of Robert's Rules of Order. These rules explain how business is conducted during the meeting. Employees become accustomed to a typical order. Meetings are formally called to order, the agenda is followed, and the meeting is concluded with adjournment. The rules explain how debate should proceed and how motions can be made to present new business, make amendments, or vote on issues at hand. Likewise, there is a formal method for keeping track of old business on the agenda until it is resolved to the satisfaction of the meeting members.

All employees should attend the scheduled monthly HIM department meetings. When employees miss a meeting, they still need to hear the information. Therefore posting or copying minutes from the meeting serves as notification for these employees. Also, employees should initial the transmittal memo attached to the minutes of the meeting, indicating that they have read the minutes.

## Agenda

> **agenda** A tool used to organize the topics to be discussed during a meeting.
> **minutes** A tool used to record the events, topics, and discussions of a meeting.

Regardless of the style of department meetings, an **agenda** is used to ensure that all of the necessary topics are covered. Although agendas vary, the example in Box 14-2 is typical for a HIM department. A meeting officially begins with the call to order, whereupon the events of the meeting begin to be recorded. Employees know that it is time to stop the chatter and begin the meeting. Minutes from the previous meeting may be reviewed, depending on the formality of the meeting. Next, any old business from the previous meeting is discussed. Occasionally, topics discussed in a meeting cannot be resolved without further investigation. Such topics will be revisited during the next meeting, when old business is discussed. Topics are typically considered old business until they are resolved, closed, or completed. The next part of the agenda is new business, during which new items may be introduced to the meeting; this is followed by items that are discussed each month, such as reports from sections within the department, quality management activities in or related to the department, safety issues, and special announcements from the administration or about the facility.

## Meeting

The HIM department meeting should be held in a location able to accommodate the number of the department's staff. In a small department the meeting may be held in the HIM office area. For a large department an alternative location may be necessary to accommodate all the employees. Management must make sure to consider the time of the meeting. If it is held during the normal hours of operation, more than one meeting may

| BOX 14-2 | HIM DEPARTMENT MEETING AGENDA |
|---|---|
| I. Call to order | |
| II. Review of minutes | |
| III. Old business | |
| IV. New business | |
| V. In-service | |
| VI. Quality improvement | |
| VII. Announcements | |
| VIII. Adjournment | |

be necessary so that employees can rotate attendance in order to cover HIM responsibilities during the meeting. Otherwise, the manager should try to find a time when the office is not too busy. In order to cover the normal business, one employee may need to remain in the department to answer requests and handle business. Another way to handle this is to have someone from another department cover the functions briefly while the employees are at the meeting. There should be a sign-in sheet for all of the employees to record their attendance at the meeting.

## Minutes

Appropriate discussion and decisions from each meeting should be recorded for future reference in the **minutes**. In preparation of minutes, the agenda should be used as a guide. This ensures that the content or discussion surrounding each topic presented at the meeting is recorded. Review the minutes shown in Figure 14-8, and notice how

**minutes** A tool used to record the events, topics, and discussions of a meeting.

Health Information Management
Department Meeting
October 30, 2012

Employees present:

Employees absent:

| Topic/Discussion | Recommendation/Action | Follow-up |
|---|---|---|
| I. Call to Order<br>The Health Information Management meeting was called to order by Michelle Parks at 2:00 PM. | | |
| II. Review of Old Minutes<br>The minutes from the September Health Information Management department meeting were reviewed and approved as presented. | | |
| III. Old Business<br>**Uniforms**<br>Employees in the department are interested in adopting a uniform as the dress code. During the previous meeting it was decided that the employees would invite three uniform companies to present at the next meeting. M & R Uniforms, Acorn Uniforms, and B & B Direct presented uniforms, pricing, and payment options to the employees. | After review of the information presented by all uniform companies the employees voted for the uniform and options presented by B & B Direct. The uniform company will return in 2 weeks to take orders and the dress code will take effect in 2 months. | 11/2012 |
| IV. New Business<br>**ICD-10 Update** | | |
| V. Report<br>Intradepartmental quality<br>Interdepartmental quality | | |
| VI. Safety/Inservice | | |
| VII. Announcements | | |
| VIII. Adjournment<br>With no further business to discuss the meeting was adjourned at 2:45 PM. | | |

Michelle Parks, RHIA _____    Date _____

**Figure 14-8** HIM department meeting minutes.

the content of the topics discussed were recorded just as they were presented at the meeting. The preparer must be careful to include only pertinent meeting information and participants' comments without mention of the participants' names in the minutes; slander, slang, and irrelevant comments by the participants should not be included in minutes.

The minutes should clearly recall the events of the meeting as presented, discussed, and decided. The topics presented are documented under the column titled "Topic/Discussion." The decision or action of the meeting members is documented under "Recommendation/Action." The final column, "Follow-up," identifies whether a topic has been closed (i.e., the business for that topic is concluded). Most important, topics that are not finalized should be recorded so they may be carried forward to the next meeting until the business is concluded.

## Meeting Records

It is important to keep a precise record of each monthly meeting. These records will support any future business, discussion, and accreditation requirements. You can set up a file folder or a binder to organize each month's meeting information. Be sure to keep a copy of the agenda, the sign-in sheet, any attachments or handouts shared with the group, and the final draft of the minutes. The records from these meetings should be kept at least 3 years, or longer if required by legal or regulatory bodies.

## WORK TEAMS

*Teamwork* is a familiar term. Basketball, football, and soccer teams must work together to accomplish a common goal. In the workplace, employees are often called upon to work together as a "team" to accomplish common goals. A common example of a health care work team is the patient care team: the employees of the health care facility who work together to treat the patient. In the emergency department (ED) the team may include emergency medical technicians (EMTs) who transport the patient into the ED, the ED physician, nurses, radiology technicians, and phlebotomists. On the rehabilitation unit the team may consist of physical therapists, occupational therapists, nurses, and physicians.

🔵 **ED** emergency department

However these are not the only employees who have to work in teams to accomplish goals. For instance, in an HIM department the coding team may have a large number of charts that must be coded for final billing. (These charts are often listed on an unbilled report). Timely and accurate coding helps the health care facility receive the appropriate reimbursement for each patient case. One single patient record can represent a large sum of reimbursement for the health care facility, consequently many charts can add up to a large sum of money. To reach the goal of coding all of the charts, the coding team and other HIM department employees must work together in an efficient manner to get the job done.

A likely game plan will involve: a team meeting to discuss the goal, a review of the list of accounts that need to be coded, division of the tasks among the team members, and then action. In larger facilities, coders are often assigned to inpatient or outpatient charts, but when the workload is exceptionally heavy, outpatient coders may be able to help with some of the less complicated charts or those with a payer other than the Centers for Medicare and Medicaid Services (CMS). Other staffers in the HIM department may be able to assist with physician communications, by researching questions, or even by looking up coding clinic guidelines.

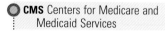
🔵 **CMS** Centers for Medicare and Medicaid Services

Achieving the goal is a rewarding experience for all of the team members. Effective teams consist of skilled and competent members, who have respect for one another and confidence in their teammates. Collaboration, communication, and cooperation are other factors that support teamwork. Successful teams have competent employees and strong leadership.

## HIT-bit

### CONFLICT MANAGEMENT

Occasionally, conflicts arise in the workplace between a supervisor and a staff member, or among two or more coworkers. Although managers may sometimes be tempted to avoid taking on conflict in the workplace, these situations can create a poor work environment and should be resolved. One effective method of addressing the conflict is to establish clear lines of communication between the employees involved. This is best done in a private setting. A supervisor may use the following procedure as one way of handling conflict:

1. Listen to each employee involved in the conflict to clearly understand each side of the conflict. Stay calm, and ensure that the other parties do as well. If the situation is tense, enlist the help of HR or another department supervisor/manager to witness and assist if necessary.
2. Ensure that each individual knows that his or her point of view is valuable. A resolution will be impossible if anyone side feels he or she is misunderstood or misrepresented.
3. After hearing both sides, assess the best method of compromise. You may need the expertise of a Human Resources manager to ensure that the best method is chosen.

## EXERCISE 14-5

### Department Meetings

1. _____ are used to record the events, topics, and discussions of a meeting.
2. A(n) _____ is used to organize the topics to be discussed during a meeting.
3. The first item on the monthly HIM department meeting agenda is:
   a. call to order.
   b. review of old business.
   c. new business.
   d. adjournment.

## LEADERSHIP

Leadership inspires others—to accomplish, to perform, or to follow—in a similar manner or on a certain course to achieve common goals for the department or organization. Sometimes people use the terms *leadership* and *management* interchangeably. However, it is possible to explain how they differ. Management can be described as the tasks, process, or tools associated with making sure the "job" is performed accurately. The skill of a leader provides support and encouragement for others to take on challenges and change with a positive, purposeful attitude. There are many styles of leadership, each with its own characteristics. Although thousands of books have been written about the qualities of an effective leadership, here are a few to consider. Leaders:

*Delegate* for several reasons: to be more efficient handling duties or responsibilities, to empower others and allow them to own a responsibility in the organization, and to create partnerships or relationships between management and staff. Delegating can allow employees to share in the department or organizations success!

*Lead* by example! In the workplace, people tend to gauge their behavior by the actions of those around them, but perhaps none more so than those of their supervisor. Exemplary behavior sets the tone, encouraging the best from the organization.

*Support* the staff: this requires both praising in public and coaching in private.

*Identify and remove* obstacles that keep staff from doing their jobs; whether ensuring the right equipment, the right workload, or the right processes, leaders are supportive in a problem-solving role.

*Are accessible*, often called having an "open door policy," which allows employees to enter the office anytime to share information and ask questions.

*Encourage* continuous improvement and provide an environment in which employees feel welcome to share their suggestions.

*Develop* the staff—an investment in an employee ensures performance, both in his or her current position and in his or her further career. Career counseling can inspire others to do their best, and advancement within the organization can create networks of individuals who have a common goal.

## EXERCISE 14-6

### Leadership

1. List the reasons a leader should delegate responsibilities to others.
2. Why is it important for an effective leader to spend time developing staff members?

## SUGGESTED READING

Burns JM: Leadership, New York, 1978, Harper & Row.

## CHAPTER ACTIVITY

### CHAPTER SUMMARY

Training and development are critical to the ongoing success of the HIM department. These efforts and activities keep HIM employees competent and abreast of all the changing technology, policy, legislative, regulatory, and accreditation requirements. New employees in the organization, whether they are HIM, medical staff, nursing, or other professionals, must be oriented to the organization and trained in HIM-related issues, including the confidentiality and security of patient information mandated by HIPAA. Training continues beyond the orientation stage; for example, employees must participate in ongoing training efforts to maintain continuing education hours, remain knowledgeable about current requirements (i.e., coding and ROI), and become skilled users of new technology that is part of their job responsibilities. Annually, the entire staff must be reminded of the requirements related to their jobs and the entire health care organization as mandated by accrediting agencies. Changes that occur as a result of quality improvement efforts are another reason for continuous training of staff. Development of the employees in the health care organization, through training, continuous education, and communication, creates an environment in which both the employees and the organization are positioned for continued success.

### REVIEW QUESTIONS

1. What is the purpose of an orientation?
2. List and briefly explain the issues discussed in the organization-wide orientation.
3. How is development different from training?
4. Identify two HIM functions that require annual (at a minimum) training of employees.
5. Explain the important items to consider in the preparation of a training presentation.
6. Explain the importance of the meeting agenda and minutes.
7. Explain three aspects of leadership and provide an example of how they can be accomplished.

## PROFESSIONAL PROFILE

### HIM Assistant Director

My name is Thomas, and I am the health information management assistant director in a 220-bed facility, Oakcrest Hospital, in the same system as Diamonte Hospital. This facility provides acute care emergency services, skilled nursing services, and ambulatory services. We have an HIM department with eight clerical and release-of-information employees under my responsibility, three coding employees with one coding supervisor, and eight transcription employees with one transcription supervisor.

In our department, things are very organized, to the credit of our department director. New employees participate in the organization orientation before reporting to our department for work. During the first few days of employment, each new employee is oriented to the department. We begin by explaining the employee's job description and expectations (performance standards). Then the new employee goes through the department, sitting with each current employee to learn about other HIM functions and how their jobs are related. Finally, the new employee is oriented to his or her new position. During this process, the employee also obtains a password for our computer systems.

I am responsible for organizing our monthly department meetings and choosing the inservice topic. I set up the agenda, copy and distribute any necessary handouts, and record the minutes. In addition, I coordinate any training required by changes in department policy, procedure, equipment, or federal and state mandates. The employees who report to me are cross-trained in several different functions so that we can cover one another for lunch, breaks, vacations, and sick leave.

I really enjoy the training and development aspect of this position. It is rewarding to see a new employee succeed in his or her position or to have an employee move up into a new position because of appropriate training and development.

### CAREER TIP

HIM professionals interact with so many people—including patients. We can no longer think of ourselves as the ones who "do not have patient contact." Our expertise and guidance are needed to help transition our patients to access their health information electronically. HIM managers can serve as leaders, providing training to patients so that meaningful uses of health information can be achieved with electronic health records!

## PATIENT CARE PERSPECTIVE

### Maria

My PCP referred me to a specialist—a cardiologist for the left bundle block that was diagnosed when I had my hysterectomy. I wanted to bring my medical records with me to the visit so I contacted the HIM department, as I have in the past, to get copies. The very nice, but insistent receptionist said they no longer make copies of records, that I would have to access my records via the patient portal. She said something about my PHR—personal health record. Since I was not happy with the receptionist's explanation, I asked to be transferred to her boss; she transferred me to Thomas, the HIM department assistant director.

## APPLICATION

### Create a Public Education Information Session

Research the current issues associated with health information. Choose a topic that requires education of the local community (the public).

Using the training session information in this chapter, perform an assessment of community education needs. In your preparation, consider the audience, the format, and the environment in which the education will be provided. Prepare a paper presentation of this information for your instructor.

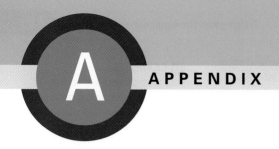

# SAMPLE PAPER RECORDS

- Inpatient Admission Form/Face Sheet
- Conditions of Admission
- Advance Directive Acknowledgement
- Emergency Department Record
- History
- Physical
- Physician's Order Form
- Physician's Progress Notes
- Informed Consent
- Consultation Record

- Medication Administration Records
- Intake/Output Record
- Nursing Progress Notes
- Operative Report Progress Notes
- Discharge Orders
- Nursing Discharge Summary
- Certificate of Live Birth
- Certificate of Death
- Report of Fetal Death

Your Hospital's Logo Here    Street Address    City, State Zip

## INPATIENT ADMISSION

| MED REC #: | ENCOUNTER #: |
|---|---|

| INSURANCE | PATIENT NAME: | SSN: | FC: | TYPE: | PHONE-HOME: | PHONE-WORK: | | | |
|---|---|---|---|---|---|---|---|---|---|
| | ADDRESS: | | | | DATE OF BIRTH: | AGE: | SEX: | RACE: | MS: |
| | | | | | MAIDEN NAME: | ETHNICITY: | | | |
| GUARANTEE NAME EMP | | | | | MAIDEN NAME: | PRIMARY LANGUAGE: | | | |
| | | | | | PHONE-HOME: | PHONE-WORK: | | | |
| NOTIFY | EMERGENCY NOTIFICATION: | RELATION: | | | PHONE-HOME: | PHONE-WORK: | | | |
| INSURANCE | INSURANCE COMPANY: | POLICY #: | | GROUP #: | CONTRACT HOLDER: | | | REL: | |

| ADMISSION | ICD9 CODE: | ADMITTING DIAGNOSIS: | | | | | | | |
|---|---|---|---|---|---|---|---|---|
| | ACCOM. ROOM | BED | SERVICE: | VIA | SRC | INFORMANT: | ADMIT BY: | ADMIT DATE: | ADMIT TIME: |
| | ADMITTING PHYSICIAN: | | ATTENDING PHYSICIAN / AHP: | | PRINCIPAL PHYSICIAN: | | | DISCHARGE DATE: | |

## NARRATIVE

**PRINCIPAL DIAGNOSIS:** THE CONDITION ESTABLISHED AFTER STUDY TO BE CHIEFLY RESPONSIBLE FOR OCCASIONING THE ADMISSION OF THE PATIENT TO THE HOSPITAL.

**OTHER DIAGNOSIS:** SEQUENCE IN ORDER OF SIGNIFICANCE TO THE CASE; INCLUDE ALL RELEVANT COMPLICATIONS AND COMORBIDITIES.
SEQ #:

TNM STAGING CLASSIFICATION: (APPLIES ONLY TO NEWLY DIAGNOSED CANCER CASES WITH SOLID TUMORS)

T _____

N _____

M _____

**PRINCIPAL PROCEDURE:** PERFORMED FOR DEFINITIVE TREATMENT, RATHER THAN FOR DIAGNOSTIC OR EXPLORATORY PURPOSES; USUALLY MOST RELATED TO PRINCIPAL DIAGNOSIS.

DATE

**OTHER DIAGNOSIS:** SEQUENCE IN ORDER OF SIGNIFICANCE TO THE CASE; INCLUDE ALL RELEVANT COMPLICATIONS AND COMORBIDITIES.
SEQ #:

DATE

CONSULTANTS:

DISPOSITION: ☐ Home ☐ SNF ☐ ICF ☐ HOME CARE ☐ OTHER HOSPITAL ☐ AMA ☐ OTHER INSTITUTION

☐ UNDER 48 HRS ☐ OVER 48 HRS    AUTOPSY: ☐ YES ☐ NO

| RESIDENT / AHP | ATTENDING PHYSICIAN | I certify that the narrative description of the principal and secondary diagnoses and the major procedures performed are accurate and complete to the best of my knowledge. |
|---|---|---|
| SIGNATURE | SIGNATURE | |
| PRINTED NAME | PRINTED NAME    DATE | CHART COPY |

## PART OF THE MEDICAL RECORD

Inpatient Admission Form/Face Sheet

PERMISSION FOR AUTOPSY

Permission is hereby given to perform an autopsy upon _____
and to remove and retain whole or parts of organs for study as necessary.

Witness _____ Signed _____ Relationship _____

_____ _____

Date _____ _____

DEPARTURE AGAINST MEDICAL ADVICE

This is to certify that I, _____, a Patient in
YOUR HOSPITAL, am leaving against the advice of the attending Physician and faculty authorities. I also acknowledge
that I have been informed of the risk involved and hereby release the attending Physician and hospital from all responsibility
for any of its effects which may result.

Witness _____ Signed _____

_____

Date _____

APPLICATION FOR ADMISSION & RELEASE OF HOSPITAL RECORDS

1. I, _____ , hereby apply for admission to YOUR HOSPITAL as a patient and request
that I be furnished appropriate hospital care and services for the condition(s) for which I am being admitted. My Physician,
Dr. _____ , is authorized to utilize the facilities of YOUR HOSPITAL on my behalf, and
I hereby authorize YOUR HOSPITAL to furnish and administer to me such diagnostic procedures, treatments, medications,
and other services as my said physician may direct.

2. I am aware that the practice of medicine and surgery is not an exact science and I acknowledge that no guarantees have
been made to me as to the result of the examination or treatment in the hospital.

3. If a health care worker is exposed significantly to my blood or body fluids, I consent to a test of my blood for hepatitis and
antibodies to the virus that causes AIDS.

4. The Hospital records concerning the patient are the property of YOUR HOSPITAL and are maintained for the benefit of
the patient, the medical staff and the Hospital. I hereby authorize YOUR HOSPITAL to release these records to the patient's
personal physician and to any other individual and private or governmental agency responsible for payment of the patient's
care and treatment.

Witness _____ Signed _____
In behalf of _____ , who is a minor and/or unable to grant permission or sign the document
and/or in need of emergency treatment, I, _____ , hereby make the aforementioned
requests and give the aforementioned authority to YOUR HOSPITAL on his/her behalf.

Signature _____ Age _____
.PERSON ACTING FOR THE PATIENT

Relationship _____
Address _____
Witness _____ Date _____ Was Hospital policy on placing patient's name on
their door explained to patient?  ☐ Yes  ☐ No

FOR CHAPLAIN'S USE

Sacraments received?  ☐ Yes  ☐ No  Date _____ Signature _____

## PART OF THE MEDICAL RECORD

Inpatient Admission Form/Face Sheet (cont'd)

DIAMONTE HOSPITAL
Diamonte, Arizona

### CONDITIONS of
### ADMISSION

**I.  LEGAL RELATIONSHIP BETWEEN DIAMONTE HOSPITAL AND PHYSICIAN**

I understand that many of the physicians on the staff of this hospital, including the attending physician(s), are not employees or agents of Diamonte Hospital but, rather, are independent contractos who have been granted privileges of using its facility for the care and treatment of their patients. I also realize that among those who attend patients at this facility are medical, nursing, and other health care professionals in training who, unless otherwise requested, may be present during patient care as part of their education.

**II.  CONSENT TO TREATMENT**

The patient, identified above, hereby consents and authorizes Diamonte Hospital and its staff and the patient's physician(s) to perform or administer the diagnostic and treatment procedures (including, but not limited to, radiology examinations, blood tests and other laboratory examinations and medication) as may be required by the Hospital or as may be ordered by the patient's physician(s). The patient acknowledges that Diamonte Hospital is a teaching institution. The patient agrees that he/she may participate as a teaching subject unless the patient otherwise notes in writing to the contrary.

**III.  RELEASE OF RECORDS**

The undersigned authorizes Diamonte Hospital to release any part or all patient medical records to such insurance company (companies), health care plan administrator, workmen's compensation carrier, welfare agency, or their respective authorized auditor or agents, or to any other person or party that is under contract or liable to Diamonte Hospital for all or any part of the hospital charges for this admission. The undersigned further authorizes Diamonte Hospital to release all or part of the patient's medical record or financial record to such physicians involved in the care of the patient, hospital committees, consultants, subsidiaries or physcian hospital organizations, including but not limited to any committee, subsidiary, or physcian hospital organization in which the pateint's physician is a member or their respective agents.

**IV.  ASSIGNMENT OF BENEFITS**

In consideration of the care and services to be provided to the patient by Diamonte Hospital, the undersigned assigns and authorizes, whether as agent or patient, direct payment to Diamonte Hospital or hospital-based physicians of all insurance and health plan benefits otherwise payable to or on behalf of the patient for this hospitalization and services. It is understood by the undersigned that he/she is finacially responsible for charges not convered by this assignment.

**V.  VALUABLES**

The undersigned understands fully that Diamonte Hospital is not responsible for the safety or security of and personal property or valuables.

**VI.  PHOTOGRAPHS**

The undersigned hereby authorizes and consents to Diamonte Hospital for the taking of photographs, images, or videotapes of such diagnostic, surgical, or treatment procedures of the patient as may be required by Diamonte Hospital or ordered by the patient's physician(s). With the exception of radiological images, Diamonte is not required to keep videotapes or photographs for any period of time if the medical record contains a record of the surgical, diagnostic, or treatment procedure. The patient hereby consents to the taking of pictures of newborns for possible purchase or for security purposes.

Conditions of Admission

DIAMONTE HOSPITAL
Diamonte, Arizona

**Advance Directive
Acknowledgment**

Instructions:   This form should be initiated upon admission to the facility and completed by the
admitting RN. All patients receive an Advance Directive Booklet upon admission

| | YES | NO |
|---|---|---|
| 1. Is the patient registering him/herself?<br><br>If NO, please give reason: | | |
| 2. Does the patient have an advance directive?<br><br>If NO, skip to question 5. | | |
| 3. Does the patient have a living will?<br><br>Has the patient supplied a copy of the living will?<br>Placed on chart by _____ Date/Time: _____ | | |
| 4. Does the patient have a durable power of attorney for health care?<br><br>Has the patient supplied a copy of the durable power of attorney for health care?<br>Placed on chart by _____ Date/Time: _____ | | |
| 5. Does the patient request additional information or wish to executre an advance directive at this time?<br><br>If YES, please consult Social Services, x 4435. | | |

Form completed by                                                                     Date   Time

Advance Directive Acknowledgement

Your
Hospital's
Logo
Here

### Hospital Dr  |  Princeton, ZZ 12345  |  T 202/555-1212  |  F 202/555-1212

# EMERGENCY
# DEPT RECORD

HOSPITAL #:

EMERGENCY ROOM #:

| PATIENT NAME: | Last | First | Middle | SEX: ☐ F  ☐ M | AGE: | ADMIN DATE: | TIME IN: |
|---|---|---|---|---|---|---|---|

| HEIGHT: | WEIGHT: | IMMUNIZATIONS CURRENT: ☐ Y  ☐ N | ALLERGIES: |
|---|---|---|---|

CONDITION ON ADMISSION:  ☐ Critical  ☐ Good  ☐ Fair  ☐ Stable  ☐ Guarded

BROUGHT IN BY:  ☐ Other_____  ☐ Self  ☐ Police  ☐ EMS  ☐ Family

BROUGHT IN BY:  ☐ Other_____  ☐ Amb  ☐ Stretcher  ☐ W/C  ☐ Parent's Arms

ER MD:                FAMILY MD:                LAST TETNUS:

| TIME: | | | | | CURRENT PRESCRIPTION MEDICATION | SIGNIFICANT MEDICAL HISTORY |
|---|---|---|---|---|---|---|
| TEMP | | | | | | |
| PULSE | | | | | | |
| RESP | | | | | | |
| B/P | | | | | | |
| PULSE OX | | | | | | PREGNANT? ☐ Y ☐ N |
| GCS | | | | | | _____ EDC  _____ FHT |
| TS | | | | | | LACTATING? ☐ Y ☐ N |

USED ANY OF THE FOLLOWING IN THE PAST 72 HRS?

| | Yes | No |
|---|---|---|
| OTC Meds | ☐ | ☐ |
| Herbs / Vitamins | ☐ | ☐ |
| Street Drugs | ☐ | ☐ |
| Alcohol | ☐ | ☐ |
| Tobacco | ☐ | ☐ |

If "Yes", name & amount:

NURSING ASSESSMENT AND HISTORY

**PHYSICAL FINDINGS**

PROBLEM ORIENTED PHYSICAL EXAM:

**LAB & X-RAY**

☐ CBC
☐ CHEM_____
☐ EKG

☐ CXR
☐ URINALYSIS  (Voided, CCMS, Cath)
☐ OTHER:

**DIAG**

**PHYSICIANS ORDERS and TX**

I _____

O _____

☐ Attending MD of Transfer / Admit
☐ Instruction Sheet Given

DISPOSITION OF CASE:
☐ Critical  ☐ Admitted:  RM#_____
☐ Guarded  ☐ Transferred _____
*FACILITY*

CONDITION ON DISCHARGE:
☐ Improved  ☐ Stable  ☐ Guarded
☐ Good  ☐ Critical  ☐ Deceased

MODE OF DISCHARGE:
☐ Ambulatory  ☐ W/C  ☐ Ambulance
☐ Parents Arms  ☐ Other_____  ☐ Stretcher

| TIME OF DISCHARGE: | PHYSICIAN'S SIGNATURE | DATE: | NURSE'S SIGNATURE: | DATE: |
|---|---|---|---|---|

**WHITE - Medical Records**          **GREEN - Family Physician**          **CANARY - Emergency Dept**

Emergency Department Record

**DIAMONTE HOSPITAL**
**Diamonte, Arizona**

**History**

(Page 1 of 2)

| | |
|---|---|
| Chief Complaint | |
| History of Present Illness | |
| History of Past Illness | |
| Family History | |
| Social History | |
| Review of Systems | |
| General | |
| Skin | |
| HEENT | |
| Neck | |
| Respiratory | |
| Cardiovascular | |
| GI | |
| GU | |
| GYN | |
| Neuropsychiatric | |
| Musculoskeletal | |

History

**DIAMONTE HOSPITAL**
**Diamonte, Arizona**

**Physical Exam**

(Page 2 of 2)

| Blood Pressure | Pulse | Resp. | Temp. | Weight |
|---|---|---|---|---|
| General | | | | |
| Skin | | | | |
| Eyes | | | | |
| Ears | | | | |
| Nose | | | | |
| Mouth | | | | |
| Throat | | | | |
| Neck | | | | |
| Chest | | | | |
| Heart | | | | |
| Abdomen | | | | |
| Genitalia | | | | |
| Lymphatic | | | | |
| Blood Vessels | | | | |
| Musculoskeletal | | | | |
| Extremities | | | | |
| Neurological | | | | |
| Rectal | | | | |
| Vaginal | | | | |
| **Diagnosis Plan of Care** | | | | |
| Signature | | | Date | |

○ *PLEASE PUNCH HERE* ○

| Diamonte Hospital<br>Phoenix, Arizona 12345-6789<br>Phone: (999) 123-XXXX Fax: (999) 123-XXXX | Patient Name Label |
|---|---|

### Physician's Order Form

| Date/<br>Time | Order | Physician's<br>Signature | Date/<br>Time | Nurse<br>Initials |
|---|---|---|---|---|
|  |  |  |  |  |
|  |  |  |  |  |
|  |  |  |  |  |
|  |  |  |  |  |
|  |  |  |  |  |

Physician's Order Form

○ *PLEASE PUNCH HERE* ○

| Diamonte Hospital<br>Phoenix, Arizona 12345-6789<br>Phone: (999) 123-XXXX Fax: (999) 123-XXXX | Patient Name Label |
|---|---|

### *Physician's Progress Notes*

| Date | Time | Progress note | Physician signature | Discipline |
|------|------|---------------|---------------------|------------|
|      |      |               |                     |            |
|      |      |               |                     |            |
|      |      |               |                     |            |
|      |      |               |                     |            |
|      |      |               |                     |            |
|      |      |               |                     |            |
|      |      |               |                     |            |
|      |      |               |                     |            |
|      |      |               |                     |            |
|      |      |               |                     |            |
|      |      |               |                     |            |
|      |      |               |                     |            |
|      |      |               |                     |            |
|      |      |               |                     |            |
|      |      |               |                     |            |
|      |      |               |                     |            |
|      |      |               |                     |            |
|      |      |               |                     |            |
|      |      |               |                     |            |

Physician's Progress Notes

**DIAMONTE HOSPITAL**
**Diamonte, Arizona**

**Informed Consent**

(example only)

**PATIENT CONSENT TO MEDICAL TREATMENT/SURGICAL PROCEDURE**
**AND ACKNOWLEDGMENT OF RECEIPT OF MEDICAL INFORMATION**

### READ CAREFULLY BEFORE SIGNING

**TO THE PATIENT:** You have been told that you should consider medical treatment/surgery. State law requires this facility to tell you (1) the nature of your condition, (2) the general nature of the procedure/treatment/surgery, (3) the risks of the proposed treatment/surgery, as defined by the state or as determined by your doctor, and (4) reasonable therapeutic alternatives and risks associated with such alternatives.

You have the right, as a patient, to be informed about your condition and the recommended surgical, medical, or diagnostic procedure to be used so that you may make the decision whether or not to undergo the procedure after knowing the risks and hazards involved.

In keeping with the State law of informed consent, you are being asked to sign a confirmation that we have discussed all these matters. We have already discussed with you the common problems and risks. We wish to inform you as completely as possible. Please read this form carefully. Ask about anything you do not understand, and we will be pleased to explain it.

1. Patient name: _____

2. Treatment/procedure:
   (a)  Description, nature of the treatment/procedure: _____
   _____
   Purpose: _____
   _____

3. Patient condition: Patient's diagnosis, description of the nature of the condition or ailment for which the medical treatment, surgical procedure, or other therapy described in Item 2 is indicated and recommended:
   _____
   _____

4. Material risks of treatment procedure:
   (a)  All medical or surgical treatment involves risks. Listed below are those risks associated with this procedure that members of this facility believe a reasonable person in your (patient's) position would likely consider significant when deciding whether to have or forego the proposed therapy. Please ask your physician if you would like additional information regarding the nature or consequences of these risks, their likelihood of occurrence, or other associated risks that you might consider significant but may not be listed below.

      - See attachment for risks identified by the State
      - See attachment for risks determined by your doctor

Page 2 of 3

    (b) Additional risks (if any) particular to the patient because of a complicating medical condition:

_____

_____

    (c) Risks generally associated with any surgical treatment/procedure, including anesthesia are death, brain damage, disfiguring scars, quadriplegia (paralysis from neck down), paraplegia (paralysis from waist down), the loss or loss of function of any organ or limb, infection, bleeding, and pain.

5. Therapeutic alternatives, risks associated therewith, and risks of no treatment:
Reasonable therapeutic alternatives and the risks associated with such alternatives:

_____

_____

**ACKNOWLEDGMENT**
**AUTHORIZATION AND CONSENT**

6. (a) No guarantees: All information given me and, in particular, all estimates made as to the likelihood of occurrence of risks of this or alternate procedures or as to the prospects of success are made in the best professional judgment of my physician. The possibility and nature of complications cannot always be accurately anticipated, and therefore there is and can be no guarantee, either express or implied, as to the success or other results of the medical treatment or surgical procedure.

    (b) Additional information: Nothing has been said to me, no information has been given to me, and I have not relied upon any information that is inconsistent with the information set forth in this document.

    (c) Particular concerns: I have had an opportunity to disclose to and discuss with the physician providing such information those risks or other potential consequences of the medical treatment or surgical procedure that are of particular concern to me.

    (d) Questions: I have had an opportunity to ask, and I have asked, any questions I may have about the information in this document and any other questions I have about the proposed treatment or procedure, and all such questions were answered in a satisfactory manner.

    (e) Authorized physician: The physician (or physician group) authorized to administer or perform the medical treatment, surgical procedures or other therapy described in Item 2 is

_____
(Name of authorized physician or group)

    (f) Physician certification: I hereby certify that I have provided and explained the information set forth herein, including any attachment, and answered all questions of the patient or the patient's representative concerning the medical treatment or surgical procedure, to the best of my knowledge and ability.

_____
(Signature of physician)                          Date                    Time

Informed Consent (cont'd)

**Consent**

I hereby authorize and direct the designated authorized physician/group, together with associates and assistants of his/her choice, to administer or perform the medical treatment or surgical procedure described in Item 2 of this consent form, including any additional procedures or services as they may deem necessary or reasonable, including the administration of any general or regional anesthetic agent, x-ray or other radiological services, laboratory services, and the disposal of any tissue removed during a diagnostic or surgical procedure, and I hereby consent thereto.

   I have read and understand all information set forth in this document, and all blanks were filled in prior to my signing. This authorization for and consent to medical treatment or surgical procedure is and shall remain valid until revoked.

   I acknowledge that I have had the opportunity to ask any questions about the contemplated medical procedure or surgical procedure described in Item 2 of this consent form, including risks and alternatives, and acknowledge that my questions have been answered to my satisfaction.

_____        _____

Witness                    Date/time          Patient or person            Date/time

                                                                           authorized to consent

If consent is signed by someone other than patient, indicate relationship: _____

Informed Consent (cont'd)

Your
Hospital's
Logo
Here

**CONSULTATION
RECORD**

| Consult Notified: | Date: _____ |
|---|---|
| TIME _____ <br> (Military Time) | Initials: _____ |
| ☐ Done by: _____ **MD** | |
| ☐ Fax: _____ | |
| ☐ Telephone: _____ | |
| ☐ Answering Svc: _____ | |

PATIENT IDENTIFICATION _____

TO CONSULTING SERVICE
AND / OR PHYSICIAN: _____

REASON FOR REQUEST _____

_____

_____    PLEASE CHECK:    ☐ **A**              ☐ **B**
SIGNATURE OF REQUESTING PHYSICIAN          DATE          WRITE ORDERS NOW    **DO NOT** WRITE ORDERS

REPORT _____

_____

_____

_____

_____

_____

_____

_____

_____

| | **DICTATED** | |
|---|---|---|
| | ☐ YES    ☐ NO | |

**TESTS, PROCEDURES, INTERVENTIONS, ETC. WHICH ARE FOR GENERAL DIAGNOSTIC USE AND WILL NOT ALTER THE
ACUTE INPATIENT MANAGEMENT, SHOULD BE PERFORMED AS AN OUTPATIENT WITH APPROPRIATE FOLLOW-UP.**

**RECOMMENDATIONS**

| INPATIENT | OUTPATIENT |
|---|---|
| | |
| | |
| | |
| | |
| | |
| | |
| | |
| | |

**IF ADDITIONAL SPACE REQUIRED, USE CONSULT ADDENDUM FORM  (S/N # 8850078)**

DATE          TIME                                    SIGNATURE OF CONSULTANT

WHITE - Medical Records          YELLOW - Attending Physician          PINK - Consultant

**PART OF THE MEDICAL RECORD**

RECOPIED BY: _____

DATE: _____

MILITARY TIME: _____

RN SIGNATURE/TITLE: _____

Page ____ of ____

ALL ENTRIES MUST BE PRINTED IN INK

Your Hospital's Logo Here

Your Hospital
Washington, DC

**MEDICATION ADMINISTRATION RECORD**

ALLERGIES

PATIENT IDENTIFICATION

| INITIAL ORDER DATE | RENEWAL DATE | MEDICATION, DOSE, FREQUENCY, ROUTE | MILITARY TIME | DATE | INITIAL | MILITARY TIME | DATE | INITIAL | DATE | MILITARY TIME | INITIAL | DATE | MILITARY TIME | INITIAL |
|---|---|---|---|---|---|---|---|---|---|---|---|---|---|---|

DATES

**SIGNATURE RECORD**

| INIT'L | SIGNATURE | TITLE | INIT'L | SIGNATURE | TITLE |
|---|---|---|---|---|---|

Medication Administration Record

## INSULIN ADMINISTRATION RECORD

### BLOOD GLUCOSE MONITORING

| DATE | TIME | LEVEL | INIT'L |
|------|------|-------|--------|
| | | | |

| INITIAL ORDER | RENEWAL DATE | MEDICATION, DOSE, FREQUENCY ROUTE | | | |
|------|------|------|------|------|------|
| | | | DATE | | |
| | | | TIME | | |
| | | | SITE | | |
| | | | INITIAL | | |

Insulin Administration Record

## ANALGESIC PAIN MANAGEMENT ASSESSMENT

| DATE | TIME | PAIN LOCATION | SEDATION RATING | PAIN SCALE | PAIN RATING | INTERVENTION | COMFORT GOAL | INIT'LS | REASSESSMENT PAIN RATING | TIME | INIT'LS |
|------|------|---------------|-----------------|------------|-------------|--------------|--------------|---------|--------------------------|------|---------|
| | | | | | | | | | | | |
| | | | | | | | | | | | |
| | | | | | | | | | | | |
| | | | | | | | | | | | |
| | | | | | | | | | | | |
| | | | | | | | | | | | |
| | | | | | | | | | | | |
| | | | | | | | | | | | |
| | | | | | | | | | | | |
| | | | | | | | | | | | |
| | | | | | | | | | | | |
| | | | | | | | | | | | |
| | | | | | | | | | | | |
| | | | | | | | | | | | |
| | | | | | | | | | | | |
| | | | | | | | | | | | |
| | | | | | | | | | | | |

ROOM #:    PATIENT Last Name:    PATIENT First Name:    Middle    DIAGNOSIS:    PHYSICIAN:

Analgesic Pain Management Assessment

**PAIN SCALES:**

**WONG-BAKER:**
*(Faces)*

0  1  2  3  4  5

**0-10 VISUAL:**
*(Numeric)*

0  1  2  3  4  5  6  7  8  9  10

**VERBAL:**

No Hurt  Hurts Little Bit  Hurts Little More  Hurts Even More  Hurts Whole Lot  Worst Pain

**NON-COGNITIVE:**

WONG-BAKER FACES PAIN SCALE from Wong DL, Hockenberry-Eaton M, Wilson D, Winkelstein ML, Ahmann E, DiVito-Thomas PA, Whaley & Wong Care of Infants & Children, 6th ed. St. Louis, MO, Mosby-Year Book Inc., 1999:1153, Copyrighted by Mosby-Year Book Inc. Reprinted with permission

**SEDATION SCALE:**

S = NORMAL SLEEP, EASY TO AROUSE, ORIENTED WHEN AWAKENED, APPROPRIATE COGNITIVE BEHAVIOR
1 = WIDE AWAKE - ALERT (OR AT BASELINE), ORIENTED, INITIATES CONVERSATION
2 = DROWSY, EASY TO AROUSE, BUT ORIENTED AND DEMONSTRATES APPROPRIATE COGNITIVE BEHAVIOR WHEN AWAKE
3 = DROWSY, SOMEWHAT DIFFICULT TO AROUSE, BUT ORIENTED WHEN AWAKE
4 = DIFFICULT TO AROUSE, CONFUSED, NOT ORIENTED
5 = UNAROUSABLE

**INTERVENTION:**

1 = Discuss Pain Management Plan with MD
2 = Pharmacological (See MED KARDEX)
3 = Non-Pharmacological
   A. Position Changed
   B. Relaxation Technique
   C. Splinting
   D. Imagery
   E. Music
   F. Education
   G. Other: _____

**FLACC SCALE:**
*(Non-Cognitive)*

1. Sum of FACE, LEGS, ACTIVITY, CRY AND CONSOLABILITY Scores = FLACC
2. Record FLACC Score using the 0-10 VISUAL (NUMERIC) Scale above

___ = FACE Score
0 = No particular expression or smile
1 = Occasional grimace or frown, withdrawn, disinterested
2 = Frequent to constant frown, clenched jaw, quivering chin

___ = LEGS Score
0 = Normal position, or relaxed
1 = Uneasy, restless, tense
2 = Kicking, or legs drawn up

___ = ACTIVITY Score
0 = Lying quietly, normal position, moves easily
1 = Squirming, shifting back and forth, tense
2 = Arched, rigid, or jerking

___ = CRY Score
0 = No crying (asleep or awake)
1 = Moans or whimpers, occasional complaint
2 = Crying steadily, screams or sobs, frequent complaints

___ = CONSOLABILITY Score
0 = Content, relaxed
1 = Reassured by touching/hugging/talking to, distractable
2 = Difficult to console or comfort

| DATE | TIME | MEDICATION | REASON FOR OMISSION | INIT'L | INIT'L |
|------|------|------------|---------------------|--------|--------|
|      |      |            |                     |        |        |
|      |      |            |                     |        |        |
|      |      |            |                     |        |        |
|      |      |            |                     |        |        |
|      |      |            |                     |        |        |
|      |      |            |                     |        |        |
|      |      |            |                     |        |        |
|      |      |            |                     |        |        |
|      |      |            |                     |        |        |
|      |      |            |                     |        |        |
|      |      |            |                     |        |        |

**SIGNATURE RECORD**

| SIGNATURE | TITLE |
|-----------|-------|
|           |       |
|           |       |
|           |       |
|           |       |

Analgesic Pain Management Assessment (cont'd)

## SINGLE ORDER / PRE-OPS

| INITIAL / ORDER DATE | MEDICATIONS / DOSE AND ROUTE OF ADMINISTRATION | SITE | GIVEN Date / Milit. Time | INIT'L |
|---|---|---|---|---|
| | | | | |
| | | | | |
| | | | | |
| | | | | |
| | | | | |
| | | | | |
| | | | | |
| | | | | |

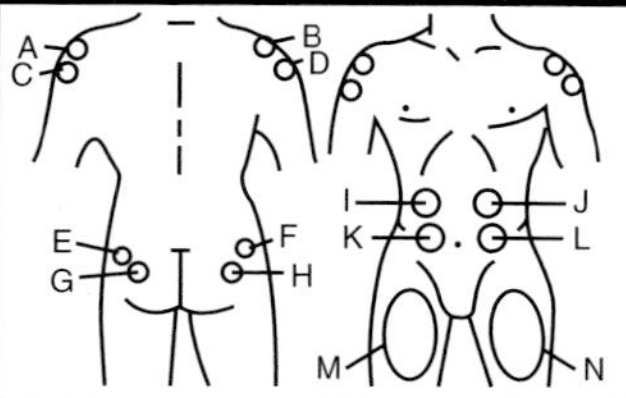
A
B
C
D
E
F
G
H
I
J
K
L
M
N

**EFFECTIVENESS:**

Y = YES N = NO

* If "NO", document interventions on Nurse's Notes

8850417 Rev. 08/06

## PRN / ANALGESIC PAIN MEDICATION ADMINISTRATION RECORD

| INITIAL | MEDICATION \| DOSAGE \| FREQUENCY ROUTE OF ADMINISTRATION | | | | | | | | | | | | | |
|---|---|---|---|---|---|---|---|---|---|---|---|---|---|---|
| Date Ord. / Exp. Date | | DATE | | | | | | | | | | | | |
| | | TIME | | | | | | | | | | | | |
| | | SITE | | | | | | | | | | | | |
| | | EFF | | | | | | | | | | | | |
| | | INIT'L | | | | | | | | | | | | |
| Date Ord. / Exp. Date | | DATE | | | | | | | | | | | | |
| | | TIME | | | | | | | | | | | | |
| | | SITE | | | | | | | | | | | | |
| | | EFF | | | | | | | | | | | | |
| | | INIT'L | | | | | | | | | | | | |
| Date Ord. / Exp. Date | | DATE | | | | | | | | | | | | |
| | | TIME | | | | | | | | | | | | |
| | | SITE | | | | | | | | | | | | |
| | | EFF | | | | | | | | | | | | |
| | | INIT'L | | | | | | | | | | | | |
| Date Ord. / Exp. Date | | DATE | | | | | | | | | | | | |
| | | TIME | | | | | | | | | | | | |
| | | SITE | | | | | | | | | | | | |
| | | EFF | | | | | | | | | | | | |
| | | INIT'L | | | | | | | | | | | | |
| Date Ord. / Exp. Date | | DATE | | | | | | | | | | | | |
| | | TIME | | | | | | | | | | | | |
| | | SITE | | | | | | | | | | | | |
| | | EFF | | | | | | | | | | | | |
| | | INIT'L | | | | | | | | | | | | |
| Date Ord. / Exp. Date | | DATE | | | | | | | | | | | | |
| | | TIME | | | | | | | | | | | | |
| | | SITE | | | | | | | | | | | | |
| | | EFF | | | | | | | | | | | | |
| | | INIT'L | | | | | | | | | | | | |
| Date Ord. / Exp. Date | | DATE | | | | | | | | | | | | |
| | | TIME | | | | | | | | | | | | |
| | | SITE | | | | | | | | | | | | |
| | | EFF | | | | | | | | | | | | |
| | | INIT'L | | | | | | | | | | | | |

Medication Administration Kardex_NURSING

Medication Administration Record (cont'd)

**DIAMONTE HOSPITAL**
Diamonte, Arizona

**Intake/Output
Record**

Date: _____

| Time AM/PM | IV Fluid/Rate | Absorbed 7AM-3PM | 3PM-11PM | 11PM-7AM | Comments: |
|---|---|---|---|---|---|
| | | | | | |
| | | | | | |
| | | | | | |
| | | | | | |
| | | | | | |
| | | | | | |
| | | | | | |
| | | | | | |
| | | | | | |
| | | | | | |
| | | | | | |
| | | | | | |

| INTAKE | | | | | | OUTPUT | | | | | |
|---|---|---|---|---|---|---|---|---|---|---|---|
| Time | Oral | Tube | IV | Blood | Total | Urine Voided | Catheter | Suction | Drains | Emesis | Total |
| 7AM-3PM | | | | | | | | | | | |
| 3PM-11PM | | | | | | | | | | | |
| 11PM-7AM | | | | | | | | | | | |
| Total | | | | | | | | | | | |

IV START/RESTART     Time: _____          IV START/RESTART     Time: _____

CATHETER SIZE# USED:          /                CATHETER SIZE# USED:          /

| TIME | APPEARANCE | SITE | |
|---|---|---|---|
| 7AM-3PM | | | |
| 3PM-11PM | | | |
| 11PM-7AM | | | |

| 7AM-3PM Shift | | 3PM-11PM Shift | |
|---|---|---|---|
| Initials | Signature/Title | Initials | Signature/Title |
| | | | |
| | | | |

| 11PM-7AM Shift | | | |
|---|---|---|---|
| Initials | Signature/Title | | |
| | | | |
| | | | |

Intake/Output Record

Your
Hospital's
Logo
Here

**NURSING PROGRESS NOTES**

**Print NAME and SIGN all entries**

Patient identification

| Abbreviations | | Date / Military Time | NOTES |
|---|---|---|---|
| DO NOT USE | USE | | |
| QD | Daily | | |
| QOD | Every other day | | |
| QID | 4 Times a day | | |
| U | Units | | |
| UG | MIcrogram | | |
| CC | mL | | |
| .2mg | 0.2 mg | | |
| 10.0mg | 10 mg | | |
| MS or MSO$_4$ | Morphine sulfate | | |
| MG or MgSO$_4$ | Magnesium sulfate | | |
| OS | Left eye | | |
| OU | Both eyes | | |
| OD | Right eye | | |
| AS | Left ear | | |
| AU | Both ears | | |
| AD | Right ear | | |

**PART OF THE MEDICAL RECORD**

Nursing Progress Notes

Operative Report Progress Notes

| Your Hospital's Logo Here | | Operative Report<br>**PROGRESS<br>NOTES**<br>**Print NAME and SIGN all entries** | | Patient identification |
|---|---|---|---|---|

| Abbreviations | | Date / Military Time | NOTES | |
|---|---|---|---|---|
| DO NOT USE | USE | | | |
| ~~QD~~ | Daily | | | |
| ~~QOD~~ | Every other day | | | |
| ~~QID~~ | 4 Times a day | | | |
| ~~U~~ | Units | | | |
| ~~UG~~ | Microgram | | | |
| ~~CC~~ | mL | | | |
| ~~.2mg~~ | 0.2 mg | | | |
| ~~10.0mg~~ | 10 mg | | | |
| ~~MS or MSO$_4$~~ | Morphine sulfate | | | |
| ~~MG or MgSO$_4$~~ | Magnesium sulfate | | | |
| ~~OS~~ | Left eye | | | |
| ~~OU~~ | Both eyes | | | |
| ~~OD~~ | Right eye | | | |
| ~~AS~~ | Left ear | | | |
| ~~AU~~ | Both ears | | | |
| ~~AD~~ | Right ear | | | |

**PART OF THE MEDICAL RECORD**

8850499 Rev. 05/05     Operative Report Progress Notes_MIH_MEDICAL AFFAIRS     PAGE 2 of 2

Operative Report Progress Notes (cont'd)

Your
Hospital's
Logo
Here

**DISCHARGE
ORDERS**

PATIENT IDENTIFICATION

DISCHARGE ORDERS FOR: _____

DISCHARGE PHYSICIAN: _____

**ACTIVITY:**  ☐ **NO RESTRICTIONS**  ☐ **RESTRICTIONS**

_____  _____

**MEDICATIONS**  Ejection Fraction: _____%  (CHF Patients only)

Ace Inhibitor: _____  _____

Beta Blocker: _____  _____

_____  _____

_____  _____

_____  _____

**TREATMENT/PAIN MANAGEMENT:**

_____  _____

_____  _____

_____  _____

**CALL YOUR DOCTOR IF YOU HAVE:**

_____  _____

_____  _____

_____  _____

**DIET:**

REGULAR _____ ** _____ CALORIE ADA _____ ** _____ Copy of diet given, as ordered by Physician

SOFT _____ ** _____ LOW SODIUM ** OTHER _____

**FOLLOW UP REFERRALS:**

Patient Education Booklet: _____

Home Care: _____

Return to MD: _____

Other: _____

**EQUIPMENT:** Supplies can be bought at: _____

**I HAVE RECEIVED THE ABOVE INSTRUCTIONS AND WAS GIVEN THE OPPORTUNITY TO ASK QUESTIONS**

_____  _____  _____

Discharging Physician's Signature    Date    Patient/Responsible Person's Signature

_____  _____

Physician's Phone    Discharging Nurse's Signature/Title

**WHITE** = Chart    **YELLOW** = Patient    **PINK** = Physician

**PART OF THE MEDICAL RECORD**

8850094 Rev. 05/05    Discharge Orders_NURSING_MEDICAL AFFAIRS    PAGE 1 of 1

Discharge Orders

**DIAMONTE HOSPITAL**
Diamonte, Arizona

**Nursing
Discharge Summary**

Patient Name:

Medical Record No.

(addressograph)

Date of discharge:_____ Time of discharge:_____ Accompanied by:_____
Disposition:_____ Home _____ Death _____Other (Please specifiy) _____
Discharged:_____ Ambulatory _____Wheelchair _____Stretcher _____Ambulance
Vital signs: Blood pressure:_____ Pulse:_____ Resp:_____ Temp:_____
Mental status:_____ Alert _____ Confused _____Other (specify)_____
Social worker: _____ Phone number: _____

<u>Services Needed</u>
**Equipment/Supplies:** Company:_____ Phone:_____
Type of service:_____ Date service is to start:_____

**Home Health:** Company:_____ Phone: _____
Type of service:_____ Date service is to start:_____

**Other:** Company:_____ Phone:_____
Type of service:_____ Date service is to start:_____

| **Medication** | **Dose** | **Time of Day** | **Special Instruction** |
|---|---|---|---|
| | | | |
| | | | |
| | | | |

_____ Medication/diet Counseling for above drugs, signature of dietitian_____ Date:_____
_____ Prescription given to patient _____ Medication from pharmacy returned_____Yes _____No

<u>Diet</u> _____Regular
_____ Other:_____ Diet Instructions: _____
_____ Signature of dietitian:_____Date:_____

<u>Treatment/Wound Care</u> _____ No treatments prescribed
Treatment/wound care
Site 1 _____
Site 2 _____
_____ Patient instructed _____Significant other Date:_____

<u>Activity</u>
_____ Special precautions: _____
_____ Gradually resume daily activities
_____ Do not lift object heavier than _____
_____ Use the following devices to move safely: _____
_____ Remain on bed rest except for: _____bathroom _____meals

<u>Follow-up</u>
_____ No appointment needed _____Patient teaching form discussed with patient/family
See doctor _____ on _____Phone _____ Appointment made: Yes/No
See doctor _____ on _____Phone _____ Appointment made: Yes/No
Call doctor if:_____
_____
I have received and understand the above instructions:
Patient signature:_____ Date:_____ Nurse signature:_____ Date:_____

Nursing Discharge Summary

TYPE/PRINT IN PERMANENT BLACK INK FOR INSTRUCTIONS SEE HANDBOOK

**CHILD**

**CERTIFIER/ATTENDANT**

DEATH UNDER ONE YEAR OF AGE
Enter State File Number of death certificate for this child

**MOTHER**

**FATHER**

**INFORMANT**

**MOTHER**

**FATHER**

MULTIPLE BIRTHS
Enter State File Number for Mates(s)
LIVE BIRTH (S)

FETAL DEATH (S)

**U.S. STANDARD**
**CERTIFICATE OF LIVE BIRTH**

LOCAL FILE NUMBER                               BIRTH NUMBER

1. CHILD'S NAME *(First, Middle, Last)* | 2. DATE OF BIRTH *(Month, Day, Year)* | 3. TIME OF BIRTH

4. SEX | 5. CITY, TOWN, OR LOCATION OF BIRTH | 6. COUNTY OF BIRTH

7. PLACE OF BIRTH: □ Hospital  □ Freestanding Birthing Center
□ Clinic/Doctor's Office        □ Residence
□ Other *(Specify)___*
8. FACILITY NAME *(If not institution, give street and number)*

9. I certify that this child was born alive at the place and time and on the date stated.
Signature ▶
10. DATE SIGNED *(Month, Day, Year)*
11. ATTENDANT'S NAME AND TITLE *(If other than certifier) (Type/Print)*
Name ___
□ M.D.  □ D.O.  □ C.N.M.  □ Other Midwife
□ Other *(Specify)___*

12. CERTIFIER'S NAME AND TITLE *(Type/Print)*
Name ___
□ M.D.  □ D.O.  □ Hospital Admin.  □ C.N.M.  □ Other Midwife
□ Other *(Specify)___*
13. ATTENDANT'S MAILING ADDRESS *(Street and Number or Rural Route Number, City or Town, State, Zip Code)*

14. REGISTRAR'S SIGNATURE ▶
15. DATE FILED BY REGISTRAR *(Month, Day, Year)*

16a. MOTHER'S NAME *(First, Middle, Last)* | 16b. MAIDEN SURNAME | 17. DATE OF BIRTH *(Month, Day, Year)*

18. BIRTHPLACE *(State or Foreign Country)* | 19a. RESIDENCE–STATE | 19B. COUNTY | 19c. CITY, TOWN, OR LOCATION

19d. STREET AND NUMBER | 19e. INSIDE CITY LIMITS? *(Yes or no)* | 20. MOTHER'S MAILING ADDRESS *(If same as residence, enter Zip Code only)*

21. FATHER'S NAME *(First, Middle, Last)* | 22. DATE OF BIRTH *(Month, Day, Year)* | 23. BIRTHPLACE *(State or Foreign Country)*

24. I certify that the personal information provided on this certificate is correct to the best of my knowledge and belief.
Signature of Parent of Other Informant ▶

INFORMATION FOR MEDICAL AND HEALTH USE ONLY

25. OF HISPANIC ORIGIN? *(Specify No or Yes—if yes, specify Cuban, Mexican, Puerto Rican, etc.)* | 26. RACE–American Indian, Black, White, etc. *(Specify below)* | 27. EDUCATION *(Specify only highest grade completed)*

| | | Elementary/Secondary (0-12) | College (1-4 or 5 +) |

25a. □ No  □ Yes  Specify: | 26a. | 27a.

25b. □ No  □ Yes  Specify: | 26b. | 27b.

28. PREGNANCY HISTORY *(Complete each section)*

| LIVE BIRTHS *(Do not include this child)* | | OTHER TERMINATIONS *(Spontaneous and induced at Any time after conception)* |

29. MOTHER MARRIED? (At birth, conception, or any time between) *(Yes or no)* | 30. DATE LAST NORMAL MENSES BEGAN *(Month, Day, Year)*

28a. Now Living  Number  □ None | 28b. Now Dead  Number  □ None | 28d.  Number  □ None

31. MONTH OF PREGNANCY PRENATAL CARE BEGAN  First, Second, Third, etc. *(Specify)* | 32. PRENATAL VISITS–Total Number *(If none, so state)*

28c. DATE OF LAST LIVE BIRTH *(Month, Year)* | 28e. DATE OF LAST OTHER TERMINATION *(Month, Year)*

33. BIRTH WEIGHT *(Specify unit)* | 34. CLINICAL ESTIMATE OF GESTATION *(Weeks)*

35a. PLURALITY- Single, Twin, Triplet, etc. *(Specify)* | 35b. IF NOT SINGLE BIRTH–Born First, Second, Third, etc. *(Specify)*

36. APGAR SCORE
36a. 1 Minute | 36b. 5 Minutes
37a. MOTHER TRANSFERRED PRIOR TO DELIVERY? □ NO  □ YES  If Yes, enter name of facility transferred from:

37b. INFANT TRANSFERRED? □ No  □ Yes  If Yes, enter name of facility transferred to:

Certificate of Live Birth

**38a. MEDICAL RISK FACTORS FOR THIS PREGNANCY**
*(Check all that apply)*

Anemia (Hct. < 30/Hgb. <101. . . . . . . . . . . . . . . . . 01 ☐
Cardiac disease . . . . . . . . . . . . . . . . . . . . . . . . . 02 ☐
Acute or chronic lung disease . . . . . . . . . . . . . . . 03 ☐
Diabetes . . . . . . . . . . . . . . . . . . . . . . . . . . . . . . 04 ☐
Genital herpes . . . . . . . . . . . . . . . . . . . . . . . . . . 05 ☐
Hydramnios/Oligohydramnios . . . . . . . . . . . . . . . 06 ☐
Hemoglobinopathy . . . . . . . . . . . . . . . . . . . . . . . 07 ☐
Hypertension, chronic . . . . . . . . . . . . . . . . . . . . 08 ☐
Hypertension, pregnancy-associated . . . . . . . . . . 09 ☐
Eclampsia . . . . . . . . . . . . . . . . . . . . . . . . . . . . . . 10 ☐
Incompetent cervix . . . . . . . . . . . . . . . . . . . . . . . 11 ☐
Previous infant 4000 + grams . . . . . . . . . . . . . . . 12 ☐
Previous preterm or small for-gestational-age
　infant . . . . . . . . . . . . . . . . . . . . . . . . . . . . . . . 13 ☐
Renal disease . . . . . . . . . . . . . . . . . . . . . . . . . . . 14 ☐
Rh sensitization . . . . . . . . . . . . . . . . . . . . . . . . . 15 ☐
Uterine bleeding . . . . . . . . . . . . . . . . . . . . . . . . . 16 ☐
None . . . . . . . . . . . . . . . . . . . . . . . . . . . . . . . . . 00 ☐
Other ＿＿＿＿＿＿＿＿＿＿＿＿＿＿＿＿ 17 ☐
　　　　　*(Specify)*

**38b. OTHER RISK FACTORS FOR THIS PREGNANCY**
*(Complete all items)*

Tobacco use during pregnancy . . . . . . . . . Yes ☐ No ☐
　Average number cigarettes per day ＿＿＿
Alcohol use during pregnancy . . . . . . . . . . Yes ☐ No ☐
　Average number drinks per week ＿＿＿
Weight gained during pregnancy ＿＿＿＿ lbs.

**39. OBSTETRIC PROCEDURES**
*(Check all that apply)*

Amniocentesis . . . . . . . . . . . . . . . . . . . . . . . . . . 01 ☐
Electronic fetal monitoring . . . . . . . . . . . . . . . . . 02 ☐
Induction of labor . . . . . . . . . . . . . . . . . . . . . . . . 03 ☐
Stimulation of labor . . . . . . . . . . . . . . . . . . . . . . 04 ☐
Tocolysis . . . . . . . . . . . . . . . . . . . . . . . . . . . . . . 05 ☐
Ultrasound . . . . . . . . . . . . . . . . . . . . . . . . . . . . . 06 ☐
None . . . . . . . . . . . . . . . . . . . . . . . . . . . . . . . . . 00 ☐
Other ＿＿＿＿＿＿＿＿＿＿＿＿＿＿＿＿ 07 ☐
　　　　*(Specify)*

**40. COMPLICATIONS OF LABOR AND/OR DELIVERY**
*(Check all that apply)*

Febrile (> 100ºF. or 38ºC.) . . . . . . . . . . . . . . . . . . 01 ☐
Meconium, moderate/heavy . . . . . . . . . . . . . . . . 02 ☐
Premature rupture of membrane (> 12 hours) . . . . 03 ☐
Abruptio placenta . . . . . . . . . . . . . . . . . . . . . . . . 04 ☐
Placenta privia . . . . . . . . . . . . . . . . . . . . . . . . . . 05 ☐
Other excessive bleeding . . . . . . . . . . . . . . . . . . 06 ☐
Seizures during labor . . . . . . . . . . . . . . . . . . . . . 07 ☐
Precipitous labor (< 3 hours) . . . . . . . . . . . . . . . 08 ☐
Prolonged labor (> 20 hours) . . . . . . . . . . . . . . . 09 ☐
Dysfunctional labor . . . . . . . . . . . . . . . . . . . . . . 10 ☐
Breech/Malpresentation . . . . . . . . . . . . . . . . . . . 11 ☐
Cephalopelvic disproportion . . . . . . . . . . . . . . . . 12 ☐
Cord prolapse . . . . . . . . . . . . . . . . . . . . . . . . . . . 13 ☐
Anesthetic complications . . . . . . . . . . . . . . . . . . 14 ☐
Fetal distress . . . . . . . . . . . . . . . . . . . . . . . . . . . 15 ☐
None . . . . . . . . . . . . . . . . . . . . . . . . . . . . . . . . . 00 ☐
Other ＿＿＿＿＿＿＿＿＿＿＿＿＿＿ 16 ☐
　　　　*(Specify)*

**41. METHOD OF DELIVERY** *(Check all that apply)*

Vaginal . . . . . . . . . . . . . . . . . . . . . . . . . . . . . . . . 01 ☐
Vaginal birth after previous C-section . . . . . . . . . . 02 ☐
Primary C-section . . . . . . . . . . . . . . . . . . . . . . . . 03 ☐
Repeat C-section . . . . . . . . . . . . . . . . . . . . . . . . 04 ☐
Forceps . . . . . . . . . . . . . . . . . . . . . . . . . . . . . . . . 05 ☐
Vacuum . . . . . . . . . . . . . . . . . . . . . . . . . . . . . . . 06 ☐

**42. ABNORMAL CONDITIONS OF THE NEWBORN**
*(Check all that apply)*

Anemia (Hct. < 39/Hgb. < 13) . . . . . . . . . . . . . . . 01 ☐
Birth injury . . . . . . . . . . . . . . . . . . . . . . . . . . . . . 02 ☐
Fetal alcohol syndrome . . . . . . . . . . . . . . . . . . . . 03 ☐
Hyaline membrane disease/RDS . . . . . . . . . . . . . 04 ☐
Meconium aspiration syndrome . . . . . . . . . . . . . 05 ☐
Assisted ventilation < 30 min . . . . . . . . . . . . . . . 06 ☐
Assisted ventilation ≥ 30 min . . . . . . . . . . . . . . . 07 ☐
Seizures . . . . . . . . . . . . . . . . . . . . . . . . . . . . . . . 08 ☐
None . . . . . . . . . . . . . . . . . . . . . . . . . . . . . . . . . 00 ☐
Other ＿＿＿＿＿＿＿＿＿＿＿＿＿＿ 09 ☐
　　　　*(Specify)*

**43. CONGENITAL ANOMALIES OF CHILD**
*(Check all that apply)*

Anencephalus . . . . . . . . . . . . . . . . . . . . . . . . . . . 01 ☐
Spina bifida/Meningocele . . . . . . . . . . . . . . . . . . 02 ☐
Hydrocephalus . . . . . . . . . . . . . . . . . . . . . . . . . . 03 ☐
Microcephalus . . . . . . . . . . . . . . . . . . . . . . . . . . 04 ☐
Other central nervous system anomalies
　*(Specify)* ＿＿＿＿＿＿＿＿＿＿＿＿ 05 ☐

Heart malformations . . . . . . . . . . . . . . . . . . . . . . 06 ☐
Other circulatory/respiratory anomalies
　*(Specify)* ＿＿＿＿＿＿＿＿＿＿＿＿ 07 ☐

Rectal atresia/stenosis . . . . . . . . . . . . . . . . . . . . 08 ☐
Tracheo-esophageal fistula/Esophageal atresia . . 09 ☐
Omphalocele/Gastoschisis . . . . . . . . . . . . . . . . . 10 ☐
Other gastrointestinal anomalies
　*(Specify)* ＿＿＿＿＿＿＿＿＿＿＿＿ 11 ☐

Malformed genitalia . . . . . . . . . . . . . . . . . . . . . . . 12 ☐
Renal agenesis . . . . . . . . . . . . . . . . . . . . . . . . . . 13 ☐
Other urogenital anomalies
　*(Specify)* ＿＿＿＿＿＿＿＿＿＿＿＿ 14 ☐

Cleft lip/palate . . . . . . . . . . . . . . . . . . . . . . . . . . 15 ☐
Polydactyly/Syndactyly/Adactyly . . . . . . . . . . . . 16 ☐
Club foot . . . . . . . . . . . . . . . . . . . . . . . . . . . . . . . 17 ☐
Diaphragmatic hernia . . . . . . . . . . . . . . . . . . . . . 18 ☐
Other musculoskeletal/integumental anomalies
　*(Specify)* ＿＿＿＿＿＿＿＿＿＿＿＿ 19 ☐

Down's syndrome . . . . . . . . . . . . . . . . . . . . . . . . 20 ☐
Other chromosomal anomalies
　*(Specify)* ＿＿＿＿＿＿＿＿＿＿＿＿ 21 ☐

None . . . . . . . . . . . . . . . . . . . . . . . . . . . . . . . . . 00 ☐
Other ＿＿＿＿＿＿＿＿＿＿＿＿＿＿ 22 ☐
　　　　*(Specify)*

Certificate of Live Birth (cont'd)

**U.S. STANDARD**
# CERTIFICATE OF DEATH

TYPE/PRINT IN PERMANENT BLACK INK FOR INSTRUCTIONS SEE HANDBOOK

LOCAL FILE NUMBER                                   STATE FILE NUMBER

**DECEDENT**

| 1. DECEDENT'S NAME *(First, Middle, Last)* | | | 2. SEX | 3. DATE OF DEATH *(Month, Day, Year)* |
|---|---|---|---|---|

| 4. SOCIAL SECURITY NUMBER | 5a. AGE–Last Birthday *(Years)* | 5b. UNDER 1 YEAR | | 5C. UNDER 1 DAY | | 6. DATE OF BIRTH *(Month, Day, Year)* | 7. BIRTHPLACE *(City and State or Foreign Country)* |
|---|---|---|---|---|---|---|---|
| | | Months | Days | Hours | Minutes | | |

| 8. WAS DECEDENT EVER IN U.S. ARMED FORCES? *(Yes or no)* | 9a. PLACE OF DEATH *(Check only one: see instructions on other side)* | | | |
|---|---|---|---|---|
| | HOSPITAL: ☐ Inpatient ☐ ER/Outpatient ☐ DOA | OTHER: ☐ Nursing Home ☐ Residence ☐ Other *(Specify)* | | |

| 9b. FACILITY NAME *(If not institution, give street and number)* | 9c. CITY, TOWN, OR LOCATION OF DEATH | 9d. COUNTY OF DEATH |
|---|---|---|

| 10. MARITAL STATUS–Married, Never Married, Widowed, Divorced *(Specify)* | 11. SURVIVING SPOUSE *(If wife, give maiden name)* | 12a. DECEDENT'S USUAL OCCUPATION *(Give kind of work done during most of working life. Do not use retired.)* | 12b. KIND OF BUSINESS/INDUSTRY |
|---|---|---|---|

**SEE INSTRUCTIONS ON OTHER SIDE**

| 13a. RESIDENCE–STATE | 13b. COUNTY | 13c. CITY, TOWN, OR LOCATION | 13d. STREET AND NUMBER |
|---|---|---|---|

| 13e. INSIDE CITY LIMITS? *(Yes or no)* | 13f. ZIP CODE | 14. WAS DECEDENT OF HISPANIC ORIGIN? *(Specify No or Yes–If yes, specify Cuban, Mexican, Puerto Rican, etc.)* ☐ No ☐ Yes Specify: | 15. RACE–American Indian, Black, White, etc. *(Specify)* | 16. DECEDENT'S EDUCATION *(Specify only highest grade completed)* |
|---|---|---|---|---|
| | | | | Elementary/Secondary (0-12) | College (1-4 or 5 +) |

**PARENTS**

| 17. FATHER'S NAME *(First, Middle, Last)* | 18. MOTHER'S NAME *(First, Middle, Last)* |
|---|---|

**INFORMANT**

| 19a. INFORMANT'S NAME *(Type/Print)* | 19b. MAILING ADDRESS *(Street and Number or Rural Route Number, City or Town, State, Zip Code)* |
|---|---|

**DISPOSITION**

| 20a. METHOD OF DISPOSITION ☐ Burial ☐ Cremation ☐ Removal from State ☐ Donation ☐ Other *(Specify)* ___ | 20b. PLACE OF DISPOSITION *(Name of cemetery, crematory, or other place)* | 20c. LOCATION–City or Town, State |
|---|---|---|

**SEE DEFINITION ON OTHER SIDE**

| 21a. SIGNATURE OF FUNERAL SERVICE LICENSEE OR PERSON ACTING AS SUCH | 21b. LICENSE NUMBER *(Of Licensee)* | 22. NAME AND ADDRESS OF FACILITY |
|---|---|---|

**PRONOUNCING PHYSICIAN ONLY**

| Complete items 23a-c only when certifying physician is not available at time of death to certify cause of death. | 23a. To the best of my knowledge, death occurred at the time, date, and place stated. Signature and Title ▶ | 23b. LICENSE NUMBER | 23c. DATE SIGNED *(Month, Day, Year)* |
|---|---|---|---|

ITEMS 24-26 MUST BE COMPLETED BY PERSON WHO PRONOUNCES DEATH

| 24. TIME OF DEATH | 25. DATE PRONOUNCED DEAD *(Month, Day, Year)* | 26. WAS CASE REFERRED TO MEDICAL EXAMINER/CORONER? *(Yes or no)* |
|---|---|---|

**CAUSE OF DEATH**

**SEE INSTRUCTIONS ON OTHER SIDE**

27. **PART I.** Enter the diseases, injuries, or complications that caused the death. Do not enter the mode of dying, such as cardiac or respiratory arrest, shock, or heart failure. List only one cause on each line.

Approximate Interval Between Onset and Death

**IMMEDIATE CAUSE** (Final deceased or condition resulting in death)

a. ___
DUE TO (OR AS A CONSEQUENCE OF:

Sequentially list conditions, if any, leading to immediate cause. Enter **UNDERLYING CAUSE** (Disease or injury that initiated events resulting in death **LAST**

b. ___
DUE TO (OR AS A CONSEQUENCE OF:

c. ___
DUE TO (OR AS A CONSEQUENCE OF:

d. ___

| PART II. Other significant conditions contributing to death but not resulting in the underlying cause given in Part I. | 28a. WAS AN AUTOPSY PERFORMED? *(Yes or no)* | 28b. WERE AUTOPSY FINDINGS AVAILABLE PRIOR TO COMPLETION OF CAUSE OF DEATH? *(Yes or no)* |
|---|---|---|

| 29. MANNER OF DEATH ☐ Natural ☐ Accident ☐ Suicide ☐ Homicide ☐ Pending Investigation ☐ Could not be Determined | 30a. DATE OF INJURY *(Month, Day, Year)* | 30b. TIME OF INJURY M | 30c. INJURY AT WORK? *(Yes or no)* | 30d. DESCRIBE HOW INJURY OCCURRED |
|---|---|---|---|---|
| | 30e. PLACE OF INJURY–At home, farm, street, factory, office building, etc. *(Specify)* | | | 30f. LOCATION (Street and Number or Rural Route Number, City or Town, State) |

**SEE DEFINITION ON OTHER SIDE**

**CERTIFIER**

31a. CERTIFIER *(Check only one)*

☐ CERTIFYING PHYSICIAN *(Physician certifying cause of death when another physician has pronounced death and completed item 23)*
To the best of my knowledge, death occurred due to the cause(s) and manner as stated.

☐ PRONOUNCING AND CERTIFYING PHYSICIAN *(Physician both pronouncing death and certifying to cause of death)*
To the best of my knowledge, death occurred at the time, date, and place, and due to the cause(s) and manner as stated.

☐ MEDICAL EXAMINER/CORONER
On the basis of examination and/or investigation, in my opinion, death occurred at the time, date, and place, and due to the cause(s) and manner as stated.

| 31b. SIGNATURE AND TITLE OF CERTIFIER ▶ | 31c. LICENSE NUMBER | 31d. DATE SIGNED *(Month, Day, Year)* |
|---|---|---|

| 32. NAME AND ADDRESS OF PERSON WHO COMPLETED CAUSE OF DEATH (ITEM 27) *(Type/Print)* |
|---|

**REGISTRAR**

| 33. REGISTRAR'S SIGNATURE ▶ | 34. DATE FILED *(Month, Day, Year)* |
|---|---|

PHS-T-003
REV. 1/89

NAME OF DECEDENT — For use by physician or institution

DEPARTMENT OF HEALTH AND HUMAN SERVICES • PUBLIC HEALTH SERVICE • NATIONAL CENTER FOR HEALTH STATISTICS • 1989 REVISION

Certificate of Death

TYPE/PRINT IN PERMANENT BLACK INK FOR INSTRUCTIONS SEE HANDBOOK

**U.S. STANDARD**
# REPORT OF FETAL DEATH

STATE FILE NUMBER

1. FACILITY NAME *(If not institution, give street and number)*

2. CITY, TOWN, OR LOCATION OF DELIVERY | 3. COUNTY OF DELIVERY | 4. DATE OF DELIVERY *(Month, Day, Year)* | 5. SEX OF FETUS

**PARENTS**

5a. MOTHER'S NAME *(First, Middle, Last)* | 5b. MAIDEN SURNAME | 7. DATE OF BIRTH *(Month, Day, Year)*

8a. RESIDENCE-STATE | 8b. COUNTY | 8c. CITY, TOWN, OR LOCATION | 8d. STREET AND NUMBER

8e. INSIDE CITY LIMITS? *(Yes or no)* | 8f. ZIP CODE | 9. FATHER'S NAME *(First, Middle, Last)* | 10. DATE OF BIRTH *(Month, Day, Year)*

| | 11. OF HISPANIC ORIGIN? *(Specify No or Yes—if yes, specify Cuban, Mexican, Puerto Rican, etc.)* | 12. RACE–American Indian, Black, White, etc. *(Specify)* | 13. EDUCATION *(Specify only highest grade completed)* Elementary/Secondary (0-12) / College (1-4 or 5 +) | 14. OCCUPATION AND BUSINESS/INDUSTRY *(Worked during last year)* Occupation / Business/Industry |

**MOTHER** | 11a. ☐ No ☐ Yes Specify: | 12a. | 13a. | 14a. | 14b.

**FATHER** | 11b. ☐ No ☐ Yes Specify: | 12b. | 13b. | 14c. | 14d.

*DEPARTMENT OF HEALTH AND HUMAN SERVICES • PUBLIC HEALTH SERVICE • NATIONAL CENTER FOR HEALTH STATISTICS • 1989 REVISION*

MULTIPLE BIRTHS Enter State File Number for Mate(s) LIVE BIRTHS

FETAL DEATH(S)

15. PREGNANCY HISTORY *(Complete each section)*

LIVE BIRTHS | OTHER TERMINATIONS *(Spontaneous and induced at Any time after conception)*

15a. Now Living Number ____ ☐ None | 15b. Now Dead Number ____ ☐ None | 15d. *(Do not include this fetus)* Number ____ ☐ None

15c. DATE OF LAST LIVE BIRTH *(Month, Year)* | 15e. DATE OF LAST OTHER TERMINATION *(Month, Year)*

16. MOTHER MARRIED? *(At delivery, conception, or any time between) (Yes or no)* | 17. DATE LAST NORMAL MENSES BEGAN *(Month, Day, Year)*

18. MONTH OF PREGNANCY PRENATAL CARE BEGAN  First, Second, Third, etc. *(Specify)* | 19. PRENATAL VISITS–Total Number *(If none, so state)*

20. WEIGHT OF FETUS *(Specify unit)* | 21. CLINICAL ESTIMATE OF GESTATION *(Weeks)*

22a. PLURALITY- Single, Twin, Triplet, etc. *(Specify)* | 22b. IF NOT SINGLE BIRTH–Born First, Second, Third, etc. *(Specify)*

**MEDICAL AND HEALTH INFORMATION**

23a. MEDICAL RISK FACTORS FOR THIS PREGNANCY *(Check all that apply)*
Anemia (Hct. < 30/Hgb. < 10). . . . . . . . . . . . . . 01 ☐
Cardiac disease . . . . . . . . . . . . . . . . . . . . . . . 02 ☐
Acute or chronic lung disease . . . . . . . . . . . . . 03 ☐
Diabetes . . . . . . . . . . . . . . . . . . . . . . . . . . . . 04 ☐
Genital herpes . . . . . . . . . . . . . . . . . . . . . . . . 05 ☐
Hydramnios/Oligohydramnios . . . . . . . . . . . . . 06 ☐
Hemoglobinopathy . . . . . . . . . . . . . . . . . . . . . 07 ☐
Hypertension, chronic . . . . . . . . . . . . . . . . . . . 08 ☐
Hypertension, pregnancy-associated . . . . . . . . . 09 ☐
Eclampsia . . . . . . . . . . . . . . . . . . . . . . . . . . . 10 ☐
Incompetent cervix . . . . . . . . . . . . . . . . . . . . .11 ☐
Previous infant 4000 + grams . . . . . . . . . . . . . 12 ☐
Previous preterm or small for-gestational-age infant . . . . . . . . . . . . . . . . . . . . . . . . . . . . 13 ☐
Renal disease . . . . . . . . . . . . . . . . . . . . . . . . 14 ☐
Rh sensitization . . . . . . . . . . . . . . . . . . . . . . . 15 ☐
Uterine bleeding . . . . . . . . . . . . . . . . . . . . . . 16 ☐
None . . . . . . . . . . . . . . . . . . . . . . . . . . . . . . 00 ☐
Other ____ 17 ☐
*(Specify)*

24. OBSTETRIC PROCEDURES *(Check all that apply)*
Amniocentesis . . . . . . . . . . . . . . . . . . . . . 01 ☐
Electronic fetal monitoring . . . . . . . . . . . . . 02 ☐
Induction of labor . . . . . . . . . . . . . . . . . . . 03 ☐
Stimulation of labor . . . . . . . . . . . . . . . . . . 04 ☐
Tocolysis . . . . . . . . . . . . . . . . . . . . . . . . . 05 ☐
Ultrasound . . . . . . . . . . . . . . . . . . . . . . . . 06 ☐
None . . . . . . . . . . . . . . . . . . . . . . . . . . . 00 ☐
Other ____ 07 ☐
*(Specify)*

25. COMPLICATIONS OF LABOR AND/OR DELIVERY *(Check all that apply)*
Febrile (> 100ºF. or 38ºC.) . . . . . . . . . . . . . 01 ☐
Meconium, moderate/heavy . . . . . . . . . . . . 02 ☐
Premature rupture of membrane (> 12 hours) . . . . 03 ☐
Abruptio placenta . . . . . . . . . . . . . . . . . . . 04 ☐
Placenta previa . . . . . . . . . . . . . . . . . . . . . 05 ☐
Other excessive bleeding . . . . . . . . . . . . . . 06 ☐
Seizures during labor . . . . . . . . . . . . . . . . . 07 ☐
Precipitous labor (< 3 hours) . . . . . . . . . . . . 08 ☐
Prolonged labor (> 20 hours) . . . . . . . . . . . . 09 ☐
Dysfunctional labor . . . . . . . . . . . . . . . . . . 10 ☐
Breech/Malpresentation . . . . . . . . . . . . . . . 11 ☐
Cephalopelvic disproportion . . . . . . . . . . . . 12 ☐
Cord prolapse . . . . . . . . . . . . . . . . . . . . . 13 ☐
Anesthetic complications . . . . . . . . . . . . . . 14 ☐
Fetal distress . . . . . . . . . . . . . . . . . . . . . . 15 ☐
None . . . . . . . . . . . . . . . . . . . . . . . . . . . 00 ☐
Other ____ 16 ☐
*(Specify)*

23b. OTHER RISK FACTORS FOR THIS PREGNANCY *(Complete all items)*
Tobacco use during pregnancy . . . . . . . . . Yes ☐ No ☐
Average number cigarettes per day ____
Alcohol use during pregnancy . . . . . . . . . . Yes ☐ No ☐
Average number drinks per week ____
Weight gained during pregnancy ____ lbs.

26. METHOD OF DELIVERY *(Check all that apply)*
Vaginal . . . . . . . . . . . . . . . . . . . . . . . . . . 01 ☐
Vaginal birth after previous C-section . . . . . . . . . . 02 ☐
Primary C-section . . . . . . . . . . . . . . . . . . . . . . 03 ☐
Repeat C-section . . . . . . . . . . . . . . . . . . . . . . 04 ☐
Forceps . . . . . . . . . . . . . . . . . . . . . . . . . . 05 ☐
Vacuum . . . . . . . . . . . . . . . . . . . . . . . . . . 06 ☐
Hysterotomy/Hysterectomy . . . . . . . . . . . . . . . 07 ☐

27. CONGENITAL ANOMALIES OF FETUS *(Check all that apply)*
Anencephalus . . . . . . . . . . . . . . . . . . . . . . . 01 ☐
Spina bifida/Meningocele . . . . . . . . . . . . . . . . 02 ☐
Hydrocephalus . . . . . . . . . . . . . . . . . . . . . . . 03 ☐
Microcephalus . . . . . . . . . . . . . . . . . . . . . . . 04 ☐
Other central nervous system anomalies *(Specify)* ____ 05 ☐
Heart malformations . . . . . . . . . . . . . . . . . . . 06 ☐
Other circulatory/respiratory anomalies *(Specify)* ____ 07 ☐
Rectal atresia/stenosis . . . . . . . . . . . . . . . . . . 08 ☐
Tracheo-esophageal fistula/Esophageal atresia . . 09 ☐
Omphalocele/Gastoschisis . . . . . . . . . . . . . . . . 10 ☐
Other gastrointestinal anomalies *(Specify)* ____ 11 ☐
Malformed genitalia . . . . . . . . . . . . . . . . . . . 12 ☐
Renal agenesis . . . . . . . . . . . . . . . . . . . . . . 13 ☐
Other urogenital anomalies *(Specify)* ____ 14 ☐
Cleft lip/palate . . . . . . . . . . . . . . . . . . . . . . . 15 ☐
Polydactyly/Syndactyly/Adactyly . . . . . . . . . . . . 16 ☐
Club foot . . . . . . . . . . . . . . . . . . . . . . . . . . 17 ☐
Diaphragmatic hernia . . . . . . . . . . . . . . . . . . 18 ☐
Other musculoskeletal/integumental anomalies *(Specify)* ____ 19 ☐
Down's syndrome . . . . . . . . . . . . . . . . . . . . . 20 ☐
Other chromosomal anomalies *(Specify)* ____ 21 ☐
None . . . . . . . . . . . . . . . . . . . . . . . . . . . . . 00 ☐
Other ____ 22 ☐
*(Specify)*

**CAUSE OF FETAL DEATH**

**Enter only one cause per line for a, b, and c.**

28.
**PART I.** Fetal or maternal condition directly causing fetal death.

{ IMMEDIATE CAUSE
a. ____ | Specify Fetal or Maternal

Fetal and/or maternal conditions, if any, giving rise to the immediate cause(s), stating the underlying cause lost.

{ DUE TO (OR AS A CONSEQUENCE OF):
b. ____ | Specify Fetal or Maternal
DUE TO (OR AS A CONSEQUENCE OF):
c. ____ | Specify Fetal or Maternal

**PART II.** Other significant conditions of fetus or mother contributing to fetal death but not resulting in the underlying cause given in Part I.

____

29. FETUS DIED BEFORE LABOR DURING LABOR OR DELIVERY, UNKNOWN *(Specify)*

30. ATTENDANT'S NAME AND TITLE *(Type/Print)*
Name ____
☐ M.D. ☐ D.O. ☐ C.N.M. ☐ Other Midwife
☐ Other *(Specify)* ____

31. NAME AND TITLE OF PERSON COMPLETING REPORT *(Type/Print)*
Name ____
Title ____

PHS-T-007

Report of Fetal Death

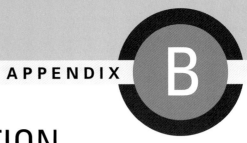

# ELECTRONIC DOCUMENTATION

## Sample Electronic Health Record

The following screen shots are examples of data collection within the electronic health record using the Web-based program Practice Fusion. This fully-functioning EHR software may be accessed by students at http://www.practicefusion.com.

- Patient demographic screen
- Allergy list
- Past medical history
- Diagnosis history
- Immunization record
- Current visit—vital signs
- SOAP note—subjective screen
- SOAP note—objective screen
- SOAP note—assessment screen
- SOAP note—plan screen
- E-prescribing
- SOAP note—finalization
- Patient visit record (migraine)
- Patient visit record (asthma)

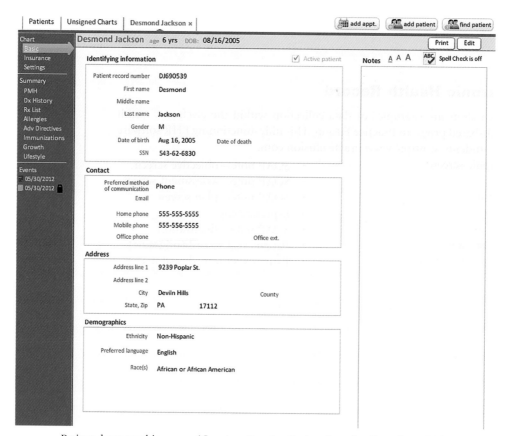

Patient demographic screen (Courtesy Practice Fusion, Inc., San Francisco, CA.)

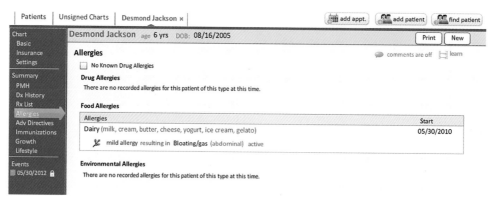

Allergy list (Courtesy Practice Fusion, Inc., San Francisco, CA.)

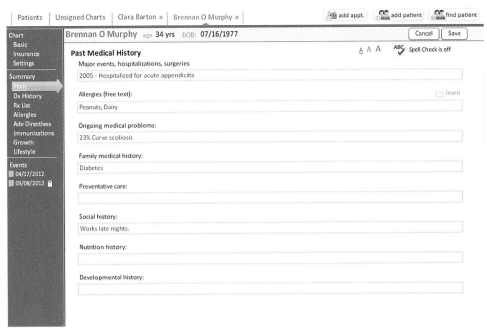

Past medical history (Courtesy Practice Fusion, Inc., San Francisco, CA.)

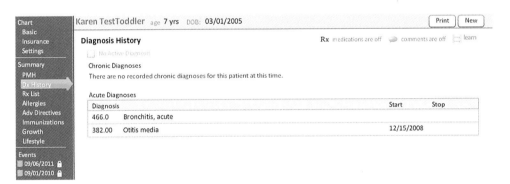

Diagnosis history (Courtesy Practice Fusion, Inc., San Francisco, CA.)

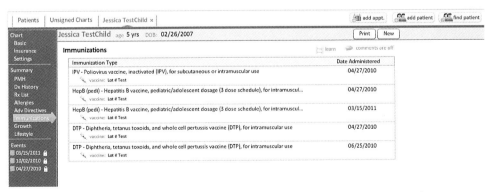

Immunization record (Courtesy Practice Fusion, Inc., San Francisco, CA.)

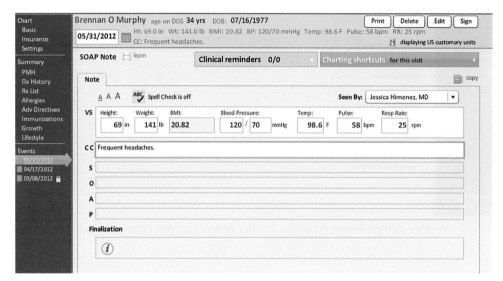

Current visit—vital signs (Courtesy Practice Fusion, Inc., San Francisco, CA.)

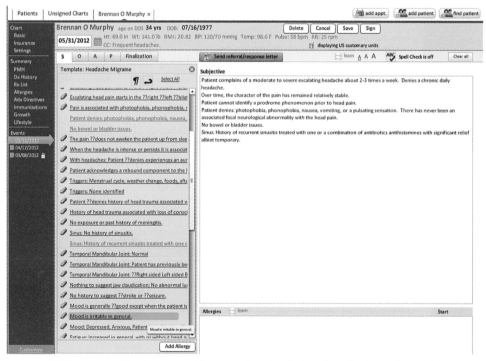

SOAP note—subjective screen (Courtesy Practice Fusion, Inc., San Francisco, CA.)

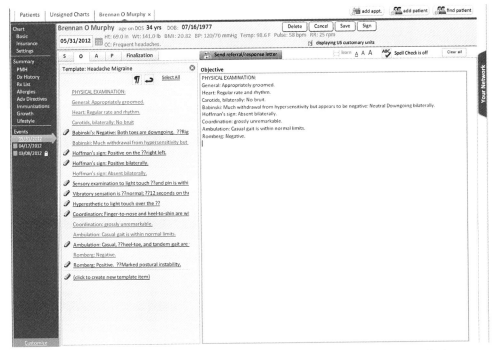

SOAP note—objective screen (Courtesy Practice Fusion, Inc., San Francisco, CA.)

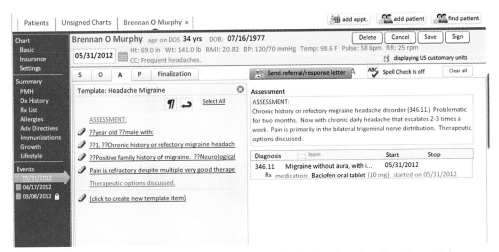

SOAP note—assessment screen (Courtesy Practice Fusion, Inc., San Francisco, CA.)

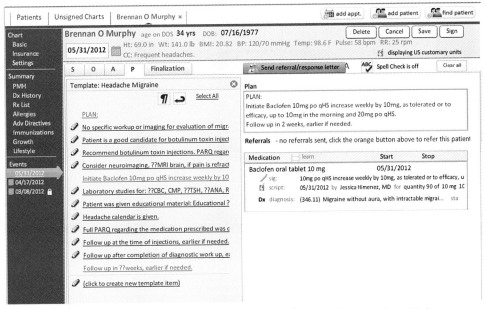

SOAP note—plan screen (Courtesy Practice Fusion, Inc., San Francisco, CA.)

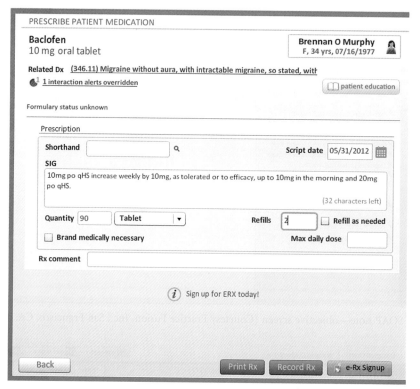

E-prescribing (Courtesy Practice Fusion, Inc., San Francisco, CA.)

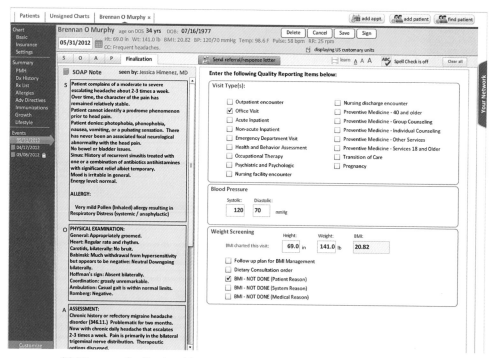

SOAP note—finalization (Courtesy Practice Fusion, Inc., San Francisco, CA.)

**Brennan Murphy (PRN: BM446656):**
**Signed SOAP Note for 05/31/2012**
Age on DOS: 34 yrs, DOB: 07/16/1977

**Diamonte Practice**
Phoenix, AZ
12345-6789

Seen by: Jessica Himenez, MD
Seen on: Thursday 31 May 2012

Signed by: Jessica Himenez, MD
Signed on: Thursday 31 May 2012 11:22 AM

**VS**

| Height: | Weight: | BMI: | Blood Pressure: | Temp: | Pulse: | Resp Rate: |
|---|---|---|---|---|---|---|
| 69.0 in | 141.0 lb | 20.8 | 120/70 mmHg | 98.6 F | 58 bpm | 25 bpm |

**CC** | Frequent headaches.

**S** | Patient complains of a moderate to severe escalating headache about 2-3 times a week.
Over time, the character of the pain has remained relatively stable.
Patient cannot identify a prodrome phenomenon prior to head pain.
Patient denies: photophobia, phonophobia, nausea, vomiting, or a pulsating sensation. There
has never been an associated focal neurological abnormality with the head pain.
No bowel or bladder issues.
Sinus: History of recurrent sinusitis treated with one or a combination of antibiotics antihistamines
with significant relief albiet temporary.
Mood is irritable in general.
Energy level: Normal.

ALLERGY:
   Very mild pollen (inhaled) allergy resulting in respiratory distress (systemic/ anaphylactic)

**O** | PHYSICAL EXAMINATION:
General: Appropriately groomed.
Heart: Regular rate and rhythm.
Carotids, bilaterally: No bruit.
Babinski: Much withdrawal from hypersensitivity but appears to be negative: Neutral Downgoing
bilaterally.
Hoffman's sign: Absent bilaterally.
Coordination: Grossly unremarkable.
Ambulation: Casual gait is within normal limits.
Romberg: Negative.

**A** | ASSESSMENT:
Chronic history or refectory migraine headache disorder (346.11.) Problematic for two months.
Now with chronic daily headache that escalates 2-3 times a week. Pain is primarily in the
bilateral trigeminal nerve distribution. Therapeutic options discussed.

DIAGNOSIS:
   Migraine without aura, with intractable migraine, so stated, without mention of status
migrainosus [346.11]

**P** | PLAN:
Initiate Baclofen 10mg po qHS increase weekly by 10mg, as tolerated or to efficacy, up to 10mg
in the morning and 20mg po qHS. Follow up in 2 weeks, earlier if needed.

MEDICATIONS:
   Baclofen oral tablet 10mg po qHS increase weekly by 10mg, as tolerated or to efficacy, up to
10mg in the morning and 20mg po qHS. (start date: 05/31/2012)
      Prescription: qty 90 of 10mg po qHS increase weekly by 10mg, as tolerated or to
efficacy, up to 10mg in the morning and 20mg po qHS. (2 refills)

Finalization
Office visit

31 May 2012 11:23 AM
page 1 of 2

Patient visit record (migraine) (Courtesy Practice Fusion, Inc., San Francisco, CA.)

**Desmond Jackson (PRN: DJ690539):**
**Signed SOAP Note for 05/30/2012**
Age on DOS: 6 yrs, DOB: 08/16/2005

**Diamonte Practice**
Phoenix, AZ
12345-6789

Seen by: Jessica Himenez, MD
Seen on: Wednesday 30 May 2012

Signed by: Jessica Himenez, MD
Signed on: Wednesday 30 May 2012 11:33 AM

**VS**

| Height: | Weight: | BMI:(%ile) | Blood Pressure: | Temp: | Pulse: | Resp Rate: |
|---|---|---|---|---|---|---|
| 48.0 in | 52.0 lb | 15.9(60%) | 120/80 mmHg | 98.6 F | 68 bpm | 20 rpm |

**CC** | Trouble breathing

**S** | Chest pain.

ALLERGY:
  Mild dairy allergy resulting in bloating/gas (abdominal)

**O** | General: Normotensive, in no acute distress.
Skin: Normal, no rashes, no lesions noted.
Head: Normacephalic, no lesions.
Ears: EAC's clear, TM's normal.
Nose: Mucosa normal, no obstruction.
Throat: Clear, no exudates, no lesions.
Neck: Supple, no masses, no thyromegaly, no bruits.
Chest: Lungs clear, no rales, no rhonchi, no wheezes.
Heart: RR, no murmurs, no rubs, no gallops.
Abdomen: Soft, no tenderness, no masses, BS normal.
Genitalia: Normal
Extremities: FROM, no deformities, no edema, no erythema.
Neuro: Physiological, no localizing findings.

**A** | DIAGNOSIS:
  Asthma, unspecified type, without mention of status asthmaticus [493.90]

**P** | MEDICATIONS:
  Proventil (albuterol) inhalation aerosol with adapter 90 mcg/inh 3 puffs as needed (start date: 05/30/2012)
        Prescription: qty 1 of 90 mcg/inh 3 puffs as needed (refill as needed)

Finalization
Outpatient encounter

Patient visit record (asthma) (Courtesy Practice Fusion, Inc., San Francisco, CA.)

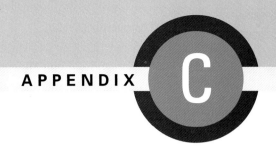

# MINIMUM DATA SET 3.0

| Overview of MDS 3.0 Items | | |
|---|---|---|
| Section | Title | Intent |
| A | Identification Information | Obtain key information to uniquely identify each resident, nursing home, and reasons for assessment. |
| B | Hearing, Speech, and Vision | Document the resident's ability to hear, understand, and communicate with others and whether the resident experiences visual, hearing, or speech limitations and/or difficulties. |
| C | Cognitive Patterns | Determine the resident's attention, orientation, and ability to register and recall information. |
| D | Mood | Identify signs and symptoms of mood distress. |
| E | Behavior | Identify behavioral symptoms that may cause distress or are potentially harmful to the resident or may be distressing or disruptive to facility residents, staff members, or the environment. |
| F | Preferences for Customary Routine and Activities | Obtain information regarding the resident's preferences for his or her daily routine and activities. |
| G | Functional Status | Assess the need for assistance with activities of daily living (ADLs), altered gait and balance, and decreased range of motion. |
| H | Bladder and Bowel | Gather information on the use of bowel and bladder appliances, the use of and response to urinary toileting programs, urinary and bowel continence, bowel training programs, and bowel patterns. |
| I | Active Disease Diagnosis | Code diseases that have a relationship to the resident's current functional, cognitive, mood or behavior status, medical treatments, nursing monitoring, or risk of death. |
| J | Health Conditions | Document health conditions that impact the resident's functional status and quality of life. |
| K | Swallowing/Nutritional Status | Assess conditions that could affect the resident's ability to maintain adequate nutrition and hydration. |
| L | Oral/Dental Status | Record any oral or dental problems present. |
| M | Skin Conditions | Document the risk, presence, appearance, and change of pressure ulcers as well as other skin ulcers, wounds or lesions. Also includes treatment categories related to skin injury or avoiding injury. |
| N | Medications | Record the number of days that any type of injection, insulin, and/or select medications was received by the resident. |
| O | Special Treatments and Procedures | Identify any special treatments, procedures, and programs that the resident received during the specified time periods. |
| P | Restraints | Record the frequency that the resident was restrained by any of the listed devices at any time during the day or night. |
| Q | Participation in Assessment and Goal Setting | Record the participation of the resident, family, and/or significant others in the assessment, and to understand the resident's overall goals. |
| V | Care Area Assessment (CAA) Summary | Document triggered care areas, whether or not a care plan has been developed for each triggered area, and the location of care area assessment documentation. |
| X | Correction Request | Indicate whether an MDS record is a new record to be added to the QIES ASAP system or a request to modify or inactivate a record already present in the QIES ASAP database. |
| Z | Assessment Administration | Provide billing information and signatures of persons completing the assessment. |

Resident _____ Identifier _____ Date _____

MINIMUM DATA SET (MDS) - Version 3.0
RESIDENT ASSESSMENT AND CARE SCREENING
*Nursing Home Comprehensive (NC) Item Set*

## Section A    Identification Information

**A0050. Type of Record**

Enter Code [ ]
1. Add new record → Continue to A0100, Facility Provider Numbers
2. Modify existing record → Continue to A0100, Facility Provider Numbers
3. Inactivate existing record → Skip to X0150, Type of Provider

**A0100. Facility Provider Numbers**

A. National Provider Identifier (NPI):
[ ][ ][ ][ ][ ]

B. CMS Certification Number (CCN):
[ ][ ][ ][ ]

C. State Provider Number:
[ ][ ][ ][ ]

**A0200. Type of Provider**

Type of provider

Enter Code [ ]
1. Nursing home (SNF/NF)
2. Swing bed

**A0310. Type of Assessment**

A. Federal OBRA Reason for Assessment

Enter Code [ ]
01. Admission assessment (required by day 14)
02. Quarterly review assessment
03. Annual assessment
04. Significant change in status assessment
05. Significant correction to prior comprehensive assessment
06. Significant correction to prior quarterly assessment
99. None of the above

B. PPS Assessment

PPS Scheduled Assessments for a Medicare Part A Stay

Enter Code [ ]
01. 5-day scheduled assessment
02. 14-day scheduled assessment
03. 30-day scheduled assessment
04. 60-day scheduled assessment
05. 90-day scheduled assessment
06. Readmission/return assessment

PPS Unscheduled Assessments for a Medicare Part A Stay
07. Unscheduled assessment used for PPS (OMRA, significant or clinical change, or significant correction assessment)

Not PPS Assessment
99. None of the above

C. PPS Other Medicare Required Assessment-OMRA

Enter Code [ ]
0. No
1. Start of therapy assessment
2. End of therapy assessment
3. Both start and end of therapy assessment
4. Change of therapy assessment

D. Is this a Swing Bed clinical change assessment? Complete only if A0200 = 2

Enter Code [ ]
0. No
1. Yes

A0310 continued on next page

---

Resident _____ Identifier _____ Date _____

## Section A    Identification Information - Continued

**A0310. Type of Assessment - Continued**

E. Is this assessment the first assessment (OBRA, Scheduled PPS, or Discharge) since the most recent admission/entry or reentry?

Enter Code [ ]
0. No
1. Yes

F. Entry/discharge reporting

Enter Code [ ][ ]
01. Entry tracking record
10. Discharge assessment-return not anticipated
11. Discharge assessment-return anticipated
12. Death in facility tracking record
99. None of the above

G. Type of discharge - Complete only if A0310 = 10 or 11

Enter Code [ ]
1. Planned
2. Unplanned

**A0410. Submission Requirement**

Enter Code [ ]
1. Neither federal nor state required submission
2. State but not federal required submission (FOR NURSING HOMES ONLY)
3. Federal required submission

**A0500. Legal Name of Resident**

A. First name:
[ ][ ][ ][ ][ ][ ][ ]

B. Middle initial: [ ]

C. Last name:
[ ][ ][ ][ ][ ][ ][ ]

D. Suffix: [ ]

**A0600. Social Security and Medicare numbers:**

A. Social Security number:
[ ][ ] - [ ][ ] - [ ][ ][ ][ ]

B. Medicare number (or comparable railroad insurance number):
[ ][ ][ ][ ][ ][ ][ ][ ][ ][ ][ ]

**A0700. Medicaid number** - Enter "+" if pending, "N" if not a Medicaid recipient
[ ][ ][ ][ ][ ][ ][ ][ ][ ][ ]

**A0800. Gender**

Enter Code [ ]
1. Male
2. Female

**A0900. Birth Date**

[ ][ ] - [ ][ ] - [ ][ ][ ][ ]
Month    Day    Year

**A1000. Race/Ethnicity**

→ Check all that apply
[ ] A. American Indian or Alaska Native
[ ] B. Asian
[ ] C. Black or African American
[ ] D. Hispanic or Latino
[ ] E. Native Hawaiian or Other Pacific Islander
[ ] F. White

Resident _____ Identifier _____ Date _____

| Section A | Identification Information |
|---|---|

**A1100. Language**

Enter Code ☐

A. Does the resident need or want an interpreter to communicate with a doctor or health care staff?
- 0. No
- 1. Yes → Specify in A1100B, Preferred language
- 9. Unable to determine

B. Preferred language: ☐☐☐☐☐☐☐☐☐☐☐

**A1200. Marital Status**

Enter Code ☐

1. Never married
2. Married
3. Widowed
4. Separated
5. Divorced

**A1300. Optional Resident Items**

A. Medical record number: ☐☐☐☐☐☐

B. Room number: ☐☐☐☐

C. Name by which resident prefers to be addressed: ☐☐☐☐☐☐☐☐

D. Lifetime occupation(s) - put "/" between two occupations: ☐☐☐☐☐☐☐☐

**A1500. Preadmission Screening and Resident Review (PASRR)**
Complete only if A0310A = 01, 03, 04, or 05

Enter Code ☐

Is the resident currently considered by the state level II PASRR process to have serious mental illness and/or intellectual disability ("mental retardation" in federal regulation) or a related condition?
- 0. No → Skip to A1550, Conditions Related to ID/DD Status
- 1. Yes → Continue to A1510, Level II Preadmission Screening and Resident Review (PASRR) Conditions
- 9. Not a Medicaid-certified unit → Skip to A1550, Conditions Related to ID/DD Status

**A1510. Level II Preadmission Screening and Resident Review (PASRR) Conditions**
Complete only if A0310A = 01, 03, 04, or 05

→ Check all that apply
- ☐ A. Serious mental illness
- ☐ B. Intellectual disability ("mental retardation" in federal regulation)
- ☐ C. Other related conditions

---

Resident _____ Identifier _____ Date _____

| Section A | Identification Information |
|---|---|

**A1550. Conditions Related to ID/DD Status**
If the resident is 22 years of age or older, complete only if A0310A = 01
If the resident is 21 years of age or younger, complete only if A0310A = 01, 03, 04, or 05

→ Check all conditions that are related to ID/DD status that were manifested before age 22 and are likely to continue indefinitely

ID/DD with Organic Condition
- ☐ A. Down syndrome
- ☐ B. Autism
- ☐ C. Epilepsy
- ☐ D. Other organic condition related to ID/DD

ID/DD without Organic Condition
- ☐ E. ID/DD with no organic condition

No ID/DD
- ☐ Z. None of the above

**A1600. Entry Date (date of this admission/entry or reentry into the facility)**

☐☐ - ☐☐ - ☐☐☐☐
Month - Day - Year

**A1700. Type of Entry**

Enter Code ☐

1. Admission
2. Reentry

**A1800. Entered From**

Enter Code ☐☐

- 01. Community (private home/apt., board/care, assisted living, group home)
- 02. Another nursing home or swing bed
- 03. Acute hospital
- 04. Psychiatric hospital
- 05. Inpatient rehabilitation facility
- 06. ID/DD facility
- 07. Hospice
- 09. Long-term care hospital (LTCH)
- 99. Other

**A2000. Discharge Date**
Complete only if A0310F = 10, 11, or 12

☐☐ - ☐☐ - ☐☐☐☐
Month - Day - Year

**A2100. Discharge Status**
Complete only if A0310F = 10, 11, or 12

- 01. Community (private home/apt., board/care, assisted living, group home)
- 02. Another nursing home or swing bed
- 03. Acute hospital
- 04. Psychiatric hospital
- 05. Inpatient rehabilitation facility
- 06. ID/DD facility
- 07. Hospice
- 08. Deceased
- 09. Long-term care hospital (LTCH)
- 99. Other

Resident _____ Identifier _____ Date _____

## Section A — Identification Information

**A2200. Previous Assessment Reference Date for Significant Correction**

Complete only if A0310A = 05 or 06

Enter Code ☐ [ ][ ] - [ ][ ] - [ ][ ][ ][ ]
Month — Day — Year

**A2300. Assessment Reference Date**

Observation end date:

[ ][ ] - [ ][ ] - [ ][ ][ ][ ]
Month — Day — Year

**A2400. Medicare Stay**

Enter Code ☐ **A. Has the resident had a Medicare-covered stay since the most recent entry?**
0. No → Skip to B0100, Comatose
1. Yes → Continue to A2400B, Start date of most recent Medicare stay

**B. Start date of most recent Medicare stay:**

[ ][ ] - [ ][ ] - [ ][ ][ ][ ]
Month — Day — Year

**C. End date of most recent Medicare stay** - Enter dashes if stay is ongoing:

[ ][ ] - [ ][ ] - [ ][ ][ ][ ]
Month — Day — Year

---

Resident _____ Identifier _____ Date _____

**Look back period for all items is 7 days unless another time frame is indicated**

## Section B — Hearing, Speech, and Vision

**B0100. Comatose**

**Persistent vegetative state/no discernible consciousness**

Enter Code ☐
0. No → Continue to B0200, Hearing
1. Yes → Skip to G0110, Activities of Daily Living (ADL) Assistance

**B0200. Hearing**

**Ability to hear** (with hearing aid or hearing appliances if normally used)

Enter Code ☐
0. **Adequate** - no difficulty in normal conversation, social interaction, listening to TV
1. **Minimal difficulty** - difficulty in some environments (e.g., when person speaks softly or setting is noisy)
2. **Moderate difficulty** - speaker has to increase volume and speak distinctly
3. **Highly impaired** - absence of useful hearing

**B0300. Hearing Aid**

**Hearing aid or other hearing appliance used** in completing B0200, Hearing

Enter Code ☐
0. No
1. Yes

**B0600. Speech Clarity**

**Select best description of speech pattern**

Enter Code ☐
0. **Clear speech** - distinct intelligible words
1. **Unclear speech** - slurred or mumbled words
2. **No speech** - absence of spoken words

**B0700. Makes Self Understood**

**Ability to express ideas and wants,** consider both verbal and non-verbal expression

Enter Code ☐
0. **Understood**
1. **Usually understood** - difficulty communicating some words or finishing thoughts **but** is able if prompted or given time
2. **Sometimes understood** - ability is limited to making concrete requests
3. **Rarely/never understood**

**B0800. Ability to Understand Others**

**Understanding verbal content, however able** (with hearing aid or device if used)

Enter Code ☐
0. **Understands** - clear comprehension
1. **Usually understands** - misses some part/intent of message **but** comprehends most conversation
2. **Sometimes understands** - responds adequately to simple, direct communication only
3. **Rarely/never understands**

**B1000. Vision**

**Ability to see in adequate light** (with glasses or other visual appliances)

Enter Code ☐
0. **Adequate** - sees fine detail, such as regular print in newspapers/books
1. **Impaired** - sees large print, but not regular print in newspapers/books
2. **Moderately impaired** - limited vision; not able to see newspaper headlines but can identify objects
3. **Highly impaired** - object identification in question, but eyes appear to follow objects
4. **Severely impaired** - no vision or sees only light, colors, or shapes; eyes do not appear to follow objects

**B1200. Corrective Lenses**

**Corrective lenses (contacts, glasses, or magnifying glass) used** in completing B1000, Vision

Enter Code ☐
0. No
1. Yes

Resident _____ Identifier _____ Date _____

| Section C | Cognitive Patterns |
|---|---|

**C0100. Should Brief Interview for Mental Status (C0200-C0500) Be Conducted?**

Attempt to conduct interview with all residents.

Enter Code ☐
- 0. **No** (resident is rarely/never understood) → Skip to and complete C0700-C1000, Staff Assessment for Mental Status
- 1. **Yes** → Continue to C0200, Repetition of Three Words

**Brief Interview for Mental Status (BIMS)**

**C0200. Repetition of Three Words**

Enter Code ☐
Ask resident: *"I am going to say three works for you to remember. Please repeat the words after I have said all three. The words are: sock, blue, and bed. Now tell me the three words."*

**Number of words repeated after first attempt**
- 0. None
- 1. One
- 2. Two
- 3. Three

After the resident's first attempt, repeat the words using cues ("Sock, something to wear; blue, a color; bed, a piece of furniture"). You may repeat the words up to two more times.

**C0300. Temporal Orientation** (orientation to year, month, and day)

Ask resident: *"Please tell me what year it is right now."*

Enter Code ☐
**A. Able to report correct year**
- 0. Missed by > 5 years or no answer
- 1. Missed by 2-5 years
- 2. Missed by 1 year
- 3. Correct

Ask resident: *"What month are we in right now?"*

Enter Code ☐
**B. Able to report correct month**
- 0. Missed by > 1 month or no answer
- 1. Missed by 6 days to 1 month
- 2. Accurate within 5 days

Ask resident: *"What day of the week is today?"*

Enter Code ☐
**C. Able to report correct day of the week**
- 0. Incorrect or no answer
- 1. Correct

**C0400. Recall**

Ask resident: *"Let's go back to an earlier question. What were those three words that I asked you to repeat?"* If unable to remember a word, give cue (something to wear; a color; a piece of furniture) for that word.

Enter Code ☐
**A. Able to recall "sock"**
- 0. No - could not recall
- 1. Yes, after cueing ("something to wear")
- 2. Yes, no cue required

Enter Code ☐
**B. Able to recall "blue"**
- 0. No - could not recall
- 1. Yes, after cueing ("a color")
- 2. Yes, no cue required

Enter Code ☐
**C. Able to recall "bed"**
- 0. No - could not recall
- 1. Yes, after cueing ("a piece of furniture")
- 2. Yes, no cue required

**C0500. Summary Score**

Enter Score ☐☐
**Add scores** for questions C0200-C0400 and fill in total score (00-15)
**Enter 99** if the resident was **unable to complete the interview**

---

Resident _____ Identifier _____ Date _____

| Section C | Cognitive Patterns |
|---|---|

**C0600. Should the Staff Assessment for Mental Status (C0700-C1000) Be Conducted?**

Enter Code ☐
- 0. **No** (resident was able to complete interview) → Skip to C1300, Signs and Symptoms of Delirium
- 1. **Yes** (resident was unable to complete interview) → Continue to C0700, Short-term Memory OK

**Staff Assessment for Mental Status**

Do not conduct if Brief Interview for Mental Status (C0200-C0500) was completed

**C0700. Short-Term Memory OK**

Enter Code ☐
Seems or appears to recall after 5 minutes
- 0. Memory OK
- 1. Memory problem

**C0800. Long-Term Memory OK**

Enter Code ☐
Seems or appears to recall long past
- 0. Memory OK
- 1. Memory problem

**C0900. Memory/Recall Ability**

→ Check all that apply
☐☐☐☐☐
- A. Current season
- B. Location of own room
- C. Staff names and faces
- D. That he or she is in a nursing home
- Z. None of the above were recalled

**C1000. Cognitive Skills for Daily Decision Making**

Enter Code ☐
Made decisions regarding tasks of daily life
- 0. **Independent** - decisions consistent/reasonable
- 1. **Modified independence** - some difficulty in new situations only
- 2. **Moderately impaired** - decisions poor; cues/supervision required
- 3. **Severely impaired** - never/rarely made decisions

**Delirium**

**C1300. Signs and Symptom of Delirium** (from CAM©)

Code after completing Brief Interview for Mental Status or Staff Assessment, and reviewing medical record

→ **Enter Codes in Boxes**

☐ **A. Inattention** - Did the resident have difficulty focusing attention (easily distracted, out of touch or difficulty following what was said)?

☐ **B. Disorganized thinking** - Was the resident's thinking disorganized or incoherent (rambling or irrelevant conversation, unclear or illogical flow of ideas, or unpredictable switching from subject to subject)?

**Coding:**
- 0. **Behavior not present**
- 1. **Behavior continuously present, does not fluctuate**
- 2. **Behavior present, fluctuates** (comes and goes, changes in severity)

**C. Altered level of consciousness** - Did the resident have altered level of consciousness (e.g., **vigilant** - startled easily to any sound or touch; **lethargic** - repeatedly dozed off when being asked questions, but responded to voice or touch; **stuporous** - very difficult to arouse and keep aroused for the interview; **comatose** - could not be aroused)?

**D. Psychomotor retardation** - Did the resident have an unusually decreased level of activity such as sluggishness, staring into space, staying in one position, moving very slowly?

**C1600. Acute Onset Mental Status Change**

Enter Code ☐
Is there evidence of an acute change in mental status from the resident's baseline?
- 0. No
- 1. Yes

Resident _____ Identifier _____ Date _____

| Section D | Mood |
|---|---|

**D0500. Staff Assessment of Resident Mood (PHQ-9-OV*)**
Do not conduct if Resident Mood Interview (D0200-D0300) was completed

**Over the last 2 weeks, did the resident have any of the following problems or behaviors?**

If symptom is present, enter 1 (yes) in column 1, Symptom Presence. Then move to column 2, Symptom Frequency, and indicate symptom frequency.

**1. Symptom Presence**
0. **No** (enter 0 in column 2)
1. **Yes** (enter 0-3 in column 2)

**2. Symptom Frequency**
0. **Never or 1 day**
1. **2-6 days** (several days)
2. **7-11 days** (half or more of the days)
3. **12-14 days** (nearly every day)

| | 1. Symptom Presence | 2. Symptom Frequency |
|---|---|---|
| ↓ Enter Scores in Boxes → | | |
| A. Little interest or pleasure in doing things | ☐ | ☐ |
| B. Feeling or appearing down, depressed, or hopeless | ☐ | ☐ |
| C. Trouble falling or staying asleep, or sleeping too much | ☐ | ☐ |
| D. Feeling tired or having little energy | ☐ | ☐ |
| E. Poor appetite or overeating | ☐ | ☐ |
| F. Indicating that s/he feels bad about self, is a failure, or has let self or family down | ☐ | ☐ |
| G. Trouble concentrating on things, such as reading the newspaper or watching television | ☐ | ☐ |
| H. Moving or speaking so slowly that other people have noticed. Or the opposite - being so fidgety or restless that s/he has been moving around a lot more than usual | ☐ | ☐ |
| I. States that life isn't worth living, wishes for death, or attempts to harm self | ☐ | ☐ |
| J. Being short-tempered, easily annoyed | ☐ | ☐ |

**D0600. Total Severity Score**
Enter Score ☐
Add scores for all frequency responses in Column 2, Symptom Frequency. Total score must be between 00 and 30.

**D0650. Safety Notification** - Complete only if D0500I1 = 1 indicating possibility of resident self-harm
Enter Code ☐
Was responsible staff or provider informed that there is a potential for resident self-harm?
0. **No**
1. **Yes**

---

Resident _____ Identifier _____ Date _____

| Section D | Mood |
|---|---|

**D0100. Should Resident Mood Interview Be Conducted?** - Attempt to conduct interview with all residents

Enter Code ☐
0. **No** (resident is rarely/never understood) → Skip to and complete D0500-D0600, Staff Assessment of Resident Mood (PHQ-9-OV)
1. **Yes** → Continue to D0200, Resident Mood Interview (PHQ-9©)

**D0200. Resident Mood Interview (PHQ-9©)**

Say to resident: *"Over the last 2 weeks, have you been bothered by any of the following problems?"*

If symptom is present, enter 1 (yes) in column 1, Symptom Presence. If yes in column 1, then ask the resident: *"About how often have you been bothered by this?"* Read and show the resident a card with the symptom frequency choices. Indicate response in column 2, Symptom Frequency.

**1. Symptom Presence**
0. **No** (enter 0 in column 2)
1. **Yes** (enter 0-3 in column 2)
9. **No response** (leave column 2 blank)

**2. Symptom Frequency**
0. **Never or 1 day**
1. **2-6 days** (several days)
2. **7-11 days** (half or more of the days)
3. **12-14 days** (nearly every day)

| | 1. Symptom Presence | 2. Symptom Frequency |
|---|---|---|
| ↓ Enter Scores in Boxes → | | |
| A. Little interest or pleasure in doing things | ☐ | ☐ |
| B. Feeling down, depressed, or hopeless | ☐ | ☐ |
| C. Trouble falling or staying asleep, or sleeping too much | ☐ | ☐ |
| D. Feeling tired or having little energy | ☐ | ☐ |
| E. Poor appetite or overeating | ☐ | ☐ |
| F. Feeling bad about yourself - or that you are a failure or have let yourself or your family down | ☐ | ☐ |
| G. Trouble concentrating on things, such as reading the newspaper or watching television | ☐ | ☐ |
| H. Moving or speaking so slowly that other people could have noticed. Or the opposite - being so fidgety or restless that you have been moving around a lot more than usual | ☐ | ☐ |
| I. Thoughts that you would be better off dead, or of hurting yourself in some way | ☐ | ☐ |

**D0300. Total Severity Score**
Enter Score ☐
Add scores for all frequency responses in Column 2, Symptom Frequency. Total score must be between 00 and 27. Enter 99 if unable to complete interview (i.e., Symptom Frequency is blank for 3 or more items).

**D0350. Safety Notification** - Complete only if D0200I1 = 1 indicating possibility of resident self-harm
Enter Code ☐
Was responsible staff or provider informed that there is a potential for resident self-harm?
0. **No**
1. **Yes**

Resident _____ Identifier _____ Date _____

| Section E | Behavior |
|---|---|

**E0100. Potential Indicators of Psychosis**

➤ Check all that apply

- A. Hallucinations (perceptual experiences in the absence of real external sensory stimuli)
- B. Delusions (misconceptions or beliefs that are firmly held, contrary to reality)
- Z. None of the above

☐ ☐ ☐

**Behavioral Symptoms**

**E0200. Behavioral Symptom - Presence & Frequency**

Note presence of symptoms and their frequency

➤ Enter Codes in Boxes

Coding:
0. Behavior not exhibited
1. Behavior of this type occurred 1 to 3 days
2. Behavior of this type occurred 4 to 6 days, but less than daily
3. Behavior of this type occurred daily

- ☐ A. Physical behavioral symptoms directed toward others (e.g., hitting, kicking, pushing, scratching, grabbing, abusing others sexually)
- ☐ B. Verbal behavioral symptoms directed toward others (e.g., threatening others, screaming at others, cursing at others)
- ☐ C. Other behavioral symptoms not directed toward others (e.g., physical symptoms such as hitting or scratching self, pacing, rummaging, public sexual acts, disrobing in public, throwing or smearing food or bodily wastes, or verbal/vocal symptoms like screaming, disruptive sounds)

**E0300. Overall Presence of Behavioral Symptoms**

Were any behavioral symptoms in questions E0200 coded 1, 2, or 3?

0. No → Skip to E0800, Rejection of Care
1. Yes → Considering all of E0200, Behavioral Symptoms, answer E0500 and E0600 below

Enter Code ☐

**E0500. Impact on Resident**

Did any of the identified symptom(s):

A. Put the resident at significant risk for physical illness or injury?
- 0. No
- 1. Yes

Enter Code ☐

B. Significantly interfere with the resident's care?
- 0. No
- 1. Yes

Enter Code ☐

C. Significantly interfere with the resident's participation in activities or social interactions?
- 0. No
- 1. Yes

Enter Code ☐

**E0600. Impact on Others**

Did any of the identified symptom(s):

A. Put others at significant risk for physical injury?
- 0. No
- 1. Yes

Enter Code ☐

B. Significantly intrude on the privacy or activity of others?
- 0. No
- 1. Yes

Enter Code ☐

C. Significantly disrupt care or living environment?
- 0. No
- 1. Yes

Enter Code ☐

Resident _____ Identifier _____ Date _____

| Section E | Behavior |
|---|---|

**E0800. Rejection of Care - Presence & Frequency**

Did the resident reject evaluation or care (e.g., bloodwork, taking medications, ADL assistance) that is necessary to achieve the resident's goals for health and well-being? Do not include behaviors that have already been addressed (e.g., by discussion or care planning with the resident or family), and determined to be consistent with resident values, preferences, or goals.

0. Behavior not exhibited
1. Behavior of this type occurred 1 to 3 days
2. Behavior of this type occurred 4 to 6 days, but less than daily
3. Behavior of this type occurred daily

Enter Code ☐

**E0900. Wandering - Presence & Frequency**

Has the resident wandered?

0. Behavior not exhibited → Skip to E1100, Change in Behavioral or Other Symptoms
1. Behavior of this type occurred 1 to 3 days
2. Behavior of this type occurred 4 to 6 days, but less than daily
3. Behavior of this type occurred daily

Enter Code ☐

**E1000. Wandering - Impact**

A. Does the wandering place the resident at significant risk of getting to a potentially dangerous place (e.g., stairs, outside of the facility)?
- 0. No
- 1. Yes

Enter Code ☐

B. Does the wandering significantly intrude on the privacy or activities of others?
- 0. No
- 1. Yes

Enter Code ☐

**E1100. Change in Behavior or Other Symptoms**

Consider all of the symptoms assessed in items E0100 through E1000

How does resident's current behavior status, care rejection, or wandering compare to prior assessment (OBRA or Scheduled PPS)?
- 0. Same
- 1. Improved
- 2. Worse
- 3. N/A because no prior MDS assessment

Enter Code ☐

Resident _____ Identifier _____ Date _____

| Section F | Preferences for Customary Routine and Activities |
|---|---|

**F0300. Should Interview for Daily and Activity Preferences Be Conducted?** - Attempt to interview all residents able to communicate. If resident is unable to complete, attempt to complete interview with family member or significant other.

Enter Code ☐
- 0. **No** (resident is rarely/never understood and family/significant other not available) → Skip to and complete F0800, Staff Assessment of Daily and Activity Preferences
- 1. **Yes** → Continue to F0400, Interview for Daily Preferences

**F0400. Interview for Daily Preferences**

Show resident the response options and say: **"While you are in this facility..."**

→ Enter Codes in Boxes

| | |
|---|---|
| ☐ | A. How important is it to you to **choose what clothes to wear?** |
| ☐ | B. How important is it to you to **take care of your personal belongings or things?** |
| ☐ | C. How important is it to you to **choose between a tub bath, shower, bed bath, or sponge bath?** |
| ☐ | D. How important is it to you to **have snacks available between meals?** |
| ☐ | E. How important is it to you to **choose your own bedtime?** |
| ☐ | F. How important is it to you to **have your family or a close friend involved in discussions about your care?** |
| ☐ | G. How important is it to you to **be able to use the phone in private?** |
| ☐ | H. How important is it to you to **have a place to lock your things to keep them safe?** |

**Coding:**
1. Very important
2. Somewhat important
3. Not very important
4. Not important at all
5. Important, but can't do or no choice
9. No response or non-responsive

**F0500. Interview for Activity Preferences**

Show resident the response options and say: **"While you are in this facility..."**

| | |
|---|---|
| ☐ | A. How important is it to you to **have books, newspapers, and magazines to read?** |
| ☐ | B. How important is it to you to **listen to music you like?** |
| ☐ | C. How important is it to you to **be around animals such as pets?** |
| ☐ | D. How important is it to you to **keep up with the news?** |
| ☐ | E. How important is it to you to **do things with groups of people?** |
| ☐ | F. How important is it to you to **do your favorite activities?** |
| ☐ | G. How important is it to you to **go outside to get fresh air when the weather is good?** |
| ☐ | H. How important is it to you to **participate in religious services or practices?** |

**Coding:**
1. Very important
2. Somewhat important
3. Not very important
4. Not important at all
5. Important, but can't do or no choice
9. No response or non-responsive

**F0600. Daily and Activity Preferences Primary Respondent**

Indicate primary respondent for Daily and Activity Preferences (F0400 and "F0500)

Enter Code ☐
1. Resident
2. Family or significant other (close friend or other representative)
9. Interview could not be completed by resident or family/significant other ("No response" to 3 or more items)

---

Resident _____ Identifier _____ Date _____

| Section F | Preferences for Customary Routine and Activities |
|---|---|

**F0700. Should the Staff Assessment of Daily and Activity Preferences Be Conducted?**

Enter Code ☐
- 0. **No** (because Interview for Daily and Activity Preferences [F0400 and F0500] was completed by resident or family/significant other) → Skip to and complete G0110, Activities of Daily Living (ADL) Assistance.
- 1. **Yes** (because 3 or more items in Interview for Daily and Activity Preferences [F0400 and F0500] were not completed by resident or family/significant other) → Continue to F0800, Staff Assessment of Daily and Activity Preferences

**F0800. Staff Assessment of Daily and Activity Preferences**

Do not conduct if Interview for Daily and Activity Preferences (F0400-F0500) was completed.

**Resident Prefers:**

→ Check all that apply.

| | |
|---|---|
| ☐ | A. Choosing clothes to wear |
| ☐ | B. Caring for personal belongings |
| ☐ | C. Receiving tub bath |
| ☐ | D. Receiving shower |
| ☐ | E. Receiving bed bath |
| ☐ | F. Receiving sponge bath |
| ☐ | G. Snacks between meals |
| ☐ | H. Staying up past 8:00 p.m. |
| ☐ | I. Family or significant other involvement in care discussions |
| ☐ | J. Use of phone in private |
| ☐ | K. Place to lock personal belongings |
| ☐ | L. Reading books, newspapers, or magazines |
| ☐ | M. Listening to music |
| ☐ | N. Being around animals such as pets |
| ☐ | O. Keeping up with the news |
| ☐ | P. Doing things with groups of people |
| ☐ | Q. Participating in favorite activities |
| ☐ | R. Spending time away from the nursing home |
| ☐ | S. Spending time outdoors |
| ☐ | T. Participating in religious activities or practices |
| ☐ | Z. None of the above |

Resident _____ Identifier _____ Date _____

| Section G | Functional Status |
|---|---|

**G0110. Activities of Daily Living (ADL) Assistance**

Refer to the ADL flow chart in the RAI manual to facilitate accurate coding

**Instructions for Rule of 3**
- When an activity occurs three times at any one given level, code that level.
- When an activity occurs three times at multiple levels, code the most dependent, exceptions are total dependence (4), activity must require full assist every time, and activity did not occur (8), activity must not have occurred at all. Example, three times extensive assistance (3) and three times limited assistance (2), code extensive assistance (3).
- When an activity occurs at various levels, but not three times at any given level, apply the following:
  ○ When there is a combination of full staff performance, and extensive assistance, code extensive assistance.
  ○ When there is a combination of full staff performance, weight-bearing assistance and/or non-weight-bearing assistance code limited assistance (2).

**If none of the above are met, code supervision.**

| **1. ADL Self-Performance** | **2. ADL Support Provided** |
|---|---|
| Code for **resident's performance** over all shifts - not including setup. If the ADL activity occurred 3 or more times at various levels of assistance, code the most dependent - except for total dependence, which requires full staff performance every time. | Code for **most support provided** over all shifts; code regardless of resident's self-performance classification |

**Coding:**

**Activity Occurred 3 or More Times**
0. **Independent** - no help or staff oversight at any time
1. **Supervision** - oversight, encouragement or cueing
2. **Limited assistance** - resident highly involved in activity; staff provide guided maneuvering of limbs or other non–weight-bearing assistance
3. **Extensive assistance** - resident involved in activity, staff provide weight-bearing support
4. **Total dependence** - full staff performance every time during entire 7-day period

**Activity Occurred 2 or Fewer Times**
7. **Activity occurred only once or twice** - activity did occur but only once or twice
8. **Activity did not occur** - activity did not occur or family non-facility staff provided care 100% of the time for that activity over the entire 7-day period

**Coding:**
0. **No setup or physical help from staff**
1. **Setup help only**
2. **One person physical assist**
3. **Two+ persons physical assist**
8. **ADL activity did not occur or family or non-facility staff provided care 100% of the time for that activity over the entire 7-day period**

| | 1. Self-Performance | 2. Support |
|---|---|---|
| | ↓ Enter Codes in Boxes → | |
| **A.** Bed mobility - how resident moves to and from lying position, turns side to side, and positions body while in bed or alternate sleep furniture | ☐ | ☐ |
| **B.** Transfer - how resident moves between surfaces including to or from: bed, chair, wheelchair, standing position (**excludes** to/from bath/toilet) | ☐ | ☐ |
| **C.** Walk in room - how resident walks between locations in his/her room | ☐ | ☐ |
| **D.** Walk in corridor - how resident walks in corridor on unit | ☐ | ☐ |
| **E.** Locomotion on unit - how resident moves between locations in his/her room and adjacent corridor on same floor. If in wheelchair, self-sufficiency once in chair | ☐ | ☐ |
| **F.** Locomotion off unit - how resident moves to and returns from off-unit locations (e.g., areas set aside for dining, activities or treatments). **If facility has only one floor,** how resident moves to and from distant areas on the floor. If in wheelchair, self-sufficiency once in chair | ☐ | ☐ |
| **G.** Dressing - how resident puts on, fastens, and takes off all items of clothing, including donning/removing a prosthesis or TED hose. Dressing includes putting on and changing pajamas and housedresses | ☐ | ☐ |
| **H.** Eating - how resident eats and drinks, regardless of skill. Do not include eating/drinking during medication pass. Includes intake of nourishment by other means (e.g., tube feeding, total parenteral nutrition, IV fluids administered for nutrition or hydration) | ☐ | ☐ |
| **I.** Toilet use - how resident uses the toilet room, commode, bedpan, or urinal; transfers on/off toilet; cleanses self after elimination; changes pad; manages ostomy or catheter; and adjusts clothes. Do not include emptying of bedpan, urinal, bedside commode, catheter bag or ostomy bag | ☐ | ☐ |
| **J.** Personal hygiene - how resident maintains personal hygiene, including combing hair, brushing teeth, shaving, applying makeup, washing/drying face and hands (**excludes** baths and showers) | ☐ | ☐ |

---

Resident _____ Identifier _____ Date _____

| Section G | Functional Status |
|---|---|

**G0120. Bathing**

How resident takes full-body bath/shower, sponge bath, and transfers in/out of tub/shower (**excludes** washing of back and hair). Code for **most dependent** in self-performance and support

Enter Code ☐

**A. Self-performance**
0. **Independent** - no help provided
1. **Supervision** - oversight help only
2. **Physical help limited to transfer only**
3. **Physical help in part of bathing activity**
4. **Total dependence**
8. **Activity itself did not occur** or family and/or non-facility staff provided care 100% of the time for that activity over the entire 7-day period

**B. Support provided**
(Bathing support codes are as defined in item G0110 column 2, ADL Support Provided, above)

Enter Code ☐

**G0300. Balance During Transitions and Walking**

After observing the resident, **code the following walking and transition items for most dependent**

→ Enter Codes in Boxes

| | |
|---|---|
| **A. Moving from seated to standing position** | ☐ |
| **B. Walking** (with assistive device if used) | ☐ |
| **C. Turning around** and facing the opposite direction while walking | ☐ |
| **D. Moving on and off toilet** | ☐ |
| **E. Surface-to-surface transfer** (transfer between bed and chair or wheelchair) | ☐ |

**Coding:**
0. **Steady at all times**
1. **Not steady, but able to stabilize without staff assistance**
2. **Not steady, only able to stabilize with staff assistance**
8. **Activity did not occur**

**G0400. Functional Limitation in Range of Motion**

Code for limitation that interfered with daily functions or placed resident at risk of injury

→ Enter Codes in Boxes

| | |
|---|---|
| **A. Upper extremity** (shoulder, elbow, wrist, hand) | ☐ |
| **B. Lower extremity** (hip, knee, ankle, foot) | ☐ |

**Coding:**
0. **No impairment**
1. **Impairment on one side**
2. **Impairment on both sides**

**G0600. Mobility Devices**

→ Check all that were normally used

☐ **A. Cane/crutch**
☐ **B. Walker**
☐ **C. Wheelchair** (manual or electric)
☐ **D. Limb prosthesis**
☐ **Z. None of the above** were used

**G0900. Functional Rehabilitation Potential** Complete only if A0310A = 01

Enter Code ☐

**A. Resident believes he or she is capable of increased independence** in at least some ADLs
0. **No**
1. **Yes**
9. **Unable to determine**

Enter Code ☐

**B. Direct care staff believe resident is capable of increased independence** in at least some ADLs
0. **No**
1. **Yes**

Resident _____ Identifier _____ Date _____

## Section I — Active Diagnoses

**Active Diagnoses in the last 7 days - Check all that apply**
Diagnoses listed in parentheses are provided as examples and should not be considered as all-inclusive lists

**Cancer**
- ☐ I0100. Cancer (with or without metastasis)

**Heart/Circulation**
- ☐ I0200. Anemia (e.g., aplastic, iron deficiency, pernicious, and sickle cell)
- ☐ I0300. Atrial Fibrillation or Other Dysrhythmias (e.g., bradycardias and tachycardias)
- ☐ I0400. Coronary Artery Disease (CAD) (e.g., angina, myocardial infarction, and atherosclerotic heart disease [ASHD])
- ☐ I0500. Deep Venous Thrombosis (DVT), Pulmonary Embolus (PE), or Pulmonary Thrombo-Embolism (PTE)
- ☐ I0600. Heart Failure (e.g., congestive heart failure [CHF] and pulmonary edema)
- ☐ I0700. Hypertension
- ☐ I0800. Orthostatic Hypotension
- ☐ I0900. Peripheral Vascular Disease (PVD) or Peripheral Arterial Disease (PAD)

**Gastrointestinal**
- ☐ I1100. Cirrhosis
- ☐ I1200. Gastroesophageal Reflux Disease (GERD) or Ulcer (e.g., esophageal, gastric, and peptic ulcers)
- ☐ I1300. Ulcerative Colitis, Crohn's Disease, or Inflammatory Bowel Disease

**Genitourinary**
- ☐ I1400. Benign Prostatic Hyperplasia (BPH)
- ☐ I1500. Renal Insufficiency, Renal Failure, or End-Stage Renal Disease (ESRD)
- ☐ I1550. Neurogenic Bladder
- ☐ I1650. Obstructive Uropathy

**Infections**
- ☐ I1700. Multidrug-Resistant Organism (MDRO)
- ☐ I2000. Pneumonia
- ☐ I2100. Septicemia
- ☐ I2200. Tuberculosis
- ☐ I2300. Urinary Tract Infection (UTI) (LAST 30 DAYS)
- ☐ I2400. Viral Hepatitis (e.g., Hepatitis A, B, C, D, and E)
- ☐ I2500. Wound Infection (other than foot)

**Metabolic**
- ☐ I2900. Diabetes Mellitus (DM) (e.g., diabetic retinopathy, nephropathy, and neuropathy)
- ☐ I3100. Hyponatremia
- ☐ I3200. Hyperkalemia
- ☐ I3300. Hyperlipidemia (e.g., hypercholesterolemia)
- ☐ I3400. Thyroid Disorder (e.g., hypothyroidism, hyperthyroidism, and Hashimoto's thyroiditis)

**Musculoskeletal**
- ☐ I3700. Arthritis (e.g., degenerative joint disease [DJD], osteoarthritis, and rheumatoid arthritis [RA])
- ☐ I3800. Osteoporosis
- ☐ I3900. Hip Fracture - any hip fracture that has a relationship to current status, treatments, monitoring (e.g., sub-capital fractures, and fractures of the trochanter and femoral neck)
- ☐ I4000. Other Fracture

**Neurological**
- ☐ I4200. Alzheimer's Disease
- ☐ I4300. Aphasia
- ☐ I4400. Cerebral Palsy
- ☐ I4500. Cerebrovascular Accident (CVA), Transient Ischemic Attack (TIA), or Stroke
- ☐ I4800. Non-Alzheimer's Dementia (e.g., Lewy body dementia, vascular or multi-infarct dementia; mixed dementia; frontotemporal dementia such as Pick's disease; and dementia related to stroke, Parkinson's or Creutzfeldt-Jakob diseases)

---

Resident _____ Identifier _____ Date _____

## Section H — Bladder and Bowel

**H0100. Appliances**

→ Check all that apply
- ☐ A. Indwelling catheter (including suprapubic catheter and nephrostomy tube)
- ☐ B. External catheter
- ☐ C. Ostomy (including urostomy, ileostomy, and colostomy)
- ☐ D. Intermittent catheterization
- ☐ Z. None of the above

**H0200. Urinary Toileting Program**

Enter Code ☐ A. Has a trial of a toileting program (e.g., scheduled toileting, prompted voiding, or bladder training) been attempted on admission/entry or reentry or since urinary incontinence was noted in this facility?
- 0. No → Skip to H0300, Urinary Continence
- 1. Yes → Continue to H0200B, Response
- 9. Unable to determine → Skip to H0200C, Current toileting program or trial

Enter Code ☐ B. Response - What was the resident's response to the trial program?
- 0. No improvement
- 1. Decreased wetness
- 2. Completely dry (continent)
- 9. Unable to determine or trial in progress

Enter Code ☐ C. Current toileting program or trial - Is a toileting program (e.g., scheduled toileting, prompted voiding, or bladder training) currently being used to manage the resident's urinary continence?
- 0. No
- 1. Yes

**H0300. Urinary Continence**

Enter Code ☐ Urinary continence - Select the one category that best describes the resident
- 0. Always continent
- 1. Occasionally incontinent (less than 7 episodes of incontinence)
- 2. Frequently incontinent (7 or more episodes of urinary incontinence, but at least one episode of continent voiding)
- 3. Always incontinent (no episodes of continent voiding)
- 9. Not rated, resident had a catheter (indwelling, condom), urinary ostomy, or no urine output for the entire 7 days

**H0400. Bowel Continence**

Enter Code ☐ Bowel continence - Select the one category that best describes the resident
- 0. Always continent
- 1. Occasionally incontinent (one episode of bowel incontinence)
- 2. Frequently incontinent (2 or more episodes of bowel incontinence, but at least one continent bowel movement)
- 3. Always incontinent (no episodes of continent bowel movements)
- 9. Not rated, resident had an ostomy or did not have a bowel movement for the entire 7 days

**H0500. Bowel Toileting Program**

Enter Code ☐ Is a toileting program currently being used to manage the resident's bowel continence?
- 0. No
- 1. Yes

**H0600. Bowel Patterns**

Enter Code ☐ Constipation present?
- 0. No
- 1. Yes

Resident _____ Identifier _____ Date _____

## Section J — Health Conditions

**J0100. Pain Management** - Complete for all residents, regardless of current pain level

At any time in the last 5 days, has the resident:

Enter Code [ ] **A. Received scheduled pain medication regimen?**
0. No
1. Yes

Enter Code [ ] **B. Received PRN pain medications OR was offered and declined?**
0. No
1. Yes

Enter Code [ ] **C. Received non-medication intervention for pain?**
0. No
1. Yes

**J0200. Should Pain Assessment Interview be Conducted?** Attempt to conduct interview with all residents. If resident is comatose, skip to J1100, Shortness of Breath (dyspnea)

Enter Code [ ] 0. **No** (resident is rarely/never understood) → Skip to and complete J0800, Indicators of Pain or Possible Pain
1. **Yes** → Continue to J0300, Pain Presence

### Pain Assessment Interview

**J0300. Pain Presence**

Ask resident: *"Have you had pain or hurting at any time in the last 5 days?"*

Enter Code [ ] 0. **No** → Skip to J1100, Shortness of Breath
1. **Yes** → Continue to J0400, Pain Frequency
9. **Unable to answer** → Skip to J0800, Indicators of Pain or Possible Pain

**J0400. Pain Frequency**

Ask resident: *"How much of the time have you experienced pain or hurting over the last 5 days?"*

Enter Code [ ] 1. Almost constantly
2. Frequently
3. Occasionally
4. Rarely
9. Unable to answer

**J0500. Pain Effect on Function**

Enter Code [ ] A. Ask resident: *"Over the past 5 days, has pain made it hard for you to sleep at night?"*
0. No
1. Yes
9. Unable to answer

Enter Code [ ] B. Ask resident: *"Over the past 5 days, have you limited your day-to-day activities because of pain?"*
0. No
1. Yes
9. Unable to answer

**J0600. Pain Intensity** - Administer **ONLY ONE** of the following pain intensity questions (A or B)

Rating [ ][ ] A. **Numeric Rating Scale (00-10).** Ask resident: "Please rate your worst pain over the last 5 days on a zero to ten scale, with zero being no pain and ten as the worst pain you can imagine." (Show resident 00 -10 pain scale). **Enter two-digit response. Enter 99 if unable to answer.**

Enter Code [ ] B. **Verbal Descriptor Scale.** Ask resident: *"Please rate the intensity of your worst pain over the last 5 days."* (Show resident verbal scale)
1. Mild
2. Moderate
3. Severe
4. Very severe, horrible
9. Unable to answer

---

Resident _____ Identifier _____ Date _____

## Section I

**Active Diagnoses**

**Active Diagnoses in the last 7 days - Check all that apply**

Diagnoses listed in parentheses are provided as examples and should not be considered as all-inclusive lists.

### Neurological - Continued

[ ][ ][ ][ ][ ][ ][ ][ ][ ]
- I4900. Hemiplegia or Hemiparesis
- I5000. Paraplegia
- I5100. Quadriplegia
- I5200. Multiple Sclerosis (MS)
- I5250. Huntington's Disease
- I5300. Parkinson's Disease
- I5350. Tourette's Syndrome
- I5400. Seizure Disorder or Epilepsy
- I5500. Traumatic Brain Injury (TBI)

### Nutritional

[ ]
- I5600. Malnutrition (protein or calorie) or at risk for malnutrition

### Psychiatric/Mood Disorder

[ ][ ][ ][ ][ ][ ]
- I5700. Anxiety Disorder
- I5800. Depression (other than bipolar)
- I5900. Manic Depression (bipolar disease)
- I5950. Psychotic Disorder (other than schizophrenia)
- I6000. Schizophrenia (e.g., schizoaffective and schizophreniform disorders)
- I6100. Post Traumatic Stress Disorder (PTSD)

### Pulmonary

[ ]
- I6200. Asthma, Chronic Obstructive Pulmonary Disease (COPD), or Chronic Lung Disease (e.g., chronic bronchitis and restrictive lung diseases such as asbestosis)

[ ]
- I6300. Respiratory Failure

### Vision

[ ]
- I6500. Cataracts, Glaucoma, or Macular Degeneration

### None of Above

[ ]
- I7900. None of the above active diagnoses within the last 7 days

### Other

I8000. Additional active diagnoses
Enter diagnosis on line and ICD code in boxes. Include the decimal for the code in the appropriate box.

A. _____ [ ][ ][ ][ ][ ][ ][ ]
B. _____ [ ][ ][ ][ ][ ][ ][ ]
C. _____ [ ][ ][ ][ ][ ][ ][ ]
D. _____ [ ][ ][ ][ ][ ][ ][ ]
E. _____ [ ][ ][ ][ ][ ][ ][ ]
F. _____ [ ][ ][ ][ ][ ][ ][ ]
G. _____ [ ][ ][ ][ ][ ][ ][ ]
H. _____ [ ][ ][ ][ ][ ][ ][ ]
I. _____ [ ][ ][ ][ ][ ][ ][ ]
J. _____ [ ][ ][ ][ ][ ][ ][ ]

Resident _____ Identifier _____ Date _____

| Section J | Health Conditions |
|---|---|

**J0700. Should the Staff Assessment for Pain Be Conducted?**

Enter Code [ ]
- 0. **No** (J0400 = 1 thru 4) → Skip to J1100, Shortness of Breath (dyspnea)
- 1. **Yes** (J0400 = 9) → Continue to J0800, Indicators of Pain or Possible Pain

**Staff Assessment for Pain**

**J0800. Indicators of Pain or Possible Pain in the last 5 days**

↳ **Check all that apply.**

[ ] A. **Non-verbal sounds** (e.g., crying, whining, gasping, moaning, or groaning)

[ ] B. **Vocal complaints of pain** (e.g., that hurts, ouch, stop)

[ ] C. **Facial expressions** (e.g., grimaces, winces, wrinkled forehead, furrowed brow, clenched teeth or jaw)

[ ] D. **Protective body movements or postures** (e.g., bracing, guarding, rubbing or massaging a body part/area, clutching or holding a body part during movement)

[ ] Z. **None of these signs observed or documented** → If checked, skip to J1100, Shortness of Breath (dyspnea)

**J0850. Frequency of Indicator of Pain or Possible Pain** in the last 5 days.

Enter Code [ ]
Frequency with which resident complains or shows evidence of pain or possible pain
- 1. Indicators of pain or possible pain observed **1 to 2 days**
- 2. Indicators of pain or possible pain observed **3 to 4 days**
- 3. Indicators of pain or possible pain observed **daily**

**Other Health Conditions**

**J1100. Shortness of Breath (dyspnea)**

↳ **Check all that apply.**

[ ] A. **Shortness of breath** or trouble breathing **with exertion** (e.g., walking, bathing, transferring)

[ ] B. **Shortness of breath** or trouble breathing **when sitting at rest**

[ ] C. **Shortness of breath** or trouble breathing **when lying flat**

[ ] Z. **None of the above**

**J1300. Current Tobacco Use**

Enter Code [ ]
**Tobacco use**
- 0. **No**
- 1. **Yes**

**J1400. Prognosis**

Enter Code [ ]
Does the resident have a condition or chronic disease that may result in a **life expectancy of less than 6 months?** (requires physician documentation)
- 0. **No**
- 1. **Yes**

**J1550. Problem Conditions**

↳ **Check all that apply.**

[ ] A. **Fever**

[ ] B. **Vomiting**

[ ] C. **Dehydrated**

[ ] D. **Internal bleeding**

[ ] Z. **None of the above**

---

Resident _____ Identifier _____ Date _____

| Section J | Health Conditions |
|---|---|

**J1700. Fall History on Admission/Entry or Reentry**

Complete only if A0310A = 01 or A0310E = 1

Enter Code [ ] A. Did the resident have a fall any time in the **last month** prior to admission/entry or reentry?
- 0. **No**
- 1. **Yes**
- 9. **Unable to determine**

Enter Code [ ] B. Did the resident have a fall any time in the **last 2-6 months** prior to admission/entry or reentry?
- 0. **No**
- 1. **Yes**
- 9. **Unable to determine**

Enter Code [ ] C. Did the resident have any **fracture related to a fall in the 6 months** prior to admission/entry or reentry?
- 0. **No**
- 1. **Yes**
- 9. **Unable to determine**

**J1800. Any Falls Since Admission/Entry or Reentry or Prior Assessment (OBRA or Scheduled PPS)**, whichever is more recent

Enter Code [ ]
Has the resident **had any falls since admission/entry or reentry or the prior assessment** (OBRA or Scheduled PPS), whichever is more recent?
- 0. **No** → Skip to K0100, Swallowing Disorder
- 1. **Yes** → Continue to J1900, Number of Falls Since Admission/Entry or Reentry or Prior Assessment (OBRA or Scheduled PPS)

**J1900. Number of Falls Since Admission/Entry or Reentry or Prior Assessment (OBRA or Scheduled PPS)**, whichever is more recent

↳ **Enter Codes in Boxes**

[ ] A. **No injury** - no evidence of any injury is noted on physical assessment by the nurse or primary care clinician; no complaints of pain or injury by the resident; no change in the resident's behavior is noted after the fall

[ ] B. **Injury (except major)** - skin tears, abrasions, lacerations, superficial bruises, hematomas and sprains; or any fall-related injury that causes the resident to complain of pain

[ ] C. **Major injury** - bone fractures, joint dislocations, closed head injuries with altered consciousness, subdural hematoma

**Coding:**
- 0. **None**
- 1. **One**
- 2. **Two or more**

Resident _____ Identifier _____ Date _____

## Section K   Swallowing/Nutritional Status

**K0100. Swallowing Disorder** - Signs and symptoms of possible swallowing disorder

↳ Check all that apply.

- A. Loss of liquids/solids from mouth when eating or drinking
- B. Holding food in mouth/cheeks or residual food in mouth after meals
- C. Coughing or choking during meals or when swallowing medications
- D. Complaints of difficulty or pain with swallowing
- Z. None of the above

**K0200. Height and Weight** - While measuring, if the number is X.1 - X.4 round down; X.5 or greater round up

A. **Height** (in inches). Record most recent height measure since the most recent admission/entry or reentry.  [inches]

B. **Weight** (in pounds). Base weight on most recent measure in last 30 days; measure weight consistently, according to standard facility practice (e.g., in a.m. after voiding, before meal, with shoes off).  [pounds]

**K0300. Weight Loss**

Enter Code [ ]   Loss of 5% or more in the last month or loss of 10% or more in last 6 months
- 0. No or unknown
- 1. Yes, on physician-prescribed weight-loss regimen
- 2. Yes, not on physician-prescribed weight-loss regimen

**K0310. Weight Gain**

Enter Code [ ]   Gain of 5% or more in the last month or gain of 10% or more in last 6 months
- 0. No or unknown
- 1. Yes, on physician-prescribed weight-gain regimen
- 2. Yes, not on physician-prescribed weight-gain regimen

**K0510. Nutritional Approaches**
Check all of the following nutritional approaches that were performed during the last 7 days.

1. **While NOT a Resident** - Performed *while NOT a resident* of this facility and within the *last 7 days.* Only check column 1 if resident entered (admission or reentry) IN THE LAST 7 DAYS. If resident last entered 7 or more days ago, leave column 1 blank

2. **While a Resident**
Performed *while a resident* of this facility and within the *last 7 days*

| | 1. While NOT a Resident | 2. While a Resident |
| --- | --- | --- |
| | ↳ Check all that apply ➤ | |
| A. Parenteral/IV feeding | [ ] | [ ] |
| B. Feeding tube - nasogastric or abdominal (PEG) | [ ] | [ ] |
| C. Mechanically altered diet - require change in texture of food or liquids (e.g., pureed food, thickened liquids) | [ ] | [ ] |
| D. Therapeutic diet (e.g., low salt, diabetic, low cholesterol) | [ ] | [ ] |
| Z. None of the above | [ ] | [ ] |

**K0700. Percent Intake by Artificial Route** - Complete K0700 only if Column 1 and/or Column 2 are checked for K0510A and/or K0510B

Enter Code [ ]   A. Proportion of total calories the resident received through parenteral or tube feeding
- 1. 25% or less
- 2. 26%-50%
- 3. 51% or more

Enter Code [ ]   B. Average fluid intake per day by IV or tube feeding
- 1. 500 cc/day or less
- 2. 501 cc/day or more

---

Resident _____ Identifier _____ Date _____

## Section L   Oral/Dental Status

**L0200. Dental**

↳ Check all that apply.

- A. Broken or loosely fitting full or partial denture (chipped, cracked, uncleanable, or loose)
- B. No natural teeth or tooth fragment(s) (edentulous)
- C. Abnormal mouth tissue (ulcers, masses, oral lesions, including under denture or partial if one is worn)
- D. Obvious or likely cavity or broken natural teeth
- E. Inflamed or bleeding gums or loose natural teeth
- F. Mouth or facial pain, discomfort, or difficulty with chewing
- G. Unable to examine
- Z. None of the above were present

Resident _____ Identifier _____ Date _____

## Section M — Skin Conditions

**Report based on highest stage of existing ulcer(s) at its worst; do not "reverse" stage**

### M0100. Determination of Pressure Ulcer Risk

Check all that apply.

- ☐ A. Resident has a stage 1 or greater, a scar over bony prominence, or a non-removable dressing/device
- ☐ B. Formal assessment instrument/tool (e.g., Braden, Norton, or other)
- ☐ C. Clinical assessment
- ☐ Z. None of the above

### M0150. Risk of Pressure Ulcers

Is this resident at risk of developing pressure ulcers?

Enter Code ☐
- 0. No
- 1. Yes

### M0210. Unhealed Pressure Ulcer(s)

Does this resident have one or more unhealed pressure ulcer(s) at Stage 1 or higher?

Enter Code ☐
- 0. No → Skip to M0900, Healed Pressure Ulcers
- 1. Yes → Continue to M0300, Current Number of Unhealed (non-epithelialized) Pressure Ulcers at Each Stage

### M0300. Current Number of Unhealed (non-epithelialized) Pressure Ulcers at Each Stage

**A. Number of Stage 1 pressure ulcers**

Stage 1: Intact skin with non-blanchable redness of a localized area usually over a bony prominence. Darkly pigmented skin may not have a visible blanching; in dark skin tones only it may appear with persistent blue or purple hues

Enter Number ☐

**B. Stage 2:** Partial thickness loss of dermis presenting as a shallow open ulcer with a red or pink wound bed, without slough. May also present as an intact or open/ruptured blister

1. Number of Stage 2 pressure ulcers - If 0 → Skip to M0300C, Stage 3

Enter Number ☐

2. Number of these Stage 2 pressure ulcers that were present upon admission/entry or reentry - enter how many were noted at the time of admission/entry or reentry

Enter Number ☐

3. Date of oldest Stage 2 pressure ulcer - Enter dashes if date is unknown:

☐☐ - ☐☐ - ☐☐☐☐
Month — Day — Year

**C. Stage 3:** Full-thickness tissue loss. Subcutaneous fat may be visible but bone, tendon, or muscle is not exposed. Slough may be present but does not obscure the depth of tissue loss. May include undermining and tunneling

1. Number of Stage 3 pressure ulcers - If 0 → Skip to M0300D, Stage 4

Enter Number ☐

2. Number of these Stage 3 pressure ulcers that were present upon admission/entry or reentry - enter how many were noted at the time of admission/entry or reentry

Enter Number ☐

**D. Stage 4:** Full-thickness tissue loss with exposed bone, tendon, or muscle. Slough or eschar may be present on some parts of the wound bed. Often includes undermining and tunneling

1. Number of Stage 4 pressure ulcers - If 0 → Skip to M0300E, Unstageable: Non-removable dressing

Enter Number ☐

2. Number of these Stage 4 pressure ulcers that were present upon admission/entry or reentry - enter how many were noted at the time of admission/entry or reentry

Enter Number ☐

**M0300 continued on next page**

---

Resident _____ Identifier _____ Date _____

## Section M — Skin Conditions

### M0300. Current Number of Unhealed (non-epithelialized) Pressure Ulcers at Each Stage - Continued

**E. Unstageable - Non-removable dressing:** Known but not stageable due to non-removable dressing/device

1. Number of unstageable pressure ulcers due to non-removable dressing/device - If 0 → Skip to M0300F, Unstageable: Slough and/or eschar

Enter Number ☐

2. Number of these unstageable pressure ulcers that were present upon admission/entry or reentry - enter how many were noted at the time of admission/entry or reentry

Enter Number ☐

**F. Unstageable - Slough and/or eschar:** Known but not stageable due to coverage of wound bed by slough and/or eschar

1. Number of unstageable pressure ulcers due to coverage of wound bed by slough and/or eschar - If 0 → Skip to M0300G, Unstageable: Deep tissue

Enter Number ☐

2. Number of these unstageable pressure ulcers that were present upon admission/entry or reentry - enter how many were noted at the time of admission/entry or reentry

Enter Number ☐

**G. Unstageable - Deep tissue:** Suspected deep tissue injury in evolution

1. Number of unstageable pressure ulcers with suspected deep tissue injury in evolution - If 0 → Skip to M0610, Dimension of Unhealed Stage 3 or 4 Pressure Ulcers or Eschar

Enter Number ☐

2. Number of these unstageable pressure ulcers that were present upon admission/entry or reentry - enter how many were noted at the time of admission/entry or reentry

Enter Number ☐

### M0610. Dimensions of Unhealed Stage 3 or 4 Pressure Ulcers or Eschar

Complete only if M0300C1, M0300D1 or M0300F1 is greater than 0

If the resident has one or more unhealed (non-epithelialized) Stage 3 or 4 pressure ulcers or an unstageable pressure ulcer due to slough or eschar, identify the pressure ulcer with the largest surface area (length x width) and record in centimeters:

**A. Pressure ulcer length:** Longest length from head to toe

☐☐.☐ cm

**B. Pressure ulcer width:** Widest width of the same pressure ulcer, side-to-side perpendicular (90-degree angle) to length

☐☐.☐ cm

**C. Pressure ulcer depth:** Depth of the same pressure ulcer from the visible surface to the deepest area (if depth is unknown, enter a dash in each box)

☐☐.☐ cm

### M0700. Most Severe Tissue Type for Any Pressure Ulcer

Select the best description of the most severe type of tissue present in any pressure ulcer bed

Enter Code ☐
1. Epithelial tissue - new skin growing in superficial ulcer. It can be light pink and shiny, even in persons with darkly pigmented skin
2. Granulation tissue - pink or red tissue with shiny, moist, granular appearance
3. Slough - yellow or white tissue that adheres to the ulcer bed in strings or thick clumps, or is mucinous
4. Necrotic tissue (eschar) - black, brown, or tan tissue that adheres firmly to the wound bed or ulcer edges, may be softer or harder than surrounding skin
9. None of the above

### M0800. Worsening in Pressure Ulcer Status Since Prior Assessment (OBRA or Scheduled PPS) or Last Admission/Entry or Reentry. Complete only if A0310E = 0

Indicate the number of current pressure ulcers that were not present or were at a lesser stage on prior assessment (OBRA or scheduled PPS) or last entry. If no current pressure ulcer at a given stage, enter 0.

Enter Number
- A. Stage 2 ☐
- B. Stage 3 ☐
- C. Stage 4 ☐

Resident _____ Identifier _____ Date _____

| Section N | Medications |
| --- | --- |

**N0300. Injections**

Enter Code ☐ **Record the number of days that injections of any type** were received during the last 7 days or since admission/entry or reentry if less than 7 days. If 0 ⟶ Skip to N0410, Medications Received

**N0350. Insulin**

Enter Code ☐ **A. Insulin injections - Record the number of days that insulin injections** were received during the last 7 days or since admission/entry or reentry if less than 7 days

Enter Code ☐ **B. Orders for insulin - Record the number of days the physician (or authorized assistant or practitioner) changed the resident's insulin orders** during the last 7 days or since admission/entry or reentry if less than 7 days.

**N0410. Medications Received**

Indicate the number of DAYS the resident received the following medications during the last 7 days or since admission/entry or reentry if less than 7 days. Enter "0" if medication was not received by the resident during the last 7 days.

Enter Code ☐ **A. Antipsychotic**

Enter Code ☐ **B. Antianxiety**

Enter Code ☐ **C. Antidepressant**

Enter Code ☐ **D. Hypnotic**

Enter Code ☐ **E. Anticoagulant** (warfarin, heparin, or low-molecular-weight heparin)

Enter Code ☐ **F. Antibiotic**

Enter Code ☐ **G. Diuretic**

---

Resident _____ Identifier _____ Date _____

| Section M | Skin Conditions |
| --- | --- |

**M0900. Healed Pressure Ulcers**

Complete only if A0310E = 0

Enter Code ☐ **A. Were pressure ulcers present on the prior assessment (OBRA or scheduled PPS)?**
  0. **No** ⟶ Skip to M1030, Number of Venous and Arterial Ulcers
  1. **Yes** ⟶ Continue to M0900B, Stage 2

Indicate the number of pressure ulcers that were noted on the prior assessment (OBRA or scheduled PPS) that have completely closed (resurfaced with epithelium). If no healed pressure ulcer at a given stage since the prior assessment (OBRA or scheduled PPS), enter 0.

Enter Code ☐ **B. Stage 2**

Enter Code ☐ **C. Stage 3**

Enter Code ☐ **D. Stage 4**

**M1030. Number of Venous and Arterial Ulcers**

Enter Code ☐ Enter the total number of venous and arterial ulcers present

**M1040. Other Ulcers, Wounds, and Skin Problems**

⟶ Check all that apply.

**Foot Problems**

☐ **A. Infection of the foot** (e.g., cellulitis, purulent drainage)

☐ **B. Diabetic foot ulcer(s)**

☐ **C. Other open lesion(s) on the foot**

**Other Problems**

☐ **D. Open lesion(s) other than ulcers, rashes, cuts** (e.g., cancer lesion)

☐ **E. Surgical wound(s)**

☐ **F. Burn(s)** (second or third degree)

☐ **G. Skin tear(s)**

☐ **H. Moisture Associated Skin Damage (MASD)** (i.e. incontinence [IAD], perspiration, drainage)

**None of the Above**

☐ **Z. None of the above** were present

**M1200. Skin and Ulcer Treatments**

⟶ Check all that apply.

☐ **A. Pressure-reducing device for chair**

☐ **B. Pressure-reducing device for bed**

☐ **C. Turning/repositioning program**

☐ **D. Nutrition or hydration intervention** to manage skin problems

☐ **E. Pressure ulcer care**

☐ **F. Surgical wound care**

☐ **G. Application of nonsurgical dressings** (with or without topical medications) other than to feet

☐ **H. Applications of ointments/medications** other than to feet

☐ **I. Application of dressings to feet** (with or without topical medications)

☐ **Z. None of the above** were provided

Resident _____ Identifier _____ Date _____

## Section O — Special Treatments, Procedures, and Programs

**O0100. Special Treatments, Procedures, and Programs** - Check all of the following treatments, procedures, and programs that were performed during the last 14 days.

1. **While NOT a Resident** - Performed *while NOT a resident* of this facility and within the *last 14 days*. Only check column 1 if resident entered (admission or reentry) IN THE LAST 14 DAYS. If resident last entered 14 or more days ago, leave column 1 blank

2. **While a Resident** - Performed *while a resident* of this facility and within the *last 14 days*

| | 1. While NOT a Resident | 2. While a Resident |
|---|---|---|
| | ↓ Check all that apply ↓ | |
| **Cancer Treatments** | | |
| A. Chemotherapy | ☐ | ☐ |
| B. Radiation | ☐ | ☐ |
| **Respiratory Treatments** | | |
| C. Oxygen therapy | ☐ | ☐ |
| D. Suctioning | ☐ | ☐ |
| E. Tracheostomy care | ☐ | ☐ |
| F. Ventilator or respirator | ☐ | ☐ |
| G. BiPAP/CPAP | ☐ | ☐ |
| **Other** | | |
| H. IV medications | ☐ | ☐ |
| I. Transfusions | ☐ | ☐ |
| J. Dialysis | ☐ | ☐ |
| K. Hospice care | ☐ | ☐ |
| L. Respite care | ☐ | ☐ |
| M. Isolation or quarantine for active infectious disease (does not include standard body/fluid precautions) | ☐ | ☐ |
| **None of the Above** | | |
| Z. None of the above | ☐ | ☐ |

**O0250. Influenza Vaccine** - Refer to current version of RAI manual for current flu season and reporting period

Enter Code ☐ A. Did the resident receive the Influenza vaccine **in this facility** for this year's Influenza season?
0. No → Skip to O0250C. If Influenza vaccine not received, state reason
1. Yes → Continue to O0250B, Date vaccine received

Enter Code ☐ B. Date vaccine received → Complete date and skip to O0300A. Is the resident's Pneumococcal vaccination up to date?
☐☐ - ☐☐ - ☐☐☐☐
Month — Day — Year

Enter Code ☐ C. If Influenza vaccine not received, state reason:
1. Resident not in facility during this year's flu season
2. Received outside of this facility
3. Not eligible - medical contraindication
4. Offered and declined
5. Not offered
6. Inability to obtain vaccine due to a declared shortage
9. None of the above

**O0300. Pneumococcal Vaccine**

Enter Code ☐ A. Is the resident's Pneumococcal vaccination up to date?
0. No → Continue to O0300B, If Pneumococcal vaccine not received, state reason
1. Yes → Skip to O0400, Therapies

Enter Code ☐ B. If Pneumococcal vaccine not received, state reason:
1. Not eligible - medical contraindication
2. Offered and declined
3. Not offered

---

Resident _____ Identifier _____ Date _____

## Section O — Special Treatments, Procedures, and Programs

**O0400. Therapies**

### A. Speech-Language Pathology and Audiology Services

1. **Individual minutes** - record the total number of minutes this therapy was administered to the resident individually in the last 7 days
   Enter Number of Minutes ☐☐☐☐

2. **Concurrent minutes** - record the total number of minutes this therapy was administered to the resident **concurrently with one other resident** in the last 7 days
   Enter Number of Minutes ☐☐☐☐

3. **Group minutes** - record the total number of minutes this therapy was administered to the resident as **part of a group of residents** in the last 7 days
   Enter Number of Minutes ☐☐☐☐

If the sum of individual, concurrent, and group minutes is zero, → skip to O0400A5, Therapy start date

4. **Days** - record the **number of days** this therapy was administered for **at least 15 minutes** a day in the last 7 days
   Enter Number of Days ☐

5. **Therapy start date** - record the date the most recent therapy regimen (since the most recent entry) started
   ☐☐ - ☐☐ - ☐☐☐☐
   Month — Day — Year

6. **Therapy end date** - record the date the most recent therapy regimen (since the most recent entry) ended - enter dashes if therapy is ongoing
   ☐☐ - ☐☐ - ☐☐☐☐
   Month — Day — Year

### B. Occupational Therapy

1. **Individual minutes** - record the total number of minutes this therapy was administered to the resident individually in the last 7 days
   Enter Number of Minutes ☐☐☐☐

2. **Concurrent minutes** - record the total number of minutes this therapy was administered to the resident **concurrently with one other resident** in the last 7 days
   Enter Number of Minutes ☐☐☐☐

3. **Group minutes** - record the total number of minutes this therapy was administered to the resident as **part of a group of residents** in the last 7 days
   Enter Number of Minutes ☐☐☐☐

If the sum of individual, concurrent, and group minutes is zero, → skip to O0400A5, Therapy start date

4. **Days** - record the **number of days** this therapy was administered for **at least 15 minutes** a day in the last 7 days
   Enter Number of Days ☐

5. **Therapy start date** - record the date the most recent therapy regimen (since the most recent entry) started
   ☐☐ - ☐☐ - ☐☐☐☐
   Month — Day — Year

6. **Therapy end date** - record the date the most recent therapy regimen (since the most recent entry) ended - enter dashes if therapy is ongoing
   ☐☐ - ☐☐ - ☐☐☐☐
   Month — Day — Year

### C. Physical Therapy

1. **Individual minutes** - record the total number of minutes this therapy was administered to the resident individually in the last 7 days
   Enter Number of Minutes ☐☐☐☐

2. **Concurrent minutes** - record the total number of minutes this therapy was administered to the resident **concurrently with one other resident** in the last 7 days
   Enter Number of Minutes ☐☐☐☐

3. **Group minutes** - record the total number of minutes this therapy was administered to the resident as **part of a group of residents** in the last 7 days
   Enter Number of Minutes ☐☐☐☐

If the sum of individual, concurrent, and group minutes is zero, → skip to O0400C5, Therapy start date

4. **Days** - record the **number of days** this therapy was administered for **at least 15 minutes** a day in the last 7 days
   Enter Number of Days ☐

5. **Therapy start date** - record the date the most recent therapy regimen (since the most recent entry) started
   ☐☐ - ☐☐ - ☐☐☐☐
   Month — Day — Year

6. **Therapy end date** - record the date the most recent therapy regimen (since the most recent entry) ended - enter dashes if therapy is ongoing
   ☐☐ - ☐☐ - ☐☐☐☐
   Month — Day — Year

**O0400 continued on next page**

Resident _____ Identifier _____ Date _____

## Section O — Special Treatments, Procedures, and Programs

### O0400. Therapies - Continued

**D. Respiratory Therapy**

Enter Number of Minutes [ ][ ][ ]
1. **Total minutes** - record the total number of minutes this therapy was administered to the resident in the last 7 days
   If zero, → skip to O0400E, Psychological Therapy

Enter Number of Days [ ][ ]
2. **Days** - record the **number of days** this therapy was administered for **at least 15 minutes** a day in the last 7 days

**E. Psychological Therapy** (by any licensed mental health professional)

Enter Number of Minutes [ ][ ][ ]
1. **Total minutes** - record the total number of minutes this therapy was administered to the resident in the last 7 days
   If zero, → skip to O0400F, Recreational Therapy

Enter Number of Days [ ][ ]
2. **Days** - record the **number of days** this therapy was administered for **at least 15 minutes** a day in the last 7 days

**F. Recreational Therapy** (includes recreational and music therapy)

Enter Number of Minutes [ ][ ][ ]
1. **Total minutes** - record the total number of minutes this therapy was administered to the resident in the last 7 days
   If zero, → skip to O0450, Resumption of Therapy

Enter Number of Days [ ][ ]
2. **Days** - record the **number of days** this therapy was administered for **at least 15 minutes** a day in the last 7 days

### O0450. Resumption of Therapy - Complete only if A0310C = 2 or 3 and A0310F = 99

Enter Code [ ]
A. **Has a previous rehabilitation therapy regimen (speech, occupational, and/or physical therapy) ended, as reported on this End of Therapy OMRA, and has this regimen now resumed at exactly the same level for each discipline?**
   0. **No** Skip to O0500, Restorative Nursing Programs
   1. **Yes**

B. **Date on which therapy regimen resumed:**
   [ ][ ] - [ ][ ] - [ ][ ][ ][ ]
   Month      Day       Year

### O0500. Restorative Nursing Programs

Record the **number of days** each of the following restorative programs was performed (for at least 15 minutes a day) in the last 7 calendar days (enter 0 if none or less than 15 minutes daily).

**Technique**

Number of days [ ][ ][ ]
A. **Range of motion (passive)**
B. **Range of motion (active)**
C. **Splint or brace assistance**

**Training and Skill Practice In:**

Number of days [ ][ ][ ][ ][ ][ ][ ]
D. **Bed mobility**
E. **Transfer**
F. **Walking**
G. **Dressing and/or grooming**
H. **Eating and/or swallowing**
I. **Amputation/prostheses care**
J. **Communication**

---

Resident _____ Identifier _____ Date _____

## Section O — Special Treatments, Procedures, and Programs

### O0600. Physician Examinations

Enter Days [ ][ ] Over the last 14 days, on how many days did the physician (or authorized assistant or practitioner) examine the resident?

### O0700. Physician Orders

Enter Days [ ][ ] Over the last 14 days, on how many days did the physician (or authorized assistant or practitioner) change the resident's orders?

## Section O — Restraints

### P0100. Physical Restraints

Physical restraints are any manual method or physical or mechanical device, material, or equipment attached or adjacent to the resident's body that the individual cannot remove easily, which restricts freedom of movement or normal access to one's body.

→ Enter Codes in Boxes

**Used in Bed**
[ ][ ][ ][ ]
A. Bed rail
B. Trunk restraint
C. Limb restraint
D. Other

**Used in Chair or Out of Bed**
[ ][ ][ ][ ]
E. Trunk restraint
F. Limb restraint
G. Chair prevents rising
H. Other

Coding:
0. **Not used**
1. **Used less than daily**
2. **Used daily**

Resident _____ Identifier _____ Date _____

## Section Q — Participation in Assessment and Goal Setting

**Q0100. Participation in Assessment**

Enter Code ☐
A. **Resident participated in assessment**
0. **No**
1. **Yes**

Enter Code ☐
B. **Family or significant other participated in assessment**
0. **No**
1. **Yes**
9. **No family or significant other available**

Enter Code ☐
C. **Guardian or legally authorized representative participated in assessment**
0. **No**
1. **Yes**
9. **No guardian or legally authorized representative available**

**Q0300. Resident's Overall Expectation** - Complete only if A0310E = 1

Enter Code ☐
A. **Select one for resident's overall goal established during assessment process**
1. Expects to be discharged to the community
2. Expects to remain in this facility
3. Expects to be discharged to another facility/institution
9. **Unknown or uncertain**

Enter Code ☐
B. **Indicate information source for Q0300A**
1. **Resident**
2. If not resident, then **family or significant other**
3. If not resident, family, or significant other, then **guardian or legally authorized representative**
9. **Unknown or uncertain**

**Q0400. Discharge Plan**

Enter Code ☐
A. **Is active discharge planning already occurring for the resident to return to the community?**
0. **No**
1. **Yes** → Skip to Q0600, Referral

**Q0490. Resident's Preference to Avoid Being Asked Question Q0500B** - Complete only if A0310A = 02, 06, or 99

Enter Code ☐
**Does the resident's clinical record document a request that this question be asked only on comprehensive assessments?**
0. **No**
1. **Yes** → Skip to Q0600, Referral
8. **Information not available**

**Q0500. Return to Community**

Enter Code ☐
B. **Ask the resident** (or family or significant other if resident is unable to respond): **"Do you want to talk to someone about the possibility of leaving this facility and returning to live and receive services in the community?"**
0. **No**
1. **Yes**
9. **Unknown or uncertain**

**Q0550. Resident's Preference to Avoid Being Asked Question Q0500B Again**

Enter Code ☐
A. **Does the resident** (or family or significant other or guardian, if resident is unable to respond) **want to be asked about returning to the community on all assessments?** (Rather than only on comprehensive assessments)
0. **No** - then document in resident's clinical record and ask again only on the next comprehensive assessment
1. **Yes**
8. **Information not available**

Enter Code ☐
B. **Indicate information source for Q0550A**
1. **Resident**
2. If not resident, then **family or significant other**
3. If not resident, family, or significant other, then **guardian or legally authorized representative**
8. **No information source available**

**Q0600. Referral**

Enter Code ☐
**Has a referral been made to the Local Contact Agency?** (Document reasons in resident's clinical record)
0. **No** - referral not needed
1. **No** - referral is or may be needed (For more information see Appendix C, Care Area Assessment Resources #20)
2. **Yes** - referral made

---

Resident _____ Identifier _____ Date _____

## Section V — Care Area Assessment (CAA) Summary

**V0100. Items from the Most Recent Prior OBRA or Scheduled PPS Assessment**
Complete only if A0310E = 0 and if the following is true for the **prior assessment**: A0310A = 01- 06 or A0310B = 01- 06

Enter Code ☐
A. **Prior Assessment Federal OBRA Reason for Assessment** (A0310A value from prior assessment)
01. **Admission** assessment (required by day 14)
02. **Quarterly** review assessment
03. **Annual** assessment
04. **Significant change in status** assessment
05. **Significant correction** to prior comprehensive assessment
06. **Significant correction** to prior quarterly assessment
99. None of the above

Enter Code ☐
B. **Prior Assessment PPS Reason for Assessment** (A0310B value from prior assessment)
01. **5-day** scheduled assessment
02. **14-day** scheduled assessment
03. **30-day** scheduled assessment
04. **60-day** scheduled assessment
05. **90-day** scheduled assessment
06. **Readmission/return** assessment
07. **Unscheduled assessment used for PPS** (OMRA, significant or clinical change, or significant correction assessment)
99. None of the above

Enter Score ☐☐ ☐☐ - ☐☐ - ☐☐☐☐
Month   Day   Year
C. **Prior Assessment Reference Date** (A2300 value from prior assessment)

Enter Score ☐☐
D. **Prior Assessment Brief Interview for Mental Status (BIMS) Summary Score** (C0500 value from prior assessment)

Enter Score ☐☐
E. **Prior Assessment Resident Mood Interview (PHQ-9©) Total Severity Score** (D0300 value from prior assessment)

Enter Score ☐☐
F. **Prior Assessment Staff Assessment of Resident Mood (PHQ-9-OV) Total Severity Score** (D0600 value from prior assessment)

Resident _____ Identifier _____ Date _____

## Section X  |  Correction Request

**Complete Section X only if A0050 = 2 or 3**
**Identification of Record to be Modified/Inactivated** - The following items identify the existing assessment record that is in error. In this section, reproduce the information EXACTLY as it appeared on the existing erroneous record, even if the information is incorrect. This information is necessary to locate the existing record in the National MDS Database.

**X0150. Type of Provider**

Enter Code [ ]   Type of provider
1. Nursing home (SNF/NF)
2. Swing Bed

**X0200. Name of Resident** on existing record to be modified/inactivated

A. First name: [_____]   B. Middle initial: [ ]

C. Last name: [_____]   D. Suffix: [ ]

**X0300. Gender** on existing record to be modified/inactivated

Enter Code [ ]
1. Male
2. Female

**X0400. Birth Date** on existing record to be modified/inactivated

[__] - [__] - [____]
Month   Day   Year

**X0500. Social Security Number** on existing record to be modified/inactivated

[___] - [__] - [____]

**X0600. Type of Assessment** on existing record to be modified/inactivated

Enter Code [ ]
A. Federal OBRA Reason for Assessment
01. Admission assessment (required by day 14)
02. Quarterly review assessment
03. Annual assessment
04. Significant change in status assessment
05. Significant correction to prior comprehensive assessment
06. Significant correction to prior quarterly assessment
99. None of the above

Enter Code [ ]
B. PPS Assessment
PPS Scheduled Assessments for a Medicare Part A Stay
01. 5-day scheduled assessment
02. 14-day scheduled assessment
03. 30-day scheduled assessment
04. 60-day scheduled assessment
05. 90-day scheduled assessment
06. Readmission/return assessment
PPS Unscheduled Assessments for a Medicare Part A Stay
07. Unscheduled assessment used for PPS (OMRA, significant or clinical change, or significant correction assessment)
Not PPS Assessment
99. None of the above

Enter Code [ ]
C. PPS Other Medicare Required Assessment - OMRA
0. No
1. Start of therapy assessment
2. End of therapy assessment
3. Both Start and End of therapy assessment
4. Change of therapy assessment

**X0600 continued on next page**

---

Resident _____ Identifier _____ Date _____

## Section V  |  Care Area Assessment (CAA) Summary

**V0200. CAAs and Care Planning**

1. Check column A if Care Area is triggered.
2. For each triggered Care Area, indicate whether a new care plan, care plan revision, or continuation of current care plan is necessary to address the problem(s) identified in your assessment of the care area. The Care Planning Decision column must be completed within 7 days of completing the RAI (MDS and CAA[s]). Check column B if the triggered care area is addressed in the care plan.
3. Indicate in the Location and Date of CAA Documentation column where information related to the CAA can be found. CAA documentation should include information on the complicating factors, risks, and any referrals for this resident for this care area.

**A. CAA Results**

| Care Area | A. Care Area Triggered | B. Care Planning Decision | Location and Date of CAA documentation |
|---|---|---|---|
|  | ► Check all that apply ► |  |  |
| 01. Delirium | [ ] | [ ] |  |
| 02. Cognitive Loss/Dementia | [ ] | [ ] |  |
| 03. Visual Function | [ ] | [ ] |  |
| 04. Communication | [ ] | [ ] |  |
| 05. ADL Functional/Rehabilitation Potential | [ ] | [ ] |  |
| 06. Urinary Incontinence and Indwelling Catheter | [ ] | [ ] |  |
| 07. Psychosocial Well-Being | [ ] | [ ] |  |
| 08. Mood State | [ ] | [ ] |  |
| 09. Behavioral Symptoms | [ ] | [ ] |  |
| 10. Activities | [ ] | [ ] |  |
| 11. Falls | [ ] | [ ] |  |
| 12. Nutritional Status | [ ] | [ ] |  |
| 13. Feeding Tube | [ ] | [ ] |  |
| 14. Dehydration/Fluid Maintenance | [ ] | [ ] |  |
| 15. Dental Care | [ ] | [ ] |  |
| 16. Pressure Ulcer | [ ] | [ ] |  |
| 17. Psychotropic Drug Use | [ ] | [ ] |  |
| 18. Physical Restraints | [ ] | [ ] |  |
| 19. Pain | [ ] | [ ] |  |
| 20. Return to Community Referral | [ ] | [ ] |  |

**B. Signature of RN Coordinator for CAA Process and Date Signed**

1. Signature _____   2. Date [__] - [__] - [____]
Month   Day   Year

**C. Signature of Person Completing Care Plan Decision and Date Signed**

1. Signature _____   2. Date [__] - [__] - [____]
Month   Day   Year

Resident _____ Identifier _____ Date _____

| Section X | Correction Request |

**X0600. Type of Assessment - Continued**

Enter Code ☐ **D. Is this a Swing Bed clinical change assessment?** Complete only if X0150 = 2
0. No
1. Yes

Enter Code ☐ **F. Entry/discharge reporting**
01. Entry tracking record
10. **Discharge assessment-return not anticipated**
11. **Discharge assessment-return anticipated**
12. Death in facility tracking record
99. **None of the above**

**X0700. Date** on existing record to be modified/inactivated - **Complete one only**

**A. Assessment Reference Date** - Complete only if X0600F = 99
☐☐ - ☐☐ - ☐☐☐☐
Month - Day - Year

**B. Discharge Date** - Complete only if X0600F = 10, 11, or 12
☐☐ - ☐☐ - ☐☐☐☐
Month - Day - Year

**C. Entry Date** - Complete only if X0600F = 01
☐☐ - ☐☐ - ☐☐☐☐
Month - Day - Year

**Correction Attestation Section** - Complete this section to explain and attest to the modification/inactivation request.

**X0800. Correction Number**

Enter Number ☐☐ **Enter the number of correction requests to modify/inactivate the existing record, including the present one.**

**X0900. Reasons for Modification** - Complete only if Type of Record is to modify a record in error (A0050 = 2)

→ **Check all that apply**
☐ **A. Transcription error**
☐ **B. Data entry error**
☐ **C. Software product error**
☐ **D. Item coding error**
☐ **E. End of Therapy - Resumption (EOT-R) date**
☐ **Z. Other error requiring modification**
If "Other" checked, please specify: _____

**X1050. Reasons for Inactivation** - Complete only if Type of Record is to inactivate a record in error (A0050 = 3)

→ **Check all that apply**
☐ **A. Event did not occur**
☐ **Z. Other error requiring inactivation**
If "Other" checked, please specify: _____

Resident _____ Identifier _____ Date _____

| Section X | Correction Request |

**X1100. RN Assessment Coordinator Attestation of Completion**

**A. Attesting individual's first name:**
☐☐☐

**B. Attesting individual's last name:**
☐☐☐☐☐

**C. Attesting individual's title:**

**D. Signature**

**E. Attestation date**
☐☐ - ☐☐ - ☐☐☐☐
Month - Day - Year

Resident _____ Identifier _____ Date _____

| Section Z | Assessment Administration |
| --- | --- |

### Z0400. Signature of Persons Completing the Assessment or Entry/Death Reporting

I certify that the accompanying information accurately reflects resident assessment information for this resident and that I collected or coordinated collection of this information on the dates specified. To the best of my knowledge, this information was collected in accordance with applicable Medicare and Medicaid requirements. I understand that this information is used as a basis for ensuring that residents receive appropriate and quality care, and as a basis for payment from federal funds. I further understand that payment of such federal funds and continued participation in the government-funded health care programs is conditioned on the accuracy and truthfulness of this information, and that I may be personally subject to or may subject my organization to substantial criminal, civil, and/or administrative penalties for submitting false information. I also certify that I am authorized to submit this information by this facility on its behalf.

| | Signature | Title | Sections | Date Section Completed |
| --- | --- | --- | --- | --- |
| A. | | | | |
| B. | | | | |
| C. | | | | |
| D. | | | | |
| E. | | | | |
| F. | | | | |
| G. | | | | |
| H. | | | | |
| I. | | | | |
| J. | | | | |
| K. | | | | |
| L. | | | | |

### Z0500. Signature of RN Assessment Coordinator Verifying Assessment Completion

A.  Signature:

B.  Date RN Assessment Coordinator signed assessment as complete:

☐☐ - ☐☐ - ☐☐☐☐
Month    Day    Year

---

Resident _____ Identifier _____ Date _____

| Section Z | Assessment Administration |
| --- | --- |

### Z0100. Medicare Part A Billing

Enter Code ☐

A.  **Medicare Part A HIPPS code** (RUG group followed by assessment type indicator):

☐☐☐☐☐

B.  **RUG version code:**

☐☐☐☐☐

C.  **Is this a Medicare Short Stay assessment?**
0. No
1. Yes

### Z0150. Medicare Part A Non-Therapy Billing

A.  **Medicare Part A non-therapy HIPPS code** (RUG group followed by assessment type indicator):

☐☐☐☐☐

B.  **RUG version code:**

☐☐☐☐☐

### Z0200. State Medicaid Billing (if required by the state)

A.  **RUG Case Mix group:**

☐☐☐☐☐

B.  **RUG version code:**

☐☐☐☐☐

### Z0250. Alternate State Medicaid Billing (if required by the state)

A.  **RUG Case Mix group:**

☐☐☐☐☐

B.  **RUG version code:**

☐☐☐☐☐

### Z0300. Insurance Billing

A.  **RUG billing code:**

☐☐☐☐☐

B.  **RUG billing version:**

☐☐☐☐☐

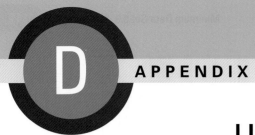

# USING MICROSOFT EXCEL TO PERFORM CALCULATIONS

When we are working with a small number of items or a simple, two-figure calculation, using a calculator is probably the easiest way to complete the computations. However, when we have a large number of figures or if we are going to be performing the same computation multiple times, it is very useful to know how to use Microsoft Excel to help with the computations.

In this Appendix, we will explain some common calculations, the purpose of the computations, and how to complete those calculations in Excel.

| | A | B | C | D | E | F |
|---|---|---|---|---|---|---|
| 1 | **Community Hospital** | | | | | |
| 2 | **First Quarter Discharges** | | | | | |
| 3 | | | | | | |
| 4 | | 19,021 | *January* | | | |
| 5 | | 18,945 | *February* | | | |
| 6 | | 21,439 | *March* | | | |
| 7 | | 59,405 | *Total First Quarter Discharges* | | | |
| 8 | | | | | | |
| 9 | The formula to obtain the total of 59,405 is: =SUM(B4:B6) | | | | | |
| 10 | This yields the same result as: =B4+B5+B6 | | | | | |
| 11 | | | | | | |
| 12 | A quarter is 1/4 of a year (3 months) | | | | | |
| 13 | A fiscal year is the organization's tax year (a business cycle) | | | | | |
| 14 | | | | | | |
| 15 | In this example, we might want to calculate the discharges, | | | | | |
| 16 | by quarter, for the entire year: | | | | | |
| 17 | | | | | | |
| 18 | On the right are the data entry and the formulas. On the left are the results. | | | | | |
| 19 | | | | | | |
| 20 | As you are preparing your worksheet, you can reveal the formulas by | | | | | |
| 21 | pressing Ctrl (The Control key and the accent grave, located to the left of | | | | | |
| 22 | the number 1 on your keyboard.) | | | | | |
| 23 | | | | | | |
| 24 | **Community Hospital** | | | | | |
| 25 | **2014 Discharges** | | | | | |
| 26 | | | | | | |
| 27 | | 19,021 | *January* | | | 19,021 |
| 28 | | 18,945 | *February* | | | 18,945 |
| 29 | | 21,439 | *March* | | | 21,439 |
| 30 | | 59,405 | *Total First Quarter Discharges* | | | =SUM(A27:A29) |
| 31 | | | | | | |
| 32 | | 18,435 | *April* | | | 18,435 |
| 33 | | 18,854 | *May* | | | 18,854 |
| 34 | | 19,146 | *June* | | | 19,146 |
| 35 | | 56,435 | *Total Second Quarter Discharges* | | | =SUM(A32:A34) |
| 36 | | | | | | |
| 37 | | 20,564 | *July* | | | 20,564 |
| 38 | | 20,437 | *August* | | | 20,437 |
| 39 | | 19,111 | *September* | | | 19,111 |
| 40 | | 60,112 | *Total Third Quarter Discharges* | | | =SUM(A37:A39) |
| 41 | | | | | | |
| 42 | | 19,021 | *October* | | | 19,021 |
| 43 | | 18,945 | *November* | | | 18,945 |
| 44 | | 21,439 | *December* | | | 21,439 |
| 45 | | 59,405 | *Total Fourth Quarter Discharges* | | | =SUM(A42:A44) |
| 46 | | | | | | |
| 47 | | 235,357 | *Total Discharges for the Year* | | | =A30+A35+A40+A45 |

| | A | B | C | D | E | F | G | H |
|---|---|---|---|---|---|---|---|---|
| 1 | **Community Hospital** | | | | | | | |
| 2 | **Health Information Department Staffing** | | | | | | | |
| 3 | | | | | | | | |
| 4 | | 75 | Total Staff | | | | | |
| 5 | | 6 | Part-time Staff | | | | | |
| 6 | | 69 | Full-time Staff | | | | | |
| 7 | Formula is: | =B4−B5 | | | | | | |
| 8 | | | | | | | | |
| 9 | | | | | | | | |
| 10 | If you are having problems understanding this calculation, you may not be using the | | | | | | | |
| 11 | correct sequence of instructions, because your calculator may require a different | | | | | | | |
| 12 | sequence of entries. Some calculators want you to enter the operation BEFORE | | | | | | | |
| 13 | the number. Other calculators want you to enter the operation AFTER the number. | | | | | | | |
| 14 | | | | | | | | |

| | A | B | C | D | E | F | G | H | I |
|---|---|---|---|---|---|---|---|---|---|
| 1 | **Community Hospital** | | | | | | | | |
| 2 | **Full-time Equivalent Staff** | | | | | | | | |
| 3 | | | | | | | | | |
| 4 | | | | | | | | | |
| 5 | | Number | Hours | Total | | | | | |
| 6 | Part-time | 6 | 20 | 120 | =B6*C6 | | | | |
| 7 | Full-time | 69 | 40 | 2760 | =B7*C7 | | | | |
| 8 | | | | | | | | | |
| 9 | Total Hours Worked | | | 2880 | =SUM(D6:D7) | | | | |
| 10 | Normal Work Hours | | | 40 | | | | | |
| 11 | Full-time Equivalents | | | 72 | =D9/D10 | | | | |
| 12 | | | | | | | | | |
| 13 | FTE = Full-time Equivalents | | | | | | | | |
| 14 | FTEs = Total number of hours worked per week, divided by number of normal work hours | | | | | | | | |
| 15 | | | | | | | | | |
| 16 | In this example, we calculated the total hours worked by the part-time employees and | | | | | | | | |
| 17 | the total hours worked by the full-time employees. We then divided the total number | | | | | | | | |
| 18 | of hours worked by all employees by the number of hours in the normal work week. This | | | | | | | | |
| 19 | calculation of Full-time Equivalents provides management with a number of employees | | | | | | | | |
| 20 | that can be compared to other departments and evaluated based on other volume | | | | | | | | |
| 21 | measurements, such as number of discharges. | | | | | | | | |

| | A | B | C | D | E | F | G |
|---|---|---|---|---|---|---|---|
| 1 | | | Community Hospital | | | | |
| 2 | | | Patient Census 12/15/14 | | | | |
| 3 | | | | | | | |
| 4 | | 175 | *Patients 12/14/14* | | | | |
| 5 | + | 3 | *Births* | | | | |
| 6 | − | 8 | *Deaths* | | | | |
| 7 | + | 11 | *Admitted* | | | | |
| 8 | − | 9 | *Discharged* | | | | |
| 9 | | 172 | *Patients 12/15/14* | | =B4+B5−B6+B7−B8 | | |
| 10 | | | | | | | |
| 11 | Be careful with the sequence of instructions in the formula. | | | | | | |
| 12 | In this sequence, the instruction to add or subtract goes BEFORE the number to be operated on. | | | | | | |

| | A | B | C | D | E | F | G |
|---|---|---|---|---|---|---|---|
| 1 | Community Hospital Cafeteria Survey | | | | | | |
| 2 | | | | | | | |
| 3 | | Total Patients Responding | Liked Food | Percent Who Liked Food | | | |
| 4 | | | | | | | |
| 5 | *2011* | 500 | 394 | 79% | =C5/B5 | | |
| 6 | *2012* | 2,000 | 1,645 | 82% | =C6/B6 | | |
| 7 | *Hospital B* | 20,011 | 15,492 | 77% | =C7/B7 | | |
| 8 | | | | | | | |
| 9 | | | | | | | |
| 10 | Percentages are useful in comparing results between different years or groups. | | | | | | |
| 11 | In this example, Community Hospital is comparing its cafeteria satisfaction between | | | | | | |
| 12 | 2011 and 2012. It is also comparing its cafeteria satisfaction with a survey taken at | | | | | | |
| 13 | another hospital (Hospital B). Because the satisfaction is expressed as a percentage, | | | | | | |
| 14 | we can easily see that Community Hospital's satisfaction results are improving and that they are superior to Hospital B. | | | | | | |
| 15 | | | | | | | |
| 16 | | | | | | | |
| 17 | Notice that the formula yields a decimal, not a percentage. In order to display the | | | | | | |
| 18 | results as a percentage, the cell must be formatted to recognize the number as a percentage. To format the cell, click on the following series of options from the main | | | | | | |
| 19 | menu at the top of the screen (Or click on the % icon on the home page, if available.) | | | | | | |
| 20 | | | | | | | |
| 21 | | Format | | | | | |
| 22 | | Cell | | | | | |
| 23 | | Number | | | | | |
| 24 | | Percentage | | | | | |
| 25 | Another way to obtain the percentage (without the % sign) is to multiply the decimal times 100; e.g. =C5/B5*100. | | | | | | |
| 26 | | | | | | | |

| | A | B | C | D | E | F | G | H | I | J | K | L | M | N | O | P | Q |
|---|---|---|---|---|---|---|---|---|---|---|---|---|---|---|---|---|---|
| 1 | | | | **Community Hospital** | | | | | | | | | | | | | |
| 2 | | | | **Length of Stay** | | | | | | | | | | | | | |
| 3 | | | | | | | | | | | | | | | | | |
| 4 | 1 | 2 | 3 | 3 | 3 | 4 | 4 | 5 | 5 | 6 | | | | | | | |
| 5 | 1 | 2 | 3 | 3 | 3 | 4 | 4 | 5 | 5 | 6 | | | | | | | |
| 6 | 1 | 2 | 3 | 3 | 4 | 4 | 4 | 5 | 5 | 6 | | | | | | | |
| 7 | 1 | 2 | 3 | 3 | 4 | 4 | 4 | 5 | 5 | 6 | | Computing the answers to | | | | | |
| 8 | 1 | 2 | 3 | 3 | 4 | 4 | 4 | 5 | 5 | 6 | | various statistical questions: | | | | | |
| 9 | 1 | 2 | 3 | 3 | 4 | 4 | 4 | 5 | 5 | 6 | | | | | | | |
| 10 | 1 | 2 | 3 | 3 | 4 | 4 | 4 | 5 | 5 | 6 | | *How many patients?* | 250 | | | | |
| 11 | 1 | 2 | 3 | 3 | 4 | 4 | 4 | 5 | 5 | 6 | | =COUNT(A4:J28) | | | | | |
| 12 | 1 | 2 | 3 | 3 | 4 | 4 | 4 | 5 | 5 | 6 | | | | | | | |
| 13 | 1 | 2 | 3 | 3 | 4 | 4 | 4 | 5 | 5 | 7 | | *What is the average length of stay?* | | | | 3.864 days | |
| 14 | 1 | 2 | 3 | 3 | 4 | 4 | 4 | 5 | 5 | 7 | | =AVERAGE(A4:J28) | | | | | |
| 15 | 1 | 2 | 3 | 3 | 4 | 4 | 4 | 5 | 5 | 7 | | (This is the mean, which could | | | | | |
| 16 | 1 | 2 | 3 | 3 | 4 | 4 | 4 | 5 | 5 | 7 | | also be calculated as | | | | | |
| 17 | 1 | 2 | 3 | 3 | 4 | 4 | 4 | 5 | 5 | 7 | | =SUM(A4:J28)/250 | | | | | |
| 18 | 1 | 2 | 3 | 3 | 4 | 4 | 4 | 5 | 5 | 7 | | | | | | | |
| 19 | 1 | 2 | 3 | 3 | 4 | 4 | 4 | 5 | 5 | 7 | | *What is the median length of stay?* | | | | 4 days | |
| 20 | 1 | 2 | 3 | 3 | 4 | 4 | 4 | 5 | 5 | 7 | | =MEDIAN(A4:J28) | | | | | |
| 21 | 1 | 2 | 3 | 3 | 4 | 4 | 5 | 5 | 5 | 7 | | | | | | | |
| 22 | 1 | 2 | 3 | 3 | 4 | 4 | 5 | 5 | 5 | 7 | | *What is the mode?* | | | | 4 days | |
| 23 | 1 | 2 | 3 | 3 | 4 | 4 | 5 | 5 | 6 | 8 | | =MODE(A4:J28) | | | | | |
| 24 | 1 | 3 | 3 | 3 | 4 | 4 | 5 | 5 | 6 | 8 | | | | | | | |
| 25 | 1 | 3 | 3 | 3 | 4 | 4 | 5 | 5 | 6 | 8 | | | | | | | |
| 26 | 1 | 3 | 3 | 3 | 4 | 4 | 5 | 5 | 6 | 8 | | | | | | | |
| 27 | 1 | 3 | 3 | 3 | 4 | 4 | 5 | 5 | 6 | 9 | | | | | | | |
| 28 | 1 | 3 | 3 | 3 | 4 | 4 | 5 | 5 | 6 | 9 | | | | | | | |

|   | A | B | C | D | E | F | G | H | I | J | K | L | M | N | O | P | Q | R | S |
|---|---|---|---|---|---|---|---|---|---|---|---|---|---|---|---|---|---|---|---|
| 1 |   |   |   |   |   |   |   |   |   |   |   |   |   |   |   |   |   |   |   |
| 2 |   |   | **Community Hospital** |   |   |   |   |   |   |   |   | Frequency distribution |   |   |   |   |   |   |   |
| 3 |   |   | **Length of Stay** |   |   |   |   |   |   |   |   |   |   |   |   |   |   |   |   |
| 4 |   |   |   |   |   |   |   |   |   |   |   | EXCEL will calculate the frequency distribution of |   |   |   |   |   |   |   |
| 5 | 1 | 2 | 3 | 3 | 3 | 4 | 4 | 5 | 5 | 6 |   | a data set. It sorts the data into class intervals that |   |   |   |   |   |   |   |
| 6 | 1 | 2 | 3 | 3 | 3 | 4 | 4 | 5 | 5 | 6 |   | we describe. In this example, we will use the individual |   |   |   |   |   |   |   |
| 7 | 1 | 2 | 3 | 3 | 4 | 4 | 4 | 5 | 5 | 6 |   | lengths of stay as our target, which EXCEL calls "BINS." |   |   |   |   |   |   |   |
| 8 | 1 | 2 | 3 | 3 | 4 | 4 | 4 | 5 | 5 | 6 |   |   |   |   |   |   |   |   |   |
| 9 | 1 | 2 | 3 | 3 | 4 | 4 | 4 | 5 | 5 | 6 |   | BINS |   |   |   |   |   |   |   |
| 10 | 1 | 2 | 3 | 3 | 4 | 4 | 4 | 5 | 5 | 6 |   | 1 |   |   |   |   |   |   |   |
| 11 | 1 | 2 | 3 | 3 | 4 | 4 | 4 | 5 | 5 | 6 |   | 2 |   |   |   |   |   |   |   |
| 12 | 1 | 2 | 3 | 3 | 4 | 4 | 4 | 5 | 5 | 6 |   | 3 |   |   | *Step 1: List the BINS in order.* |   |   |   |   |
| 13 | 1 | 2 | 3 | 3 | 4 | 4 | 4 | 5 | 5 | 6 |   | 4 |   |   | *(THIS BINS ARRAY IS LOCATED* |   |   |   |   |
| 14 | 1 | 2 | 3 | 3 | 4 | 4 | 4 | 5 | 5 | 7 |   | 5 |   |   | *IN CELLS L10 THROUGH L18.)* |   |   |   |   |
| 15 | 1 | 2 | 3 | 3 | 4 | 4 | 4 | 5 | 5 | 7 |   | 6 |   |   |   |   |   |   |   |
| 16 | 1 | 2 | 3 | 3 | 4 | 4 | 4 | 5 | 5 | 7 |   | 7 |   |   |   |   |   |   |   |
| 17 | 1 | 2 | 3 | 3 | 4 | 4 | 4 | 5 | 5 | 7 |   | 8 |   |   |   |   |   |   |   |
| 18 | 1 | 2 | 3 | 3 | 4 | 4 | 4 | 5 | 5 | 7 |   | 9 |   |   |   |   |   |   |   |
| 19 | 1 | 2 | 3 | 3 | 4 | 4 | 4 | 5 | 5 | 7 |   |   |   |   |   |   |   |   |   |
| 20 | 1 | 2 | 3 | 3 | 4 | 4 | 4 | 5 | 5 | 7 |   |   |   |   |   |   |   |   |   |
| 21 | 1 | 2 | 3 | 3 | 4 | 4 | 4 | 5 | 5 | 7 |   | BINS |   |   |   |   |   |   |   |
| 22 | 1 | 2 | 3 | 3 | 4 | 4 | 5 | 5 | 5 | 7 |   | 1 | =FREQUENCY(A5:J29,L10:L18) |   |   |   |   |   |   |
| 23 | 1 | 2 | 3 | 3 | 4 | 4 | 5 | 5 | 5 | 7 |   | 2 |   |   |   |   |   |   |   |
| 24 | 1 | 2 | 3 | 3 | 4 | 4 | 5 | 5 | 6 | 8 |   | 3 |   |   |   |   |   |   |   |
| 25 | 1 | 3 | 3 | 3 | 4 | 4 | 5 | 5 | 6 | 8 |   | 4 |   |   | *Step 2: Enter the formula.* |   |   |   |   |
| 26 | 1 | 3 | 3 | 3 | 4 | 4 | 5 | 5 | 6 | 8 |   | 5 |   |   | *Specify the range for the data; press Enter.* |   |   |   |   |
| 27 | 1 | 3 | 3 | 3 | 4 | 4 | 5 | 5 | 6 | 8 |   | 6 |   |   | *Specify the range for the BINS.* |   |   |   |   |
| 28 | 1 | 3 | 3 | 3 | 4 | 4 | 5 | 5 | 6 | 9 |   | 7 |   |   |   |   |   |   |   |
| 29 | 1 | 3 | 3 | 3 | 4 | 4 | 5 | 5 | 6 | 9 |   | 8 |   |   |   |   |   |   |   |
|   |   |   |   |   |   |   |   |   |   |   |   | 9 |   |   |   |   |   |   |   |

Lower section:

| | L | M | N O P Q R S |
|---|---|---|---|
| | BINS | | |
| | 1 | | =FREQUENCY(A5:J29,L10:L18) |
| | 2 | | |
| | 3 | | *Step 3: Click and drag to highlight the* |
| | 4 | | *entire area in which you wish to display* |
| | 5 | | *the results, including the formula cell.* |
| | 6 | | |
| | 7 | | |
| | 8 | | |
| | 9 | | |

| | L | M | N O P Q R S |
|---|---|---|---|
| | BINS | | |
| | 1 | 25 | |
| | 2 | 20 | *Step 4: Press F2. Then, press and hold:* |
| | 3 | 57 | *Ctrl   Shift   Enter* |
| | 4 | 65 | |
| | 5 | 52 | *The frequencies of each BIN will appear next* |
| | 6 | 15 | *to the BIN they represent. These frequencies* |
| | 7 | 10 | *can then be used to prepare informative* |
| | 8 | 4 | *tables and graphs.* |
| | 9 | 2 | |

|  | A | B | C | D | E | F |
|---|---|---|---|---|---|---|
| 1 | | | | | | |
| 2 | | **Community Hospital** | | | | |
| 3 | | **Length of Stay** | | | | |
| 4 | | | | | | |
| 5 | | *Frequencies:* | | *Percentage:* | | |
| 6 | | 1 | 25 | 10% | =C6/$C$15 | |
| 7 | | 2 | 20 | 8% | =C7/$C$15 | |
| 8 | | 3 | 57 | 23% | =C8/$C$15 | |
| 9 | | 4 | 65 | 26% | =C9/$C$15 | |
| 10 | | 5 | 52 | 21% | =C10/$C$15 | |
| 11 | | 6 | 15 | 6% | =C11/$C$15 | |
| 12 | | 7 | 10 | 4% | =C12/$C$15 | |
| 13 | | 8 | 4 | 2% | =C13/$C$15 | |
| 14 | | 9 | 2 | 1% | =C14/$C$15 | |
| 15 | | **Total** | 250 | | | |
| 16 | | | =SUM(C6:C14) | | | |
| 17 | | | | | | |
| 18 | | Notice that we anchored the total in the percentage formula | | | | |
| 19 | | by placing a dollar sign in front of each element of the cell. | | | | |
| 20 | | | | | | |
| 21 | | | | | | |
| 22 | | The graph below is a "Scatter" graph with a line | | | | |
| 23 | | connecting the dots. It represents the data fields | | | | |
| 24 | | **B6:B14, D6:D14.** | | | | |

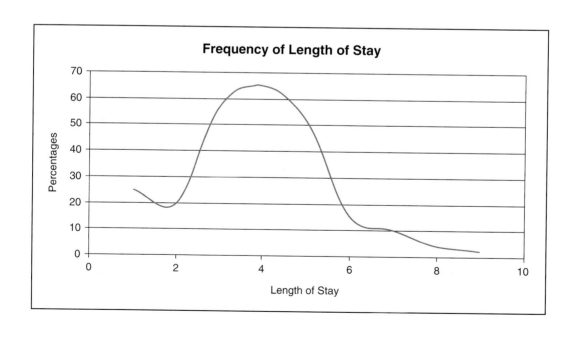

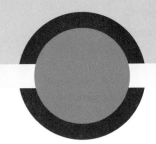

# GLOSSARY

## A

**Abstract** A summary of the patient record.

**Abstracting** The recap of selected fields from a health record to create an informative summary; also refers to the activity of identifying such fields and entering them into a computer system.

**Access** The ability to learn the contents of a record by obtaining it or having the contents revealed.

**Accounting of disclosures** The listing of the identities of those to whom certain protected health information has been disclosed.

**Accreditation** Voluntary compliance with a set of standards developed by an independent agent, who periodically performs audits to ensure compliance.

**Accreditation Association for Ambulatory Health Care (AAAHC)** An organization that accredits ambulatory care facilities.

**Activities of daily living** Refers to self-care, such as bathing, as well as cooking, shopping, and other routines requiring thought, planning, and physical motion.

**Acute care facility** A health care facility in which patients have an average length of stay less than 30 days and that has an emergency department, operating suite, and clinical departments to handle a broad range of diagnoses and treatments.

**Admission** The act of accepting a patient into care in a health care facility, including any nonambulatory care facility. Admission requires a physician's order.

**Admission consent form** A form signed by the patient in an inpatient facility granting permission to the hospital to provide general diagnostic and therapeutic care as well as to release patient information to a third party payer, if applicable. Also known as a *general consent form.*

**Admission denial** Occurs when the payer or its designee (such as utilization review staff) will not reimburse the facility for treatment of the patient because the admission was deemed unnecessary.

**Admission record** The demographic, financial, socioeconomic, and clinical data collected about a patient at registration. Also refers to the document in a paper record that contains these data.

**Admitting diagnosis** The reason given by the physician for initiating the order for the patient to be placed into care in a hospital.

**Admitting physician** The physician who gives the order to observe or admit a patient.

**Advance directive** A written document, such as a living will, that specifies a patient's wishes for his or her care and dictates power of attorney, for the purpose of providing clear instructions in the event the patient is unable to do so.

**Agenda** A tool used to organize the topics to be discussed during a meeting.

**Aggregate data** A group of like data elements compiled to provide information about the group.

**Algorithm** A procedure (set of instructions) for accomplishing a task.

**Allied health professionals** Health care professionals who support patient care in a variety of disciplines, including occupational therapy and physical therapy.

**Ambulatory care** Care provided on an outpatient basis, in which the patient is not admitted; arriving at a facility, receiving treatment, and leaving within one day.

**Ambulatory care facility** An outpatient facility, such as an emergency department or physician's office, in which treatment is intended to occur within 1 calendar day.

**Ambulatory payment classifications (APCs)** A prospective payment system for ambulatory care based on medically necessary services.

**Ambulatory surgery** Surgical procedures performed on an outpatient basis; the patient returns home after the procedure is performed. Also called *same day surgery.*

**Ambulatory surgery center (ASC)** A surgical facility that performs procedures that do not require an inpatient stay.

**Amendment** A change to the original document.

**American College of Surgeons (ACS)** A national professional organization that supports surgeons, to encourage higher quality of care for surgical patients.

**American Health Information Management Association (AHIMA)** A professional organization supporting the health care industry by promoting high-quality information standards through a variety of activities, including but not limited to accreditation of schools, continuing education, professional development and educational publications, and legislative and regulatory advocacy.

**American Medical Association (AMA)** National professional organization involved in supporting all medical decision makers; the AMA also owns and maintains the Current Procedural Terminology (CPT) code set.

**American Psychiatric Association (APA)** National professional organization involved in supporting licensed psychiatrists; maintains the *Diagnosis and Statistical Manual* *of Mental Disorders,* Fourth Edition (DSM-IV) Behavioral Health code set.

**American Recovery and Reinvestment Act (ARRA)** Also called the "stimulus bill." Federal legislation (2009) providing many stimulus opportunities in different areas. The portion of the law that finds and sets mandates for health information technology is called the Health Information Technology for Economic and Clinical Health (HITECH) Act.

**Analysis** The review of a record to evaluate its completeness, accuracy, or compliance with predetermined standards or other criteria.

**Anesthesia report** An anesthesiologist's documentation of patient evaluations before, during, and after surgery, including the specifics of the administration of anesthesia.

**Arithmetic mean** Also called the "average" or just "mean". Expresses the typical value in a set; computed by dividing the sum of the values in the set by the number of values in the set.

**Assembly** The reorganization of a paper record into a standard order.

**Assessment** An evaluation. In medical decision making, the physician's evaluation of the subjective and objective evidence. Also refers to the evaluation of a patient by any clinical discipline.

**Assisted living** A type of long-term care in which the resident is significantly independent in activities of daily living and does not need high levels of skilled nursing.

**Attending physician** The physician who is primarily responsible for coordinating the care of the patient in the hospital; it is usually the physician who ordered the patient's admission to the hospital.

**Audit trail** Software that tracks and stores information related to the activity of users in the system.

**Authenticate** To assume responsibility for data collection or the activities described by the data collection by signature, mark, code, password, or other means of identification.

**Average length of stay (ALOS)** The arithmetic mean of the lengths of stay of a group of inpatients.

## B

**Bar code** The representation of data using parallel lines or other patterns in a way readable to a machine, such as an optical bar code scanner or a smartphone.

**Bar graph** A chart that uses bars to represent the frequencies of items in the specified categories of a variable.

**Baseline** A beginning value; the value at which an activity is originally measured, such as the first blood pressure reading at an initial physician's office visit.

**Batch control form** A listing of charts in process, postdischarge, that identifies which steps have been completed.

**Bed control** The function of assigning beds in an acute care facility.

**Bed count** The actual number of beds that a hospital has staffed, equipped, and otherwise made available for occupancy by patients for each specific operating day.

**Behavioral health facility** An inpatient or outpatient health care facility that focuses on the treatment of psychiatric conditions. Also called a *mental health* or *psychiatric facility.*

**Benchmarking** An improvement technique that compares one facility's process with that of another facility that has been noted to have superior performance.

**Billing** The process of submitting health insurance claims or rendering invoices.

**Brainstorming** A data-gathering quality improvement tool used to generate information related to a topic.

**Business associate** Under the Health Insurance Portability and Accountability Act (HIPAA), a contracted vendor that uses confidential health information to perform a service on behalf of a covered entity.

**Business record rule** An exception to the hearsay rule. Allows health records to be admitted as evidence in legal proceedings because they are kept in the normal course of business, are recorded concurrently with the events that they describe, and are recorded by individuals who are in a position to know the facts of the events that are described.

## C

**Cancer treatment center** A facility that specializes in cancer treatment and management.

**Capital budget** Money set aside for larger purchases, usually over a certain dollar amount, whose use will span multiple fiscal years.

**Capitation** A uniform reimbursement to a health care provider based on the number of patients contractually in the physician's care, regardless of diagnoses or services rendered.

**Case management** The coordination of the patient's care and services, including reimbursement considerations.

**Case mix** Statistical distribution of patients according to their utilization of resources. Also refers to the grouping of patients by clinical department or other meaningful distribution, such as health insurance type.

**Case mix index** The arithmetic average (mean) of the relative diagnosis related group (DRG) weights of all health care cases in a given period.

**Census** The actual number of inpatients in a facility at a point in time, for comparative purposes, usually midnight.

**Centers for Disease Control and Prevention (CDC)** A federal agency that collects health information to provide research for the improvement of public health.

**Centers for Medicare and Medicaid Services (CMS)** The division of the U.S. Department of Health and Human Services that administers Medicare and Medicaid.

**Central limit theorem** The tendency of a large number of means to distribute symmetrically, approaching a normal distribution.

**Certification** Approval by an outside agency, such as the federal or state government, indicating that the health care facility has met a set of predetermined standards. In litigation, the custodian's authentication that the copies of medical records used are true and complete.

**Certification Commission for Health Information Technology (CCHIT)** A nonprofit organization that seeks to advance health information technology by defining and certifying electronic health record (EHR) technology.

**Chain of command** The formal authority and decision-making structure within an organization.

**Character** A single letter, number, or symbol.

**Charge capture** The systematic collection of specific charges for services rendered to a patient.

**Chargemaster** The database that contains the detailed description of charges related to all potential services rendered to a patient.

**Charges** Fees or costs for services rendered.

**Chart locator system** A system for locating records within a facility.

**Chief complaint** The main reason a patient has sought treatment.

**Children's hospital** A specialty facility that focuses on the treatment of children.

**Claim** The application to an insurance company for reimbursement of services rendered.

**Class intervals** Groups, categories, or tiers of the highest and lowest values that are meaningful to the user.

**Classification** Systematic organization of elements into categories. ICD-10-CM is a classification system that organizes diagnoses into categories, primarily by body system.

**Clinic** A facility-based ambulatory care department that provides general or specialized outpatient services, such as those provided in a physician's office.

**Clinical data** All of the medical data that have been recorded about the patient's stay or visit, including diagnoses and procedures.

**Clinical decision-making system (CDS)** A computer application that compares two or more items of patient data in order to advise clinicians on the treatment of that specific patient.

**Clinical pathway** A predetermined standard of treatment for a particular disease, diagnosis, or procedure designed to facilitate the patient's progress through the health care encounter.

**Cloud computing** A computing architecture in which the resources, software, and application data are Internet based rather than existing on a local system.

**Coding** The assignment of alphanumerical values to a word, phrase, or other nonnumerical expression. In health care, coding is the assignment of alphanumerical values to diagnosis and procedure descriptions.

**Coding compliance plan** The development, implementation, and enforcement of policies and procedures to ensure that coding standards are met.

**Cognitive remediation** A type of therapy for judgment, reasoning, perception, or memory impairments.

**Co-insurance** A type of third party payer arrangement in which an individual is responsible for a percentage of the amount owed to the provider.

**Commission on Accreditation for Health Informatics and Information Management (CAHIIM)** The organization that accredits and sets quality and educational standards for HIM higher education programs.

**Commission on Accreditation of Rehabilitation Facilities (CARF)** An organization that accredits behavioral health and rehabilitation facilities.

**Community Health Accreditation Program (CHAP)** An organization that accredits home health care agencies.

**Comorbidity** A condition that affects the patient's care and/or length of stay and exists at the same time as the principal diagnosis.

**Competency** The ability to successfully complete a task or skill.

**Completeness** The data quality of existence. If a required data element is missing, the record is not complete.

**Compliance** Meeting standards. Also, the development, implementation, and enforcement of policies and procedures that ensure that standards are met.

**Complication** A condition that arises during hospitalization or as a result of the health care encounter.

**Computer output to laser disk (COLD)** Forms or reports generated from computer output transferred for storage on laser disk.

**Computerized physician order entry (CPOE)** A health information system in which physicians enter orders electronically. Includes decision support and alerts.

**Concurrent analysis** Any type of record analysis performed during the patient's stay (i.e., after admission but before discharge).

**Concurrent coding** Coding performed during the patient's stay (i.e., after admission but before discharge); this process is performed to obtain the working diagnosis related group (DRG).

**Concurrent review** Review occurring during the act or event (i.e., a chart review during the patient's stay in the facility).

**Conditions of admission** The legal agreement between the health care facility and a patient (or the patient's legal agent) to perform routine services. May also include the statement of the patient's financial responsibility and prospective consent for release of information and examination and disposal of tissue.

**Conditions of participation (COP)** The terms under which a facility is eligible to receive reimbursement from Medicare.

**Confidential communications** The sharing of patient health information protected from disclosure in court, such as patient/physician. Also refers to transmission of information so as to minimize the risk of inadvertent disclosure, such as patient requesting mailing to an alternative address.

**Confidentiality** Discretion regarding the disclosure of information.

**Consent** An agreement or permission to receive health care services.

**Consultant** A medical professional who provides clinical expertise in a specialty at the request of the attending physician.

**Consultation** The formal request by a physician for the professional opinion or services of another health care professional, usually another physician, in caring for a patient. Also refers to the opinion or services themselves as well as the activity of rendering the opinion or services.

**Continued stay denial** Similar to *admission denial*; however, it is the additional payment for the length of stay that is not approved rather than the entire admission.

**Continuing education (CE)** Education required after a person has attained a position, credential, or degree, intended to keep the person knowledgeable in his or her profession.

**Continuity of care** The coordination among caregivers to provide, efficiently and effectively, the broad range of health care services required by a patient during an illness or for an entire lifetime. May also refer to the coordination of care provided among caregivers / services within a health care organization. Also called *continuum of care*.

**Continuum of care** See *continuity of care*.

**Cooperating Parties** The four organizations responsible for maintaining the ICD-10-CM: Center for Medicare and Medicaid Services (CMS), National Center for Health Statistics (NCHS), American Hospital Association (AHA), and American Hospital Information Management Association (AHIMA).

**Copay** A fixed amount paid by the patient at the time of service.

**Corrective controls** Procedures, processes, or structures that are designed to fix errors when they are detected. Because errors cannot always be fixed, corrective controls also include the initiation of investigation into future error prevention or detection.

**Correspondence** Mailing or letters exchanged between parties.

**Countersignature** See *countersigned*.

**Countersigned** Evidence of supervision of subordinate personnel, such as physician residents.

**Court order** The direction of a judge who has made a decision that an order to produce information (on the record) is necessary.

**Covered entity** Under Health Insurance Portability and Accountability Act (HIPAA) and Health Information Technology for Economic and Clinical Health (HITECH) Act provisions, any organization that collects and manages health information.

**Credentials** An individual's specific professional qualifications. Also refers to the acronym or abbreviation representing a degree or certification that a professionally qualified person is entitled to list after his or her name.

**Cross-training** Training of employees for additional jobs or functions within the department so that they can help with those jobs when necessary.

**Current Procedural Terminology (CPT)** A nomenclature and coding system developed and maintained by the American Medical Association (AMA) to facilitate billing for physicians and other services.

**Custodian** The person entrusted with the responsibility for the confidentiality, privacy, and security of medical records.

# D

**Data** The smallest elements or units of facts or observations. Also refers to a collection of such elements.

**Data accessibility** Data can be obtained when needed by authorized individuals.

**Data accuracy** The quality that data are correct.

**Data analytics** The process of analyzing data and exploring them to create information.

**Data collection devices** Paper forms designed to capture data elements in a standardized format, or the physical computer hardware that facilitates the data collection process.

**Data consistency** Data is the same wherever it appears.

**Data dictionary** A list of details that describe each field in a database.

**Data Elements for Emergency Department Systems (DEEDS)** Minimum data set for emergency services.

**Data entry** The process of recording elements into a collection device. Generally refers to the recording of elements into a computer system.

**Data repository** Where data is stored from different, unrelated software programs.

**Data set** A group of data elements collected for a specific purpose.

**Data validity** The quality that data reflect the known or acceptable range of values for the specific data.

**Data warehouse** Where information from different databases is collected and organized to be used for ad hoc reports and analytical research.

**Database** An organized collection of data.

**Date-oriented record** See *integrated record*.

**Decision matrix** A quality improvement tool used to narrow focus or choose between two or more related possible decisions.

**Deductible** A specified dollar amount for which the patient is personally responsible before the payer reimburses for any claims.

**Deemed status** The Medicare provision that an approved accreditation is sufficient to satisfy the compliance audit element of the Conditions of Participation.

**Defendant** The party or parties against whom the plaintiff has initiated litigation.

**Deficiencies** Required elements that are missing from a record.

**Deficiency system** The policies and procedures that form the corrective control of collecting the missing data identified in quantitative analysis. Includes the recording and reporting of deficiencies. Also called an *incomplete system*.

**Delegation** The transfer of a responsibility, task, or project from a manager to a lower-level employee.

**Delinquent** Status accorded to a record that has not been completed within a specified time frame, such as within 30 days of discharge.

**Demographic data** Identification: those elements that distinguish one patient from another, such as name, address, and birth date.

**Department of Health and Human Services (DHHS)** The United States agency with regulatory oversight of American health care, which also provides health services to certain populations through several operating divisions.

**Designated record set** A specific portion of the patient's health information, consisting of medical records, reimbursement and payer information, and other information used to make health care decisions, all of which may be accessed by the patient under Health Insurance Portability and Accountability Act (HIPAA) provisions.

**Detective controls** Procedures, processes, or structures that are designed to find errors after they have been made.

**Diagnosis** Literally, "complete knowledge"; refers to the name of the patient's condition or illness or the reason for the health care encounter.

**Diagnosis related groups (DRGs)** A collection of health care descriptions organized into statistically similar categories.

***Diagnostic and Statistical Manual of Mental Disorders, Fifth Edition (DSM-5)*** Used for coding behavior and mental health care encounters in a structured format.

**Dialysis** The extracorporeal elimination of waste products from bodily fluids (e.g., blood).

**Dialysis center** An ambulatory care facility that specializes in blood-cleansing procedures to treat, for example, chronic kidney (renal) failure.

**Digital Imaging and Communications in Medicine (DICOM)** A standard that enables the storage and use of clinical digital imaging, making their exchange among physicians and other providers possible.

**Digital signature** An electronic means to identify the authenticity and integrity of the user's identification.

**Digitized signature** An original signature on a report that is then scanned into an electronic document.

**Direct admission** An expedited inpatient admission arranged in advance by a physician's office or other entity due to a patient's urgent medical condition.

**Discharge** When the patient leaves the care of the facility to go home, for transfer to another health care facility, or expires (dies). Also refers to the status of a patient.

**Discharge planning** The multidisciplinary, coordinated effort to ensure that a patient is discharged to the appropriate level of care and with the appropriate support.

**Discharge register (discharge list)** A list of all patients discharged on a specific date or during a specific period.

**Discharge summary** The recap of an inpatient's stay, usually dictated by the attending physician and transcribed into a formal report.

**Disclosure** When patient health information is given to someone.

**Discounted fee for service** The exchange of cash for professional services rendered, at a rate less than the normal fee for the service.

**Discovery** The process of investigating the circumstances surrounding a lawsuit.

**Discrete data** Named and identifiable pieces of data that can be queried and reported in a meaningful way.

**Document imaging** Scanning or faxing of printed papers into a computer system or optical disk system. See also *computer output to laser disk.*

**Dual governance** In hospitals, a shared organization structure consisting of the administration, headed by the Chief Executive Officer, and the medical staff, headed by the Chief of Medical Staff.

## E

**Electronic data interchange (EDI)** A standard in which data can be transmitted, communicated, and understood by the sending and receiving computer systems, allowing the exchange of information.

**Electronic document management system (EDMS)** Computer software and hardware, typically scanners, that allow health record documents to be stored, retrieved, and shared.

**Electronic health record (EHR)** A secure real-time, point-of-care, patient centric information resource for clinicians allowing access to patient information when and where needed and incorporating evidence-based decision support.

**Electronic signature** When the authenticator uses a password or personal identification number (PIN) to electronically sign a document.

**Emancipation** Consideration of a patient as an adult even though the patient is younger than the statutory age.

**Encounter** A patient's interaction with a health care provider to receive services; a unit of measure for the volume of ambulatory care services provided.

**Encounter form** A data collection device that facilitates the accurate capture of ambulatory care diagnoses and services.

**Encryption** A security process that blocks unauthorized access to patient information.

**Enterprise master patient index (EMPI)** A master patient index shared across a multihospital system, such as a health information exchange (HIE).

**Entitlement programs** In health care, government-sponsored programs that pay for certain services on the basis of an individual's age, condition, employment status, or other circumstances.

**e-PHI** Under the Health Insurance Portability and Accountability Act (HIPAA), protected health information in electronic format.

**Epidemiology** The study of morbidity (disease) trends and occurrences.

**Ergonomics** Alignment of the work environment to accommodate the employee's job function.

**Error report** An electronically generated report that lists deficient or erroneous data.

**Ethics** A system of beliefs about acceptable behavior; a standard of moral excellence that all health information management professionals must uphold while managing patient information.

**Etiology**  The cause or source of the patient's condition or disease.

**Evidence-based decision support**  Information systems that provide clinical best-knowledge practices to make decisions about patient care.

**Evidence-based medicine (EBM)**  Health care delivery that uses clinical research to make decisions in patient care.

**Exception report**  See *error report*.

**Exceptions**  In the Health Insurance Portability and Accountability Act (HIPAA), uses and disclosures of protected health information for certain public priorities without patient authorization.

## F

**Face sheet**  The first page in a paper record. Usually contains at least the demographic data and contains space for the physician to record and authenticate the discharge diagnoses and procedures. In many facilities, the admission record is also used as the face sheet.

**Family unit numbering system**  A numerical identification system to identify an entire family's health record using one number and modifiers.

**Federal Drug and Alcohol Abuse Regulations**  Regulations at the national level addressing requirements for disclosure of chemical and alcohol abuse patient information.

*Federal Register*  The publication of the proceedings of the United States Congress.

**Fee for service**  The exchange of monies for professional services rendered at a specific rate, typically determined by the provider and associated with specific activities (such as a physical examination).

**Fee schedule**  The list of charges that a physician expects to be paid for services rendered. Also, a list of the amounts a payer will remit for certain services.

**Field**  A collection or series of related characters. A field may contain a word, a group of words, a number, or a code, for example.

**File**  Numerous records of different types of related data. Files can be large or small, depending on the number of records they contain.

**File folder**  The physical container used to store the health record in a paper-based system.

**Financial data**  Elements that describe the payer. For example, the name, address, and telephone number of the patient's insurance company, as well as the group and member numbers the company has assigned to the patient.

**Fiscal intermediaries**  Organizations that administer the claims and reimbursements for the funding agency. Medicare uses fiscal intermediaries to process its claims and reimbursements.

**Flexible benefit account**  A savings account in which health care and certain child-care costs can be set aside and paid using pretax funds.

**Frequency distribution**  The grouping of observations into a small number of categories.

**Full-time equivalent (FTE)**  A unit of staffing that equals the regular 32 to 40 hour work week as defined by the organization.

## G

**General consent form**  A form signed by the patient in an acute care facility granting permission to the hospital to provide general diagnostic and therapeutic care, as well as to release patient information to a third party payer, if applicable. Also known as an *admission consent form*.

**Goals**  Desired achievements.

**Granularity**  The level of detail with which data is collected, recorded, or calculated.

**Graph**  An illustration of data.

**Group plan**  A pool of covered individuals that averages the risk for a third party payer, used to leverage lower premiums for the group as a whole.

**Group practice**  Multiple physicians who share facilities and resources and may also cooperate in rendering patient care.

**Group practice model HMO**  A health maintenance organization (HMO) that contracts with a group or network of physicians and facilities to provide health care services.

**Grouper**  The software used to derive the diagnosis related group (DRG) from the ICD-10-CM diagnoses and procedures.

**Guarantor**  The individual or organization that promises to pay for the rendered health care services after all other sources (such as insurance) are exhausted.

## H

**Health Care Quality Improvement Program (HCQIP)**  A quality initiative established by the Balanced Budget Act (1997) that administers various review processes in order to identify and improve care outcomes for Medicare beneficiaries.

**Health data**  Elements related to a patient's diagnosis and procedures as well as factors that may affect the patient's condition.

**Health information**  Organized data that have been collected about a patient or a group of patients. Sometimes used synonymously with *health data*.

**Health information exchange (HIE)**  The database of a network of health care providers (physicians, hospitals, laboratories, and public health organizations) allowing access to patient records within the network from approved points of care.

**Health information management (HIM)**  The profession that manages the sources and uses of health information, including the collection, storage, retrieval, and reporting of health information.

**Health information technology (HIT)**  The specialty in the field of health information management that focuses on the day-to-day activities of health information management that support the collection, storage, retrieval, and reporting of health information.

**Health Information Technology for Economic and Clinical Health (HITECH) Act**  A subset of the American

Recovery and Reinvestment Act (2009) legislation providing federal funding and mandates for the use of technology in health care.

**Health Insurance Portability and Accountability Act (HIPAA)** Public law 104-191, federal legislation passed in 1996 that outlines the guidelines of managing patient information in terms of privacy, security, and confidentiality. The legislation also outlines penalties for noncompliance.

**Health Level Seven (HL7)** A health information systems compliance organization whose goal is to standardize the collection of patient information in the electronic health care record.

**Health maintenance organization** Managed care organization characterized by the ownership or employer control over the health care providers.

**Health record** Contains all of the data collected for an individual patient. Also called *record* or *medical record*.

**Healthcare Common Procedure Coding System (HCPCS)** The Centers for Medicare and Medicaid Services (CMS) coding system, of which CPT-4 (Current Procedural Terminology) is level one. Used for physician services, drugs, equipment, supplies, and other auxiliary health care services rendered.

**Healthcare Effectiveness Data and Information Set (HEDIS)** A performance measure data set published by health insurance companies that employers use to establish health care contracts on behalf of their employees.

**Hearsay rule** The court rule that prohibits most testimony regarding events by parties who were not directly involved in the event.

**HIPAA *Official Guidelines for Coding and Reporting*** Annually updated instructions for the use of ICD-10 codes.

**Histogram** A modified bar graph representing continuous data. Each bar represents a class interval; the height of the bar represents the frequency of observations.

**History** The physician's record of the patient's chief complaint, history of present illness, pertinent family and social history, and review of systems.

**History and physical (H&P)** Health record documentation comprising the patient's history and physical examination; a formal, dictated copy must be included in the patient's health care record within 24 hours of admission for inpatient facilities.

**Home health care** Health care services rendered in the patient's home; an agency that provides such services.

**Hospice** Palliative health care services rendered to the terminally ill, their families, and their friends.

**Hospital** An organization having permanent facilities that delivers inpatient health care services through 24-hour nursing care, an organized medical staff, and appropriate ancillary departments.

**Hospitalist** A physician employed by a hospital, whose medical practice is focused primarily on patient care situations specific to the acute care setting.

**Hybrid record** A record in which both electronic and paper media are used.

**I**

**ICD-9-CM** International Classification of Diseases, Ninth Revision—Clinical Modification. The United States' version of the ICD-9, maintained and updated by the Cooperating Parties.

**ICD-10-CM** International Classification of Diseases, Tenth Revision—Clinical Modification. The United States clinical modification of the World Health Organization ICD-10 morbidity and mortality data set. ICD-10-CM is mandated by HIPAA for reporting diagnoses and reasons for healthcare encounters in all settings.

**ICD-10-PCS** International Classification of Diseases, Tenth Revision, Procedural Coding System. A unique classification system, developed in the U.S., for reporting procedures performed in inpatient settings. It is a HIPAA mandated code set.

**ICD-O** International Classification of Diseases—Oncology. The coding system used to record and track the occurrence of neoplasms (i.e., malignant tumors, cancer).

**Incidence** Number of occurrences of a particular event, disease, or diagnosis or the number of new cases of a disease.

**Incomplete system** See *deficiency system*.

**Indemnity insurance** Assumption of the payment for all or part of certain, specified services. Characterized by out-of-pocket deductibles and caps on total covered payments.

**Independent practice association (IPA) model HMO** A Health Maintenance Organization (HMO) that contracts with individual physicians, a portion of whose practices is devoted to the HMO.

**Index** A system to identify or name a file or other item so that it can be located; a system that places specific data items within a frame of reference, creating collections of patient data (or a database) specific to a diagnosis, procedure, physician, or action such as admission or discharge.

**Indexing** The process of sorting a record by the different report types, making the viewing of the record uniform.

**Information** Processed data (i.e., data that are presented in an appropriate frame of reference).

**Informed consent** A permission given by a competent individual, of legal age, with full knowledge or understanding of the risks, potential benefits, and potential consequences of the permission.

**Infrastructure** The interrelated components of a system.

**Inpatient** An individual who is admitted to a hospital with the intention of staying overnight.

**Inpatient service day (IPSD)** A measure of the use of hospital services, representing the care provided to one inpatient during a 24-hour period.

**Inservice** Training provided to employees of an organization for continued or reinforced education.

**Institutional Review Board (IRB)** A committee within a facility charged with ensuring that research conducted within conforms to all applicable rules and regulations.

**Insurance** A contract between two parties in which one party assumes the risk of loss on behalf of the other party in return for some, usually monetary, compensation.

**Insurer** The party that assumes the risk of paying some or all of the cost of providing health care services in return for the payment of a premium by or on behalf of the insured.

**Integrated delivery system** A health care organization that provides services through most or all of the continuum of care.

**Integrated record** A paper record in which the pages are organized sequentially, in the chronological order in which they were generated; also known as *date-oriented record* or *sequential record*.

**Integrity** The data quality characteristic displayed when alteration of a finalized document is not permitted.

**Intensity of service (IS)** In utilization review, a type of criteria consisting primarily of monitoring and diagnostic assessments that must be met in order to qualify a patient for inpatient admission.

**Interactive map-assisted generation of ICD-10-CM Codes (I-MAGIC) algorithm** An algorithm used to map electronic health record (EHR)–generated SNOMED-CT codes to the more specific ICD-10-CM code set, seeking input from a coder to supply missing information as necessary.

**Interdepartmental** Relationship between two or more departments (e.g., HIM and the business office).

**Interface** Computer configuration allowing information to pass from one system to another.

**International Health Terminology Standards Development Organisation (IHTSDO)** A multinational organization the supports the standardized exchange of health information through the development of clinical terminologies, notably SNOMED-CT.

**Interoperability** The ability of different software and computer systems to communicate and share data.

**Intradepartmental** Occurrence or relationship within a department (e.g., assembly and analysis within health information management).

### J

**Job analysis** Review of a function to determine all of the tasks or components that make up an employee's job.

**Job description** A list of the employee's responsibilities.

**Joint Commission (TJC)** See *The Joint Commission*.

**Jurisdiction** The authority of a court to decide certain cases. May be based on geography, money, or type of case.

### L

**Laboratory** The physical location of the specialists who analyze body fluids.

**Laboratory tests** Procedures for analysis of body fluids.

**Length of stay (LOS)** The duration of an inpatient visit, measured in whole days: the number of whole days between the inpatient's admission and discharge.

**Licensed beds** The maximum number of beds that a facility is legally permitted to have, as approved by state licensure.

**Licensure** The mandatory government approval required for performing specified activities. In health care, the state approval required for providing health care services.

**Line graph** A chart that represents observations over time or between variables by locating the intersection of the horizontal and vertical values and connecting the dots signifying the intersections.

**Litigation** The term used to indicate that a matter must be settled by the court and the process of engaging in legal proceedings.

**Local coverage determination (LCD)** A list of diagnostic codes used by Medicare contractors to determine medical necessity.

**Longitudinal record** The compilation of information from all providers over the span of a patient's care, potentially from birth to death, which is facilitated by the electronic flow of information among providers.

**Long-term care (LTC) facility** A hospital that provides services to patients over an extended period; an average length of stay is in excess of 30 days. Facilities are characterized by the extent to which nursing care is provided.

**Loose sheets** In a paper health record, documents that are not present when the patient is discharged. These documents must be accumulated and filed with the record at a later date. Also called *loose reports*.

### M

**Major diagnostic categories (MDCs)** Segments of the diagnosis related group (DRG) assignment flowchart (grouper).

**Managed care** A type of insurer (payer) focused on reducing health care costs, controlling expensive care, and improving the quality of patient care provided.

**Marketing** Promoting products or services in the hope that the consumer chooses them over the products or services of a competitor.

**Master forms file** A file containing blank copies of all current paper forms used in a facility.

**Master patient index (MPI)** A system containing a list of patients who have received care at the health care facility and their encounter information, often used to correlate the patient with the file identification.

**Matrix reporting** An employee reports to more than one manager.

**Maximization** The process of determining the highest possible diagnosis related group (DRG) payment.

**Mean** The measure of central tendency that represents the arithmetic average of the observations.

**Meaningful use** A set of measures to gauge the level of health information technology used by a provider and required, in certain stages, in order to receive financial incentives from the Centers for Medicare and Medicaid Services (CMS).

**Median** The measure of central tendency that represents the observation that is exactly halfway between the highest and lowest observations.

**Medicaid** A federally mandated, state-funded program providing access to health care for the poor and the medically indigent.

**Medicaid Integrity Contractor (MIC)** A contractor who works with the Centers for Medicare and Medicaid Services (CMS) to identify fraud and waste through claims audits and other data collection activities.

**Medical record** See *health record; record.*

**Medical record number (MR#)** A unique number assigned to each patient in a health care system; this code will be used for the rest of the patient's encounters with that specific health system.

**Medical specialty** The focus of a physician's practice, such as pediatrics or oncology. Specialties are represented by Boards, which certify physicians in the specialties.

**Medicare** Federally funded health care entitlement program for older adults and for certain categories of chronically ill patients.

**Medicare administrative contractor (MAC)** Regional, private contractor who processes reimbursement claims for the Centers for Medicare and Medicaid Services (CMS).

**Medicare Code Editor (MCE)** A part of grouping software that checks for valid codes in claims data.

**Medication** Chemical substance used to treat disease.

**Medication administration** Clinical data including the name of the medication, dosage, date and time of administration, method of administration, and the nurse who administered it.

**Memorandum (memo)** A communication tool used to inform members of an organization.

**Mental health facility** See *behavioral health facility.*

**Microfiche** An alternative storage method for paper records on plastic sheets.

**Microfilm** An alternative storage method for paper records on plastic film.

**Middle-digit filing system** A modification of the terminal-digit filing system in which the patient's medical record number is separated into sets for filing and the first set of numbers is called *secondary,* the second set of numbers is called *primary,* and the third set is called *tertiary.*

**Minimum data set (MDS 3.0)** The detailed data collected about patients receiving long-term care. It is collected several times, and it forms the basis for the Resource Utilization Group.

**Minimum necessary** A rule requiring health providers to disclose only the minimum amount of information necessary to accomplish a task.

**Minutes** A tool used to record the events, topics, and discussions of a meeting.

**Mission statement** The strategic purpose of the organization documented in a formal statement.

**Mobile diagnostics** An alternate health care setting providing convenient access to patient testing and diagnostics, offering services such as diagnostic imaging and some types of laboratory screenings.

**Mode** The measure of central tendency that represents the most frequently occurring observation.

**Modifier** A two-digit addition to a CPT or HCPCS code that provides additional information about the service or procedure performed.

**Morbidity** A disease or illness.

**Morbidity rate** The rate of disease that can complicate a condition for which the patient is seeking health care services; or, the prevalence of a particular disease within a population.

**Mortality** Refers to death.

**Mortality rate** The frequency of death.

**Multi-axial** A code structure in which the position of a character has a specific meaning.

**Multispecialty group** In ambulatory care, a group practice consisting of physicians with different specialties.

## N

**National Cancer Institute's Surveillance, Epidemiology and End Results (SEER)** The National Cancer Institute's program collecting cancer statistics using the ICD-O-3 code set.

**National Center for Health Statistics (NCHS)** A division of the U.S. Centers for Disease Control and Prevention (CDC) that collects and analyzes vital statistics. Acts as one of the ICD-10-CM Cooperating Parties.

**National Center for Injury Prevention and Control (NCIPC)** A component of the U.S. Centers for Disease Control and Prevention (CDC) that focuses on reducing injuries and the diseases associated with, death from, and sequelae of injuries.

**National Committee for Quality Assurance (NCQA)** A nonprofit entity focusing on quality in health care delivery that accredits managed care organizations.

**National coverage determination (NCD)** A process using evidence-based medicine to determine whether Medicare will cover an item or service on the basis of medical necessity.

**National Drug Codes (NDCs)** A transaction code set used to identify drugs by the firm, labeler, and batch.

**National Integrated Accreditation for Healthcare Organizations (NIAHO)** A compliance and accreditation entity partnered with the Centers for Medicare and Medicaid Services (CMS) to ensure quality and standards in acute care settings. Facilities maintaining NIAHO accreditation receive *deemed status* from the CMS.

**National Library of Medicine (NLM)** The medical library operated by the U.S. government under the National Institutes of Health. Serves as representative for the United States in the International Health Terminology Standards Development Organisation (IHTSDO).

**National Patient Safety Goals** Guidance created by The Joint Commission (TJC) to recommend patient safety measures in accredited facilities.

**Nationwide Health Information Network (NHIN)** A system of nationally shared health data, composed of a network of providers, consumers, and researchers, that aims to improve health care delivery through the secure exchange of information.

**Network** A group of providers serving the members of a managed care organization; the payer will generally not cover health care services from providers outside the network.

**Nomenclature** In medical coding, a systematic assignment of a name to a diagnosis or procedure and associating that name with a numeric or alphanumeric value.

**Nonrepudiation** A process that provides a positive identification of the user.

**Normal curve** The symmetrical distribution of observations around a mean, usually in the shape of a bell.

**Nosocomial infection** A hospital-acquired infection.

**Notice of Privacy Practices** A notice, written in clear and simple language, summarizing a facility's privacy policies and the conditions for use or disclosure of patient health information.

**Nurse** A medical professional who has satisfied the academic, professional, and legal requirements to care for patients at state-specified levels. Although usually delivering patient care at the direction of physicians, nurse practitioners may also deliver care independently.

**Nursing assessment** The nurse's evaluation of the patient.

**Nursing progress notes** Routine documentation of the nurse's interaction with a patient.

## O

**Objective** In the SOAP format for medical decision making, the physician's observations and review of diagnostic tests.

**Objectives** Directions for achieving a goal.

**Occupancy** In a hospital, the percentage of available beds that have been used over time.

**Office of the National Coordinator of Health Information Technology (ONC)** An executive division of the U.S. Department of Health and Human Services that coordinates and promotes the national implementation of technology in health care.

**Open access** The physician's office scheduling method that allows for patient visits without an appointment. Some versions of open access focus on group visits for certain types of routine care.

**Operation** Surgery; an operation consists of one or more surgical procedures.

**Operational budget** Costs related to the operation of the health information department, such as utilities and supplies.

**Operative report** The surgeon's formal report of surgical procedure(s) performed. Often dictated and transcribed into a formal report.

**Optical disk** Electronic storage medium; a disk used to store digital data.

**Optimization** The process of determining the most accurate diagnosis related group (DRG) payment.

**Organization chart** An illustration used to describe the relationships among departments, positions, and functions within an organization.

**Orientation** Training to familiarize a new employee with the job.

**ORYX** A data set collection tool used by The Joint Commission (TJC) to measure the quality of patient care in hospitals.

**Outcome** The result of a patient's treatment.

**Outcome and Assessment Information Set (OASIS)** Data set most associated with home health care. This data set monitors patient care by identifying markers over the course of patient care.

**Outguide** A physical file guide used to identify another location of a file in the paper-based health record system.

**Outlier** A patient whose length of stay or cost is far lower or higher than the average expected by the prospective payment system, notably the diagnosis related group (DRG).

**Outlier payment** An unusually high payment within a given case-mix group.

**Out-of-pocket** Payment from personal funds.

**Outpatient** A patient whose health care services are intended to be delivered within 1 calendar day or, in some cases, a 24-hour period.

**Outpatient Prospective Payment System (OPPS)** A Medicare prospective payment system (PPS) used to determine the amount of reimbursement for outpatient services.

**Outsourcing** Services that are provided by external organizations or individuals who are not employees of the facility for which the services are being provided.

## P

**Pain management treatment center** A specialty setting that provides care and intervention procedures to alleviate acute and chronic pain.

**Palliative care** Health care services that are intended to soothe, comfort, or reduce symptoms but are not intended to cure.

**Patient account number** A numerical identifier assigned to a specific encounter or health care service received by a patient; a new number will be assigned to each encounter, but the patient will retain the same medical record number.

**Patient Assessment Instrument (PAI)** A tool used to identify patients with greater needs, and for the treatment of whom the long-term care or skilled nursing facility will receive higher reimbursement.

**Patient care plan** The formal directions for treatment of the patient, which involves many different individuals, including the patient. It may be as simple as instructions to "take two aspirins and drink plenty of fluids," or it may be a multiple-page document with delegation of responsibilities. Care plans may also be developed by discipline, such as nursing.

**Patient financial services** The department in a health care facility that is responsible for submitting bills or claims for reimbursement. Also called *patient accounts* or *patient accounting*.

**Payer** The individual or organization that is primarily responsible for the reimbursement for a particular health care service. Usually refers to the insurance company or third party.

**Per diem** Each day, daily. Usually refers to all-inclusive payments for inpatient services.

**Percentage** Standardization of data so that unlike groups can be compared. Can be calculated by dividing the observations in the category by the total observations and multiplying by 100.

**Performance improvement (PI)** Also known as *quality improvement (QI)* or *continuous quality improvement (CQI)*. Refers to the process by which a facility reviews its services or products to improve quality.

**Performance improvement plan (PIP)** A plan to explain the required responsibilities and competencies expected of an employee's job performance.

**Performance standards** Set guidelines explaining how much work an employee must complete.

**Permitted disclosure** Disclosure authorized by the patient, or allowed for treatment, payment, or health care operations.

**Personal health record (PHR)** A patient's own copy of health information documenting the patient's health care history and providing information on continuing patient care.

**Personal identification number (PIN)** A unique set of characters that a computer system recognizes as belonging to a previously registered individual.

**Physiatrist** A physician who specializes in physical medicine and rehabilitation.

**Physical examination** The physician's record of examination of the patient.

**Physician** A medical professional who has satisfied the academic, professional, and legal requirements to diagnose and treat patients at state-specified levels and within a declared specialty.

**Physician-patient privilege** The legal foundation that private communication between a physician and a patient is confidential. Only the patient has the right to give up this privilege.

**Physician's office** A setting for providing ambulatory care in which the primary provider is the physician.

**Physician's orders** The physician's directions regarding the patient's care. Also refers to the data collection device on which these elements are captured.

**Picture archiving and communication system (PACS)** A system that allows many different kinds of diagnostic images (e.g., radiographs, magnetic resonance images, ultrasound scans, computed tomography scans) produced by many different kinds of machines to be archived and accessed from any computer terminal in the network.

**Pie chart** A circular chart in which the frequency of observations is represented as a wedge of the circle.

**Plaintiff** The party who initiates litigation.

**Plan of treatment** In the SOAP format for medical decision making, the diagnostic, therapeutic, or palliative measures that are taken to investigate or treat the patient's condition or disease.

**Point-of-care documentation** Clinical data recorded at the time the treatment is delivered to the patient.

**Policy** A statement of something that is done or expected in an organization.

**Population** An entire group.

**Postdischarge processing** The procedures designed to prepare a health record for retention.

**Potentially compensable event (PCE)** An event that could cause the facility a financial loss or lead to litigation.

**Power of attorney** The legal document that identifies someone as the legal representative to make decisions for the patient when the patient is unable to do so.

**Preemption** The legal principle supporting the Health Insurance Portability and Accountability Act (HIPAA) stipulation that when the privacy regulations conflict with state law, the regulation or law that gives the patient more rights or is more restrictive should prevail.

**Preferred provider organization (PPO)** A managed care organization that contracts with a network of health care providers to render services to its members.

**Premiums** Periodic payments to an insurance company made by the patient for coverage (an insurance policy).

**Prevalence** Rate of incidence of an occurrence, disease, or diagnosis or the number of existing cases.

**Preventive controls** Procedures, processes, or structures that are designed to minimize errors at the point of data collection.

**Primary care physician (PCP)** In insurance, the physician who has been designated by the insured to deliver routine care to the insured and to evaluate the need for referral to a specialist, if applicable. Colloquial use is synonymous with "family doctor."

**Primary caregiver** The individual who is principally responsible for the daily care of a patient at home; usually a friend or family member.

**Primary data** Data taken directly from the patient or the original source. The patient's health record contains primary data.

**Principal diagnosis** According to the Uniform Hospital Discharge Data Set (UHDDS), the condition that, after study, is determined to be chiefly responsible for occasioning the admission of the patient to the hospital for care.

**Principal procedure** According to the Uniform Hospital Discharge Data Set (UHDDS), the procedure that was performed for definitive treatment, rather than one performed for diagnostic or exploratory purposes, or that was necessary to take care of a complication. If two procedures appear to meet this definition, then the one more related to the principal diagnosis should be selected as the principal procedure.

**Privacy** The right of an individual to control access to medical information.

**Privacy officer** The designated official in the health care organization who oversees privacy compliance and handles complaints.

**Problem list** A chronological summary of the patient's conditions and treatments.

**Problem-oriented record** A paper record with pages organized by diagnosis.

**Procedure** A process that describes how to comply with a policy. Also, a medical or surgical treatment. Also refers to the processing steps in an administrative function.

**Productivity** The amount of work produced by an employee in a given time frame.

**Progress notes** The physician's record of each interaction with the patient.

**Prospective consent** Permission given prior to having knowledge of the event to which the permission applies. For example, a permission to release information before the information is gathered (i.e., before admission).

**Prospective payment** Any of several reimbursement methods that pay an amount predetermined by the payer on the basis of the diagnosis, procedures, and other factors (depending on setting) rather than actual, current resources expended by the provider.

**Prospective Payment System (PPS)** A system used by payers, primarily the Centers for Medicare and Medicaid Services (CMS), for reimbursing acute care facilities on the basis of statistical analysis of health care data.

**Prospective Payment System (PPS) blended rate** A weighted component of Medicare Severity Diagnosis Related Group (MS-DRG) assignment that consists of the hospital-specific rate and additional factors such as regional labor costs and graduate medical education.

**Protected health information (PHI)** Individually identifiable health information that is transmitted or maintained in any form or medium by covered entities or their business associates.

**Protocol (order set)** A predetermined plan of care that guides the health care professional toward best practices in diagnosing or treating the condition.

**Provider number** The number assigned to a participating facility by Medicare for identification purposes.

**Psychiatrist** A physician who specializes in the diagnosis and treatment of patients with conditions that affect the mind.

**Public priority exception** Permitted disclosure in which authorization is not required as long as state law allows the exception.

## Q

**Qualitative analysis** Review of the actual content of the health record to ensure that the information is correct as it pertains to the patient's care.

**Quality assurance (QA)** A method for reviewing health care functions to determine their compliance with predetermined standards that requires action to correct noncompliance and then follow-up review to ascertain whether the correction was effective.

**Quality Improvement Organization (QIO)** An organization that contracts with payers, specifically Medicare and Medicaid, to review care and reimbursement issues.

**Quantitative analysis** The process of reviewing a health record to ensure that the record is complete according to organization policies and procedures for a complete medical record.

**Query** To question the database for specific elements, information, or a report.

**Queue** Electronic work area.

## R

**Radiology** Literally, the study of radiographs. In a health care facility, the department responsible for maintaining radiological and other types of diagnostic and therapeutic equipment as well as analyzing diagnostic films.

**Radiology examination** The examination of internal body structures using radiographs and other imaging technologies.

**Random selection** In sampling of a population, a method that ensures that all cases have equal chances of being selected and that the cases are selected in no particular order or pattern.

**Reciprocal services** Professional services exchanged instead of paid for in cash.

**Record** A collection of related fields. Also refers to all of the data collected about a patient's visit or all of the patient's visits (see also *health record*).

**Record retention schedule** The length of time that a record must be retained.

**Recovery Audit Contractors (RACs)** Entities contracting with the Centers for Medicare and Medicaid Services (CMS) that audit providers, using diagnosis related group (DRG) assignment and other data to identify overpayments and underpayments.

**Redact** To remove patient-identifying information from a health record.

**Redundant array of independent disks (RAIDs)** "Stacked" hard drives that split up and duplicate data to enable larger capacities and faster access.

**Referral** The act or documentation of one physician's request for an opinion or services from another health care professional, often another physician, for a specific patient regarding specific signs, symptoms, or diagnosis.

**Registry** A database of health information specific to disease, diagnosis, or implant used to improve the care provided to patients with that disease, diagnosis, or implant.

**Rehabilitation facility** A health care facility that delivers services to patients whose activities of daily living are impaired by their illness or condition. May be inpatient, outpatient, or both.

**Reimbursement** The amount of money that the health care facility receives from the party responsible for paying the bill; health care services are paid after services have been rendered.

**Relative weight (RW)** A number assigned yearly by the Centers for Medicare and Medicaid Services (CMS) that is applied to each diagnosis related group (DRG) and used to calculate reimbursement. This number represents the comparative difference in the use of resources by patients in each DRG.

**Release of information (ROI)** The health information management (HIM) department function that provides disclosure of patient health information.

**Reliability** A characteristic of quality exhibited when codes are consistently assigned by one or more coders for similar or identical cases.

**Report** The result of a query. A list from a database.

**Request for proposal (RFP)** A document composed from provider's list of system requirements used to explain to electronic health record (EHR) vendors what the health care organization intends to accomplish and requires of an EHR product.

**Required disclosure** A disclosure to the patient and to the U.S. Secretary of the Department of Health and Human Services for compliance auditing purposes.

**Research** The systematic investigation into a matter to find fact.

**Resident** A person who, after attending college and medical school, performs professional duties under the supervision of a fully qualified physician.

**Resident Assessment Instrument (RAI)** A data set collected by skilled nursing facilities (SNFs) that includes elements of Minimum Data Set (MDS) 3.0, along with information on patient statuses and conditions in the facility.

**Resident Assessment Protocols (RAPs)** A detailed, individualized evaluation and plan for patients in long-term care.

**Resource intensity (RI)** A weight of the resources used for the care of an inpatient in an acute care setting that result in a successful discharge.

**Resource Utilization Groups (RUGs)** These constitute a prospective payment system for long-term care. Current Medicare application is a per diem rate based on the RUG III grouper.

**Resource-based relative value system (RBRVS)** The system used to determine reimbursements to physicians for the treatment of Medicare patients.

**Respite care** Services rendered to an individual who is not independent in activities of daily living, for the purpose of temporarily relieving the primary caregiver.

**Restriction** Under the Health Insurance Portability and Accountability Act (HIPAA) Privacy Rule, the right of patients to limit the use of their protected health information.

**Retail care** Preventive health services and treatment for minor illnesses offered in large retail stores, supermarkets, and pharmacies.

**Retention** The procedures governing the storage of records, including duration, location, security, and access.

**Retrospective consent** Permission given after the event to which the permission applies. For example, permission to release information after the information is gathered (i.e., after discharge).

**Retrospective review** Review occurring after the act or event (i.e., after the patient is discharged).

**Revenue code** A chargemaster code required for Medicare billing.

**Revenue cycle** The groups of processes that identify, record, and report the financial transactions that result from the facility's clinical relationship with a patient.

**Revenue cycle management (RCM)** All the activities that connect the services being rendered to a patient with the provider's reimbursement for those services.

**Right to complain** The patient's right to discuss his or her concerns about privacy violations.

**Right to revoke** The right to withdraw consent or approval for a previously approved action or request.

**Risk** The potential exposure to loss, financial expenditure, or other undesirable events; used to determine potential reimbursement of health care services.

**Risk management** The coordination of efforts within a facility to prevent and control inadvertent occurrences.

**Root cause analysis (RCA)** The process of determining the cause of an error.

**Rule out** The process of systematically eliminating potential diagnoses. Also refers to the list of potential diagnoses.

## S

**Sample** A small group within a population.

**Scanner** A machine, much like a copier, used to turn paper-based records into digital images for a computerized health record.

**Secondary data** Data taken from the primary source document for use elsewhere.

**Security** The administrative, physical, and technological safeguards used to protect patient health information.

**Self-pay** A method of payment for health care services in which the patient pays the provider directly, without the involvement of a third party payer (e.g., insurance).

**Sequential record** See *integrated record.*

**Serial numbering system** A numerical patient record identification system in which the patient is given a new number for each visit and each file folder contains separate visit information.

**Serial-unit numbering system** A numerical patient record identification system in which the patient is given a new number for each visit; however, with each new admission, the previous record is retrieved and filed in the folder with the most recent visit.

**Severity of illness (SI)** In utilization review, a type of criteria based on the patient's condition that is used to screen patients for the appropriate care setting.

**Skewed** Frequency distributions that are not symmetrical, sometimes because of a small sample.

**Skilled nursing facility (SNF)** A long-term care facility providing a range of nursing and other health care services to patients who require continuous care, typically those with a chronic illness.

**SOAP format** Subjective, Objective, Assessment, and Plan: the medical decision-making process used by physicians to assess the patient at various intervals.

**Socioeconomic data** Elements that pertain to the patient's personal life and personal habits, such as marital status, religion, and culture.

**Source-oriented record** A paper record in which the pages are organized by discipline, department, and/or type of form.

**Span of control** The number of employees who report to one supervisor, manager, or administrator.

**Staff model HMO** A Health Maintenance Organization that owns the facilities, employs the physicians, and provides essentially all the health care services.

**Stakeholder** Regarding electronic health record (EHR) implementation and selection, an individual or department with an interest in the process, in either the implementation or the outcome.

**Standard deviation** A measure of the average distance of observations from a mean.

**Standards for code sets** Standards that must be used under the Health Insurance Portability and Accountability Act (HIPAA) for the electronic exchange of data for certain transactions, namely encounter and payment data.

**Standards of Ethical Coding** Guidelines from the American Health Information Management Association (AHIMA) to guide professional coders toward ethical decisions.

**Statistics** Analysis, interpretation, and presentation of information in numerical or pictorial format derived from the numbers.

**Statute** A law that has been passed by the legislative branch of government.

**Storage area network (SAN)** The use of redundant arrays of independent disks (RAIDs) and other storage technologies over a network.

**Straight numerical filing** Filing folders in numerical order.

**Subjective** In the SOAP format of medical decision making, the patient's description of the symptoms or other complaints.

**Subpoena** A direction from an officer of the court.

**Subpoena ad testificandum** A direction from an officer of the court to provide testimony.

**Subpoena duces tecum** A direction from an officer of the court to provide documents.

**Substance Abuse and Mental Health Services Administration (SAMHSA)** An agency under the U.S. Department of Health and Human Services (DHHS) facilitating research and care for the treatment of patients with substance abuse and mental health problems.

**Super user** An individual trained in all aspects of a computer system who can offer on-site support to others.

**Superbill** An ambulatory care encounter form on which potential diagnoses and procedures are preprinted for easy check-off at the point of care.

**Surgeon** A physician who specializes in diagnosing and treating diseases with invasive procedures.

**Survey** A data-gathering tool for capturing the responses to queries. May be administered verbally or by written questionnaire. Also refers to the activity of querying, as in "taking a survey."

**Symptom** The patient's report of physical or other complaints, such as dizziness, headache, and stomach pain.

**System development life cycle (SDLC)** The process of planning, designing, implementation, and evaluation used in updating and improving, or implementing a new health information system.

**Systemized Nomenclature of Medicine—Clinical Terms (SNOMED-CT)** Systematized nomenclature of human and veterinary medicine clinical terms; a reference terminology that, among other things, links common or input medical terminology and codes with the output reporting systems in an electronic health record.

## T

**Table** A chart organized in rows and columns to organize data.

**Tax Equity and Fiscal Responsibility Act of 1982 (TEFRA)** A federal law with wide-reaching provisions, one of which was the establishment of Medicare prospective payment systems (PPSs).

**Telemedicine** Care provided through the use of mobile technology, which allows care providers to view and consult patient from satellite locations.

**Terminal-digit filing system** A system in which the patient's medical record number is separated into sets for filing, and the first set of numbers is called *tertiary*, the second set of numbers is called *secondary*, and the third set of numbers is called *primary*.

**The Joint Commission (TJC)** An organization that accredits and sets standards for acute care facilities, ambulatory care networks, long-term care facilities, and rehabilitation facilities, as well as certain specialty facilities, such as hospice and home care. Facilities maintaining TJC accreditation receive *deemed status* from the Centers for Medicare and Medicaid Services (CMS).

**Third party payer** An entity that pays a provider for part or all of a patient's health care services; often the patient's insurance company.

**Timeliness** The quality of data's being obtained, recorded, or reported within a predetermined time frame.

**Title IX of the Social Security Act** Amendment to the Social Security Act that established Medicaid.

**Title XVIII of the Social Security Act** Amendment to the Social Security Act that established Medicare.

**Tort** Harm, damage, or wrongdoing that entitles the injured party to compensation.

**Tracer methodology** The Joint Commission (TJC) method of onsite review of open records in which the surveyors follow the actual path of documentation from start to finish.

**Training** Education in, instruction in, or demonstration of how to perform a job.

**Transaction code set** A code set, established by Health Insurance Portability and Accountability Act (HIPAA) guidelines, to be used in electronic data transfer to ensure that the information transmitted is complete, private, and secure.

**Treatment** A procedure, medication, or other measure designed to cure or alleviate the symptoms of disease.

**Trend** The way in which a variance of values behaves over time.

**Triage** In emergency services, the system of prioritizing patients by severity of illness.

**TRICARE** A U.S. program of health benefits for military personnel, their families, and military retirees, formerly called *CHAMPUS*.

## U

**Uniform Ambulatory Care Data Set (UACDS)** The mandated data set for ambulatory care patients.

**Uniform Bill (UB-04)** The standardized form used by hospitals for inpatient and outpatient billing to the Centers for Medicare and Medicaid Services (CMS) and other third-party payers.

**Uniform Hospital Discharge Data Set (UHDDS)** The mandated data set for hospital inpatients.

**Unit numbering system** A numerical patient record identification system in which the patient record is filed under the same number for all visits.

**Unity of command** Sole management of one employee by one manager.

**Universal chart order** Pertaining to a paper health record, the maintenance of the same page organization both before and after discharge.

**Urgent Care Association of America (UCAOA)** A professional organization representing those working in urgent care settings, serving as an advocate for the role of urgent care facilities in health care delivery.

**Urgent care center** A facility that treats patients whose illness or injury requires immediate attention but that is not life threatening.

**Use** Employ PHI for a purpose.

**Usual and customary fees (UCFs)** Referring to health care provider fees, the rates established by an insurance company on the basis of the regional charges for particular services.

**Utilization review (UR)** The process of evaluating medical interventions against established criteria, on the basis of the patient's known or tentative diagnosis. Evaluation may take place before, during, or after the episode of care for different purposes.

## V

**Validity** The data quality characteristic of a recorded observation falling within a predetermined size or range of values.

**Verification** Confirming accuracy.

**Vision** The goal of the organization, above and beyond the mission.

**Visit** In ambulatory care, a unit of measuring the number of patients who have been served.

**Vital statistic** Public health data collected through birth certificates, death certificates, and other data-gathering tools.

## W

**Workers' compensation** An employer's coverage of an employee's medical expenses due to a work-related injury or illness.

**Workflow** The process of work flowing through a set of procedures to complete the health record.

**Workflow analysis** A careful examination of how work is performed in order to identify inefficiencies and make changes.

**Working DRG** The concurrent diagnosis related group (DRG). The DRG that reflects the patient's current diagnosis and procedures while still an inpatient.

**World Health Organization (WHO)** An agency under the United Nations establishing focus areas for international public health policy. The WHO maintains the ICD-10 classification system.

**Wraparound policies** Insurance policies that supplement Medicare coverage. Also called *secondary insurance*.

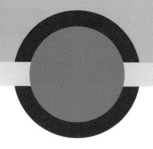

# INDEX

Page numbers followed by *b* indicate boxes; *f*, figures; *t*, tables.

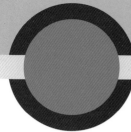

# ABBREVIATION LIST

| | |
|---|---|
| **AAAHC** | Accreditation Association for Ambulatory Health Care |
| **AAMRL** | American Association of Medical Record Librarians |
| **AAPC** | American Academy of Professional Coders |
| **ABN** | Advance Beneficiary Notice |
| **ACO** | Accountable Care Organization |
| **ACS** | American College of Surgeons |
| **ADA** | Americans with Disabilities Act |
| **ADLs** | activities of daily living |
| **AHA** | American Hospital Association |
| **AHIMA** | American Health Information Management Association |
| **AHRQ** | Agency for Healthcare Research and Quality |
| **AKA** | also known as |
| **ALOS** | average length of stay |
| **AMA** | against medical advice |
| **AMA** | American Medical Association |
| **AMRA** | American Medical Record Association |
| **AOA** | American Osteopathic Association |
| **APA** | American Psychiatric Association |
| **APC** | Ambulatory Payment Classification |
| **AP-DRG** | All Patient Diagnosis Related Groups |
| **APR-DRG** | All Patient Refined Diagnosis Related Groups |
| **APRN** | Advanced Practice Registered Nurse |
| **AR** | accounts receivable |
| **ARLNA** | Association of Record Librarians of North America |
| **ARRA** | The American Recovery and Reinvestment Act |
| **ASC** | ambulatory surgery center |
| **ATS** | American Trauma Society |
| **BCBSA** | Blue Cross and Blue Shield Association |
| **BMI** | Body Mass Index |
| **BMV** | bedside medication verification |
| **CABG** | coronary artery bypass graft |
| **CAC** | computer-assisted coding |
| **CAHIIM** | Commission on Accreditation of Health Informatics and Information Management |
| **CAP** | College of American Pathologists |
| **CARF** | Commission on Accreditation of Rehabilitation Facilities |
| **CBC** | complete blood count |
| **CC** | comorbidity or complication |
| **CCA** | Certified Coding Associate |
| **CCC** | convenient care clinic |
| **CCHIIM** | Commission on Certification for Health Informatics and Information Management |
| **CCHIT** | Commission on the Certification for Health Information Technology |
| **CCI** | Correct Coding Initiative |
| **CCI** | Canadian Classification of Interventions |
| **CCS** | Certified Coding Specialist |
| **CCS-P** | Certified Coding Specialist—Physician-based |
| **CCU** | coronary care unit |
| **CDC** | Centers for Disease Control and Prevention |
| **CDI** | Clinical Documentation Improvement |
| **CDIP** | Clinical Documentation Improvement Professional |
| **CDM** | Charge Description Master |
| **CDS** | clinical decision-making system |
| **CDT** | Current Dental Terminology |
| **CE** | continuing education |
| **CEO** | Chief Executive Officer |
| **CEU** | continuing education unit |
| **CFO** | Chief Financial Officer |
| **CFR** | Code of Federal Regulations |
| **CHAMPUS** | Civilian Health and Medical Program for the Uniformed Services |
| **CHAMPVA** | Civilian Health and Medical Program of the Veterans Administration |
| **CHAP** | Community Health Accreditation Program |
| **CHDA** | Certified Health Data Analyst |
| **CHF** | congestive heart failure |
| **CHP** | Certified in Healthcare Privacy |
| **CHPS** | Certified in Healthcare Privacy and Security |
| **CHS** | Certified in Healthcare Security |
| **CIO** | Chief Information Officer |
| **CLIA** | Clinical Laboratory Improvement Amendment |
| **CMAT** | Case Mix Assessment Tool |
| **CMG** | case mix group |
| **CMI** | case mix index |
| **CMS** | Centers for Medicare and Medicaid Services |

| | |
|---|---|
| **CNA** | Certified Nursing Assistant |
| **CNO** | Chief Nursing Officer |
| **COO** | Chief Operating Officer |
| **COLD** | Computer Output to Laser Disk |
| **COP** | Conditions of Participation (Medicare) |
| **CPC** | Certified Professional Coder |
| **CPC-H** | Certified Professional Coder—Hospital-based |
| **CPOE** | Computerized Physician Order Entry |
| **CPT** | Current Procedural Terminology |
| **CQI** | continuous quality improvement |
| **CQM** | Clinical Quality Measure |
| **CRNA** | Certified Registered Nurse Anesthetist |
| **CT** | computed tomography |
| **CTR** | Certified Tumor Registrar |
| **CY** | calendar year |
| **DD** | date dictated |
| **DEEDS** | Data Elements for Emergency Department Systems |
| **DHHS** | Department of Health and Human Services |
| **DICOM** | Digital Imaging and Communications in Medicine |
| **DMADV** | Definition, Measurement, Analysis, Design, Verification |
| **DMAIC** | Definition, Measurement, Analysis, Improvement, and Control |
| **DME** | durable medical equipment |
| **DNFB** | Discharged No Final Bill/Discharged Not Final Billed |
| **DNR** | do not resuscitate |
| **DNV** | Det Norske Veritas |
| **DO** | Doctor of Osteopathy |
| **DOA** | dead on arrival |
| **DOB** | date of birth |
| **DRG** | diagnosis related groups |
| **DSM-IV** | *Diagnostic and Statistical Manual of Mental Disorders, 4th edition* |
| **DSM-5** | *Diagnostic and Statistical Manual of Mental Disorders, 5th edition* |
| **DT** | date transcribed |
| **DTR** | Dietetic Technician, Registered |
| **EBM** | evidence-based medicine |
| **ED** | emergency department |
| **EDI** | Electronic Data Interchange |
| **EDMS** | Electronic Document Management System |
| **EEG** | electroencephalography |
| **EEOC** | Equal Employment Opportunity Commission |
| **EHR** | electronic health record |
| **EKG** | electrocardiography |
| **EMDS** | Emergency Medical Data Set |
| **EMPI** | Enterprise master patient index |
| **EMTALA** | Emergency Medical Treatment and Active Labor Act |
| **e-PHI** | electronic protected health information |
| **ESRD** | end-stage renal disease |
| **FAHIMA** | Fellow of the American Health Information Management Association |
| **FDA** | Food and Drug Administration |
| **FL** | Form Locator |
| **FLSA** | Fair Labor Standards Act |
| **FTE** | full-time equivalent |
| **FY** | fiscal year |
| **GLOS** | geometric length of stay |
| **GMLOS** | geometric mean length of stay |
| **GUI** | graphical user interface |
| **H&P** | History and Physical |
| **HCA** | Home Care Aide |
| **HCAHPS** | Hospital Consumer Assessment of Healthcare Providers and Systems |
| **HCFA** | Health Care Financing Administration (now CMS) |
| **HCO** | Health Care Organization |
| **HCPCS** | Healthcare Common Procedure Coding System |
| **HCQIP** | Health Care Quality Improvement Program |
| **HEDIS** | Healthcare Effectiveness Data and Information Set |
| **HFAP** | Healthcare Facilities Accreditation Program Language |
| **HH PPS** | Home Health Prospective Payment System |
| **HHRG** | Home Health Resources Group |
| **HIAA** | Health Insurance Association of America |
| **HIE** | health information exchange |
| **HIM** | health information management |
| **HIMSS** | Health Information Management Systems Society |
| **HIPAA** | Health Insurance Portability and Accountability Act |
| **HIT** | Health Information Technology |
| **HITECH** | Health Information Technology for Economic and Clinical Health (Act) |
| **HL7** | Health Level 7 |